IMAGING *in* ONCOLOGY

IMAGING *in* ONCOLOGY

Edited by

Janet E. S. Husband

Academic Department of Diagnostic Radiology
The Royal Marsden NHS Trust, London, UK

and

Rodney H. Reznek

Academic Department of Radiology
St. Bartholomew's Hospital, London, UK

Medical illustration by
Dee McLean

I S I S
MEDICAL
MEDIA
—
Oxford

© 1998 by Isis Medical Media Ltd.
59 St Aldates
Oxford OX1 1ST, UK

First published 1998

British Library Cataloguing in Publication Data.
A catalogue record for this title is available from
the British Library

ISBN 1 899066 48 9

Husband, J (Janet)
Imaging in Oncology (Volume 2)
Janet E. S. Husband and Rodney H. Reznek (eds)

Always refer to the manufacturer's Prescribing
Information before prescribing drugs cited in this book.

Page layout and design
The EDI Partnership, UK

Image reproduction
Track Direct, UK

Isis Medical Media staff
Commissioning Editor: John Harrison
Editor: Catherine Rickards
Production Manager: Julia Savory

Produced by Phoenix Offset, HK
Printed in China

Distributed in the USA by
Mosby-Year Book, Inc, 11830 Westline Industrial Drive
St Louis MO 63145, USA

Distributed in the rest of the world by
Plymbridge Distributors Ltd, Estover Road,
Plymouth, PL6 7PY, UK

Contents

PART I: GENERAL PRINCIPLES

1 An overview of imaging in oncology   3
Janet Husband and Rodney Reznek

2 Trends in cancer incidence, survival and mortality   11
Michel Coleman and Jacques Estève

3 Staging of cancer   23
Anthony Neal

4 Principles of treatment   33
Alan Horwich

PART II: PRIMARY TUMOUR EVALUATION AND STAGING

5 Lung cancer   45
Julian Hanson and Peter Armstrong

6 Mediastinal tumours   67
Janet Kuhlman

7 Pleural tumours   79
Sujal Desai and David Hansell

8 Oesophageal cancer   93
Sheila Rankin

9 Gastric cancer   111
Alison McLean

10 Colorectal cancer   129
Dennis Balfe and Michelle Semin

11 Pancreatic cancer   151
Rodney Reznek and David Stephens

12 Primary tumours of the liver and bile ducts   169
Richard Baron

13 Renal tumours   191
Rodney Reznek

14 Bladder cancer   215
Janet Husband

15 Prostate cancer   239
Gerrit Jager and Jelle Barentsz

16 Testicular germ cell tumours   259
Janet Husband and David MacVicar

17 Ovarian cancer   277
Syed Sohaib, Rodney Reznek and Janet Husband

18 Uterine and cervical tumours   309
Jane Hawnaur

19 Primary retroperitoneal tumours   329
Jeremiah Healy, Rodney Reznek and Janet Husband

20 Primary bone tumours   351
Dennis Stoker

21 Soft tissue sarcomas   377
Eleanor Moskovic

22 Breast cancer   395
David MacVicar

23 Paranasal sinus tumours   415
Sheila Rankin

24 Tumours of the pharynx, tongue and mouth   429
Michael King

25 Laryngeal tumours   457
Michael Lev, Paul Silverman and Hugh Curtin

26 Thyroid cancer   481
Hero Hussain, Keith Britton, Ashley Grossman and Rodney Reznek

27 Primary tumours of the central nervous system   515
Juliet Britton and Jane Evanson

Contents

PART III: HAEMATOLOGICAL MALIGNANCY

28 Lymphoma — 583
Rodney Reznek and Janet Husband

29 Multiple myeloma — 625
Conor Collins

30 Leukaemia — 635
Janet Husband

PART IV: PAEDIATRICS

31 General principles in paediatric oncology — 661
Helen Carty

32 Wilms' tumour and associated neoplasms of the kidney — 671
Helen Carty

33 Neuroblastoma — 691
Claire Dicks-Mireaux

34 Uncommon paediatric neoplasms — 707
Marilyn Siegel

PART V: METASTASES

35 Lymph nodes — 729
Bernadette Carrington

36 Lung — 749
Anwar Padhani

37 Bone — 765
Anwar Padhani and Janet Husband

38 Liver — 787
Philip Robinson

39 Metastatic effects on the nervous system — 811
David MacVicar

40 Adrenal glands — 831
Delia Peppercorn and Rodney Reznek

41 Peritoneum — 841
Jeremiah Healy and Rodney Reznek

42 Radiological investigation of carcinoma of unknown primary site — 853
Christopher Gallagher, Rodney Reznek and Janet Husband

PART VI: TREATMENT EVALUATION

43 Radiological intervention in oncology — 861
Anthony Lopez

44 Imaging for radiotherapy treatment planning — 889
Jane Dobbs and Ann Barrett

45 Assessment of response to treatment and detection of relapse — 899
Janet Husband and David MacVicar

46 Radiological manifestations of acute complications of treatment — 925
Louise Wilkinson, David MacVicar and Janet Husband

47 Second malignancies — 945
James Malpas

PART VII: EFFECTS OF TREATMENT ON NORMAL TISSUE

48 Thorax — 955
Herman Libshitz, Revathy Iyer and Evelyne Loyer

49 Bone and bone marrow — 967
Lia Moulopoulos

50 Abdomen and pelvis — 975
Richard Johnson, Bernadette Carrington and Paul Hulse

PART VIII: AIDS-RELATED TUMOURS

51 Chest — 1003
Janet Kuhlman

52 Abdomen and pelvis — 1019
Alec Megibow

Peter Armstrong
Professor, Department of Academic Radiology, St. Bartholomew's Hospital, London, EC1A 7BE, UK

Dennis M. Balfe
Professor, Mallinckrodt Institute of Radiology, Washington University School of Medicine, 510 South Kingshighway Boulevard, St. Louis, MO 63110, USA

Jelle O. Barentsz
Department of Diagnostic Radiology, University Hospital Nijmegen, P.O. Box 9101, 6500 HB Nijmegen, The Netherlands

Richard L. Baron
Professor and Chairman, Department of Radiology, University of Pittsburgh Medical Center, 200 Lothrop Street, Pittsburgh, PA 15213-2582, USA

Ann Barrett
Professor of Radiation Oncology, Beatson Oncology Centre, Weston Infirmary, Glasgow GL11 6NT, UK

Juliet A. Britton
Consultant Neuroradiologist, Atkinson Morley's Hospital, Wimbledon, London SW20 0NE, UK

Keith E. Britton
Professor of Nuclear Medicine, St. Bartholomew's and the Royal London School of Medicine and Dentistry, Queen Mary Westfield College, University of London EC1A 7BE, UK

Bernadette M. Carrington
Department of Radiology, Christie Hospital, Wilmslow Road, Withington, Manchester, M20 4BX, UK

Helen Carty
Professor of Paediatric Radiology, University of Liverpool; Consultant Radiologist, Department of Radiology, Alder Hey Children's Hospital, Eaton Road, Liverpool, L12 2AP, UK

Michel P. Coleman
Professor of Epidemiology and Vital Statistics; Head, Cancer and Public Health Unit, London School of Hygiene and Tropical Medicine, Keppel Street, London, WC1E 7HT and Deputy Chief Medical Statistician, Office for National Statistics, 1 Drummond Gate, London SW1V 2QQ, UK

Conor D. Collins
Consultant Radiologist, Department of Diagnostic Radiology, Christie Hospital NHS Trust, Wilmslow Road, Manchester M20 4BX, UK

Hugh D. Curtin
Chief of Radiology, Department of Radiology, Massachusetts Eye and Ear Infirmary, Boston, MA 02114, USA

Sujal R. Desai
Clinical Research Fellow (Imaging), Royal Brompton Hospital, Sydney Street, London SW3 6NP, UK

Claire M. F. Dicks-Mireaux (deceased)
Consultant Paediatric Radiologist, Department of Radiology, The Hospital for Sick Children, Great Ormond Street, London, WC1N 3JH, UK

H. Jane Dobbs
Consultant in Clinical Oncology, Guy's and St. Thomas' Cancer Centre, St. Thomas' Hospital, Lambeth Palace Road, London SE1 7EH, UK

Jacques Estève
Professor of Biostatistics, University Claude Bernard, Lyon, France

Jane Evanson
Consultant Neuroradiologist, Department of Neuro X-ray, Royal London Hospital, Whitechapel Road, London E1 1BB, UK

Christopher J. Gallagher
Senior Lecturer and Honorary Consultant in Medical Oncology, Department of Medical Oncology, St. Bartholomew's Hospital, West Smithfield, London, EC1A 7BE, UK

Ashley B. Grossman
St. Bartholomew's Hospital, London EC1A 7BE, UK

Julian Hanson
Department of Radiology, St. Bartholomew's Hospital, London EC1A 7BE, UK

Jane Hawnaur
Senior Lecturer and Honorary Consultant (Central Manchester Healthcare Trust), Department of Diagnostic Radiology, University of Manchester, Oxford Road, Manchester M13 9PT, UK

David M. Hansell
Consultant Radiologist, Department of Radiology, Royal Brompton Hospital, Sydney Street, London SW3 6NP, UK

Jeremiah C. Healy
Department of Radiology, Chelsea and Westminster Hospital, Fulham Road, London SW10 9NH, UK

Jay Heiken
Mallinckrodt Institute of Radiology, 510 South Kingshighway Boulevard, St. Louis, Missouri 63110, USA

Alan Horwich
Professor, Department of Radiotherapy, The Royal Marsden NHS Trust, Downs Road, Sutton, Surrey SM2 5PT, UK

Paul Hulse
Senior Registrar in Diagnostic Radiology, University of Manchester, UK

Janet E. S. Husband
Department of Diagnostic Radiology, The Royal Marsden NHS Trust, Downs Road, Sutton, Surrey SM2 5PT, UK

Hero K. Hussain
Senior Registrar in Radiology, Department of Diagnostic Radiology, St. Bartholomew's Hospital, West Smithfield, London EC1A 7BE, UK

Revathy B. Iyer
Assistant Professor, Department of Radiology, M. D. Anderson Cancer Center, 1515 Holcombe Boulevard, Houston, Texas 77030, USA

Gerrit J. Jager
Department of Diagnostic Radiology, University Hospital Nijmegen, P.O. Box 9101, 6500 HB Nijmegen, The Netherlands

Richard Johnson
Director of Diagnostic Radiology, Department of Radiology, Christie Hospital, Wilmslow Road, Withington, Manchester, M20 4BX, UK

D. Michael King
Consultant Radiologist, Department of Radiology, The Royal Marsden NHS Trust, Fulham Road, London SW6 3JJ, UK

Janet E. Kuhlman
Professor of Radiology, Chief of Thoracic Imaging, Department of Radiology, University of Wisconsin Medical School, E3/311 Clinical Science Center, 600 Highland Avenue, Madison, WI 53792-3252, USA

Michael H. Lev
Director of Emergency Radiology, Massachusetts General Hospital; Staff Radiologist, Massachusetts Eye and Ear Infirmary, Boston, MA 02114, USA

Herman I. Libshitz
Professor, Department of Radiology, M. D. Anderson Hospital, 1515 Holcombe Boulevard, Houston, Texas 77030, USA

Anthony J. Lopez
Consultant Radiologist, Department of Radiology, The Royal Surrey County Hospital and St. Luke's Cancer Centre, Guildford, Surrey GU2 5XX, UK

Evelyne M. Loyer
Assistant Professor, Department of Radiology, M. D. Anderson Cancer Center, 1515 Holcombe Boulevard, Houston, Texas 77030, USA

David MacVicar
Consultant Radiologist, Department of Diagnostic Radiology, The Royal Marsden NHS Trust, Downs Road, Sutton, Surrey, SM2 5PT, UK

Alison M. McLean
Consultant Radiologist, Department of Diagnostic Radiology, St. Bartholomew's Hospital, West Smithfield, London, EC1A 7BE, UK

James S. Malpas
Emeritus Professor of Medical Oncology, ICRF Department of Medical Oncology, St. Bartholomew's Hospital, West Smithfield, London EC1A 7BE, UK

Alec J. Megibow
Professor of Radiology, Director of Abdominal Imaging, Department of Radiology, New York University Medical Center, 560 First Avenue, New York, NY 10016, USA

Eleanor C. Moskovic
Consultant Radiologist, Department of Radiology, The Royal Marsden NHS Trust, Downs Road , Sutton, Surrey SM2 5PT, UK

Lia A. Moulopoulos
Adjunct Assist Professor, M. D. Anderson Cancer Center; Instructor in Radiology, Department of Radiology, Areteion Hospital, University of Athens, 76 Vas. Sophias Avenue, 11528 Athens, Greece

Anthony Neal
Department of Radiotherapy, The Royal Marsden NHS Trust, Downs Road, Sutton, Surrey, SM2 5PT, UK

Anwar R. Padhani
Senior Lecturer, Honorary Consultant Radiologist, Department of Diagnostic Radiology, The Royal Marsden NHS Trust, Downs Road, Sutton, Surrey, SM2 5PT, UK

P. Delia Peppercorn
Department of Radiology, St. Bartholomew's Hospital, West Smithfield, London EC1A 7BE, UK

Sheila C. Rankin
Consultant Radiologist, Department of Radiology, Guy's Hospital, St. Thomas Street, London, SE1 9RT, UK

Rodney H. Reznek
Department of Radiology, St. Bartholomew's Hospital, West Smithfield, London, EC1A 7BE, UK

Philip J. Robinson
Consultant Radiologist, St. James' University Hospital, Leeds LS9 7TF, UK

Michelle D. Semin
Instructor, Mallinckrodt Insitute of Radiology, Washington University School of Medicine, 510 South Kingshighway Boulevard, St. Louis, MO 63110, USA

Marilyn J. Siegel
Professor of Radiology and Pediatrics, Edward Mallinckrodt Institute of Radiology, Washington University School of Medicine, 510 South Kingshighway Boulevard, St. Louis, Missouri 63110, USA

Paul M. Silverman
Department of Radiology and Medical Oncology, Division of Abdominal Imaging, Georgetown University School of Medicine, 3800 Reservoir Road NW, Washington DC 20007, USA

Syed A. A. Sohaib
Department of Radiology, St. Bartholomew's Hospital, West Smithfield, London EC1A 7BE, UK

P. Som
Department of Radiology, New York University Medical Center, 560 First Avenue, New York, NY 10016, USA

David H. Stephens
St. Bartholomew's Hospital, London EC1A 7BE, UK

Dennis J. Stoker
Consultant Radiologist (Emeritus), London Bone Tumour Service, Royal National Orthopaedic Hospital, 45–51 Bolsover Street, London W1P 8AQ, UK

Louise Wilkinson
Department of Diagnostic Radiology, The Royal Marsden NHS Trust, Downs Road, Sutton, Surrey SM2 5PT, UK

Foreword

In the past 30 years, advances in the technology of medical imaging have provided radiologists with an ever increasing range of powerful methods for examining the human body. Application of the new technologies has led to major advances in both the diagnosis and management of patients. One of the challenges for radiologists and clinicians flowing from these advances is for them to learn how to deploy the increasing number of technologies most efficiently and effectively. All investigations have costs as well as benefits and it is important to remember that costs are not just financial. There are also costs for patients. Most examinations in an X-ray department are uncomfortable, some are painful and a few may be hazardous, quite apart from the risks of X-irradiation. Radiologists, therefore, have to learn how to use best the available imaging techniques to maximise benefit to an individual patient in a particular clinical situation. This question is not always emphasised in textbooks of radiology, yet it lies at the heart of patient care.

Radiology is usually concerned with making a diagnosis and choosing an appropriate method for doing this is usually straightforward. When the diagnosis is known but radiology is needed to support management, the choice of imaging strategy can be more difficult, not least because it depends on understanding the questions being asked by the clinician. The problem is not likely to cause much difficulty for a radiologist working closely with clinical colleagues in a specialist department. A radiologist working in a less specialised environment or working with colleagues in many different departments will have more difficulty. This is especially so in relation to specialties in which treatment is continually advancing and raising different questions requiring different imaging strategies. Nowhere is this problem illustrated more clearly than in the management of different types of cancer.

Professor Husband and Professor Reznek have recognised this problem and this book is the welcome result. Both of them have deep and long experience of imaging in oncology and they have gathered a team of distinguished contributors, mainly from the UK but with a substantial proportion from Europe and the USA. The main part of the book consists of chapters describing the role of imaging in the management of individual primary tumours. These accounts are not only authoritative but are also set out clearly and are splendidly illustrated. Non-specialists will appreciate the four introductory chapters describing the principles underlying the treatment of cancer. There is also a useful section reminding radiologists of the principles involved in determining the accuracy and clinical value of an investigative technique.

The book is aimed at non-specialist radiologists but where there is cancer there will be few radiologists or clinicians, specialist or non-specialist, who will not welcome the opportunity to refer to 'Husband & Reznek'.

Dr. Ian Kelsey-Fry

Preface

During recent years enormous strides have been made in understanding the basic mechanisms of cancer and in developing effective therapies. These advances, together with the ever increasing sophistication of imaging technology, have changed the role of the radiologist working with cancer patients. Today the radiologist plays a pivotal role within a multi-disciplinary team of medical oncologists, radiotherapists, surgeons and pathologists, frequently providing crucial information on which major management decisions are made. Furthermore, in the light of the complex array of imaging methods currently available, the radiologist can guide the clinical team so that the most appropriate investigation is performed according to the clinical circumstances.

In order to meet the challenges of this new role the radiologist requires an in-depth knowledge of imaging findings in the many different tumour types as well as an understanding of the patterns of tumour spread, tumour staging methods, patterns of recurrence and modern approaches to therapy. *Imaging in Oncology* has been written in an attempt to meet these needs and is intended for all radiologists whose daily work includes the management of cancer patients, as well as those working as dedicated oncology radiologists in specialised cancer centres.

Imaging in Oncology comprises two volumes and is divided into eight sections. The first section provides a general overview of cancer and discusses imaging strategies in oncology, cancer incidence, staging methods and principles of treatment. While the diagnosis of cancer is of critical importance this task usually falls within the context of general radiology and for this reason investigations leading to the diagnosis of cancer and its differential diagnosis are not considered in detail in this text. In *Imaging in Oncology* emphasis has been placed on image interpretation for tumour staging and follow-up.

Where relevant, each chapter is accompanied by colour diagrams of tumour staging, anatomy or other aspects of tumour imaging. These illustrations have been produced by Dee McLean to whom we are indebted for her beautiful work. In this text MR images have been annotated according to the sequence used but the precise detailed sequence information including repetition time and echo time has not been included as a general rule. This is a decision based on the fact that *Imaging in Oncology* represents a multi-modality approach to cancer imaging and therefore we did not wish to enter into a detailed discussion of magnetic resonance techniques, a topic considered in detail in the numerous textbooks dedicated to magnetic resonance imaging which are available today. In each chapter we have highlighted the text with a system of key points as well as a summary of the salient issues covered. The new 1997 UICC TNM Staging Classification of Malignant Tumours has been used throughout the book.

We would like to acknowledge all those who have worked so hard to bring the concept of *Imaging in Oncology* to fruition. Mrs. Maureen Watts, Mrs. Julie Jessop and Miss Paula Taylor have all spent many hours typing the manuscript and deciphering the Editors' often illegible handwriting! Mrs. Maureen Watts has co-ordinated the whole project for Janet Husband and Mrs. Julie Jessop for Rodney Reznek, and Miss Paula Taylor has also typed numerous editions of different chapters emanating from the Royal Marsden Hospital. Mrs. Janet Macdonald has worked tirelessly to produce an enormous number of illustrations. We would also like to thank the Medical Illustration Department of St. Bartholomew's Hospital for their meticulous high quality work.

We are most grateful to all our contributors who have found the time within a busy working schedule to provide us with excellent accounts of their own special expertise in imaging individual cancers. It is not possible to mention everyone by name but we would like to say a special thank you to Dr. Marilyn Siegel for her help and advice in aspects of imaging in paediatric cancer and Dr. Scott Barrett for reviewing the manuscripts from the point of view of a general radiologist working with cancer patients.

Finally, we were immensely saddened by the sudden tragic death of Dr. Claire Dicks-Mireaux shortly before publication of the book and wish to extend our deepest sympathies to her family and colleagues at Great Ormond Street Hospital for Sick Children.

We hope that *Imaging in Oncology* will make a useful contribution to the radiological literature and will allow those working with cancer to have a greater understanding of imaging within this complex and rapidly changing specialty. There is no doubt that oncological radiology is developing as an important sub-specialty of radiology and we therefore hope that within this new arena, *Imaging in Oncology* will provide the specialist radiologist with the foundations on which further knowledge and future experience can be based and will also provide the general radiologist with a useful and informative text.

Janet E. S. Husband
Rodney H. Reznek

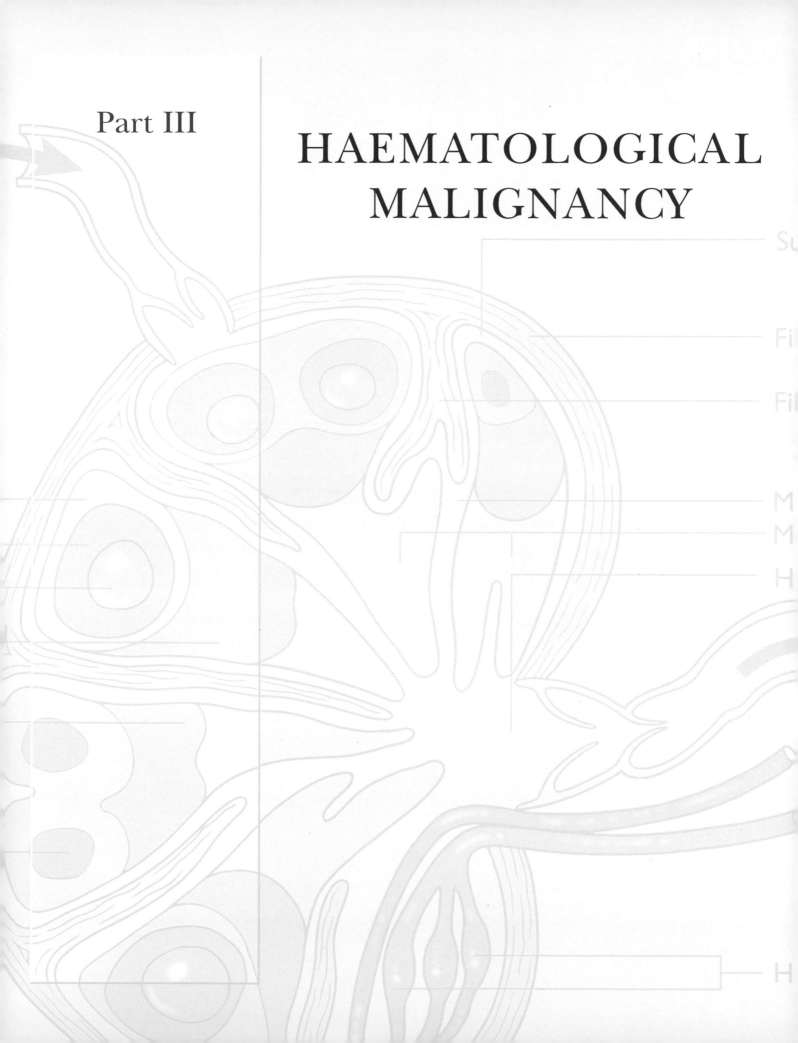

Part III

HAEMATOLOGICAL MALIGNANCY

Chapter 28

Lymphoma

Rodney Reznek and Janet Husband

INTRODUCTION

The lymphomas, Hodgkin's disease (HD) and non-Hodgkin's lymphoma (NHL) are a diverse group of neoplasms which vary widely in age of presentation, patterns of tumour growth and survival rates. Hodgkin's disease was first described by Thomas Hodgkin in 1832 but it is only during the last two decades that the prognosis has improved so that currently Hodgkin's disease is curable in the majority of patients. Non-Hodgkin's lymphoma (NHL) has a variable course, ranging from slow and indolent to aggressive and rapidly fatal. As in Hodgkin's disease, improvements in survival are attributed to advancements in therapy but the use of modern imaging methods to delineate the extent of disease with a high degree of accuracy is also an important factor.

In the lymphomas, imaging plays a vital role in the correct deployment of combined modality treatment at the time of diagnosis and staging, in monitoring response to therapy and in the detection of relapse.

The objectives of initial staging are to define as accurately as possible the local extent of clinically overt disease and to search for occult disease elsewhere with a full knowledge of the likely pattern of tumour spread.[1] The choice of the appropriate imaging method requires an appreciation of:

- The likelihood of particular sites being affected
- The sensitivity and specificity of particular tests chosen to investigate those sites
- The likely impact of a positive result on treatment choice

INCIDENCE

Lymphoma accounts for 5–6% of malignancy in adults in the UK and about 10% of all childhood cancers.[2,3] In the USA it is estimated that there will be 61,100 new cases of lymphoma in 1997 (53,600 NHL and 7500 HD), with an estimated number of total deaths of 25,280 of which 23,800 will be due to NHL and 1,480 to HD.[4] The annual incidence of NHL and HD in the south east of England is similar to that of the USA;

11.2 per 100,000 for males and 10 per 100,000 for females in NHL and 4 per 100,000 for males and 3 per 100,000 for females in HD.[2] Men are affected slightly more often than females in both types of lymphoma:

- Hodgkin's disease M1·4:F1
- Non-Hodgkin's lymphoma M1·1:F1

While the incidence of Hodgkin's disease has decreased over the last 30 years, that of NHL has risen by approximately 60% in the USA since 1960 and in the south east of England the incidence is expected to have doubled by the year 2010.[5]

Hodgkin's disease shows a bimodal peak distribution, the first in the third decade of life and the second between 65 and 75 years of age; however NHL is a disease mainly of the elderly with an increasing incidence over the age of 50 years.[6]

Key points: incidence

- The incidence of NHL has increased by 60% over the last 2 decades in the USA and UK, while the incidence of HD is decreasing

- HD has a peak incidence between the ages of 30 and 40 years and also in those aged over 65 years. NHL is seen in children and in those over 50 years of age

- There is a link between the Epstein–Barr virus (EBV) and HD as well as NHL. Genetic dysfunction is an important aetiological factor

AETIOLOGY

There is an association between the Epstein–Barr virus (EBV) and HD but debate continues regarding the exact aetiological role of EBV in this disease. It is interesting that the suggestion of infection having a causal relationship with HD was first made by Hodgkin himself at the time of his first description of the morbid anatomy of the condition. Patients with HD have a higher antibody titre to the EBV viral capsular antigen than normal adults and there is also an increased risk of HD amongst patients who have had infectious mononucleosis.[7]

Genetic studies have revealed the importance of mutation, altered expression and loss of function of genes in the development and progression of NHL, largely accounting for the diversity of clinical presentations and course of this disease.[8] In NHL immunosuppression is an important aetiological factor, the disease having a high incidence in patients with auto-immune deficiency syndrome (AIDS) and those on long-term immunosuppressant therapy, for example, following renal transplantation.[9,10] Epstein–Barr virus may be an important aetiological factor in Burkitt's lymphoma and the HTLV-1 retrovirus is known to have a causal relationship with adult T-cell leukaemia/lymphoma.[8,11]

PATHOLOGY

Classification

The importance of any classification is first its clinical relevance and second its translatability to allow communication of new knowledge and comparison of clinical results.[12] In this context, the reproducibility and widespread use of the Rye modification of the Luke–Butler classification introduced in 1966 has proved to be reliable (Table 28.1).[13,14] This contrasts greatly with the profusion of classifications for NHL, although since its introduction in 1982, the working formulation has resulted in some degree of consensus.[15] In 1994, a new classification (REAL) was proposed and is now being introduced into clinical practice.[16]

Hodgkin's disease

The demonstration of Reed–Sternberg cells is central to the diagnosis of HD (Fig. 28.1). The subclassification of HD into four subgroups is based on the proportion of lymphocytes in the relation to the number of atypical mononuclear cells, Reed–Sternberg cells and the type of connective tissue background.

In lymphocytic-predominant HD, atypical cells and Reed–Sternberg cells are sparse and difficult to identify, and lymphocytes predominate. At the other end of the spectrum in lymphocyte depletion, Reed–Sternberg cells are plentiful and lymphocytes sparse. Lymphocyte depleted HD is mainly found in elderly men with advanced disease; there are two subtypes, diffuse fibrosis and reticular. The diffuse form is extremely aggressive and carries a very poor prognosis. In nodular-sclerosing HD, nodules of lymphoid tissue are separated by dense bands of collagen. This is the most frequent subgroup of HD and occurs most commonly in young women who present with mediastinal lymphadenopathy. Mixed cellularity HD is composed of a mixed cellular picture including histiocytes, eosinophils, plasma cells, lymphocytes

Table 28.1. *Rye classification of Hodgkin's disease with approximate distribution of frequency*[13,14]

Histology	Frequency (%)
Lymphocyte predominance	5
Nodular sclerosis	65
Mixed cellularity	25
Lymphocyte depletion	5

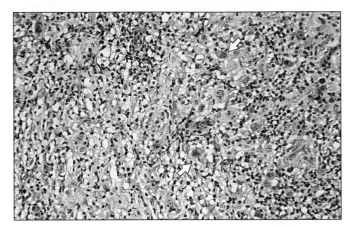

Figure 28.1. *Histological section of mixed cellularity HD showing Reed–Sternberg cells (arrows), lymphocytes and neutrophils.*

and neutrophils. This subgroup predominantly affects males and is the commonest type to be found in the infradiaphragmatic area, including the spleen.

Non-Hodgkin's lymphoma

The functional anatomy of the lymph node and its relationship to lymphoma is shown in Fig. 28.2. The recognition that most NHLs arise from the cells of the germinal follicle of the lymph node led to the development of a Working Formulation of NHL for clinical usage (Table 28.2).[15] This classification is widely employed and completely superseded the plethora of previous classifications which were largely unsatisfactory.[17,18]

Non-Hodgkin's lymphomas are developmentally arrested clonal expansions of B or T lymphocytes.[19] The Working Formulation is based on the point at which normal maturation of the lymphocyte is arrested. B lymphocytes (bone marrow derived) are concerned with antibody production and develop into plasma cells that produce immunoglobulin. If normal maturation is prevented the arrested cell multiplies resulting in lymphoma; the type and grade of lymphoma which results depends on the stage of maturation at the time of insult. T lymphocytes (thymic derived) do not contain immunoglobulin but are also concerned with immune response. T-cell lymphomas are either central T-cell lymphomas which are immature (e.g. diffuse lymphoblastic lymphoma), or those derived from more mature T lymphocytes, which are termed peripheral T-cell lymphomas. Histiocytic lymphomas do not fall into either of these categories and as yet their derivative cells are not completely defined.

The majority of NHLs (over 90%) are B-cell lymphomas. Non-Hodgkin's lymphomas which arise at stages of development which occur within the germinal centre of the node have a follicular pattern, whereas lymphomas which arise outside the germinal centre have a diffuse architectural pattern. The Working Formulation designates each lymphoma according to characteristics of the cell type at the time of arrested maturation and overall divides NHL into low-grade, intermediate and high-grade tumours. The 'miscellaneous' group do not fulfil all the requirements of the main three categories.[4]

The Working Formulation has important practical implications:

- Therapy is based on the grade of lymphoma
- The grade of lymphoma carries important prognostic significance
- The classification of lymphoma predicts possible transformation into a higher grade
- The detailed subclassification of lymphomas allows standardization of therapies and comparison of results from different centres

Improvement in the understanding of NHL and the recognition of new clinical/pathological entities has resulted in the introduction of a new classification by the International Lymphoma Study Group called the Revised European-American Lymphoma (REAL) classification which is now being adopted internationally (Table 28.3).[16] Even more recently a committee appointed by the World Health Organization has met in an attempt to resolve the confusion arising from this plethora of classifications of NHL. The resulting report has yet to be published.

STAGING CLASSIFICATIONS

The Ann Arbor staging system was introduced for HD in 1970 and takes into account the extent of nodal disease and the presence of extranodal extension. However, an increasing recognition of the influence of tumour bulk as an independent prognostic indicator within each stage, and the routine application of new diagnostic techniques, such as computed tomography (CT) or magnetic resonance imaging, (MRI) led to a modification of the Ann Arbor classification in 1989, known as the Cotswolds classification (Table 28.4).[20] This system is similar to the Ann Arbor classification but Stage III is subdivided and an additional qualifier 'X' denotes bulky

Table 28.2. *A working formulation of non-Hodgkin's lymphoma for clinical usage*[15]

Low grade	
A	Small lymphocytic
	Consistent with chronic lymphocytic leukaemia or with plasmacytoid features
B	Follicular, small cleaved cell
C	Follicular, mixed small cleaved and large cell
Intermediate grade	
D	Follicular, large cell
E	Diffuse, small cleaved cell
F	Diffuse, mixed small and large cell
G	Diffuse, large cell
High grade	
H	Large cell immunoblastic
I	Lymphoblastic (convoluted or non-convoluted)
J	Small non-cleaved cell (Burkitt or non-Burkitt type)
Miscellaneous	
Composite	
Histiocytic	
Mycosis fungoides	
Extramedullary plasmacytoma	
Hairy cell	
Unclassifiable	

disease. Both the Ann Arbor and Cotswold systems are applied to NHL, but are of less value, as in NHL the prognosis is more dependent on histological grade and other parameters, such as tumour bulk and specific organ involvement, than on stage.[21,22] In NHL the critical question is whether or not disease is limited and therefore potentially treatable with radiotherapy or whether it is disseminated.

Childhood NHL exhibits a clinical spectrum somewhat different to adult lymphoma with more frequent extranodal involvement, there being a very high incidence of lymphoma in the gastro-intestinal tract, solid abdominal viscera including the kidneys and pancreas, and extranodal sites in the head and neck.[23,24] The staging system of Murphy is most widely used (Table 28.5).

CLINICAL FEATURES

Hodgkin's disease and NHL are both diseases of the lymph nodes, both may present as truly localized processes involving a single nodal group or organ, or both may present as widely

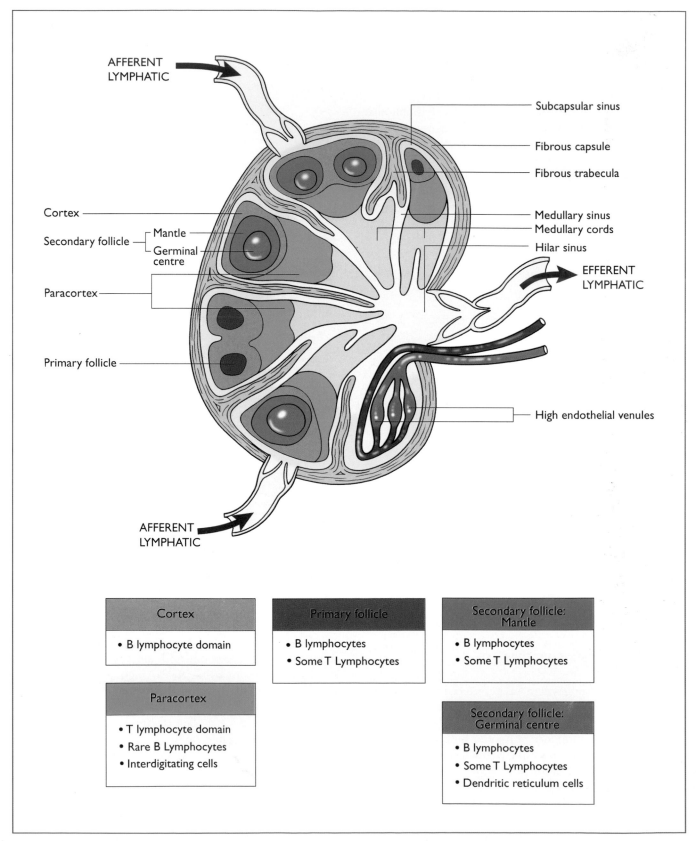

Figure 28.2. *Relationship of functional lymph node anatomy to normal cell type and lineage of the non-Hodgkin's lymphomas.*

Table 28.3 *The REAL classification*

B cell	T cell	Others
Precursor B lymphoblastic	Precursor T lymphoblastic	Composite lymphoma (types specified)
Small lymphocytic (CLL)	T cell chronic lymphocytic leukaemia	Unclassifiable, high grade
Lymphoplasmacytic	Large granular lymphocyte leukaemia	Unclassifiable, high grade
Mantle cell	Mycosis fungoides	Unclassifiable
Follicle centre lymphoma	Peripheral T cell, unspecified	
Follicular	Medium sized	
Grades 1, 2 and 3	Mixed medium and large cell	
	Large cell	
	Lymphoepithelioid	
	Hepatosplenic	
	Subcutaneous panniculitic	
Follicle centre lymphoma	Angioimmunoblastic	
Diffuse		
Marginal zone B-cell,	Angiocentric, nasal	
MALT type		
Marginal zone, B-cell, nodal	Intestinal	
Marginal zone, B-cell, splenic	Adult T-cell lymphoma/ leukaemia	
Hairy cell leukaemia	Anaplastic large cell	
Plasmacytoma	Anaplastic large cell	
	Hodgkin's like	
Diffuse large B-cell	Unclassifiable, low grade	
Diffuse mediastinal large B cell	Unclassifiable, high grade	
Burkitt's		
High grade B-cell, Burkitt-like		
Unclassified, low grade		
Unclassified, high grade		

Table 28.4. *Staging of lymphoma (Cotswolds classification)*[20]

Stage	Area of involvement
I	One lymph node region or extralymphatic site
II	Two or more lymph node regions on the same side of the diaphragm
III	Involvement of lymph node region or structures on both sides of diaphragm, subdivided thus:
III(1*)	With involvement of spleen and/or splenic hilar, coeliac and portal nodes
III(2*)	With para-aortic, iliac or mesenteric nodes
IV	Extranodal sites beyond those designated E
Additional qualifiers	
A	No symptoms
B	Fever, sweats, weight loss (to 10% of body weight)
E	Involvement of single extranodal site, contiguous in proximity to a known nodal site
X*	Bulky disease Mass >1/3 thoracic diameter at T5 Mass >10 cm maximum dimension
CE*	Clinical stage
PS*	Pathological stage: PS at a given site denoted by a subscript (i.e. M = marrow, H = liver, L = lung, O = bone, P = pleural, D = skin)

*Modifications from Ann Arbor system

disseminated disease. However, recognizable differences distinguish the clinical presentation in the two diseases.

Hodgkin's disease

Most patients with HD present with painless asymmetrical lymph node enlargement which may be accompanied with sweats, fever, weight loss and pruritus in about 40% of patients. Alcohol-induced pain is a rare complaint.

On clinical examination the commonest nodal site of involvement is the cervical region which is seen in 60–80% of patients. Axillary nodal involvement is also common, occurring in 6–20% of patients, and inguinal/femoral nodal disease is seen in 6–15%. Exclusive infradiaphragmatic lymphadenopathy only occurs in less than 10% of patients at diagnosis. Splenomegaly is found on clinical examination in about a third of patients.

Table 28.5. *Murphy's staging system for childhood non-Hodgkin's lymphoma*

Stage	Criteria for extent of disease
I	A single tumour (extranodal) or single anatomical area (nodal) with the exclusion of the mediastinum or abdomen
II	A single tumour (extranodal) with regional nodal involvement
	Two or more nodal areas on the same side of the diaphragm
	Two single (extranodal) tumours with or without regional node involvement of the same side of the diaphragm
	A primary gastro-intestinal tract tumour, usually in the ileocaecal area, with or without involvement of associated mesenteric nodes only, grossly completely resected
III	Two single tumours (extranodal) on opposite sides of the diaphragm
	Two or more nodal areas above and below the diaphragm
	ALL primary intrathoracic tumours (mediastinal, pleural, thymic)
	ALL extensive primary intra-abdominal disease, unresected
	ALL paraspinal or epidural tumours, regardless of other tumour site(s)
IV	Any of the above with initial central nervous system (CNS) and/or bone marrow involvement

Hodgkin's disease tends to spread in a contiguous fashion from one lymph node group to the next adjacent group. Primary extranodal Hodgkin's disease is very rare and can only be diagnosed after a thorough search for disease in other sites.

Non-Hodgkin's lymphoma

As in Hodgkin's disease, the majority of patients with NHL present with nodal enlargement.

In low-grade lymphoma lymphadenopathy may be intermittent and the median age at diagnosis is between 55 and 60 years. They are rarely diagnosed under the age of 30 years and account for 30–45% of all the lymphomas.

Intermediate grade lymphoma usually includes both follicular and diffuse forms. The diffuse large-cell lymphoma is the most common NHL subtype and usually presents with rapidly enlarging lymph nodes. Together with follicular large-cell lymphoma, these tumours comprise 50% of all lymphomas. They usually present between the ages of 50 and 55 years and may be associated with extranodal disease at presentation.

High-grade lymphomas are the most aggressive tumour subtype but most patients have apparently localized disease at the time of presentation. Overall, approximately 20% of patients with NHL have systemic symptoms, such as fever, sweats and weight loss, compared with 40%

of patients with HD. Non-Hodgkin's lymphoma is a disseminated disease involving lymph node groups haphazardly, multiple organs may be involved as well as the bone marrow.[25]

Key points: clinical aspects

■ The majority of patients with HD and NHL present with painless enlargement of a group of lymph nodes

■ In HD, most patients present with Stage-I or -II disease and in NHL the majority of patients have Stage-III or -IV disease at diagnosis

■ Systemic symptoms are seen more frequently in HD than NHL

■ Ten-year survival rates of over 90% are achieved in Stage-I and -II HD treated with radiotherapy. Hodgkin's disease is also highly chemosensitive; fifty to eighty percent of patients achieving complete remission in advanced HD

■ Multi-agent chemotherapy is the mainstay of treatment of NHL but radiotherapy and surveillance also have a role in management

PROGNOSIS AND TREATMENT OPTIONS

Hodgkin's disease

The prognosis of HD depends upon a number of factors.[7] These include:

- Age. Older patients have a worse prognosis
- Tumour subtype. Mixed cellularity and lymphocyte depletion have a worse prognosis than nodular sclerosis and lymphocyte-predominant HD
- Raised erythrocyte sedimentation rate (ESR)
- Multiple sites of involvement
- Bulky mediastinal disease
- Systemic symptoms

The standard treatment for early-stage HD is radiotherapy to the involved nodes as well as the adjacent lymph node chains. These tumours are highly radiosensitive and can be cured by radiotherapy alone.[20] Mantle radiotherapy for cervical lymphadenopathy has stood the test of time and includes irradiation to the bilateral cervical nodes, the supraclavicular and axillary nodes, together with mediastinal nodes, extending down to the lower border of the vertebral body of T10.

Until relatively recently, staging laparotomy was routinely undertaken in patients with HD to identify splenic involvement and intra-abdominal lymph node spread.

Although it is known that the spleen is involved in about 30% of patients with Stage-I and Stage-II HD, the technique has been abandoned for the following reasons:

- Even if the laparotomy is negative, relapse in the abdomen is common following mantle radiotherapy
- Combination chemotherapy is more frequently used in the treatment of HD thereby obviating the need for splenectomy
- Patients with undiagnosed infradiaphragmatic disease who are treated with mantle radiotherapy can be salvaged with subsequent chemotherapy
- Staging laparotomy is a major procedure and splenectomy increases the risk of infection and may have a causal relationship with the subsequent development of leukaemia[26]

Hodgkin's disease is chemosensitive and chemotherapy combined with radiotherapy is widely used in patients with adverse prognostic indicators in early-stage disease, for example, those presenting with bulky mediastinal masses or multiple sites of involvement. Chemotherapy with or without irradiation is also the standard approach for the treatment of Stage-III and -IV disease.

Major developments in treatment have been aimed to reduce toxicity while at the same time maintaining efficacy. The different regimes have different side-effects ranging from nausea, vomiting, and hair loss to bone marrow suppression, sterility and leukaemogenesis.[27–29] The overall 10-year survival in patients with Stage-I and -II HD treated with radiotherapy is greater than 90%.[30,31]

In patients with more advanced disease (bulky Stage II, Stage III and IV), overall, between 50 and 80% will achieve complete remission following multi-agent chemotherapy, but of these between 30 and 50% will subsequently relapse within 5 years.[20] Combination chemotherapy for recurrence after primary treatment with radiotherapy alone is successful in achieving a prolonged second remission.[32] Patients failing initial chemotherapy for advanced HD have a poor prognosis but high-dose chemotherapy with haemopoietic stem-cell rescue is being increasingly employed although its long-term benefits are not yet established.[33]

Non-Hodgkin's lymphoma

The prognosis of NHL varies tremendously. Low-grade follicular lymphomas, although incurable, often have a prolonged indolent course. Low-grade lymphoma, for example, follicular small cell lymphoma, is slowly progressive and has a tendency to become more diffuse with a greater number of large cells. Such transformation has important implications for prognosis and therefore an impact on treatment strategy. Intermediate and high-grade lymphomas carry a worse prognosis, especially those with larger cells and blast forms. In these patients, how-ever, cure is possible with advanced chemotherapeutic regimens.

The treatment of NHL depends on the grade of lymphoma at presentation as well as the sites of involvement. At one end of the scale, patients presenting with low-grade lymphomas who are asymptomatic may simply be followed without treatment until symptoms develop or transformation occurs. At the other end of the scale, patients presenting with high-grade disease may be successfully treated with multi-agent chemotherapy with most attaining a remission and up to 50% of patients achieving long-term disease-free survival.[34] However, once relapse occurs, particularly if remission is short, further response to salvage chemotherapy is difficult to sustain. Current investigation is directed towards high-dose therapy with autologous bone marrow transplant.[35]

Radiotherapy has a role in low and intermediate-grade NHL but is usually inappropriate for treatment of high-grade lymphomas which are frequently widely disseminated tumours.

Overall, 10-year survival in patients treated with radiotherapy for Stage-I and -II disease are in the order of 90%.[30,31]

The major differences between the clinical features of HD and NHL are shown in Table 28.6.

Broadly, NHL is disseminated at presentation more frequently than HD and, although the majority of adult patients with NHL present with superficial lymphadenopathy, involvement of the viscera is more common in all types of NHL than it is in HD.

NODAL DISEASE

Lymph node enlargement tends to be greater in NHL than HD but both types may produce huge conglomerate tumour masses or may not produce any significant nodal enlargement. In nodular sclerosing HD and lymphocyte-depleted HD, involved nodes tend to be normal in size or are only moderately enlarged. Typically, low-grade NHL produces large-volume nodal disease. A characteristic feature of lymphoma is that involved nodes tend to displace structures rather than invade them and in this respect they differ from carcinomas; an exception being the large cell high-grade lymphomas which are often locally invasive.

Imaging techniques

The ability of computed tomography to demonstrate enlarged lymph nodes throughout the body, detect associated pathology in soft tissue structures, together with its reproducibility, have all contributed to CT becoming the modality of choice for the staging and follow-up of lymphoma. Ultrasound will readily show lymph node enlargement in the coeliac region, splenic hilum and porta hepatis.[36,37] Frequently, however, the

Table 28.6. *Key differences between the clinical features of Hodgkin's disease and non-Hodgkin's lymphoma*

	Hodgkin's disease	Non-Hodgkin's lymphoma
Clinical features		
Fever, night sweats, loss of weight	40%	20%
Spread	Tends to be by contiguity	Multiple remote nodal groups are often involved
Age	Uncommon in childhood	More frequent 40–70 yrs
Nodal groups		
Thoracic	65–85%	25–40%
Para-aortic	25–35%	45–55%
Mesenteric	5%	50–60%
Extranodal disease		
Central nervous system	<1%	2%
Gastro-intestinal tract	<1%	5–15%
Genito-urinary tract	<1%	1–5%
Bone marrow	3%	20–40%
Lung parenchyma	8–12%	3–6%
Bone	<1%	1–2%
Stage at diagnosis	>80% Stage I–II	>85% Stage III–IV

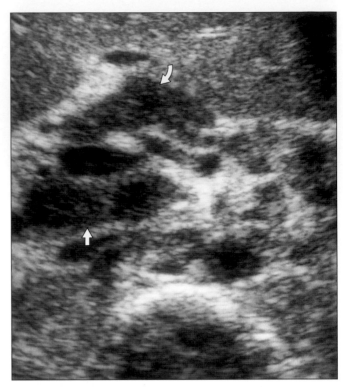

Figure 28.3. *Nodal enlargement on ultrasound. A transverse scan through the upper abdomen showing multiple hypoechoic lobulated masses consistent with lymph node enlargement located between the inferior vena cava and portal vein (arrow) and within the porta hepatis (curved arrow).*

entire retroperitoneum cannot be shown, limiting its value in staging. Typically, lymphomatous nodal involvement produces uniformly hypoechoic, lobulated masses, appearances that are non-specific (Fig. 28.3). The main value of ultrasound in lymphoma lies not in routine staging,[38] for which it is not sufficiently reliable, but in confirming that a palpable mass is in fact nodal or in solving specific problems in the liver, spleen or kidneys.[39] Although the accuracy of MRI in detecting lymph node involvement is equal to that of CT,[40–42] it has no particular advantage over CT, and its role is essentially adjunctive, used to solve problems in the identification of lymph node pathology or in monitoring response to treatment.[43] On MRI, lymph nodes are easily identified as relatively low/intermediate signal intensity masses on T1-weighted images and are of intermediate/high signal in T2-weighted images (Fig. 28.4). On short tau inversion recovery (STIR) sequences, enlarged nodes may have a very high signal intensity. Treated nodes, particularly in nodular sclerosing HD, may become necrotic and the nodes then have a signal intensity similar to that of fluid (Fig. 28.5). Calcification may occasionally develop following treatment for HD which is clearly seen on CT. On MRI the signal intensity of calcified nodes is reduced.

Radio-isotope studies using Ga-67 and the positron emitter 2-[F-18] fluoro-2-deoxy-D-glucose can also demonstrate viable tumour cells within nodes with high sensitivity.[44,45] Neither are primary staging techniques and they are best used in the detection of residual masses after treatment. The accuracy of Ga-67 is dependent on several factors including cell type, and the location and size of the lesions. Its accuracy is greater for HD and histiocytic lymphoma than for other forms; its accuracy decreases when the lesion exceeds 5 cm and it is poor below the diaphragm.

During the 1980s, several studies showed that lymphangiography was equal to or slightly superior to CT for detecting nodal lymphoma.[46–53] However, lymphangiography does have several disadvantages, most significant are its inability to demonstrate lymph nodes above the level of the second lumbar vertebra and outside the retroperitoneum as well as the true extent of a nodal mass once it is has broken through the lymph node capsule (Fig. 28.6). Its advantages have become limited due to the development of newer generation CT scanners which permit the detection of smaller degrees of lymphadenopathy. Another important factor is the increasing efficacy of chemotherapy which is now able to salvage patients with apparent early stage supradiaphragmatic disease, but who

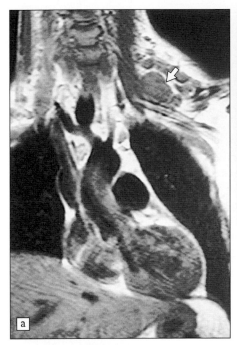

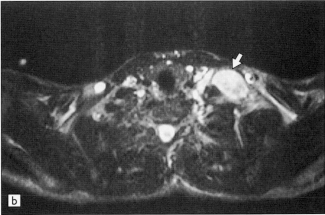

Figure 28.4. *MR images in a patient with HD showing enlarged lymph nodes in the left supraclavicular fossa. (a) T1-weighted paracoronal image showing the involved nodes (arrowed) as low signal intensity masses; (b) an axial T2-weighted image shows that the enlarged nodes have a high signal intensity (arrowed). Note a high signal intensity 1 cm node is also visible on the right.*

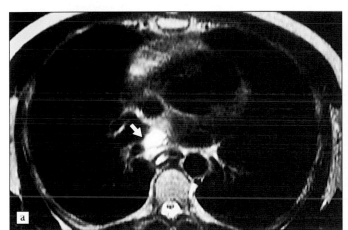

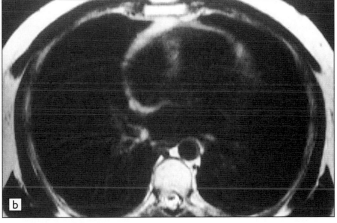

Figure 28.5. *MR images of a patient with HD. (a) Pretreatment turbo spin-echo T2-weighted image shows a high signal intensity residual lymph node in the subcarinal space* (arrowed). *No further treatment was given; (b) a follow-up examination 4 months later shows complete resolution of the node presumed to be necrotic.*

actually harbour microscopic foci of tumour in the spleen and/or infradiaphragmatic nodes. Thus although lymphan–giography remains the only imaging method which visualizes nodal architecture, the complementary yield of lymphangiography over CT in HD is negligible and it is estimated that in only 5% of cases of HD will lymphangiography show abnormalities in lymph nodes smaller than 1 cm. Another problem with lymphangiography is the general lack of expertise currently available both in carrying out the procedure and in interpretation of the results. Even with lymphangiography, false-negative examinations are inevitable due to microscopic

deposits in normal sized nodes, but in addition false-positive examinations result from nodal enlargement due to benign hyperplasia.[54] Although some specialized centres continue to undertake lymphangiography in HD, it is generally only recommended when immediate detection of tumour in a normal sized retroperitoneal node is considered essential for patient management and local expertise is available.[54]

Nodal disease in HD and NHL may involve any site where lymph nodes are found anatomically but for convenience this description is divided into the following sections neck, thorax, abdomen and pelvis.

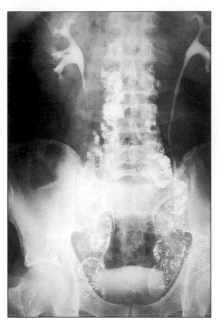

Figure 28.6. *A lymphogram combined with an intravenous urogram in a patient with widespread abdominal and pelvic nodal NHL. In the lower abdomen and pelvis the nodes are grossly enlarged; the true extent of disease can only be inferred by the extent of abnormal contrast enhancement. Disease has clearly spread beyond the capsule of the involved nodes.*

Neck

A group of enlarged lymph nodes in the neck is the commonest presentation in HD seen in 60–80% of cases and may also be the presenting feature in NHL. Hodgkin's disease typically involves the internal jugular chain of nodes first, but further spread is to the spinal accessory chain and the transverse cervical chain, these nodes forming the deep lymphatic chains of the neck.[55] The internal jugular chain follows the course of the internal jugular vein, the spinal accessory nodes are found between the sternocleidomastoid and trapezius muscles in the posterior triangle and the transverse cervical nodes join the internal jugular and spinal accessory nodes in

the lower neck (Fig. 28.7). Nodes in the submandibular, submental, parotid and retropharyngeal regions are occasionally involved. The pattern of NHL is more haphazard than HD and is more likely to be associated with extranodal disease.

Lymph nodes greater than 1 cm in diameter are generally considered enlarged on CT. Minimally enlarged discrete lymph nodes seen in the neck in patients with lymphoma usually have a well defined contour, but once the tumour has broken beyond the confines of the node, the fat planes between the nodal mass and adjacent structures is lost. Fibrosis following radiotherapy may also eliminate the fat planes making post-treatment assessment difficult on clinical examination. Central necrosis within a lymph node is rarely seen in the lymphomas, a striking contrast to the typical features seen in squamous carcinoma nodal metastasis on contrast enhanced CT.

Imaging, particularly CT, has a useful role in evaluating the neck in patients with lymphoma as it may:

- Identify involved nodes which are clinically impalpable
- Assess treatment response, particularly in patients treated with radiotherapy
- Identify recurrence in patients with thickened tissues due to previous radiotherapy (Fig. 28.8)

Magnetic resonance imaging may be particularly useful for defining the extent of lymphomatous masses in the lower neck and supraclavicular fossa (Fig. 28.9).

Thorax

The frequency and distribution of intrathoracic lymph node involvement in HD and NHL differ, although the appearances on imaging are similar. As in the neck, lymph nodes

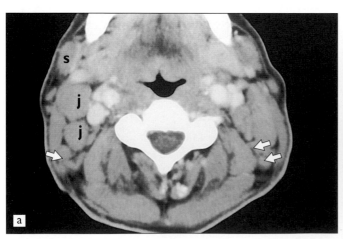

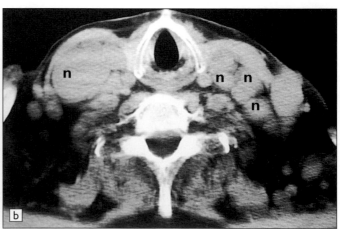

Figure 28.7. *NHL involving lymph nodes in the neck.(a) Contrast-enhanced CT scan shows discrete enlargement of lymph nodes bilaterally at presentation (arrowed). The involved nodes are larger on the right. Submandibular node (s), jugular node (j);*

(b) unenhanced CT in a patient with intermediate grade NHL showing bilateral involvement of midjugular nodes (n). The sternocleidomastoid muscle on the right is displaced by a node measuring 3 × 2 cm in diameter.

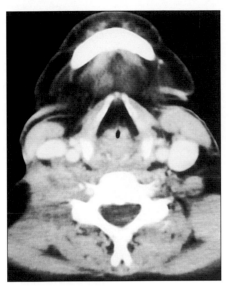

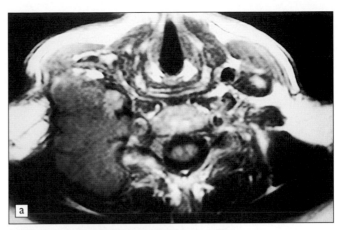

Figure 28.8.
Recurrent low-grade NHL. A nodal mass on the right side of the neck is seen on contrast-enhanced CT which has an ill-defined contour and is closely applied to the sternocleidomastoid muscle. The patient had previously been treated with radiotherapy.

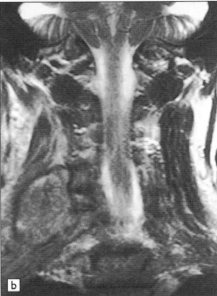

Figure 28.9.
MR images in a patient with NHL showing a large mass in the right lower neck extending into the supraclavicular fossa. (a) A turbo spin-echo T1-weighted image clearly shows the lobulated low signal intensity mass on the right side of the neck; (b) a turbo spin-echo T2-weighted image shows that the mass has a heterogeneous intermediate/high signal intensity. The mass is surrounded by a well-defined low signal intensity rim.

greater than 1 cm in diameter are considered enlarged both on CT and MRI. However, account should also be given to the number of nodes present; multiple nodes, although less than 1 cm in diameter within the anterior mediastinum, should certainly be regarded as suspicious (Fig. 28.10). Nodes within the thorax are involved at the time of presentation in 60–85% of patients with HD and 25–40% of patients with NHL.[22,56–58] Any intrathoracic group of nodes may be involved in patients with lymphoma, but all the mediastinal sites are more frequently involved by HD than NHL, except the paracardiac and posterior mediastinal nodes. The frequency of nodal involvement in HD is as follows:[57]

- Prevascular and paratracheal (84%)
- Hilar (28%)
- Subcarinal (22%)
- Other sites (approx. 5%)
  - Aortopulmonary window
  - Anterior diaphragmatic
  - Internal mammary
  - Posterior mediastinal

The frequency of intrathoracic nodal involvement in NHL has recently been analysed by Castellino et al:[59]

- Superior mediastinal (34%)
- Hilar (9%)
- Subcarinal (13%)
- Other sites (up to 10%)

In most cases lymphadenopathy is bilateral but asymmetric. Almost all patients with nodular sclerosing HD have disease in the anterior mediastinum.[58] The great majority of cases of HD show enlargement of two or more nodal groups, whereas only

one nodal group is involved in up to half of the cases of NHL. Hilar nodal enlargement is rare without associated mediastinal involvement, particularly in HD. The posterior mediastinum is infrequently involved but if disease is present in the lower part of the mediastinum contiguous retrocrural disease is likely.[60] Although paracardiac nodes are rarely involved at presentation, they become important as sites of recurrence as they may not be included in the radiation field.[61]

On CT, enlarged nodes may be discrete or matted together, and usually show only minor enhancement after injection of intravenous contrast medium (Fig. 28.11). Calcification prior to therapy is extremely rare,[58,62] but is seen occasionally following therapy. Cystic degeneration may be seen rarely in both HD and NHL, which may persist following therapy when the rest of the nodal masses shrink away[63] (Fig. 28.5).

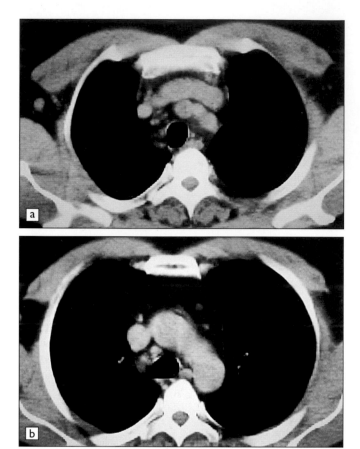

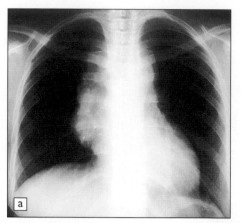

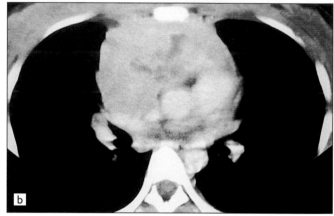

Figure 28.10. *(a, b) NHL. Multiple prominent nodes are seen in the prevascular space and in the pretracheal retrocaval space. All these nodes measure less than 1 cm in diameter but the number of lymph nodes raise suspicion of involvement. Note a 1 cm diameter node in the right axilla.*

Figure 28.11. *Massive lymph node enlargement in a patient presenting with HD. (a) Plain chest radiograph; (b) contrast-enhanced CT scan showing anterior mediastinal lymph node mass. Note low density area centrally, probably representing necrosis.*

In about 10% of patients with HD, CT demonstrates enlarged mediastinal nodes despite a normal chest radiograph[57] (Fig. 28.12).

Even in patients with bulky disease, CT frequently provides additional information such as:

- The inferior extent of the mass and its relationship to the heart
- Pericardial thickening and effusion which can be distinguished from lymphadenopathy

Large anterior mediastinal masses usually represent thymic infiltration as well as a nodal mass[64] (Fig. 28.13a). Enlarged nodes can usually be distinguished from a thymic mass but on occasion thymic involvement can only be definitely recorded on evaluation of follow-up studies after treatment when the thymus has resumed its normal shape in up to 30% of patients[65] (Fig. 28.13b). Thymic infiltration may be seen in both HD and NHL. Although the thymus is usually seen on CT as a homogeneous soft tissue mass, cystic areas within the mass may be identified both on CT and MRI (Fig. 28.13). These cysts are more frequently detected on MRI.[66]

Impalpable axillary nodal enlargement is also frequently detected on CT in HD and NHL, and may be unilateral or bilateral (Figs. 28.10a and 28.12b). Occasionally nodes contain fat centrally which is helpful in distinguishing those involved by lymphoma from those with enlargement due to benign hyperplasia.

Magnetic resonance imaging of the chest may provide additional information to CT in a problem-solving role, for example in the demonstration of nodal enlargement in areas where evaluation with CT is difficult, such as the subcarinal space and aortopulmonary window. Magnetic resonance imaging is also helpful for defining the full extent of disease, for example infiltration of the chest wall (Fig. 28.14).

When reporting thoracic CT for staging HD or NHL, it is always important to check all possible sites of involvement

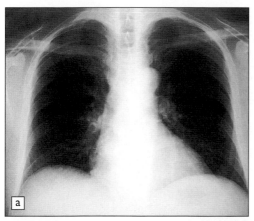

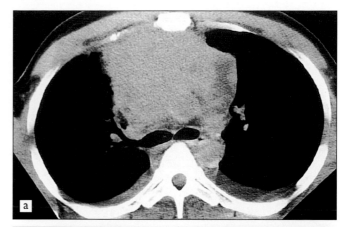

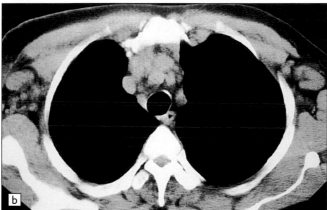

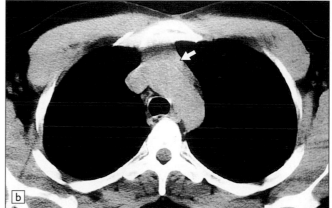

Figure 28.12. *(a) Plain chest radiograph and (b) CT scan in a patient with NHL. The plain chest radiograph appears normal but CT shows multiple enlarged lymph nodes in the mediastinum indicating intrathoracic disease. Note left internal mammary and bilateral axillary lymph node enlargement.*

Figure 28.13. *CT scan in a patient with HD. (a) Before treatment there is a large anterior mediastinal mass probably involving the thymus. Note an area of low density within the mass on the left which either represents necrosis or cystic change; (b) following treatment the mass has shown an excellent response to treatment and the thymus has resumed its normal shape (arrowed), indicating that the mass almost certainly represented thymic infiltration. (From ref. 66, with permission)*

because minimally enlarged nodes in such sites as the internal mammary group or diaphragmatic nodes are easily overlooked (Fig. 28.15).

Abdomen and pelvis

At presentation, the retroperitoneal nodes are involved in 25–35% of patients with HD, and 45–55% of patients with NHL.[67–69] Mesenteric lymph nodes are involved in more than half of patients with NHL and <5% of patients with HD.[67–70] Other sites, as in the porta hepatis and around the splenic hilum, are also less frequently involved in HD than NHL. In HD, nodal spread is predictably from one lymph node group to contiguous groups.[71,72] In this context, the term 'contiguous' does not mean physical contiguity but through directly connected lymphatic pathways. Nodes are frequently of normal size or only minimally enlarged.[53] In NHL, nodal involvement is frequently non-contiguous, bulky and is more frequently associated with extranodal disease.

In HD the coeliac axis, splenic hilar and porta hepatis nodes are involved in about one-third of patients and splenic hilar nodal involvement is al-most always associated with diffuse splenic infiltration (Fig. 28.16 a,b,c). In the porta hepatis an important node is the node of the foramen of Winslow (portocaval node) which lies between the portal vein and inferior vena cava (Fig. 28.17). This node has a triangular or lozenge shape; its normal transverse diameter is up to 3 cm in diameter and in the anterioposterior plane is approximately 1 cm.[73] Enlargement of its portocaval node is easily overlooked which is particularly important if it is the only site of relapse. Spread from the mediastinum occurs through lymphatic vessels to the retrocrural nodes, coeliac axis and so on. In the coeliac axis, multiple normal-sized nodes may be seen which can be difficult to evaluate because involved normal-sized nodes are frequent in HD.[53]

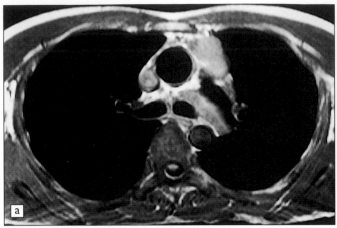

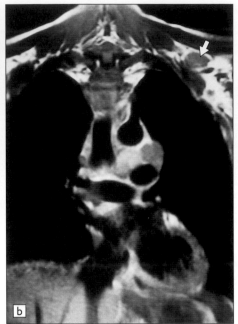

Figure 28.14. *MR images in a patient with HD showing nodal enlargement in the anterior mediastinum and aortopulmonary window. Turbo spin-echo T1-weighted images: (a) axial; (b) coronal. The enlarged nodes have an intermediate signal intensity lower than that of fat but higher than that of muscle. Note an enlarged lymph node in the left supraclavicular fossa (arrowed).*

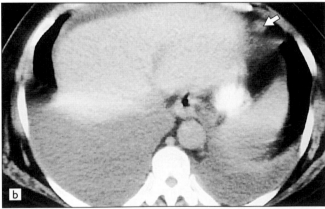

Figure 28.15. *CT scan in a patient with NHL showing (a) an enlarged left internal mammary lymph node. Note an enlarged pretracheal lymph node. (b) CT scan of a patient with NHL with bilateral pleural effusions. There is a 1 cm diaphragmatic lymph node adjacent to the left cardiac border (arrowed).*

Key points: supradiaphragmatic nodal disease

- 60–80% of patients with HD present with enlarged neck nodes. It is also a common presentation in NHL

- 60–80% of patients with HD have prevascular and paratracheal lymphadenopathy at diagnosis

- 10% of patients with HD have enlarged nodes detected on CT but a normal chest radiograph

- Hilar lymphadenopathy is rarely seen in isolation

- A large anterior mediastinal mass may represent lymphomatous infiltration of the thymus

- Enlarged axillary nodes are found in 6–20% of patients with HD at diagnosis

In NHL, nodal involvement is frequently non-contiguous and bulky. Discrete mesenteric nodal enlargement or masses may be seen with or without retroperitoneal nodal enlargement (Fig. 28.18). Large volume nodal disease in both the mesentery and retroperitoneum, may give rise to the so called 'hamburger' sign in which a loop of bowel is compressed between the two large nodal masses (Fig. 28.18c). In NHL, regional nodal involvement is frequently seen in patients with primary extranodal lymphoma involving an abdominal viscera.

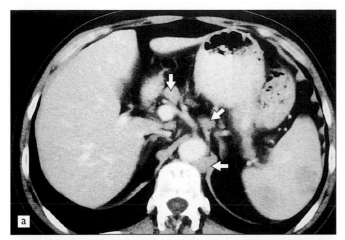

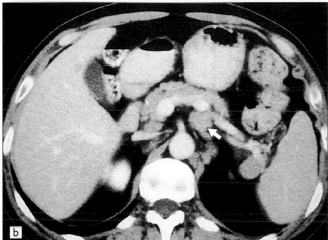

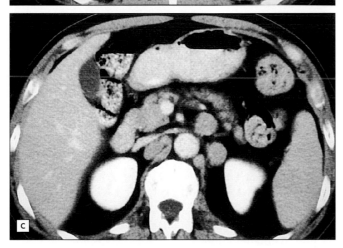

Figure 28.16. *HD. CT scans showing involvement of (a) coeliac axis lymph nodes and a retrocrural lymph node on the left (arrowed). Note focal deposits in the spleen; (b) at a lower level there is an enlarged lymph node at the splenic hilum and a further enlarged node is seen in the superior mesenteric group (arrowed). The portal node is prominent but not enlarged on CT criteria; (c) at the level of the upper poles of the kidneys, enlarged retroperitoneal lymph nodes are seen.*

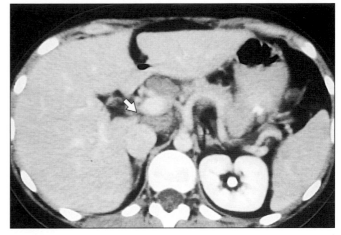

Figure 28.17. *A patient with NHL showing an enlarged portocaval lymph node (arrowed). There is also an enlarged node anterior to the portal vein in the porta hepatis.*

Key points: abdominal nodal disease

■ Retroperitoneal lymphadenopathy is more commonly seen in NHL than HD

■ In NHL, mesenteric lymphadenopathy is seen in greater than 50% of cases

■ In HD, the coeliac, splenic hilar and porta hepatis nodes are most frequently involved

■ Splenic hilar lymphadenopathy is almost invariably accompanied by splenic infiltration

In the pelvis all nodal groups may be involved in both HD and NHL (Fig. 28.19). Presentation of enlarged inguinal/femoral lymphadenopathy is seen in less than 20% of HD but when it does occur, careful attention must be paid to the evaluation of pelvic nodes on imaging as these will be the next contiguous sites of tumour spread. In patients with massive pelvic disease, MRI is helpful for delineating the full extent of tumour in the coronal and axial planes.

EXTRANODAL DISEASE

In about 40% of cases, lymphoma arises in extranodal sites, the vast majority of these are NHL.[74] There is a propensity for lymphomas associated with immunodeficiency and also those which develop in childhood to arise extranodally. Secondary extranodal lymphoma occurs due to spread of lymph node disease into adjacent structures and organs and may be seen in both HD and NHL.

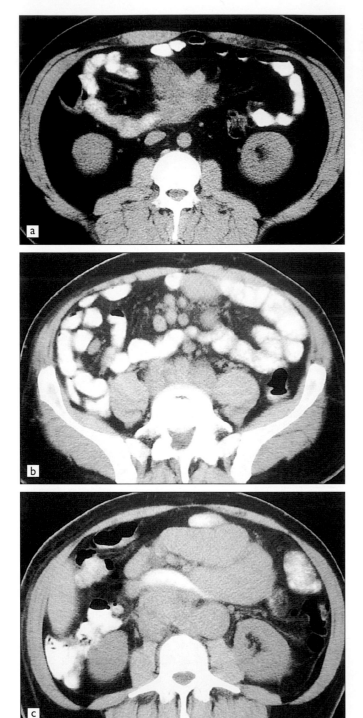

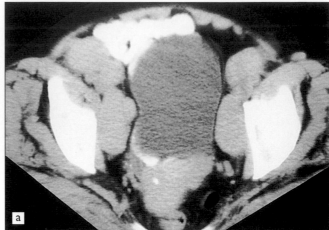

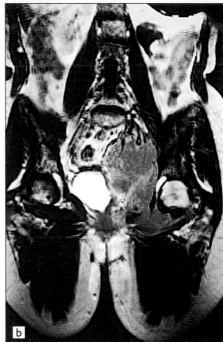

Figure 28.19. *Pelvic lymph node involvement in NHL. (a) Gross bilateral enlargement of external iliac and obturator lymph nodes; (b) coronal contrast enhanced T1-weighted MR image showing an extensive left-sided lymph mass.*

Figure 28.18. *CT scans in three different patients with NHL: (a) shows a large mesenteric mass without evidence of retroperitoneal lymph node involvement; (b) discrete nodal enlargement of mesenteric lymph nodes associated with retroperitoneal lymphadenopathy; (c) a large mass in the mesentery associated with a mass of retroperitoneal lymph nodes. These masses compress on opacified loop of bowel giving rise to the 'hamburger' sign.*

Thorax

The lung

Secondary involvement of the lung parenchyma at presentation in HD is most commonly by direct invasion from involved hilar and mediastinal nodes. However, peripheral subpleural masses or consolidations without visible connection to enlarged nodes in the mediastinum or hilar also occur in both HD and NHL. On chest radiography, lung parenchymal involvement is seen three times more frequently in HD (12%) than in NHL[54,58,74] (Fig. 28.20). Parenchymal involvement in HD is almost invariably accompanied by intrathoracic adenopathy, whereas in NHL pulmonary or pleural lesions may be seen without mediastinal or hilar lymphadenopathy.[76] However, if the mediastinal and hilar nodes have been previously irradiated, recurrence

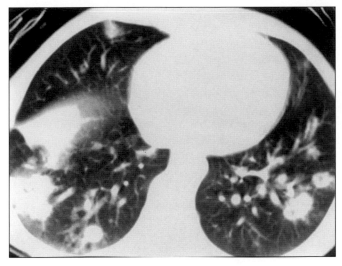

Figure 28.20. *CT scan showing pulmonary involvement in a patient with HD. There are multiple ill-defined nodules, several of which show cavitation, particularly those at the left lung base.*

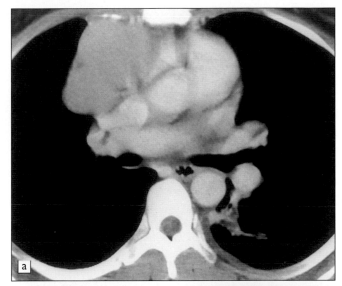

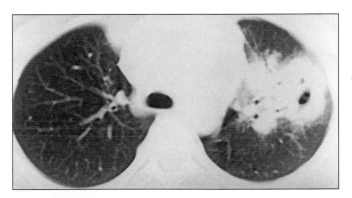

Figure 28.21. *Pulmonary involvement in a patient with high-grade NHL. The CT scan shows consolidation with air bronchograms and cavitation.*

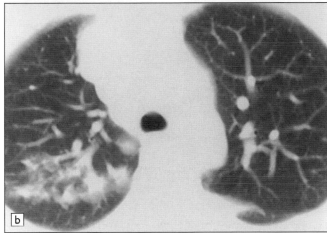

Figure 28.22. *Pulmonary involvement in a patient with HD: (a) shows a predominantly right-sided anterior mediastinal mass; (b) a CT scan showing peribronchial pulmonary nodules extending from the hila.*

confined to the lungs is seen in both HD and NHL.[77] Thus, in a patient with HD who has not received radiotherapy, in whom there is no evidence of hilar or mediastinal disease, pulmonary abnormality probably represents pathology other than HD.[58,76]

The radiographic changes in both HD and NHL are varied and difficult to characterize. Pulmonary involvement is frequently perihilar or juxtamediastinal.[78] The most common pattern is one or more discrete nodules resembling primary or metastatic carcinoma, but usually less well-defined, which may also cavitate (Fig. 28.20).[56,79,80] Rounded or segmental consolidation with visible air bronchograms is another common pattern (Fig. 28.21). Peribronchial pulmonary nodules (Fig. 28.22) extending from the hila, or focal streak shadowing, also peribronchial, may be seen in

association with the consolidation, reflecting spread along the peribronchial lymphatics (Fig. 28.22). The least common pattern is widespread reticulonodular (lymphangitic) shadowing. This is sufficiently rare in HD to necessitate other conditions causing interstitial lung disease to be excluded. Endobronchial disease causing atelectasis is extremely rare, but is still more likely than extrinsic occlusion by neighbouring lymph node enlargement.[81]

Primary (or isolated) pulmonary lymphoma is usually due to NHL. Low-grade B-cell lymphomas comprise the majority of primary NHL of the lung. These are neoplasms of small lymphoid cells that have been classified as malignant lymphoma — small lymphocytic type, or malignant lymphoma — small lymphocytic plasmacytoid type, according to the 'Working Formulation'. Currently, most of the low-grade lymphomas of the lung are believed to represent lymphomas of mucosa (or bronchus) associated lymphoid tissue (MALT or BALT).[82,83] These low-grade lymphomas occur most frequently in patients in the fifth to sixth decade, the clinical course is indolent, and there is an 80–90% survival at 5 years. The radiographic findings are non-specific. Solitary nodules are identified on chest radiographs in >50% of cases, ranging from 2–20 cm. Multiple nodules may occur, or there may be localized or multiple areas of consolidation.[84] Hilar or mediastinal lymph nodes are rarely involved.

Although MALT constitute the majority of primary pulmonary lymphomas, high-grade NHL accounts for the remaining 15–20% of primary lung lymphomas.[84] These patients are usually symptomatic, and solitary or multiple nodules are the most common radiographic pattern. Primary pulmonary HD is an extremely rare entity.[84]

The diverse appearances of pulmonary lymphoma provide a particular challenge to diagnosis because many of these patients have other reasons for developing lung disease, such as:

- Opportunistic infection either following or during chemotherapy
- Pneumonitis following radiotherapy
- Drug-related pulmonary fibrosis

Thus, the differential diagnosis is difficult and the diagnosis of pulmonary lymphoma, particularly in previously treated patients, must be made in the light of full clinical information.

Pleural disease

Pleural effusions due to lymphoma are nearly always accompanied by mediastinal lymph node enlargement and sometimes by pulmonary involvement, visible on a chest radiograph.[55] Most effusions are unilateral, are usually exudates and may disappear with irradiation of mediastinal nodes. Such effusions probably result from venous or lymphatic obstruction by enlarged mediastinal nodes, rather than direct neoplastic involvement, and may be detected on CT in over 50% of patients with mediastinal nodal involvement (Fig. 28.23).[80] Chylothorax is only occasionally encountered. Solid soft tissue pleural masses are rare and usually seen in recurrent disease.

Chest wall

Involvement of the chest wall occurs most commonly in HD as a result of direct extension from an anterior mediastinal mass. Less commonly, large masses of NHL may arise primarily in the soft tissues of the thoracic wall. Both direct invasion and primary chest wall lymphoma are better demonstrated on MRI than CT. T2-weighted images are preferable to T1-weighted images because tumour is seen as a high signal intensity mass, well contrasted against the low signal intensity of the normal muscles of the chest wall.[85]

Pericardium and heart

Pericardial effusions are seen on CT in 6% of patients with HD at presentation.[86] Effusions are presumptive evidence of pericardial involvement and in all such patients there is coexistent large mediastinal adenopathy extending over the cardiac margins.[56] Pericardial effusions are not infrequently seen in patients undergoing therapy for HD and NHL. They are usually distinguishable from pericardial lymphomatous involvement (Fig. 28.23) because they develop when the patient is on chemotherapy, are usually small and resolve spontaneously.

Direct invasion of the heart may be seen in patients with aggressive bulky mediastinal masses and in this rare situation MRI is probably the best technique for defining the presence and extent of cardiac involvement.[87]

Thymus

Thirty to fifty percent of patients with newly diagnosed HD have thymic involvement.[64] It may be impossible to distinguish the enlarged thymus on CT or MRI from adjacent lymphadenopathy, which is usually but not invariably present (Fig. 28.13). On CT, the gland may be of homogeneous soft tissue density, similar to adjacent lymph nodes. On MRI too the signal intensity on both T1- and T2-weighted images is similar to that of enlarged nodes. Cysts and calcification may be seen within the enlarged gland, either at presentation or during follow-up on both CT and MRI.[65,66] Cysts are better appreciated on MRI but calcification is more easily recognized on CT.[66]

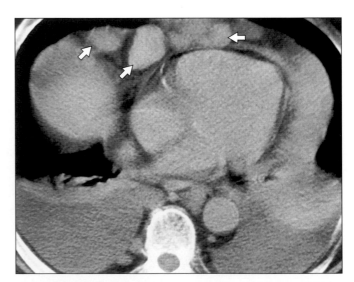

Figure 28.23. *Pericardial involvement in a high-grade NHL. The CT scan shows massive pericardial disease with a large soft tissue mass encasing the pericardium. There is also discrete paracardiac lymph node enlargement (arrows). Note too, the bilateral pleural effusions.*

Mycosis fungoides

Mycosis fungoides is a cutaneous T-cell lymphoma, that occurs in middle-aged adults and may disseminate to multiple sites, most frequently the lungs.[87] On chest radiographs the lungs may show solitary or multiple nodules, multiple areas of consolidation, or bilateral reticulonodular shadowing.[88] Hilar and mediastinal lymphadenopathy are usually present.[88] Detection of visceral involvement, particularly the lungs, portends a poor prognosis and influences treatment decisions.[84]

Key points: extranodal thoracic disease

- Secondary involvement of the lung parenchyma is seen three times more frequently in HD than NHL. Lung involvement in HD is almost invariably associated with mediastinal lymphadenopathy

- Most primary low-grade lymphomas of the lung are believed to represent MALT or BALT tumours

- Pleural effusions are associated with mediastinal lymphadenopathy in over 50% of cases

- Chest wall invasion occurs most commonly in HD by direct extension of a mediastinal mass

- Thymic infiltration occurs in 30–50% of newly diagnosed patients with HD

- The lungs are a frequent site of dissemination of disease in mycosis fungoides

Breast

Primary breast lymphoma is rare, accounting for less than 1% of all breast tumours. Mammographically, features are relatively non-specific, being those of a well circumscribed soft tissue mass without calcification and with little, if any, architectural distortion. Multiple nodules or a more diffuse pattern is occasionally seen.[89]

Abdomen

Spleen

The spleen is involved in 30–40% of patients with HD[68,90] In the majority of cases this occurs in the presence of nodal disease above and below the diaphragm,[91] but it is the sole abdominal focus of disease in 10% of adults presenting with HD clinically confined to sites above the diaphragm. To date, all imaging techniques have been unreliable in the detection of splenic involvement, partly because in the vast majority of cases of splenic HD, nodules are less than 1 cm in size. An enlarged spleen is not a reliable indicator of disease; one-third of patients with HD and splenomegaly do not have enlargement of the spleen; however, one-third of normal-sized spleens in patients with either HD or NHL are found to contain tumour at laparotomy.[69]

Occasionally, focal splenic nodules are seen exceeding 1 cm on cross-sectional imaging (Fig. 28.24). These lesions have a non-specific appearance, are usually hypoechoic on ultrasound, isodense on unenhanced CT and enhance to a lesser extent than normal parenchyma following intravenous injection of contrast medium (Fig. 28.16). The sensitivity of ultrasound in demonstrating splenic involvement is thus extremely low and does not exceed 35%.[36,48,50]

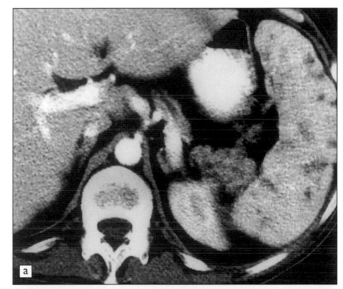

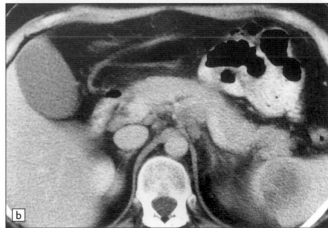

Figure 28.24. *Splenic involvement in lymphoma. (a) Postcontrast CT scan showing multiple small focal abnormalities of similar size within the spleen. The patient had HD; (b) CT scan showing a solitary large focal abnormality within the spleen in a patient with NHL. Note too, the presence of paracoeliac lymph node enlargement.*

Although this low accuracy for the detection of splenic involvement on imaging is disappointing, failure to detect splenic infiltration in HD is now of less clinical disadvantage than before. This is because patients with early-stage disease who relapse due to untreated splenic infiltration can be salvaged by multi-agent chemotherapy, following primary treatment with radiotherapy. This has also resulted in the cessation of staging laparotomy for Stages-I and -II HD in most European centres.

Key points: splenic involvement

- In 10% of HD, the spleen is the only site of diaphragmatic disease

- An enlarged spleen is not a reliable indicator of disease

- Staging laparotomy is no longer undertaken because early relapse due to undetected splenic involvement can be salvaged by treatment with chemotherapy

Liver

In HD, nearly 5% of patients have liver involvement, nearly always associated with splenic involvement.[91,92] In NHL about 15% of patients have hepatic infiltration. True primary lymphoma of the liver is extremely rare but may be indistinguishable radiologically from other forms of hepatic malignancy such as hepatocellular carcinoma or metastatic disease.

As with splenic disease, in untreated patients, liver lymphoma usually occurs as microscopic or small macroscopic foci of tumour confined to the portal triad.

Detection of liver involvement by cross-sectional imaging is usually difficult. Large focal areas of involvement, detectable on ultrasound, CT or MRI, are seen in only 5–10% of patients with liver disease and resemble metastatic disease from other sources (Fig. 28.25). In both HD and NHL the lesions are well-defined, frequently large, hypoechoic on ultrasound and hypodense relative to the normal parenchyma on both enhanced and unenhanced CT scans (Fig. 28.25). As in metastatic disease, on T1-weighted MR images, the lesions are hypointense and on T2-weighted images they are hyperintense relative to the liver. As in the detection of other focal liver pathology, it has been suggested that MRI may be more sensitive than CT in the detection of focal hepatic pathology.[93] Occasionally, especially in children, a form of liver infiltration is demonstrated as low density soft tissue infiltrating the porta hepatis and along the margins of the portal veins.[24]

Cross-sectional imaging is relatively insensitive to the detection of the more common diffuse microscopic liver infiltration. However, in contradistinction to the unreliability of splenomegaly, liver enlargement is strongly suggestive of infiltration in NHL particularly. To date, despite initial enthusiasm,[94] attempts to detect the diffuse form on MRI have not been successful.[95,96]

Involvement of the bile ducts and gall bladder is rare, but has been described in AIDS-related lymphoma (see section on AIDS).

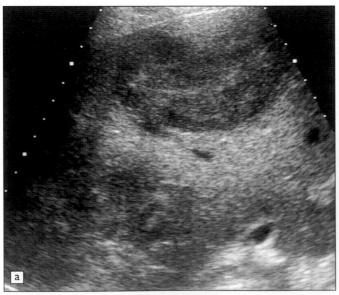 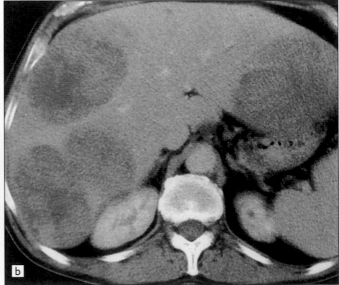

Figure 28.25. *Liver involvement in a patient with NHL. (a) Transverse ultrasound scan showing multiple large inhomogeneous focal abnormalities of varying echogenicity;* *(b) postcontrast CT scan in the same patient also showing multiple focal partially enhancing lesions of decreased echogenicity within the liver.*

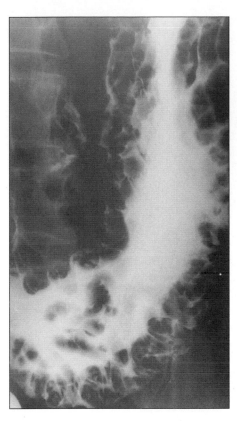

Figure 28.26.
Stomach involvement in NHL. The barium meal shows diffuse enlargement of the gastric folds due to submucosal infiltration.

- Absence of superficial or intrathoracic lymph nodes
- Normal white cell count
- No involvement of liver or spleen
- Lymph node involvement if present must be confined to the drainage area of the involved segment of gut[98]

Secondary gastro-intestinal involvement is common because of the frequent origin of lymphoma in the mesenteric or retroperitoneal nodes. Typically, multiple sites are involved.

In both the primary and secondary forms, the stomach is the most commonly involved organ (51%), followed by the small bowel (33%), the large bowel (16%), and the oesophagus (<1%). In 10–50% of cases the involvement is multicentric.[97] In children, the disease appears almost exclusively in the ileum and ileocaecal region.

Stomach

Primary lymphoma of the stomach accounts for about 2–5% of gastric tumours.[97,99] Radiologically, the appearances reflect the gross pathological findings: common appearances are multiple nodules, some with central ulceration, seen readily at endoscopy or barium meal or a large fungating lesion with or without ulceration. About a third of cases present with diffuse infiltration with marked thickening of the wall and narrowing of the lumen, sometimes with extension into the duodenum, indistinguishable from scirrhous carcinoma. Only about one-tenth are characterized by diffuse enlargement of the gastric folds (Fig. 28.26), similar to the pattern seen in hypertrophic gastritis and Menetrier's disease.

Because the disease originates in the submucosa, these signs are best demonstrated endoscopically or on barium studies, but do not reflect the extent of the disease (Fig. 28.26). Computed tomography has proved particularly valuable, often showing extensive gastric wall thickening with a smoothly lobulated border. Unlike gastric carcinoma, the walls of the stomach are usually clearly separable from the surrounding organs (Fig. 28.27).[100]

Key points: liver involvement

■ Liver involvement is almost invariably associated with splenic infiltration

■ Only 5–10% of patients with liver disease have focal lesions detectable on cross-sectional imaging

■ Enlargement of the liver is a strong indicator of lymphomatous infiltration

Gastro-intestinal tract

The gastro-intestinal tract is the most common site of primary extranodal lymphoma, being the initial site of involvement in 5–10% of adult patients.[97] Hodgkin's disease of the gastro-intestinal tract is extremely rare.

Primary gastro-intestinal lymphomas develop from the lymphoid elements in the lamina propria and constitute about 1% of gastro-intestinal tumours, occurring most frequently in two age-related peaks, the first below the age of 10 years and a second between 50 and 60 years of age (mean 53 years). Primary lymphomas of the gastro-intestinal tract usually involve only one site. The criteria for the diagnosis of primary gastro-intestinal lymphoma include:

Small bowel

Lymphoma accounts for up to 50% of all primary tumours of the small bowel,[98] occurring most frequently in the terminal ileum and becoming less frequent proximally. Multifocal disease is present in up to 50% of cases. As it usually originates in the lymphoid follicles, mural thickening is typical and results in constriction of segments of bowel with obstructive symptoms which are common at presentation. Thickening of the bowel is well demonstrated on CT (Figs. 28.28 and 28.29) with displacement of adjacent loops. As the tumour spreads through the submucosa and muscularis propria, it creates a tube-like segment which ultimately becomes aneurysmal, presumably because of destruction of

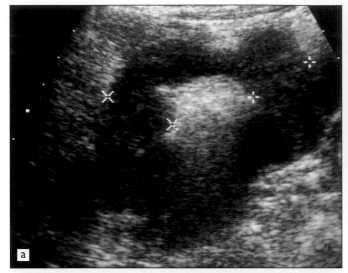

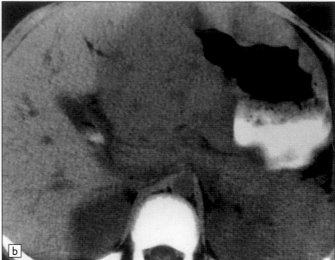

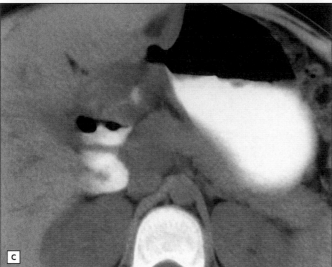

Figure 28.27. *Burkitt's lymphoma of the stomach in a child. (a) Transverse ultrasound scan showing massive thickening of the wall of the body of the stomach; (b) CT scan correlating with the ultrasound appearances in (a). Again showing massive thickening of the wall which is clearly separable from the surrounding organs; (c) follow-up CT scan following chemotherapy 2 months after (b) showing an excellent response to chemotherapy. Only a minor amount of thickening of the wall of the gastric antrum persists.*

ution of nodules 0.2–2 cm in diameter, typically with the mucosa intact (Fig. 28.28). A focal form appears as a large polypoid mass, often in the caecum, and is indistinguishable from colonic cancer, unless there is concomitant involvement of the terminal ileum which is more suggestive of lymphoma. The mass may have a large intraluminal component.

the muscularis and autonomic plexus in the affected segment. Alternating areas of dilatation and constriction are the most common manifestation.[98] Occasionally, the lymphomatous infiltration is predominantly submucosal, resulting in multiple nodules or polyps of varying size, scattered throughout the small bowel but predominantly in the terminal ileum. This form is particularly prone to intussusception which is a classical mode of presentation (Fig. 28.30). Secondary invasion of the small bowel by large mesenteric lymph node masses causing displacement, encasement or compression may also be seen.

Colon and rectum
Primary lymphoma accounts for only 0.05% of all colonic neoplasms and usually involves the caecum and rectum rather than other parts of the colon. Conversely, secondary involvement is usually widely distributed and multicentric. The most common form of the disease is a diffuse or segmental distrib-

Key points: gastro-intestinal tract

■ The stomach is the most frequent site of gastro-intestinal lymphoma and may be primary or secondary

■ Lymphoma accounts for up to 50% of all primary tumours of the small bowel and is multifocal in 50% of cases

■ Intussusception is a characteristic feature at presentation with predominantly submucosal nodular/polypoid lymphoma

■ Involvement of the colon and rectum accounts for only 0.5% of colonic neoplasms

■ Pancreatic lymphoma is usually secondary due to invasion by adjacent lymph node masses

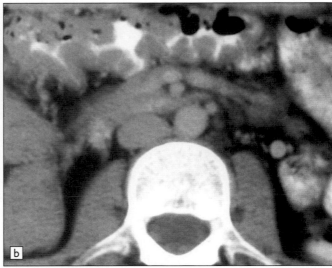

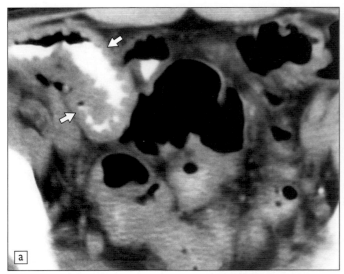

Figure 28.28. *Involvement of the bowel by NHL. (a) This shows marked uniform thickening of the wall of a loop of ileum in the right iliac fossa (arrows); (b) CT scan of the same* *patient showing diffuse uniform thickening of the transverse colon due to infiltration by NHL.*

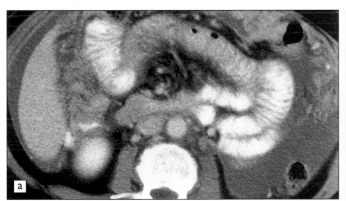

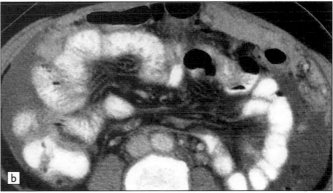

Figure 28.29. *Small bowel infiltration in NHL. (a) Marked thickening of the valvulae conniventes in a loop of jejunum; (b) CT scan performed slightly inferior to (a) also shows* *thickening of the valvulae in the ileum. Note in (a) and (b) the extensive infiltration of the omentum, perivascular thickening and thickening of the peritoneum.*

In very advanced disease, there may be marked thickening of the colonic or rectal folds resulting in focal strictures or ulcerative masses with fistula formation (Fig. 28.31).

Intrinsic oesophageal involvement is extremely uncommon, usually involves the distal third of the oesophagus and can result in a smooth tapered narrowing. Occasionally, both the fundus and distal oesophagus are involved by a bulky fungating tumour.

Pancreas

Primary pancreatic lymphoma is extremely rare and accounts for only 1.3% of all cases of pancreatic malignancy.[101] Secondary pancreatic involvement usually occurs in association with disease elsewhere, most commonly due to direct infiltration from adjacent nodal masses.[102] Intrinsic involvement of the pancreas most commonly results in a solitary mass lesion, indistinguishable from a primary adenocarcinoma on ultrasound, CT or MRI (Fig. 28.32).[102] Less commonly diffuse palpable masses or diffuse uniform enlargement of the pancreas is seen. Involvement is far more common in NHL than HD.

Genito-urinary tract

The genito-urinary tract is very rarely involved at the time of presentation, although in end-stage disease more than 50% of cases will have involvement of some part of the genito-urinary tract. The testicle is the most commonly involved organ, followed by the kidney and perirenal space. Involvement of the bladder, prostate, uterus, vagina and ovaries is extremely rare.[103]

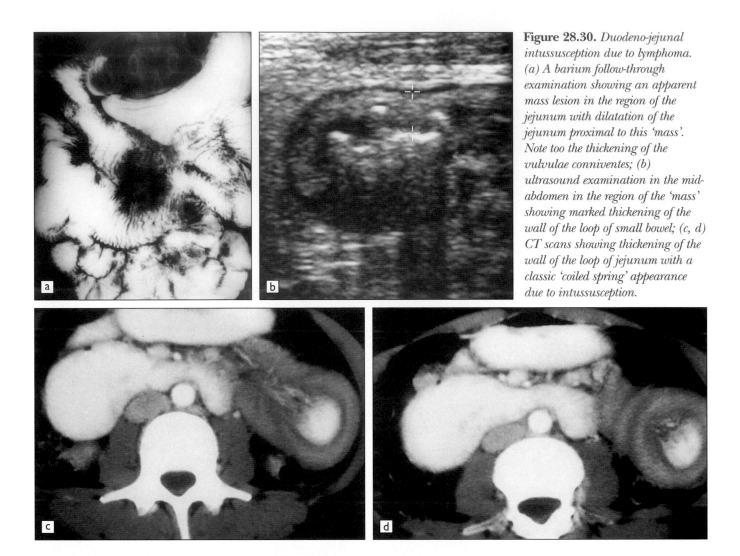

Figure 28.30. *Duodeno-jejunal intussusception due to lymphoma. (a) A barium follow-through examination showing an apparent mass lesion in the region of the jejunum with dilatation of the jejunum proximal to this 'mass'. Note too the thickening of the vulvulae conniventes; (b) ultrasound examination in the mid-abdomen in the region of the 'mass' showing marked thickening of the wall of the loop of small bowel; (c, d) CT scans showing thickening of the wall of the loop of jejunum with a classic 'coiled spring' appearance due to intussusception.*

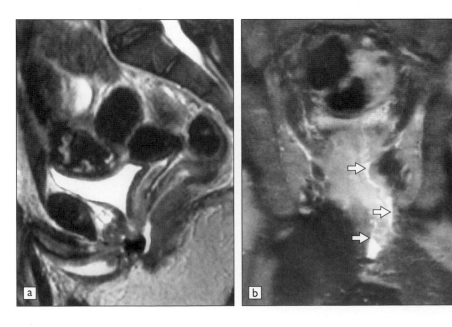

Figure 28.31. *Rectal involvement in a patient with lymphoma and AIDS. (a) A sagittal fast spin-echo T2-weighted MR image showing thickening of the rectal wall and a high-signal intensity fistula extending into the perineum; (b) a coronal STIR image in the same patient showing the marked thickening and marked increase in signal intensity of the rectal wall. This scan also shows the high-signal intensity of the complex fistula extending from the left side of the rectal wall into the perineum (arrowed).*

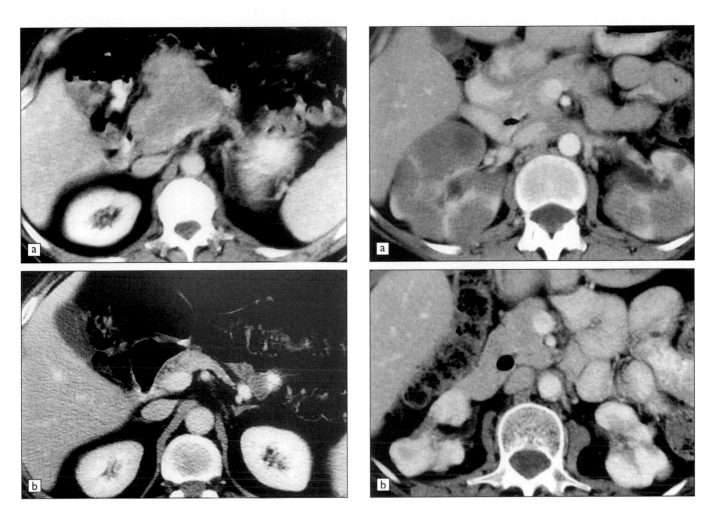

Figure 28.32. *Primary pancreatic lymphoma. (a) Note a large mass of decreased attenuation following contrast medium replacing the normal body and head of the pancreas due to primary pancreatic NHL; (b) a CT scan performed 3 months following chemotherapy shows complete resolution of the lymphomatous mass with marked atrophy of the remaining pancreas.*

Figure 28.33. *Renal lymphoma. (a) CT scan showing multiple masses enhancing less than the adjacent renal parenchyma following intravenous injection of contrast medium. Note the absence of retroperitoneal lymph node enlargement; (b) CT scan performed 4 months after (a) following chemotherapy shows complete resolution of the multiple renal masses with marked scarring of the kidneys following treatment.*

Kidney

Renal involvement is detected in about 3% of all patients undergoing abdominal scans for the staging of lymphoma.[104–106] Although CT is more sensitive in identifying lymphomatous renal masses than ultrasound or urography, a large discrepancy exists between the radiological detection and incidence at autopsy, presumably because renal involvement is a late phenomenon. It is extremely unusual for the detection of renal involvement to alter the disease stage, close to 90% of cases are due to high-grade NHL, renal function is usually normal and in more than 40% of patients the disease occurs at the time of recurrence only.[104]

Multiple masses is the most frequent pattern of disease which on CT may show a typical 'density reversal pattern'

before and after contrast administration, with the lesion being more dense than the surrounding parenchyma before contrast medium administration and less dense after (Fig. 28.33).[104]

Solitary masses occur less frequently and may be indistinguishable from renal cell carcinoma.[104] An important feature of renal masses occurring in NHL is that in over 50% of cases there is no evidence of retroperitoneal lymph node enlargement on CT, suggesting that the kidneys are involved by haematogenous spread.

Direct infiltration of the kidney is the second most common type of renal involvement. Not infrequently, a soft tissue mass is seen in the perirenal space, occasionally encasing the kidney without evidence on CT of invasion of the parenchyma (Fig. 28.34).

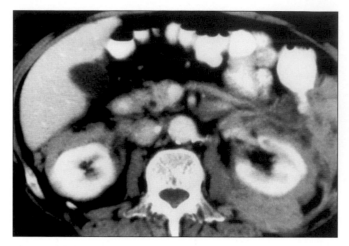

Figure 28.34. *Perirenal lymphomatous infiltration. CT scan following intravenous injection of contrast medium shows low-density masses infiltrating the perirenal and pararenal space bilaterally, with thickening of Gerota's fascia. The renal parenchyma appears normal bilaterally. Note the absence of retroperitoneal (para-aortic) lymph node enlargement.*

Diffuse infiltration of the kidneys (Fig. 28.35) with global renal enlargement without focal nodules is a less common manifestation, usually without lymph node enlargement. The appearance after intravenous contrast medium injection is variable, but usually the normal parenchymal enhancement replaced by homogeneous non-enhancing tissue.

Bladder and prostate

Although primary lymphoma of the bladder is extremely rare, secondary lymphoma of the bladder is more common and is found in 10–15% of patients with lymphoma at autopsy.[103,107] Such secondary involvement can affect the wall of the bladder intrinsically or in contiguity from the adjacent involved nodes. Microscopic involvement is far more common than gross involvement, but this too can be associated with haematuria. The appearances on CT are non-specific (Fig. 28.36) with either diffuse widespread thickening of the bladder wall or a large nodular mass — both patterns indistinguishable from transitional cell carcinoma.

Unlike primary lymphoma of the bladder, where the response to chemotherapy/radiotherapy is good, lymphomatous involvement of the prostate carries a poor prognosis. Solitary nodules are uncommon and in the majority of cases involvement is extrinsic, with infiltration throughout the prostate and periprostatic tissue. Secondary involvement of the prostate is far more common than primary prostatic involvement and direct extension into the prostate from pelvic lymph nodes is often seen in very advanced disease.

Testis

Testicular lymphoma is the most common testicular tumour over the age of 60, but accounts for only 5% of all testicular neoplasms.[108] At presentation it is seen in about 1% of men with NHL (more commonly in Burkitt's lymphoma) but is practically non-existent in HD. As in other sites of lym-

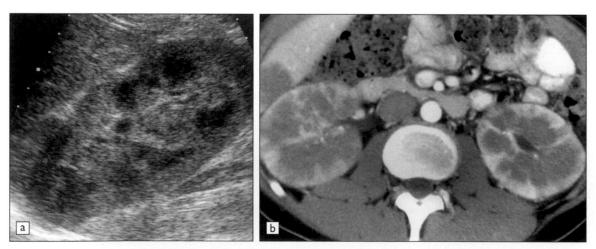

Figure 28.35. *Diffuse lymphomatous infiltration of the kidney in a patient with high-grade non-Hodgkin's lymphoma. (a) Longitudinal ultrasound scan through the right kidney showing marked enlargement of the kidney (the right kidney measures 16 cm, the left 16.5 cm). There is diffuse increased reflectivity of the renal parenchyma with resultant prominent lucency of the renal papillae. The normal outline of the kidney is preserved; (b) CT scan following intravenous injection of contrast medium in the same patient as (a), showing diffuse infiltration of both kidneys by lymphomatous tissue. There is preservation of a rim of normal renal parenchyma. Note the absence of retroperitoneal lymph node enlargement and the presence of a focal lesion in the inferior aspect of the right lobe of the liver.*

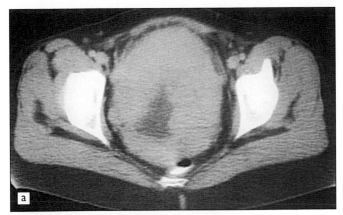

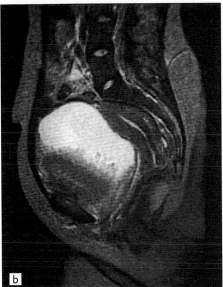

Figure 28.36.
NHL of the bladder. (a) CT scan showing large soft tissue mass occupying a major part of the base of the bladder; (b) sagittal spin-echo T2-weighted MR image showing extensive involvement of the anterior abdominal wall in the same patient.

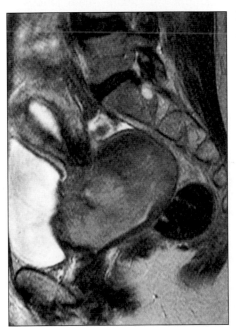

Figure 28.37.
Primary NHL of the cervix. Sagittal fast spin-echo T2-weighted MR image showing a very large mass in the uterine cervix due to high-grade NHL. There was no evidence of disease elsewhere in this patient.

phomatous involvement of the genito-urinary tract, the frequency of involvement discovered at autopsy is much higher: 18% of men with NHL.

On ultrasound, the lesions usually have a non-specific appearance, with focal areas of decreased echogenicity. However, a well-recognized pattern is a diffuse decrease in reflectivity of the testicle without any focal abnormality. As involvement is bilateral in 10–25% of cases, it is extremely important to examine the contralateral side.

Female genitalia

In advanced, widespread lymphomatous disease, the female genital organs are frequently secondarily involved.[17] However, isolated lymphomatous involvement is rare, accounting for approximately 1% of extranodal NHL. The tumours originate predominantly in the uterine cervix where on CT and MRI a large mass can be seen (Fig. 28.27). Involvement of the uterine body usually produces diffuse enlargement, often with a lobular contour similar to a fibroid. Similarly, primary lymphoma of the cervix and/or vagina is characterized by a large soft tissue mass. Involvement of these gynaecological organs is best demonstrated by MRI, since masses are seen as high signal intensity lesions on T2 weighting and are therefore clearly distinguished from the surrounding normal tissues, including the uterus, cervix and vaginal wall (Fig. 28.37).[109] Ovarian lymphoma is less common and carries a worse prognosis than uterine lymphoma because the tumours are more advanced at the time of discovery. The appearance on cross-sectional imaging is indistinguishable from primary ovarian carcinoma.[110]

Key points: genito-urinary tract

- Renal involvement is seen in about 3% of cases undergoing abdominal CT

- Lymphomatous involvement of the kidneys is not usually associated with renal impairment

- Primary lymphoma of the prostate carries a poor prognosis whereas primary lymphoma of the bladder has a good prognosis

- The testes is the most frequent site of involvement of the genito-urinary tract with lymphoma

- Lymphoma of the testis accounts for only 5% of all testicular tumours

- Primary lymphoma of the female genital tract is rare and is best demonstrated on MRI

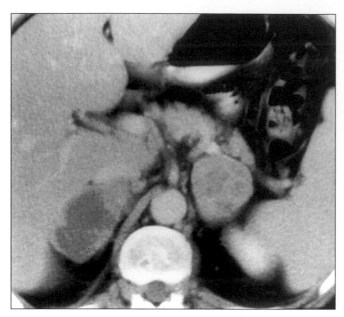

Figure 28.38. *Adrenal lymphoma. CT scan performed following intravenous injection of contrast medium showing bilateral adrenal masses that enhance slightly, are inhomogeneous and irregular in outline.*

Adrenal glands

Involvement of the adrenal glands in lymphoma is usually demonstrated on routine abdominal CT for staging (where it is seen in about 6% of cases of NHL) as presentation with adrenal insufficiency is extremely rare.[103,110] Involvement is usually bilateral and the appearances are indistinguishable from bilateral metastases, but readily distinguishable from adenomas (Fig. 28.38). Non-lymphomatous bilateral hyperplasia of the adrenal glands has been described.[111] The reason for this is unclear.

Key point: adrenal glands

■ Lymphoma of the adrenal glands is usually secondary and asymptomatic

Central nervous system
Primary
Primary CNS lymphoma is initially localized to the CNS at presentation. It occurs almost exclusively within the brain, as the spinal cord is only very rarely the site of origin (<1%).[112,113] Although in the mid-1980s, primary lymphoma accounted for only 1.5% of all brain tumours, its frequency is increasing which is in part due to an association with immunosuppressive therapy following cardiac or renal

transplants and immunodeficiency. Cases of primary CNS lymphoma have been reported from the age of 2 months to 90 years, but presentation between the fourth and sixth decades appears to be the most frequent. There is a separate peak in the first decade of life.

Key points: central nervous system

■ Primary CNS lymphoma almost exclusively involves the cerebral white matter

■ Primary cerebral lymphoma is increasing in incidence

■ Secondary lymphoma preferentially involves the extracerebral spaces and the spinal epidural and subarachnoid spaces

■ Spinal cord compression results from nodal spread through the intervertebral neural foramina in both HD and NHL

■ NHL is the most common primary orbital malignancy in adults

On CT or MRI, more than 50% of lesions occur within the cerebral white matter, close to or within the corpus callosum.[113] In about 15% of cases, the deep cortical grey matter of the basal ganglia, thalamus and hypothalamus are involved. In 11% of cases, lymphoma develops in the posterior fossa and is multifocal in about 15% of cases. On CT, the tumour mass is typically of increased density on unenhanced CT and the majority of lesions enhance homogeneously after intravenous injection of contrast medium. Only about 10% of lesions do not enhance.[112] On MRI, the typical appearance is of a tumour mass hypo- or isointense, relative to the surrounding normal tissue on T1-weighted sequences. As after injec-tion of X-ray contrast medium, intravenous injection of gadolinium-DTPA also results in enhancement on T1-weighted sequences (Fig. 38.39). The appearance of primary and secondary lymphoma within the brain is essentially similar on CT and MRI.

Secondary
Cerebral involvement occurs in 10–15% of patients with NHL at some time during the course of their disease,[114,115] whereas it is so rare in HD that a space-occupying lesion in the brain of a patient with known HD should prompt a second diagnosis.[116] Secondary lymphoma is distinguishable from the primary form, to some extent by its propensity to involve the extracerebral spaces (epidural, subdural and subarachnoid) (Fig. 28.40) and the spinal epidural and subarachnoid spaces.[112] Magnetic resonance imaging with direct multiplanar imaging, is ideal for detecting extracerebral plaque-like tumour deposits in the subdural or epidural spaces. Typically,

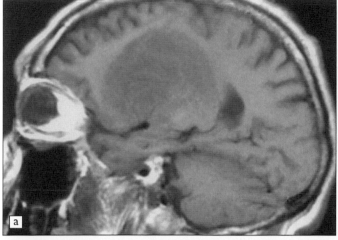

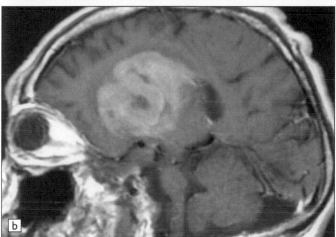

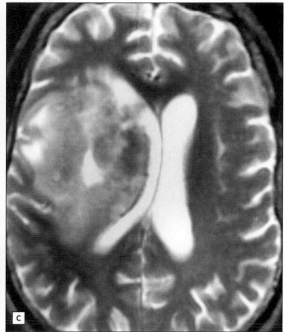

Figure 28.39. *Primary cerebral NHL of the parietal lobe. (a) A fast spin-echo T1-weighted sagittal MR image showing a hypointense mass in the parietal lobe; (b) following intravenous administration of gadolinium-DTPA, the mass enhances intensely; (c) an axial fast spin-echo T2-weighted MR image showing a typical parietal lobe mass resulting in marked mass effect with compression of the right lateral ventricle.*

these plaques are hypo- to isodense on all pulse sequences, but they are made more obvious on gadolinium-DTPA enhanced T1-weighted images (Fig. 28.40). Computed tomography is less sensitive, not only in the detection of these extracerebral lesions, but also in demonstrating leptomeningeal deposits of lymphoma coating the cranial nerves,[117] particularly when resulting in cranial nerve palsies.

Gadolinium-enhanced MRI is also a relatively sensitive, non-invasive method for demonstrating spinal leptomeningeal involvement by lymphoma and involvement of the spinal cord and nerve roots. Epidural extension of tumour into the spinal canal from a paravertebral nodal mass may also be elegantly demonstrated on MRI. Although extension through the intervertebral foramina may also be clearly depicted on CT, subtle disease is easily missed (Fig. 28.41).[118]

Compression of the spinal cord or cauda equina due to lymphomatous disease is a late manifestation of HD, but is often an earlier manifestation of NHL. In both types of lymphoma, extension of nodal spread through the intervertebral neural foramina is the most common cause. Tumour compresses the dura, but the dura itself usually acts as an

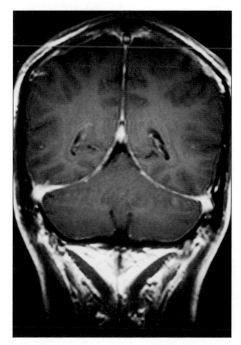

Figure 28.40. *NHL showing meningeal disease on a coronal MR image using a T1-weighted sequence following injection of intravenous contrast medium (gadolinium-DTPA). Note intense enhancement of the thickened meninges over the cerebral hemispheres, cerebellum and tentorium.*

effective barrier to the intrathecal spread of tumour. Vertebral collapse with cord compression may be seen in some of the aggressive forms of NHL, but it is less common than compression due to an epidural mass (Fig. 28.41).

The orbit

Non-Hodgkin's lymphoma is the most common primary orbital malignancy in adults and accounts for 10–15% of orbital masses.[112] Primary orbital lymphomas occur most commonly in patients between 40 and 70 years of age, and most typically present as a slow-growing, diffusely infiltrative tumour for which the main differential diagnosis is from the non-malignant condition known as 'orbital pseudotumour'.

Retrobulbar lymphoma infiltrates around and through the extraocular muscles causing proptosis and ophthalmoplegia, however, visual acuity is rarely disturbed. In patients with an orbital lymphomatous mass, about half will be found to have an extracentral nervous system primary site of origin. Secondary orbital involvement occurs in approximately 3.5–5% of both HD and NHL. In both the primary and secondary forms, the clinical manifestations will depend on the site of involvement. Involvement of the lachrymal glands is frequently bilateral, the presenting features are those of bilateral masses with downward displacement of the globe (Fig. 28.42). Involvement of the eyelids and subconjunctival spaces is readily assessed on clinical examination.

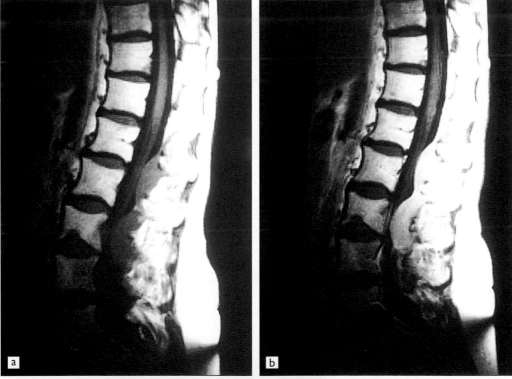

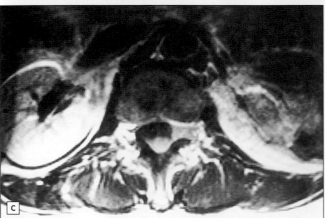

Figure 28.41. *T1-weighted MR images showing extradural disease in a patient with NHL; (a) precontrast, (b, c) postcontrast. In the sagittal plane, the extradural mass is clearly shown on both the pre- and postcontrast images extending from the level of the first lumbar vertebra to the level of the fourth lumbar vertebra. In the axial plane (c), extension of enhancing tissue into the spinal canal is clearly seen.*

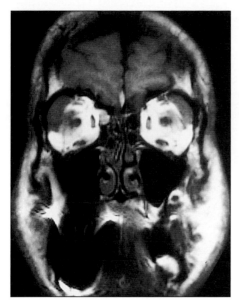

Figure 28.42.
Orbital lymphoma. T1-weighted coronal MR image. There are bilateral orbital masses of homogeneous low signal intensity. The masses are symmetrical and occupy the superolateral orbital compartments. There is no evidence of bone erosion.

Head and neck lymphoma

Although HD typically involves the cervical lymph nodes as the presenting feature, true extranodal involvement of sites in the head and neck region is rare. Extension from nodal masses in the neck to Waldeyer's ring may occur, but this is seen in less than 1% of patients.

In NHL, extranodal head and neck tumour involvement is relatively common and indeed 10% of patients present with extranodal disease in the head and neck; on investigation about half will have disseminated lymphoma. Extranodal NHL accounts for approximately 5% of head and neck cancers.[119]

Waldeyer's ring is the commonest site of head and neck lymphoma and there is a close link with involvement of the gastro-intestinal tract which may be synchronous or metachronous. Waldeyer's ring comprises of lymphoid tissue in the nasopharynx, oropharynx, the faucal and palatine tonsil and the lingual tonsil on the posterior third of the tongue. Whilst paranasal sinus involvement often presents with acute facial swelling and pain, and disease often spreads from one sinus to the other in a contiguous fashion, bony destruction is considerably less marked than in squamous cell carcinomas.[120]

Magnetic resonance is the preferred imaging technique for evaluating head and neck lymphoma due to high tissue contrast between tumour adjacent to normal structures and its multiplanar capability allowing clear demonstration of the full extent of disease within the intricate anatomy of the facial region. It also permits detection of tumour spread into the cranial cavity from the infratemporal fossa orbit and soft tissue of the face.

Salivary glands

All the salivary glands may be involved in lymphoma but the parotid gland is the most frequent.[121] The patient presents with single or multiple well defined masses which are of higher density than the surrounding gland on CT, hypoechoic on ultrasound, and of intermediate signal intensity on T1- and T2-weighted MRI sequences.

Thyroid

Non-Hodgkin's lymphoma accounts for 2% of malignant tumours of the thyroid.[122] Direct spread of tumour beyond the gland and involvement of adjacent lymph nodes is common. On CT these masses usually have a lower attenuation than the normal gland and they may show peripheral enhancement following injection of intravenous contrast medium (Fig. 28.43).

Key points: head and neck

- ◼ Extranodal NHL accounts for approximately 5% of all head and neck cancers

- ◼ Waldeyer's ring is the most common site of head and neck lymphoma

- ◼ The parotid is the most frequent salivary gland involved by lymphoma

- ◼ Non-Hodgkin's lymphoma accounts for 2% of all malignant thyroid tumours

Musculoskeletal system

Skeletal involvement may occur in both HD and NHL. Since the bone marrow is an integral part of the reticulo-endothelial system, lymphomas may arise within the marrow as a true primary disease. It is then categorized as Stage-IE disease. More often, however, the marrow is involved as part of a disseminated process. In this instance bone marrow involvement is categorized as Stage-IV disease. The majority of 'apparent' primary lymphomas usually have widespread disease and are therefore in reality secondary lymphomas. This is particularly true in children.

Bone and bone marrow are important sites of disease relapse and any skeletal symptoms following previous treatment for lymphoma should raise the suspicion of bone disease. Involvement of osseous bone is less widespread, does not necessarily imply bone marrow involvement,[123] and skeletal radiography has no predictive value in determining marrow involvement. Infiltration of bone may also occur by direct invasion of adjacent soft tissue masses. This is designated with the suffix 'E' after the appropriate stage of disease elsewhere, e.g. Stage IIE. For the purposes of clarity, involvement of the bone is distinguished from diffuse involvement of the bone marrow.

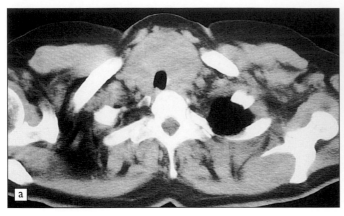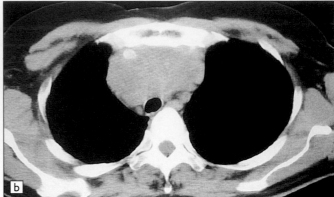

Figure 28.43. *(a, b) CT scans showing primary lymphoma of the thyroid. On staging, no other evidence of disease was found in this patient with biopsy-proven disease.*

Bone

Primary lymphoma of bone is almost exclusively due to NHL as primary HD of bone is extremely rare. The criteria for the diagnosis of primary lymphoma require that:

- Only a single bone is involved
- Unequivocal histological evidence of lymphoma
- Other disease is limited to regional areas at the time of presentation
- The primary tumour precedes metastasis by at least 6 months

The average age at presentation is 24 years; 50% of cases occur in patients between 10–30 years. Primary lymphoma affects the appendicular skeleton involving the femur, tibia and humerus, in descending order of frequency. Primary lymphoma of bone accounts for about 1% of all NHL.[124]

Secondary involvement of bones is present in 5–6% of patients with NHL,[123,124] although less present with symptoms due to a skeletal lesion. Bone involvement is more frequent in children with NHL.[24] Radiographic evidence of bone involvement is present in 20% of patients, with HD appearing in 4% as the initial presentation.[123] Systemic (secondary) NHL involves the axial skeleton more frequently than the appendicular skeleton.

Appearances

Primary NHL of bone is roentgenographically indistinguishable from systemic NHL, HD and other bone tumours. However, whereas the bone lesions in NHL (primary or secondary) are usually permeative osteolytic (77%) (Fig. 28.44), sclerotic in only 4% and mixed in 16%, bony involvement in HD typically gives sclerotic or mixed sclerotic and lytic (86%) and infrequently lytic (14%).[125]

In HD, soft tissue disease typically may involve adjacent bones; anterior mediastinal and paravertebral masses not infrequently invade the sternum and vertebrae, respectively, resulting either in destruction or scalloping. A classic finding is the sclerotic 'ivory vertebra'. Direct invasion of bone by local lymph node disease is denoted by the suffix 'E' added to the appropriate stage.

Because of the relatively low incidence of bone lesions at presentation, screening for bone involvement is not routine but is reserved for patients with specific complaints. Bone scintigraphy has a sensitivity of close to 95% in the detection of bone involvement,[126] but is relatively nonspecific so that plain films are used to investigate areas that are positive on the bone scans.

Bone marrow

Involvement of the bone marrow indicates Stage-IV disease. It is rare at presentation in HD but is found in 20–40% of patients with NHL at presentation[71,127–129] and is associated with a worse prognosis than involvement of the liver, lung or osseous bone.[130] During the course of HD, marrow involvement occurs in 5–15% of patients.[131]

Because of these figures, bone marrow biopsies are not indicated as part of the initial staging of HD, but the high incidence in NHL justifies its use as a staging procedure,[132] increasing the stage in up to 30% of cases, mainly from Stage II to Stage IV.[132] Bone marrow involvement in low-grade NHL is typically diffuse but in intermediate- and high-grade lymphoma it is more likely to be focal. Therefore, not surprisingly, the performance of bilateral rather than single-site biopsies increases the pick-up rate substantially.[133] Magnetic resonance imaging is undoubtedly an extremely sensitive technique in the demonstration of bone marrow involvement (Fig. 28.45). On T1-weighted images, tumour infiltration is of low signal (Figs. 28.44 and 28.45).[133] and of high signal intensity on STIR.[134] However, its precise role in the staging of patients with lymphoma has not yet been defined, given the obvious need to examine the cytology of bone marrow in these patients.

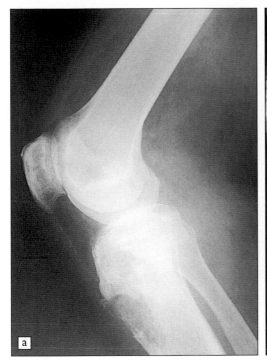

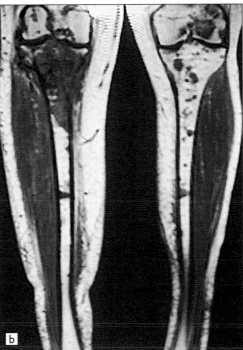

Figure 28.44. *NHL of upper tibia. (a) Lateral plain radiograph showing a destructive lesion in the upper aspect of the tibia; (b) coronal T1-weighted MR image showing a large area of abnormal low signal intensity in the upper tibia which corresponds to the abnormal bone on the plain radiograph. However, in addition, multiple lesions of low signal intensity are seen throughout both femoral condyles and tibiae, indicating much more extensive disease than had been appreciated clinically and on skeletal radiographs.*

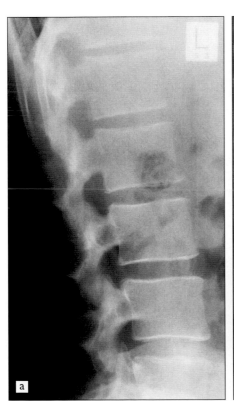

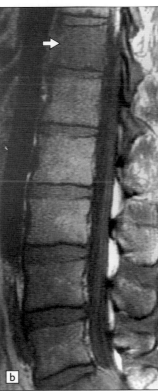

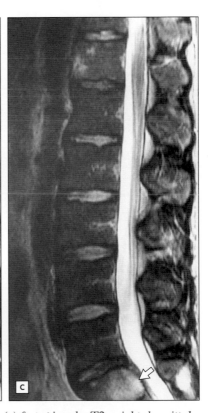

Figure 28.45. *Bone involvement in a patient with NHL. (a) Normal skeletal radiograph in a patient with NHL and back pain. The radio-isotope scan was also normal; (b) T1-weighted sagittal MR image showing loss of the normal high-signal intensity of fat in the body of L1 (arrowed); (c) fast spin-echo T2-weighted sagittal MR image showing areas of high-signal intensity within the body of L1 vertebra and also the body of S1 (arrowed). A bone biopsy of S1 showed involvement of the cortical bone as well as of the bone marrow.*

Key points: bone and bone marrow

■ Primary lymphoma of bone accounts for only 1% of all cases of NHL, whereas secondary involvement is seen in 5–6% of cases

■ Secondary bone involvement is seen in 20% of patients with HD. Primary HD of bone is extremely rare

■ In HD, soft tissue disease may invade adjacent bone but this is rare in NHL

■ Bone scintigraphy has a sensitivity approaching 95% but is relatively non-specific

■ Bone marrow involvement indicates Stage-IV disease and is present in 20–40% of patients with NHL at presentation

■ Bone marrow biopsy in NHL increases the stage of disease in up to 30% of cases (Stage II to Stage IV)

■ In HD, bone marrow involvement occurs in 5–15% of patients during the course of disease

■ Burkitt's lymphoma is an aggressive variant of NHL which most frequently involves the mandible and maxilla

■ MRI is the method of choice for detecting soft tissue lymphomatous masses which are usually due to secondary NHL

Soft tissues

Soft tissue masses may develop in both HD and NHL either as tumour extension from bone involvement, or as an isolated mass within the muscles. Primary muscle lymphoma is extremely rare and is based on the absence of clinical or imaging features of lymphoma elsewhere. Patients with soft tissue lymphoma usually present with pain or neurological deficit, but occasionally a palpable mass may be present.[137] Without question, MRI is the technique of choice for investigating patients with persistent pain, and even though a mass may be detected in retrospect on CT, the lack of contrast between the mass and adjacent muscle groups may lead to difficulties in diagnosis (Fig. 28.46).

BURKITT'S LYMPHOMA

Burkitt's lymphoma is a variant of NHL and is subdivided as follows:

• Endemic African type[135]
• Non-endemic non-African type[136]

They both usually occur in childhood and present as aggressive, rapidly growing extranodal masses. Prognosis is generally poor although response to treatment is initially good. The mandible and maxilla are the most common sites of involvement in the African type and may produce the characteristic 'floating tooth' appearance. Other sites which may be involved include the pelvis, long bones and small bones of the hands and feet.

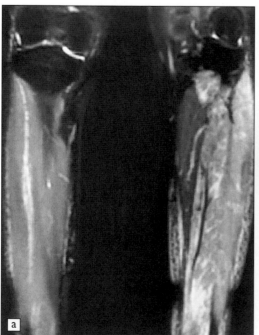

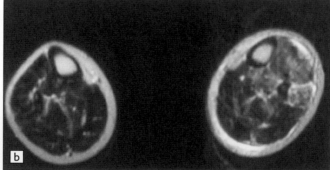

Figure 28.46. *Soft tissue involvement by lymphoma. (a) Coronal STIR MR image showing marked thickening and increased signal intensity of the muscles of the lateral aspect of the leg due to diffuse infiltration by NHL; (b) fast spin-echo T2-weighted axial MR image of the same patient as (a) showing increased signal intensity of the involved muscles on the left and providing the exact distribution of muscle involvement.*

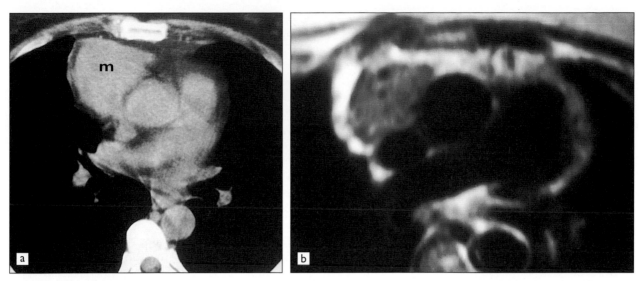

Figure 28.47. *A residual mediastinal mass in a patient treated for HD. (a) CT scan; (b) conventional spin-echo T2-weighted MR image. The residual mass (m) measures approximately 5 × 5 cm in diameter and has a homogeneous intensity, suggesting that the mass is inactive. A CT-guided core biopsy was obtained. On histological examination there was no evidence of active HD.*

POST-TREATMENT EVALUATION

Imaging plays an extremely important role in monitoring response to therapy. Also, once treatment is com-pleted, periodic surveillance studies help in detection of potential relapse. In clinical evidence of relapse, imaging studies are performed to evaluate the extent of the disease.

Monitoring response to therapy

Achievement of a complete remission following treatment is the most important factor for prolonged survival in both HD and NHL.[116] 'Complete remission' is diagnosed only when no abnormality is seen at the site of previously demonstrated disease. The chest radiograph is useful in assessing response when there is intrathoracic disease and is repeated at each monthly visit. Although the chest radiograph will show response early in the treatment, changes due to radiotherapy often make the mediastinum difficult to assess. Other mediastinal changes associated with treatment such as rebound hyperplasia or thymic cyst formation cannot be reliably identified on the chest radiograph and therefore response cannot be monitored reliably. A CT scan therefore remains essential in the monitoring of response to treatment for mediastinal disease. In patients with intra-abdominal disease, serial CT is essential in monitoring response.

The optimal and exact timing of such scans for reassessment has not been widely investigated.[138,139] In many centres, the practice is to assess patients fully 1 month after completion of therapy. Others favour an interim CT study during initial chemotherapy for lymphoma after two cycles of chemotherapy; the timing will often depend on local clinical practice and on the availability of resources. The speed of modern CT scanners has largely removed the need for limited scans advocated by some. We do not routinely administer intravenous contrast medium for follow-up scans, reserving its administration for those situations where the unenhanced scans are in any way equivocal.

Assessment of residual masses

Although successfully treated enlarged nodes often return to normal, in HD and NHL a residual mass of 'sterilized' fibrous tissue can persist. On a chest radiograph such a residual mass may remain following treatment in 12–88% of patients.[38,140] Such residual masses occur more frequently in patients with bulky rather than non-bulky disease, at least in HD. Determining the nature of such residual masses and excluding the possibility of active disease by imaging is one of the major challenges in oncological radiology today.

On CT, residual masses may be seen in sites of previously demonstrated disease. When these are less than 1 cm, they are designated 'incomplete imaging remission' or 'complete remission — unconfirmed', whereas masses >1 cm in diameter are designated 'residual masses'.[140] Computed tomography cannot distinguish between fibrotic tissue and residual active disease on the basis of density alone. Nevertheless, serial CT performed every 2–3 months is the most widely used method of determining the true nature of a residual mass. Masses which remain static after 1 year are considered inactive, whereas any increase in size is highly suggestive of relapse.

Ga-67 scanning can be helpful. If no uptake is shown in a mass that initially showed substantial activity, it can be inferred that it represents residual fibrosis with over 80% specificity.[141–143] Conversely, persistent positive uptake usually indicates persistent active neoplasm. However, the sensitivity of Ga-67 in the initial detection of lymphoma will depend on cell type, location, and size of the lesion; sensitivity is lower in lymphocytic lymphoma, in masses less than 2.5 cm, and in those masses below the diaphragm. Its value in monitoring response is therefore diminished by these factors. Absence of activity on a Ga-67 scan, without a pretreatment scan, is also of limited value.[42]

Key points: post-treatment evaluation

■ Achievement of complete remission following treatment is the most important prognostic indicator in both HD and NHL

■ Relapse following initial treatment occurs in 40% of patients with HD and over 50% of patients with NHL

■ Relapse usually occurs within the first 2 years following treatment of HD

■ Residual masses in HD and NHL may contain active malignancy which cannot yet be reliably detected on imaging

There is now substantial data investigating the value of MRI in identifying residual active neoplasm within residual masses.[42,144–146] In general, a reduction in signal intensity on T2-weighted images is seen during or following successful treatment. A high signal intensity on T2-weighted sequences following treatment appears to have a high specificity and positive predictive value for residual active disease.[42] False-positives do arise due to inflammatory oedema or cyst formation. However, not surprisingly, the sensitivity for the detection of active disease is low, as small foci of persistent tumour within a low signal intensity mass cannot be identified reliably on T2-weighted images.[42]

Positron emission tomography (PET) using 2-[F-18]fluoro-2-deoxy-D-glucose (18-FDG-PET) has also been investigated.[44] Whether this will prove to be more reliable in identifying residual active disease than available imaging strategies will be the aim of future research.

Relapse following satisfactory response to initial treatment occurs in 10–40% of patients with HD and in over 50% of patients with NHL.[71] In HD, relapse usually occurs within the first 2 years following treatment and patients are followed-up closely during this period, although CT examinations are not usually required unless clinical features suggest the possibility of recurrence.

Strategies for follow-up with imaging vary between institutions and in addition in patients with residual masses in HD and NHL, follow-up depends on the size of the mass, the sites of involvement, and the extent of disease; it is therefore impossible to define strict guidelines for each clinical situation.

The role of percutaneous biopsy
Percutaneous core biopsy using imaging guidance is now established as a valuable method of determining the nature of soft tissue masses in lymphoma. The indications for its use include:

- Defining the nature of a residual mass following treatment
- Detection of transformation of NHL to a higher grade
- Primary diagnosis in patients who present with unusual manifestations of disease

Summary

■ NHL and HD are a heterogeneous diverse group of malignancies which predominantly involve the lymph nodes.

■ In HD, most patients present with early-stage malignancy whereas in NHL, most patients present with advanced disease.

■ The incidence of NHL is increasing but the incidence of HD is decreasing.

■ In NHL, the prognosis varies widely according to tumour grade and stage at diagnosis.

■ HD tends to spread from one lymph node to the next in a contiguous manner, whereas NHL spreads in a more haphazard manner.

■ Involvement of intrathoracic lymph nodes is more common in HD than NHL.

■ Involvement of retroperitoneal and mesenteric nodes is more common in NHL than HD.

■ Extranodal sites of involvement are more common in NHL than HD.

■ Spleen is involved in 10% of patients with HD as isolated infradiaphragmatic disease.

■ Splenomegaly is an unreliable indicator of splenic lymphoma.

■ Primary extranodal lymphoma is almost exclusively seen in NHL.

REFERENCES

1. Reznek R H, Richards M A. The radiology of lymphoma. Clin Haematol 1987; 1: 77–107
2. Cancer in South East England 1991. Cancer incidence, prevalence and survival in the District Health Authorities in South East England. Thames Cancer Registry, 1994
3. Callender S T, Vancghan R I. The lymphomas. In: Weatherall D J, Ledingham J G, Warrell D A (eds). Oxford Textbook of Medicine (1st ed). Oxford: Oxford University Press, 1983: 160–174
4. Cancer Facts and Figures, 1997. Atlanta: American Cancer Society, Inc., 1997
5. Cancer in South East England, 1993. Thames Cancer Registry
6. Barnes N, Cartwright R A, O'Brien C et al. Rising incidence of lymphoid malignancies. Br J Cancer 1986; 53: 393–398
7. Horwich A. Hodgkin's disease. In: Horwich A (ed). Oncology: A Multidisciplinary Textbook. London: Chapman and Hall, 1995: 235–250
8. Magrath I T. The Non-Hodgkin's Lymphomas. London: Edward Arnold, 1990.
9. Ballerini P, Gaidano G, Gong J Z et al. Multiple genetic lesions in acquired immuno-deficiency syndrome-related non-Hodgkin's lymphoma. Blood 1993; 81: 166–176
10. Cleary ML, Sklar J. Lympho-proliferative disorders in cardiac transplant patients are multiclonal lymphomas. Lancet 1994; ii: 489–493
11. Kuefler P R, Bunn P A. Adult T cell leukemia/lymphoma. Clin Haematol 1986; 15: 695–726
12. Osborne B M. Contextual diagnosis of Hodgkin's disease and non-Hodgkin's lymphoma. Radiologic Clin North Am 1990; 28: 669–682
13. Lukes R J, Butler J J. The pathology and nomenclature of Hodgkin's disease. Cancer Res 1966; 26: 1063
14. Lukes R J, Craver L F, Hall T C et al. Report of the nomenclature committee. Cancer Res 1966; 26: 1311
15. National Cancer Institute. Study of classifications of non-Hodgkin's lymphomas. Cancer 1982; 49: 2112–2135
16. Harris N L, Stein H, Banks P M et al. A revised European-American classification of lymphoid neoplasms: a proposal from the International Lymphoma Study Group. Blood 1994; 84(5): 1361–1392
17. Rosenberg S, Diamond H D, Jaslowitz B, Craver L F. Lymphosarcoma: A review of 1269 cases. Medicine 1961; 40: 31–84
18. Rappaport H. Tumours of the haematopoietic system. In: Atlas of Tumour Pathology (Section 2, Fascicle no 8). Washington D C: Armed Forces Institute of Pathology, 1966
19. Cossman J, Uppenkamp M, Sundeen J et al. Molecular genetics and the diagnosis of lymphoma. Arch Pathol Lab Med 1988; 112: 117
20. Lister T A, Crowther D M, Sutcliffe S B et al. Report of a Committee convened to discuss the evaluation and staging of patients with Hodgkin's disease; Cotswolds Meeting. J Clin Oncol 1989 7: 1630–1636 [erratum]. J Clin Oncol 1990; 1602

21. Carbanillas F, Fuller L M. The radiologic assessment of the lymphoma patient from the standpoint of the clinician. Radiologic Clin North Am 1990; 28: 683–695

22. Marglin S I, Castellino R A. Selection of imaging studies for the initial staging of patients with Hodgkin's disease. Semi Ultrasound C T and M R 1985; 6: 380–393

23. Murphy S. Childhood non-Hodgkin's lymphoma. N Engl J Med 1978; 299: 1446–1448

24. Ng Y Y, Healy J C, Vincent J M et al. The radiology of non-Hodgkin's lymphoma in childhood: a review of 80 cases. Clin Radiol 1994; 49: 594–600

25. Price C G A. Non-Hodgkin's lymphoma. In: Price C, Sikora K (eds). Treatment of Cancer (3rd ed). London: Chapman and Hall Medical, 1995: 881–897

26. Gupta R K, Lister T A. Hodgkin's disease. In: Price C, Sikora K (eds). Treatment of Cancer (3rd ed). London: Chapman and Hall Medical, 1995: 851–880

27. DeVita V T, Serpick A A, Carbone P P. Combination chemotherapy in the treatment of advanced Hodgkin's disease. Ann Intern Med 1970; 73: 881–895

28. Bonadonna G, Santoro A, Bonfante V, Valagussa P. Cyclic delivery of MOPP and ABVD combinations in stage IV Hodgkin's disease: rationale, background studies and recent results. Cancer Treatment Report 1982; 66: 881–887

29. Canellos G P, Anderson J R, Propert K J et al. Chemotherapy of advanced Hodgkin's disease with MOPP, ABVD, or MOPP alternating with ABVD. N Engl J Cancer 1992; 327: 1478–1484

30. Hellman S, Mauch P. Role of radiation therapy in the treatment of Hodgkin's disease. Cancer Treatment Report 1982; 66: 915–923

31. Tubiana M, Henry-Amwar M, Carde P et al. Toward comprehensive management tailored to prognostic factors of patients with clinical stages I and II in Hodgkin's disease. The EORTC Lymphoma Group controlled clinical trials 1964–1987. Blood 1989; 73: 47–56

32. Healey E A, Tarbell N J, Kalish L A et al. Prognostic factors for patients with Hodgkin's disease in first relapse. Cancer 1993; 71: 2613–2620

33. Desch C E, Lasala M R, Smith T J, Hillner B E. The optimal timing of autologous bone marrow transplantation in Hodgkin's disease patients after a chemotherapy relapse. J Clin Oncol 1992; 10: 200–209

34. Dyer M J. Non-Hodgkin's lymphoma: In: Horwich A (ed). Oncology: A Multidisciplinary Textbook (3rd ed). London: Chapman and Hall, 1995: 251–259

35. Goldstone A H, McMillan A K, Chopra R. High-dose therapy for the treatment of non-Hodgkin's lymphoma. In: Armitage J O, Antman K H (eds). High-dose Cancer Therapy. Pharmacology, Hematopoietins, Stem cells. Baltimore: Williams and Wilkins, 1992

36. Carroll B A. Ultrasound of lymphoma. Semin Ultrasound 1982; III(2): 114–122

37. Beyer D, Peters D. Real-time ultrasonography: an efficient screening method for abdominal and pelvic lymphadenopathy. Lymphology 1980; 13: 142–149

38. Neumann C H, Robert N J, Rosenthal D, Canellos G. Clinical value of ultrasonography for the management of non-Hodgkin's lymphoma patients as compared with abdominal computed tomography. J Comput Assist Tomogr 1983; 7: 666–669

39. Reznek R H, Husband J E. The radiology of lymphoma. Curr Imag 1990; 2: 9–17

40. Lee J K T, Heiken J P, Ling D et al. Magnetic resonance imaging of abdominal and pelvic lymphadenopathy. Radiology 1984; 153: 181–188

41. Dooms G C, Hricak H, Crooks L E, Higgins C B. Magnetic resonance imaging of the lymph nodes. Comparison with C T. Radiology 1984; 153: 719–728

42. Greco A, Jeliffe A M, Maher J E, Leung A W L. M R imaging of lymphomas: impact on therapy. J Comput Assist Tomogr 1988; 19: 785–791

43. Hill M, Cunningham D, MacVicar D et al. Role of magnetic resonance imaging in predicting relapse in residual masses after treatment of lymphoma. J Clin Oncol 1993; 11: 2273–2278

44. Front D, Bar-Shalom R, Epelbaum R et al. Early detection of lymphoma recurrence with gallium-67 scintigraphy. J Nucl Med 1993; 34: 2101–2104

45. Newman J S, Francis I R, Kaminski M S, Wahl R L. Imaging of lymphoma with PET with 2-(F-18)-fluoro-2-deoxy-D-glucose: Correlation with C T. Radiology 1994; 190: 111–116

46. Lee J K T, Stanley R J, Sagel S S, Levitt R G. Accuracy of computed tomography in detecting intra-abdominal and pelvic adenopathy in lymphoma. Am J Roentgenol 1978; 131: 311–315

47. Best J J K, Blackledge G St C, Forbes W et al. Computed tomography of the abdomen in the staging and clinical management of lymphoma. Br Med J 1978; ii: 1675–1677

48. Earl H M, Sutcliffe S B J, Kelsey Fry I et al. Computerised tomographic (CT) abdominal scanning in Hodgkin's disease. Clin Radiol 1980; 31: 149–153

49. Marglin S, Castellino R. Lymphographic accuracy in 632 consecutive, previously untreated cases of Hodgkin's disease and non-Hodgkin's lymphoma. Radiology 1981; 140: 351–353

50. Castellino R A, Hoppe R T, Blank N et al. Computed tomography, lymphography and staging laparotomy: Correlations in initial staging of Hodgkin's disease. Am J Roentgenol 1984; 143: 37–41

51. Enig B, Jensen B, Madsen E et al. Detection of neoplastic lymph nodes in Hodgkin's disease and non-Hodgkin's lymphoma. Acta Radiol Oncol 1985; 24. Fasc 6:

52. Strijk S P. Lymphography and abdominal computed tomography in the staging of non-Hodgkin's lymphoma. Acta Radiol 1987; 28. Fasc 3: 263–269

53. Stomper P C, Cholewinski S P, Park J et al. Abdominal staging of thoracic Hodgkin disease: CT-lymphangiography-Ga-67 scanning correlation. Radiology 1993; 187: 381–386

54. Libson E, Polliack A, Bloom R A. Value of lymphangiography in the staging of Hodgkin lymphoma. Radiology 1994; 193: 757–759

55. DePeña C A, van Tassel P, Ya-Yen L. Lymphoma of the head and neck. In: Libshitz H (ed). The Radiologic Clinics of North America: Imaging the Lymphomas. Philadelphia: W. B. Saunders Co., 1990: 723–743

56. Filly R, Blank N, Castellino R A. Radiographic distribution of intrathoracic disease in previously untreated patients with Hodgkin's disease and non-Hodgkin's lymphoma. Radiology 1976; 120: 277–281

57. Castellino R A, Blank N, Hoppe R T, Cho C. Hodgkin's disease: contribution of chest CT in the initial staging evaluation. Radiology 1986; 160: 603–605

58. Bragg D G. Radiology of the lymphomas. Curr Prob Diagnost Radiol 1987; 16: 183–206

59. Castellino R A, Hilton S, O'Brien J P, Portlock C S. Non-Hodgkin's lymphoma: contribution of chest CT in the initial staging evaluation. Radiology 1996; 199: 129–131

60. Grossman H, Winchester P H, Bragg D G et al. Roentgenographic changes in childhood Hodgkin's disease. Am J Roentgenol 1970; 108: 354–364

61. Jochelson M S, Balikian J P, Mauch P et al. Peri- and paracardial involvement in lymphoma in a radiographic study of 11 cases. Am J Roentgenol 1983; 140: 483–488

62. Strijk S P. Lymph node calcification in malignant lymphoma: Presentation of nine cases and a review of the literature. Acta Radiol Diagn (Stockh) 1985; 26: 427–431

63. Hopper K D, Diehl L F, Cole B A et al. Significance of necrotic mediastinal lymph nodes on CT in patients with newly diagnosed Hodgkin disease. Am J Roentgenol 1990; 155: 267–270

64. Heron C W, Husband J E, Williams M P. Hodgkin's disease: CT of the thymus. Radiology 1988; 167: 647–651

65. Wernecke K, Vassallo P, Rutsch F et al. Thymic involvement in Hodgkin disease. CT and sonographic findings. Radiology 1992; 181: 375–383

66. Spiers A S D, Husband J E S, MacVicar A D. Magnetic resonance imaging of treated thymic lymphoma — a comparison with computed tomography. Radiology 1997; 203: 369–376

67. Harel G S, Breiman R S, Glatstein E J et al. Computed tomography of the abdomen in the malignant lymphomas. Radiol Clin North Am 1977; 15: 391–400

68. Kadin M E, Glastein E J, Dorfman R E. Clinicopathologic studies in 117 untreated patients subject to laparotomy for the staging of Hodgkin's disease. Cancer 1977; 27: 1277–1294

69. Castellino R A, Marglin S, Blank N. Hodgkin's disease, the non-Hodgkin's lymphomas and the leukaemias in the retroperitoneum. Semin Roentgenol 1980; 15: 288–301

70. Goffinet D R, Warnke R, Dunnick N R et al. Clinical and surgical (laparotomy) evaluation of patients with non-Hodgkin's lymphomas. Cancer Treat Rep 1977; 61:981–992

71. Rosenberg S A, Kaplan H S. Evidence for an orderly progression in the spread of Hodgkin's disease. Cancer Res 1966; 26: 1225–1231

72. Urba W J, Longo D L. Hodgkin's disease. [Review]. N Engl J Med 1992; 326: 678–687

73. Weinstein J B, Heiken J P, Lee J K T et al. High resolution CT of the porta hepatis and hepatoduodenal ligament. Radiographics 1986; 6: 55–74

74. Kilgore T L, Chasen M H. Endobronchial non-Hodgkin's lymphoma. Chest 1983; 84: 58–61

75. Chabneer B A, Fisher R I, Young R C, DeVita V T. Staging of non-Hodgkin's lymphoma. Semin Oncol 1980; 7: 285–291

76. Kaplan H S. Contiguity and progression in Hodgkin's disease. Cancer Res 1971; 31: 1811–1813

77. Cobby M, Whipp E, Bullimore J et al. CT appearances of relapse of lymphoma in the lung. Clin Radiol 1990; 41: 232–238

78. MacDonald J B. Lung involvement in Hodgkin's disease. Thorax 1977; 32: 664–667

79. Burgener F A, Hamlin D J. Intrathoracic histiocytic lymphoma. Am J Roentgenol 1981; 136: 499–504

80. Lewis E R, Caskey C, Fishman E K. Lymphoma of the lung: CT findings in 31 patients. Am J Roentgenol 1991; 156: 711–714

81. Isaacson P G, Norton A J. General features of extranodal lymphoma. In: Extranodal Lymphomas. London: Churchill Livingstone, 1994: 1–14

82. Cordier J F, Chailleux E, Lauque D et al. Primary pulmonary lymphomas: a clinical study of 70 cases in nonimmunocompromised patients. Chest 1993; 103: 201–208

83. Peterson H, Snider H L, Yam L T et al. Primary pulmonary lymphoma: A clinical and immunohistochemical study of six cases. Cancer 1985; 56: 805–813

84. Murray K A, Chor P J, Turner J F. Intrathoracic lymphoproliferative disorders and lymphoma. Curr Prob Diagnos Radiol 1996; XXV: 77–108

85. Bergin C J, Healy M V, Zincone G E et al. MR evaluation of chest wall involvement in malignant lymphoma. J Comput Assist Tomogr 1990; 14: 928–932

86. North L B, Libshitz H I, Lorigan J G. Thoracic lymphoma. In: Libshitz H I (ed). Radiologic Clinics of North America: Imaging the Lymphomas. Philadelphia: W. B. Saunders Co., 1990: 745–762

87. Abel E A, Wood G S, Hoppe R T. Mycosis fungoides: Clinical and histologic features, staging, evaluation, and approach to treatment. CA Cancer J Clin 1993; 43: 93–115

88. Rubin D L, Blank N. Rapid pulmonary dissemination in mycosis fungoides simulating pneumonia: a case report and review of the literature. Cancer 1985; 56: 649–651

89. Paulus D D. Lymphoma of the breast. In: Libshitz H (ed). The Radiologic Clinics of North America: Imaging the Lymphomas. Philadelphia: W. B. Saunders Co., 1990: 833–840

90. Thomas J L, Bernadino M E, Vermess M et al. EOE-13 in the detection of hepatosplenic lymphoma. Radiology 1982; 145: 629–634

91. Bonadonna G, Santoro A. Clinical evolution and treatment of Hodgkin's disease. In: Wiernik P H, Canellos G, Kyle R A, Schiffer C A (eds). Neoplastic Disease of the Blood. Edinburgh: Churchill Livingstone, 1985: 789

92. Kaplan H S, Dorfman R F, Nelson T S, Rosenberg S A. Analysis of indications and patterns of involvement in 285 consecutive unselected patients. International Symposium of Hodgkin's Disease. Natl Cancer Inst Monogr 1973; 36: 291

93. Weissledeer R, Stark D D, Elizondo G et al. MRI of hepatic lymphoma. Mag Res Imag 1988; 6: 675–681

94. Richards M A, Webb J A W, Reznek R H et al. Detection of spread of malignant lymphoma to the liver at low field strength magnetic resonance imaging. Br Med J 1986; 293: 1126–1128

95. Weinreb J C, Brateman L, Maravilla K R. Magnetic resonance imaging of hepatic lymphoma. Am J Roentgenol 1984; 143: 1211–1214

96. Nyman R S, Rehn S M, Ericsson A et al. An attempt to characterise malignant lymphoma in spleen, liver and lymph nodes with magnetic resonance imaging. Acta Radiol 1987; 28: 527–533

97. Brady L W, Asbell S O. Malignant lymphoma of the gastrointestinal tract. Radiology 1980; 137: 291–298

98. Dodd G D. Lymphoma of the hollow abdominal viscera. Radiol Clin North Am 1990; 28: 771–783

99. Dragosick S B, Bauer P, Radaszkiewicz T U S. Primary gastrointestinal non-Hodgkin's lymphomas: a retrospective clinicopathologic study of 150 cases. Cancer 1984; 152: 291–296

100. Megibow A J, Balthazar E J, Naidich D P et al. Computed tomography of gastrointestinal lymphoma. Am J Roentgenol 1983; 141: 541–543

101. Reed K, Vose P C, Jarstfer B S. Pancreatic cancer: 30 year review (1947 to 1977). Am J Surg 1979; 138: 929–933

102. Shirkhoda A, Ros P R, Farah J, Staab E. Lymphoma of the solid abdominal viscera. Radiol Clin North Am 1990; 28: 785–799

103. Charnsangavej C. Lymphoma of the genitourinary tract. Radiologic Clin North Am 1990; 28: 865–877

104. Reznek R H, Mootoosamy I, Webb J A W, Richards M A. CT in renal and perirenal lymphoma: a further look. Clin Radiol 1990; 42: 233–238

105. Hartman D S, Davis C J, Golman S M et al. Renal lymphoma: radiologic-pathologic correlation of 21 cases. Radiology 1982; 144: 759–766

106. Heiken J P, Gold R P, Schnur M J et al. Computed tomography of renal lymphoma with ultrasound correlation. J Comput Assist Tomogr 1983; 7: 245–250

107. Aigen A B, Phillips M. Primary malignant lymphoma of the urinary bladder. Urology 1986; 28: 235–237

108. Mostofi F K. Testicular tumors: epidemiologic, etiologic and pathologic features. Cancer 1973; 32: 1186–1201

109. Jenkins N, Husband J, Sellars N et al. MRI in primary non-Hodgkin's lymphoma of the vagina associated with a uterine congenital anomaly: a case report. Br J Radiol 1997; 70: 219–222

110. Glazer H S, Lee J K T, Balfe D M et al. Non-Hodgkin lymphoma: computed tomographic demonstration of unusual extranodal involvement. Radiology 1983; 149: 211–217

111. Vincent J M, Morrison I D, Armstrong P, Reznek R H. Computed tomography of diffuse, non-metastatic enlargement of the adrenal glands in patients with malignant disease. Clin Radiol 1994; 49: 456–460

112. Zimmerman R A. Central nervous system lymphoma. Radiologic Clin North Am 1990; 28: 697–721

113. Hobson D E, Anderson B A, Carr I, West M. Primary lymphoma of the central nervous system: Manitoba experience and review of literature. Can J Neurol Sci 1986; 13: 55–61

114. Greco A, Jelliffe A M, Maher J, Leung A W L. MR imaging of lymphomas: impact on therapy. J Comput Assist Tomogr 1988; 12: 785–791

115. Heerman T S, Hammond N, Jones S E et al. Involvement of the CNS by non-Hodgkin's lymphoma. The Southwestern Oncology Group experience. Cancer 1979; 43: 390–397

116. Bragg D G, Colby T H, Ward J H. New concepts in the non-Hodgkin's lymphomas: radiologic implications. Radiology 1986; 159: 289–304

117. Chamberlain M C, Sandy A D, Press G A. Leptomeningeal metastasis: a comparison of gadolinium-enhanced MR and contrast enhanced CT of brain. Neurology 1990; 40: 435–438

118. MacVicar A D, Williams M P. CT scanning in epidural lymphoma. Clin Radiol 1991; 43: 95–102

119. Evans C. A review of non-Hodgkin's lymphomata of the head and neck. Clin Oncol 1981; 7: 23–31

120. Robbins K T, Fuller L M Vlasak M et al. Primary lymphomas of the paranasal sinuses. Cancer 1985; 56: 814–819

121. Shikhani A, Samara M, Allam C et al. Primary lymphoma in the salivary glands: report of five cases and review of the literature. Laryngoscope 1987; 97: 1438–1442

122. Takashima S, Izezoe J, Morimoto S et al. Primary thyroid lymphoma: evaluation with CT. Radiology 1988; 168: 765–768

123. Braunstein E M. Hodgkin's disease of bone: radiographic correlation with the histological classification. Radiology 1980; 137: 643–646

124. Cooley B L, Higinbotham N L, Groesbeck H P. Primary reticulum cell sarcoma of bone: summary of 37 cases. Radiology 1950; 55: 641–658

125. Ngan H, Preston B J. Non-Hodgkin's lymphoma presenting with osseous lesions. Clin Radiol 1975; 26: 351–356

126. Anderson K C, Kaplan W D, Leonard R C F et al. Role of [99m]Technetium-methylene diphosphonate bone imaging in the management of lymphoma. Cancer Treat Rep 1985; 69: 1347–1351

127. Castellino R A, Goffinet D R, Blank N et al. The role of radiography in the staging of non-Hodgkin's lymphoma with laparotomy correlation. Radiology 1974; 110: 329–338

128. Chabner B A, Johnson R E, Young R C et al. Sequential nonsurgical and surgical staging of non- Hodgkin's lymphoma. Ann Intern Med 1976; 85: 149–154

129. Glastein E, Guernsey A M, Rosenberg S A, Kaplan H S. The value of laparotomy and splenectomy in the staging of Hodgkin's disease. Cancer 1969; 24: 709–718

130. Kaplan H S. Essentials of staging and management of the malignant lymphomas. Semin Roentgenol 1980; 15: 219–226

131. Linden A, Zankovich R, Theissen R, Diehl V, Schicha H. Malignant lymphoma: bone marrow imaging versus biopsy. Radiology 1989; 173: 335–339

132. Pond G D, Castellino R A, Horning S, Hoppe R T. Non-Hodgkin's lymphoma: influence of lymphography, CT and bone marrow biopsy on staging and management. Radiology 1989; 170: 159–164

133. Dohner H, Guckel F, Knauf W et al. Magnetic resonance imaging of bone marrow in lymphoproliferative disorders: correlation with bone marrow biopsy. Br J Haematol 1989; 73: 12–17

134. Hoane B R, Shields A F, Porter B A, Shulman H M. Detection of lymphomatous bone marrow involvement with magnetic resonance imaging. Blood 1991; 78: 728–738

135. Burkitt D P. A sarcoma involving the jaws in African children. Br J Surg 1968; 46: 218–223

136. O'Connor G T, Rappaport H, Smith E B. Childhood lymphoma resembling 'Burkitt tumour' in the United States. Cancer 1965; 18: 411–417

137. Williams M P, Olliff J. Magnetic resonance imaging of extra nodal pelvic lymphoma. Clin Radiol 1990; 42: 264–268

138. De Vita V T, Hellman S, Rosenberg S A (eds). Cancer — Principles and Practice of Oncology. Toronto: J B Lippincott Co, 1981: 1354

139. North L B, Fuller L M, Sullivan-Halley J A, Hagemeister F B. Regression of mediastinal Hodgkin disease after therapy: evaluation of time interval. Radiology 1987; 164: 599–602

140. Radford J A, Cowan R A, Flanagan M et al. The significance of residual mediastinal abnormality on the chest radiograph following treatment for Hodgkin's disease. J Clin Oncol 1988; 6: 940–946

141. Drossman S R, Schiff R G, Kronfeld G D et al. Lymphoma of the mediastinum and neck: evaluation with Ga-67 imaging and CT correlation. Radiology 1990; 174: 171–175

142. Israel O, Front D, Epelbaum R. Residual mass and negative gallium scintigraphy in treated lymphoma. J Nucl Med 1990; 31: 365–368

143. Weiner M, Leventhal B, Cantor A et al. Gallium-67 scans as an adjunct to computed tomography scans for the assessment of a residual mediastinal mass in pedia-tric patients with Hodgkin's disease. Cancer 1991; 68: 2478–2480

144. Nyman R S, Rehn S M, Glimelius B L G et al. Residual mediastinal masses in Hodgkin disease: Prediction of size with MR imaging. Radiology 1989; 170: 435–440

145. Rahmouni A, Tempany C, Jones R et al. Lymphoma: monitoring tumour size and signal intensity with MR imaging. Radiology 1993; 188: 445–451

146. Hill M, Cunningham D, MacVicar D. The role of magnetic resonance imaging in predicting relapse in residual masses after treatment of lymphoma. J Clin Oncol 1994; 11: 2273–2278

Chapter 29

Multiple myeloma

Conor Collins

INTRODUCTION

Multiple myeloma is the most common primary tumour arising in bone accounting for 10% of haematological malignancy and 1% of all malignant disease. In the UK the annual incidence is approximately 4 per 100,000 with a 2 to 1 male predominance. The disease occurs twice as frequently in African Americans as in white Americans and Europeans and is much lower amongst Chinese and Japanese populations. The median age at diagnosis is 69 years but it is extremely rare in patients under 40 years whilst the incidence climbs to over 30 per 100,000 in those aged over 80 years.[1]

Multiple myeloma is due to uncontrolled proliferation of a single clone of plasma cells, the cells of the bone marrow that make immunoglobulins. As a result, a monoclonal protein in the form of an intact immunoglobulin (Ig) is produced and secreted (M protein). Immunoglobulin (Ig)G paraprotein is present in 60% of patients, IgA in 20–25% and free immunoglobulin light chains alone in 15–20% of patients. The latter are detectable in the urine as Bence–Jones protein, the former are demonstrable by serum protein electrophoresis. The malignant transformation of a single clone of plasma cells is manifest as a monoclonal gammopathy and demonstrable by serum protein electrophoresis.

CLINICAL FEATURES

Bone destruction is a characteristic resulting from increased osteoclastic bone resorption (manifest as hypercalcaemia) and impaired osteoblastic bone formation. There is abnormal bone remodelling with a marked predisposition to pathological fractures. Accumulation of plasma cells within bone marrow leads to anaemia and production of the M protein may lead to hyperviscosity or renal failure (due to tubular protein deposition). Production of normal immunoglobulin is impaired making the patient susceptible to recurrent infection.

The most common presenting complaint is back pain although symptoms of anaemia, renal failure and infection are also frequent. Symptoms associated with hyperviscosity (impaired vision, purpura, neuropathy), spinal cord compression, hypercalcaemia or amyloidosis are less common. About 30% of patients are asymptomatic and diagnosis results from routine investigations.[2] The disease is characterized by the classic triad of:

- Bone marrow infiltration by plasma cells
- Lytic bone deposits on plain film radiography
- The presence of M protein in the serum or urine

TREATMENT OPTIONS

Treatment strategy is directed towards adequate analgesia, rehydration, management of hypercalcaemia and renal impairment, and treatment of infection. Chemotherapy in the form of oral melphalan and prednisolone produces a greater than 50% reduction in M protein concentration in 50% of patients. Combination regimens are more effective in younger patients and may produce a higher response rate (up to 70% of patients). Younger patients may also benefit from high-dose melphalan and autologous stem-cell transplantation as a second-line treatment but it should be remembered that this is not a curative procedure.[1] In most patients a stable plateau response occurs which may be prolonged by maintenance interferon alpha or bisphosphonate treatment. Radiotherapy is the treatment of choice for patients with evidence of spinal cord compression. Ultimately, the prognosis is poor with a 5-year survival of only 20%. Death results from bacterial infection, renal insufficiency and thromboembolism.

Key points: general features

■ Multiple myeloma is an uncontrolled proliferation of a single clone of plasma cells

■ Myeloma is characterized by: (a) plasma cell infiltration of the bone marrow, (b) lytic bone lesions and (c) myeloma protein in the serum or urine

STAGING

The staging system devised by Durie and Salmon is the most widely used.[3] This is based on the serum concentrations of haemoglobin, calcium and paraprotein, urinary Bence–Jones protein excretion and the number of skeletal lesions seen on plain radiographs.

RADIOLOGY AND CROSS-SECTIONAL IMAGING

The role of radiology and cross-sectional imaging is staging (assessment of disease extent and severity), monitoring treatment response and detection of disease relapse and complications. The various imaging techniques employed and their associated findings are described more fully below.

Detection and staging
Plain film radiography

Almost 80% of patients with multiple myeloma will have radiological evidence of skeletal involvement and the plain radiograph (skeletal survey) is the best method of identifying lytic deposits within bone.[4,5] Due to diffuse involvement of the marrow, bony abnormalities usually occur at multiple sites including:

- Vertebrae in 66% of patients
- Ribs (45%)
- Skull (40%)
- Shoulder (40%)
- Pelvis (30%)
- Long bones (25%)

The skeletal survey should therefore include radiographs of skull, chest, upper humeri, thoracic and lumbar spine, pelvis and upper femora.

Myeloma lesions are sharply defined, small lytic areas (average size 20 mm) of bone destruction with no reactive bone formation. The pattern of destruction may be geographic, moth-eaten or permeated.[6] Involvement may be so diffuse that the bones will be simply osteopenic or even normal in radiographic appearance. The differential diagnosis may be difficult especially in an elderly female patient as males aged between 50 and 70 years rarely show extensive idiopathic osteoporosis. Myelomatous lesions may be expansile, break through the cortex and form large extra-osseous soft tissue masses. Pathological fractures are common (Fig. 29.1).

Scintigraphy

The technetium-99m labelled diphosphonate bone scan is typically normal or may show areas of decreased uptake (photopenia). These areas represent destruction and replacement

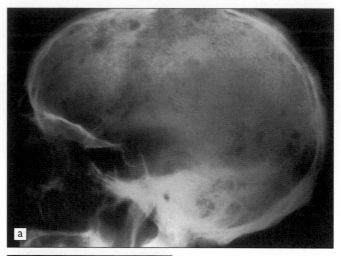

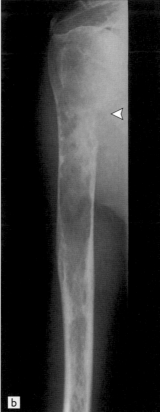

Figure 29.1. *(a) Lateral radiograph of skull demonstrating multiple lytic lesions. (b) Anteroposterior (AP) radiograph of right humerus demonstrating expansion of proximal shaft and destruction of medial cortical margin (arrowhead). A pathological fracture is imminent. (c) Posteroanterior (PA) view of chest demonstrating an expansile lytic deposit affecting 6th left posterior rib with destruction of the inferior cortical margin (arrowhead). (d) and (e) AP and lateral views of lower dorsal spine demonstrating multiple compression fractures. Note intact pedicles. (f) AP radiograph of pelvis demonstrating a large lytic deposit within right ischium (arrowhead).*

of bone by myeloma tissue without an accompanying osteoblastic bone reaction. In a study comparing radionuclide images and plain radiographs the bone scan failed to show radiographically evident disease or underestimated its extent at 27% of anatomical sites. The scintigraphic abnormality preceded the radiographic abnormality in less than 1% of cases.[7] When the bone scan is positive before the radiograph shows evidence of myeloma it may subsequently revert to normal in the presence of an abnormal radiograph. As a result bone scintigraphy is of little value in evaluating osseous myeloma lesions because

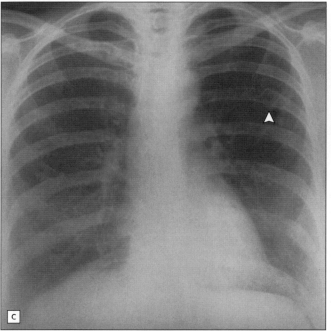

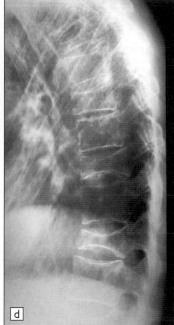

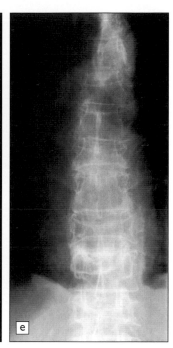

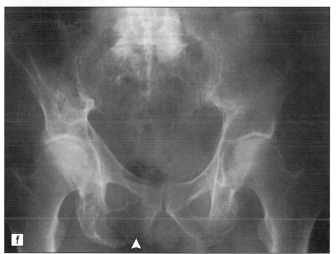

Key points: radiological features

- Up to 80% of patients with myeloma have radiographic evidence of skeletal disease

- 66% of patients have vertebral deposits

- Bone lesions are typically sharply defined small lytic deposits with no reactive bone formation

- Technetium-99m diphosphonate bone scans are usually normal or show areas of decreased uptake

- FDG PET may be a useful imaging technique

of the many false-negative radionuclide scans.[8,9] Scintigraphy, however, may detect lesions in regions where plain film radiography is less efficient, e.g. the ribs. More recent reports in the literature describe increased isotope uptake within osseous myelomatous deposits using 2-[F-18] fluoro-2 deoxy-D-glucose (FDG) positron emission tomography (PET) imaging and technetium-99m sestamibi.[10,11]

Multiple myeloma versus bone metastases

Several differential points may help distinguish between multiple myeloma and lytic bone metastases. These features by themselves do not always provide the answer and need to be taken in conjunction with all other evidence present (Table 29.1).

Cross-sectional imaging

Computed tomography

Prior to the advent of magnetic resonance imaging (MRI), computed tomography (CT) was valuable in patients with normal radiographs and bone pain. Findings on CT include the presence of multiple lytic lesions with cortical disruption and in the spine there is often an associated paravertebral soft tissue mass[12] (Fig. 29.2). The main role of CT is:

- To evaluate for the presence or absence of bony lesions
- Aid in performing biopsy
- To demonstrate disseminated disease in a patient with an apparently solitary plasmacytoma

Table 29.1. *Durie and Salmon staging system for multiple myeloma*

Stage*	Criteria
I	All of the following: Haemoglobin value >10 g/dl (100 g/l) Normal serum calcium value <12 mg/dl (3 mmol/l) At radiography, normal bone structure or solitary bone plasmacytoma only Low M component production rates IgG value: <5 g/dl (50 g/l) IgA value: <3 g/dl (30 g/l) Urine light chain M component at electrophoresis: <4 g/24 h
II	Fitting neither Stage I nor stage III
III	One or more of the following: Haemoglobin value <8.5 g/dl (85 g/l) Serum calcium value >12 mg/dl (2 mmol/l) Advanced lytic bone lesion High M component production rates IgG value: >7 g/dl (70 g/l) IgA value: >5 g/dl (50 g/l) Urine light chain M component at electrophoresis >12 g/24 h

*Subclassifications: A = relatively normal renal function (serum creatinine value <2.0 mg/dl [175 mmol/l]). B = abnormal renal function (serum creatinine value >2.0 mg/dl [175 mmol/l])

Table 29.2. *Multiple myeloma versus bone metastases*

Radiological features	Multiple myeloma	Bone metastases
Involvement of intervertebral discs	Yes	No
Involvement of mandible	Yes	No
Involvement of vertebral pedicles	No	Yes
Associated paraspinal soft tissue mass	Yes	No
Isotope bone scan	Frequently negative	Frequently positive

Magnetic resonance imaging

As a result of its ability to directly visualize bone marrow and its increased sensitivity, MRI is routinely used in many centres as a diagnostic technique for patients with multiple myeloma. In patients with suspected epidural involvement it is the examination of first choice.[13,14] Bone lesions have been shown by MRI in about 50% of asymptomatic myeloma patients with normal plain radiographs.[15,16] Nonetheless, a recent study involving 41 patients suggested that it was more practical to screen all bone areas with plain

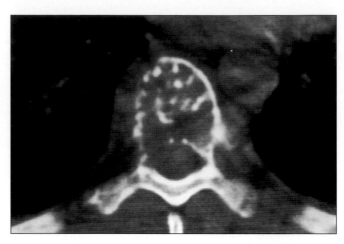

Figure 29.2. *CT scan of T8 vertebral body (axial view). There is extensive infiltration of the marrow with cortical destruction and an associated paravertebral soft tissue mass bilaterally.*

film radiography initially and perform MRI of the thoracolumbar spine using a phase-array spine coil in patients who have normal radiographs.[17]

Multiple myeloma gives a variable appearance on MRI due to the fact that marrow infiltration takes two forms; diffuse infiltration, with mixing of myeloma cells and haematopoietic cells, and tumour nodules composed entirely of myeloma cells.[18]

The patterns are reflected in the MRI appearances with diffuse or focal changes in marrow signal intensity on T1- and T2-weighted images. These findings, however, are not specific and do not distinguish multiple myeloma from other infiltrative processes in the bone marrow.[19,20] With multiple myeloma detection of diffuse infiltration is dependent on knowledge of the normal range of the appearance of bone marrow for the age of the patient.[21,22]

Haematopoietic marrow in adults between 40 and 70 years old is composed of approximately 20–25% bone substance, 40–45% fat, 30–35% cellular marrow (see Chapter 37).[23] The appearance of the marrow is dependent not only on the extent of disease but also on the extent of fatty replacement which varies considerably even in people of similar age. In addition, difficulties may arise in the interpretation of the observations themselves.

In the early stages of marrow infiltration monoclonal plasma cells arrange themselves so as not to displace the fat cells. Normal haematopoiesis is thought to be impaired due to the production of an inhibitory growth factor resulting in a relative increase in the fat component. As a result, in cases with minor marrow infiltration no signal alterations on MRI may be present.[14,19,24]

A diffuse infiltration pattern in multiple myeloma has been described but it may be difficult to diagnose as no normal marrow is preserved for comparison.[13,14,19,24,25] It has been

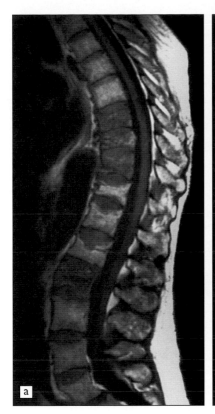
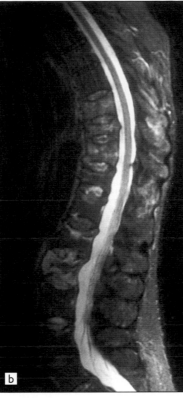

Figure 29.3. *MR images of thoracic and lumbar spine prior to treatment (sagittal view using a phase array coil). (a) T1-weighted spin-echo sequence (TR400/TE15); (b) fat suppression short tau inversion recovery (STIR) sequence (TR4900/TE60). There is partial collapse of several thoracic and lumbar vertebrae, many of which have a low signal intensity on T1 and a high signal intensity on STIR, representing active disease.*

shown recently that when signal intensity enhances greater than 40% over baseline following intravenous contrast medium injection (Gd-DTPA), an intermediate or high degree of diffuse plasma cell infiltration is present.[24] This allows an objective assessment of the degree of marrow infiltration.

Focal areas of marrow abnormality are more frequently observed and usually demonstrate low signal intensity on T1-weighted spin-echo images[13,14,19,24–26] but they can be isointense or hyperintense compared with surrounding marrow (Fig. 29.3a).[24,26] On T2-weighted spin-echo images variable signal intensity patterns have been reported[13] but in general the lesions show high signal intensity.[13,19,26,27] However, as this sequence also shows fat as relatively high signal intensity it has a limited usefulness in assessing myeloma. This problem can be overcome by combining a fast spin-echo T2-weighted sequence with fat suppression (Fig. 29.3b).[26,28] Use of intravenous contrast medium confers no extra benefit in the detection of extra lesions using spin-echo sequences.[26]

Normal haematopoietic marrow has low signal intensity on opposed phase gradient recalled echo (GRE) images.[29] In multiple myeloma tumour foci demonstrate increased signal intensity on opposed phase GRE images making them easy to visualize. In patients with diffuse infiltration of the marrow the signal intensity is low but where diffuse and focal infiltration coexist there are areas of high signal intensity on a background of low signal intensity. However, in marrow, where there has been an increase in fat cells, distinction may be difficult on GRE images. In such a situation use of intravenous contrast medium may enable differentiation between the various infiltration patterns.[24]

The inability to identify multiple myeloma with MRI in all cases makes it difficult to distinguish benign from malignant causes of vertebral compression fractures. This problem is compounded by the significant osteoporosis often present in multiple myeloma. In one study marrow abnormalities were seen in only 50% of vertebral bodies which had evidence of collapse.[19] This refuted the suggestion that complete replacement of the bone marrow of a vertebral body by tumour at MRI would permit differentiation between pathological and osteoporotic compression fractures. More recently, however, differentiation of myelomatous from osteoporotic causes of vertebral body collapse has been demonstrated on the basis of an increase in signal intensity on postcontrast T1-weighted spin-echo and T2-weighted spin-echo images in vertebrae with myelomatous infiltration.[30]

Non-secretory myeloma is characterized by involvement of the bone marrow but there is no evidence of abnormal protein in the blood or urine.[31] It is likely that MRI will prove to be the most useful non-invasive method of assessing the course of disease in these patients. When solitary plasmacytoma is present, MRI can detect or exclude additional marrow abnormalities.[32]

Key points: MRI

- MRI shows bone abnormalities in 50% of asymptomatic patients with normal plain radiographs

- Bone marrow lesions on MRI are either diffuse or focal

- MRI appearances on T1- and T2-weighted images are variable and non-specific

- Intravenous contrast enhancement greater than 40% over baseline indicates an intermediate or high degree of diffuse infiltration

- Intravenous contrast enhancement helps to distinguish benign from malignant vertebral collapse

Assessment of response

A skeletal survey should be repeated following completion of treatment. Shrinking or sclerosing lesions indicate partial or complete resolution. New or enlarging lesions indicate progressive disease. These features also apply to bone lesions being monitored with CT. Although bone scintigraphy is not helpful in detecting myelomatous bone lesions, an abnormal bone scan following treatment indicates residual disease.[9]

On MRI, decreased signal intensity on T2-weighted spin-echo images has been observed after radiotherapy. As a result, it was postulated that MRI could be used to differentiate lesions stabilized by radiotherapy from lesions of progressive myelomatous bone disease.[14]

Rahmouni et al.[33] described different patterns of response on follow-up MRI of treated patients. Before treatment all lesions had high signal intensity on T2-weighted spin-echo images. On T1-weighted spin-echo images the nodules had a low signal intensity and all enhanced following intravenous contrast medium. Following treatment, all nodules remained hypointense on T1-weighted spin-echo images but changes in signal intensity on T2-weighted spin-echo images and on postcontrast T1-weighted spin-echo images occurred in 78% of patients. Three different patterns following administration of intravenous contrast medium were described as below:

- The first pattern (rim enhancement or no enhancement) represented MRI criteria of a good response to treatment (decreased serum myeloma protein by 50%, decreased urinary myeloma protein by 75%)
- The second pattern (arterial and complete enhancement associated with rim enhancement or no enhancement) correlated with good or partial response to treatment (decreased serum protein less than 50%, decreased urinary myeloma protein less than 75%)
- The third pattern (no changes in signal intensity on spin-echo images and arterial enhancement of the lesions) usually represented evidence of progressive disease

Although different therapies were utilized, lack of enhancement of tumour was seen in responding patients treated by chemotherapy only and in responding patients who received both chemotherapy and radiotherapy.[33]

In another study involving 20 patients, before and after chemotherapy MRI patterns of marrow involvement were classified as focal, diffuse or variegated. Patterns of complete response (disappearance of serum myeloma protein with immunofixation tests) included complete resolution of marrow abnormality or persistent abnormality without enhancement or with peripheral rim enhancement. Conversion of a diffuse to a variegated or focal pattern and a decrease in the amount of marrow abnormality with persistent enhancement were observed in patients who showed a partial response (decrease of serum myeloma protein by greater than 50%).[34]

A persistently high signal intensity on T2-weighted images post-treatment does not necessarily imply active tumour because necrosis and inflammation may prolong T2-weighting (Fig. 29.4). Focal myelomatous lesions may remain hyperintense in both responding and non-responding patients.[33] In focal myeloma dense, nodular plasma-cell aggregates may destroy normal bony substrate and cause permanent fibrotic change. This is reflected by an increased frequency of lytic lesions on plain radiographs of the spine in patients with a focal pattern and by the lack of complete resolution of the pretreatment MRI findings, even among patients who achieve a complete remission. In patients with variegated or diffuse patterns of infiltration, abnormal cells are interspersed in normal marrow so focal aggregates may not be large enough to produce changes on plain radiographs.[34] In such cases the tumour may resolve without evidence of residual abnormality on MRI.

On MRI absence of enhancement or peripheral rim enhancement may suggest treated inactive tumour.[33] In complete responders with focal lesions, persistent inhomogeneous enhancement was seen only with new compression fractures or lesions within irradiated vertebrae.[34] The effect of treatment on focal lesions in irradiated or collapsed vertebrae can be difficult to assess with MRI because persistent enhancement in such cases may not necessarily indicate resistant disease.

Back pain that increases in severity during remission is a distressing symptom for patients with multiple myeloma. In one study 35% of patients experienced new or increasing back pain during treatment.[34] Virtually all of these patients had new or progressive compression fractures demonstrated

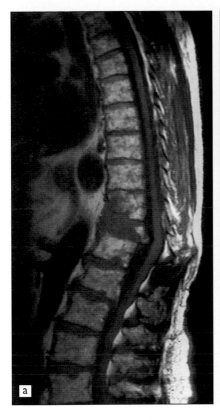 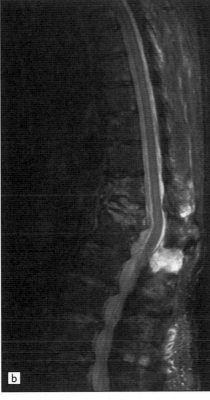

Figure 29.4. *MR images of the thoracic and lumbar spine following chemotherapy (sagittal view using a phase array coil). T1-weighted spin-echo sequence (TR400/TE15) (a) and fat suppression STIR sequence (TR4900/TE60) (b). There is a complete collapse of T11 vertebral body associated with posterior displacement of the spinal cord. The increased signal intensity on the STIR sequence within T10, T11 and T12 indicates active disease in this region. The lack of increased signal within the remaining vertebrae indicates inactive disease.*

on follow-up MRI. All fractures involved vertebrae that had extensive marrow disease prior to treatment. With response to treatment there was resolution of the tumour mass that had replaced the bony trabeculae resulting in collapse of the unsupported vertebral body. Magnetic resonance imaging may help to clarify the cause of the fracture and guide choice of therapy in such cases.

Key points: post-treatment evaluation

■ Shrinking or sclerosing lesions on skeletal survey on completion of treatment indicates partial or complete resolution

■ Abnormal bone scintigraphy following treatment indicates residual disease

■ Changes in signal intensity on T2-weighted spin-echo sequences are observed in response to treatment

■ A persistent high signal intensity on T2-weighted images may represent necrosis and inflammation as well as persistent tumour

■ Contrast-enhanced MRI shows different patterns which correlate well with clinical assessment of response

Relationship of radiology to laboratory values and prognosis

In devising their clinical staging system for multiple myeloma Durie and Salmon[3] found that the extent of radiographic changes showed the closest correlation with measured cell mass and survival. However, this finding was not confirmed in other studies.[35,36] In the largest published series, involving 172 patients, it was demonstrated that anaemia was more common, hypercalcaemia less common and survival time shorter among patients with normal radiographs than in patients with abnormal radiographic findings.[37]

It was subsequently demonstrated that patients with diffuse myeloma had fewer abnormal radiographs of the spine than did those with focal disease. A paradoxical finding was the combination of a normal skeletal survey and an MRI pattern of diffuse infiltration being indicative of more advanced disease. Conversely, lytic lesions on plain radiographs did not necessarily imply an adverse prognosis for patients with multiple myeloma.[34]

Correlation between MRI patterns of marrow involvement and haemoglobin and bone marrow plasmacytosis values has been demonstrated with diffuse and focal patterns of infiltration lesions being associated with more pronounced laboratory abnormalities.[25] In a study examining changes in MRI appearances pre- and post-treatment the patterns on MRI correlated with haematological and urinary protein parameters.[33] MRI is also useful for assessing the response to treatment when the myeloma is non-secretory or when a discrepancy exists between the clinical and haematological status of the patient.

At present, the clinical implications of early demonstration of myeloma foci detectable by MRI but not by plain film radiography, are not clear. It has been reported that patients with a negative MRI examination have a more favourable early course of the disease than those with changes detected by MRI or plain film radiography.[15] In another study assessing prognosis in newly diagnosed asymptomatic multiple myeloma, marrow abnormalities were demonstrated in half of patients on MRI with asymptomatic myeloma and normal skeletal radiographs.[16] The presence of marrow involvement on MRI, particularly the presence of diffuse or focal MRI patterns, appeared to identify asymptomatic patients at higher risk for early disease progression. Postponement of treatment can therefore be considered in those patients with a normal MRI examination. Elsewhere, MRI of the bone marrow has been demonstrated as an independent factor in the prediction of disease progression in patients with Stage I multiple myeloma.[38]

Investigative work has been performed on quantification of marrow involvement using T1- and T2-weighted sequences in patients suffering from myeloproliferative diseases.[39] Recent work has shown that using results from qualitative and quantitative measurements of marrow involvement on MRI correlated significantly with staging and survival.[24]

Key points: laboratory tests and MRI

■ The presence of marrow involvement on MRI may identify asymptomatic patients at higher risk for early disease progression

■ Correlation between MRI patterns of marrow involvement, haemoglobin and bone marrow plasmacytosis has been demonstrated

■ Serum β_2 microglobulin levels are probably the single most powerful determinant of outcome

■ There is no apparent correlation between serum β_2 microglobulin levels and MRI patterns of involvement

Serum β_2 microglobulin levels are probably the single most powerful determinant of outcome.[18] However, no correlation between serum β_2 microglobulin levels and appearances on MR images has been demonstrated.[19,25] Likewise, no definite correlation has been demonstrated between scintigraphic findings and haematological measurements of myeloma activity.[8]

Long-term prospective studies are required to establish the significance and prognostic value of the different MRI patterns of marrow involvement and their correlation with various laboratory values.

COMPLICATIONS ASSOCIATED WITH MULTIPLE MYELOMA

Complications of multiple myeloma are summarized below:

• Spinal cord compression
• Pathological fractures
• Secondary amyloidosis
• Renal impairment
• Predilection for recurrent pneumonia due to leucopenia
• Thromboembolism

A pathological fracture affects about 50% of patients at some time with many of the fractures affecting the vertebral bodies. It is not surprising therefore that spinal cord compression resulting from vertebral body collapse may occur in up to 25% of patients and has been described as a presenting feature in 12% of patients.[40,41] Early recognition of back pain and neurological symptoms is essential. Magnetic resonance is the imaging investigation of choice (Fig. 29.4).

Fractures of the tubular bones heal readily with normal amounts of callus but extensive fractures may require insertion of intramedullary nails.

Secondary amyloid occurs in approximately 10% of cases and in the early stages ultrasound demonstrates enlarged kidneys with increased cortical reflectivity. Amyloid protein is deposited mainly in the cortex so that corticomedullary differentiation is preserved and the pyramids are of normal size.[42] Unfortunately, imaging with iodine labelled serum amyloid P component has not been particularly successful in identifying renal amyloid, unlike amyloid deposition elsewhere.[43]

Patients with myeloma have a predilection for recurrent pneumonia due to associated leucopenia. These patients can be assessed using plain chest radiography and thin-section CT.

As stated previously the major causes of death are recurrent infection, renal impairment, and thrombo-embolism.

UNCOMMON VARIANTS OF MYELOMA

Extra-osseous myeloma
Clinical manifestations of extra-osseous myeloma are rare occurring in less than 5% of patients with multiple myeloma. Infiltration of adjacent organs, resulting from

direct spread, has been demonstrated at postmortem in 66% of patients with the liver, spleen and lymph nodes being most frequently involved.[44] Extra-osseous myeloma is more aggressive, occurs in a younger age group (average age 50 years) and is associated with a median survival of 1.5 months.[45]

Sclerotic myeloma

Examples of purely sclerotic myeloma have occasionally been reported and in one series occurred in approximately 3% of patients.[46] It may take the form of diffuse osteosclerosis, patchy sclerotic areas throughout the skeleton, or very small numbers of focal sclerotic lesions.

Summary

■ Multiple myeloma is characterized by the classic triad of bone marrow infiltration by plasma cells, lytic bone deposits on plain film radiographs (skeletal survey) and the presence of M protein in serum or urine.

■ The staging system devised by Durie and Salmon is based on serum haematological, urinary Bence–Jones protein and skeletal survey findings.

■ 80% of patients have identifiable lytic deposits on skeletal survey.

■ Several differential points help distinguish the lytic deposits of multiple myeloma from bone metastases.

■ Although MRI is more sensitive than the plain radiograph in identifying marrow lesions, imaging of the thoracolumbar spine with MRI should only be performed following normal plain film radiography.

■ Multiple myeloma may appear as nodules or diffuse infiltration on MRI.

■ On MRI multiple myeloma demonstrates low signal intensity on T1-weighted and high signal intensity on T2-weighted sequences. Use of a T2-weighted fat-suppression sequence helps differentiate myeloma deposits from marrow fat.

■ Patients responding to chemotherapy demonstrate a decrease in signal intensity on T2-weighted sequences.

■ Extent of changes on skeletal survey do not correlate with survival; serum β_2 microglobulin levels are probably the single most powerful determinant of outcome and are independent of appearances on MRI.

■ Spinal cord compression, resulting from vertebral body collapse, occurs in up to 25% of patients and as a presenting feature in 12% of patients.

REFERENCES

1. Singer C R J. Multiple myeloma. Br Med J 1997; 314: 960–963

2. Riccardi A, Gobbi P G, Ucci G et al. Changing clinical presentation of multiple myeloma. Eur J Cancer 1991; 27: 1401–1405

3. Durie B G M and Salmon S E. A clinical staging system for multiple myeloma correlation of measured myeloma cell mass with presenting clinical features response to treatment and survival. Cancer 1975; 36: 842–854

4. Kyle R A. Multiple myeloma: review of 869 cases. Mayo Clin Proc 1975; 50: 29–40

5. Ludwig H, Tscholakoff, Neuhold A et al. MRI of the spine in multiple myeloma. Lancet 1987; 15: 364–366

6. Longo D L. Plasma cell disorders. In: Wilson J D, Braunwald E, Isselbacher K J et al. (eds). Harrisons Principles of Internal Medicine (12th ed). New York: McGraw Hill, 1991; 1412–1416

7. Wahner H W, Kyle R A, Beabout J W. Scintigraphic evaluation of the skeleton in multiple myeloma. Mayo Clin Proc 1980; 55: 739–746

8. Woolfenden J M, Pitt M J, Durie B G M, Moon T E. Comparison of bone scintigraphy and radiography in multiple myeloma. Radiology 1980; 134: 723–728

9. Bataille R, Chevalier J, Rossie M, Sany J. Bone scintigraphy in plasma cell myeloma. A prospective study of 70 patients. Radiology 1982; 145: 801–804

10. Sasaki M, Ichiya Y, Kuwabara Y et al. Fluorine-18-fluorodeoxyglucose positron emission tomography in technetium-99m-hydroxymethlyenediphosphate negative bone tumours. J Nucl Med 1993; 34: 288–290

11. Adams B K, Fataar A, Nizami M A. Technetium-99m sestamibi uptake in myeloma. J Nucl Med 1996; 37: 1001–1002

12. Schreiman J S, McLeod R A, Kyle R A, Beabout J W. Multiple myeloma: evaluation by CT. Radiology 1985; 154: 483–486

13. Daffner R N, Lupetin A R, Dash N et al. MRI in the detection of malignant infiltration of bone marrow. Am J Roentgenol 1986; 146: 353–358

14. Fruehwald F X J, Tscholakoff D, Schwaighofer B et al. Magnetic resonance imaging of the lower vertebral column in patients with multiple myeloma. Invest Radiol 1988; 23: 193–199

15. Dimopoulos M A, Mouloupoulos L A, Smith T et al. Risk of disease progression in asymptomatic multiple myeloma. Am J Med 1993; 94: 57–61

16. Mouloupoulos L A, Dimopoulos M A, Smith T L et al. Prognostic significance of magnetic resonance imaging in patients with asymptomatic multiple myeloma. J Clin Oncol 1995; 13: 251–256

17. Tertti R, Alanen A, Remer K. The value of magnetic resonance imaging in screening myeloma lesions of the lumbar spine. Br J Haematol 1995; 91: 658–660

18. Galton D A G. Myelomatosis. In: Hoffbrand A V, Lewis S M, (eds). Postgraduate Haematology (3rd ed). Oxford: Heinemann, 1989; 474–501

19. Libshitz H I, Malthouse S R, Cunningham D et al. Multiple myeloma: appearance at MR imaging. Radiology 1992; 182: 833–837

20. Vosler J B, Murphy W A. Bone marrow imaging. Radiology 1988; 168: 679–693

21. Weinreb J C. MR imaging of bone marrow: a map could help. Radiology 1990; 177: 23–24

22. Ricci C, Cova M, Kang Y S. Rahmouni A et al. Normal age related patterns of cellular and fatty bone marrow distribution in the axial skeleton: MR imaging study. Radiology 1990; 177: 83–88

23. Bartl R, Frisch B, Fateh-Moghadam A et al. Histological classification and staging of multiple myeloma. Am J Clin Pathol 1987; 87: 342–355

24. Stabler A, Baur A, Bartl R et al. Contrast enhancement and quantitative signal analysis in MR imaging of multiple myeloma: assessment of focal and diffuse growth patterns in marrow correlated with biopsies and survival rates. Am J Roentgenol 1996; 167: 1029–1036

25. Mouloupoulos L A, Varma D G, Dimopoulos M A et al. Multiple myeloma: spinal MR imaging in patients with untreated newly diagnosed disease. Radiology 1992; 185: 833–840

26. Rahmouni A, Divine M, Mathieu D et al. Detection of multiple myeloma involving the spine: efficacy of fat suppression and contrast enhanced MR imaging. Am J Roentgenol 1993; 160: 1049–1052

27. Siegal T, Siegal T. Spinal epidural involvement in haematological tumours: clinical features and therapeutic options. Leuk Lymphoma 1991; 5: 101–110

28. Dwyer A J, Frank S L, Sank V J et al. Short T1 inversion recovery pulse sequence: analysis and initial experience in cancer imaging. Radiology 1988; 168: 827–836

29. Wismer G L, Rosen B R, Buxton R et al. Chemical shift imaging of bone marrow: preliminary experience. Am J Roentgenol 1985; 145: 1031–1037

30. Cuenod C A, Laredo J D, Chevret S et al. Acute vertebral collapse due to osteoporosis or malignancy: appearance on unenhanced and gadolinium enhanced MR images. Radiology 1996; 199: 541–549

31. Drecier R, Alexanian R. Non-secretory myeloma. Am J Haematol 1982; 13: 313–316

32. Mouloupoulos L A, Dimopoulos M A, Weber D et al. Magnetic resonance imaging in the staging of solitary plasmacytoma of bone. J Clin Oncol 1993; 11: 1311–1315

33. Rahmouni A, Divine M, Mathieu D et al. MR appearance of multiple myeloma before and after treatment. Am J Roentgenol 1993; 160: 1053–1057

34. Mouloupoulos L A, Dimopoulos M A, Alexanian R et al. Multiple myeloma: MR patterns of response to treatment. Radiology 1994; 193: 441–446

35. Gompels B M, Votaw M L. Martel W. Correlation of radiological manifestation of multiple myeloma with immunoglobulin abnormalities and prognosis. Radiology 1972; 104: 509–514

36. de Gramont A, Benitez O, Brissand P et al. Quantification of bone lytic lesions and prognosis in myelomatosis. Scand J Haematol 1985; 34: 78–82

37. Smith D B, Scarffe J H, Eddleston B. The prognostic significance of X-ray changes at presentation and reassessment in patients with multiple myeloma. Haematol Oncol 1988; 6: 1–6

38. VandeBerg B C, Lecouvet F E, Michaux L et al. Stage I multiple myeloma: value of MR imaging of the bone marrow in the determination of prognosis. Radiology 1996; 201: 243–246

39. Jenkins J P R, Stehling M, Sivewright G. et al. Quantitative magnetic resonance imaging of vertebral bodies: a T1 and T2 study. Mag Res Imag 1989; 7: 17–23

40. Woo E, Yu Y L, Ng M et al. Spinal cord compression in multiple myeloma. Who gets it? Aust NZ J Med 1986; 16: 671–675

41. Speiss J L, Adelstein D J, Hines F D. Multiple myeloma presenting with spinal cord compression. Oncology 1988; 45: 88–92

42. Subramanyam B R. Renal amyloidosis — sonographic features. Am J Roentgenol 1981; 136: 411–412

43. Saile R, Deveaux M, Hachulla E et al. Iodine-123 labelled serum amyloid P component scintigraphy in amyloidosis. Eur J Nucl Med 1993; 20: 130–137

44. Kapadia S B. Multiple myeloma: a clinicopathological study of 32 consecutively autopsied cases. Medicine 1980; 59: 380–392

45. Mouloupoulos L A, Granfield C A, Dimoploulos M. A. et al. Extraosseous multiple myeloma: imaging features. Am J Roentgenol 1993; 161: 1083–1087

46. Evison G, Evans K T. Bone sclerosis in multiple myeloma. Br J Radiol 1967; 40: 81–89

Chapter 30

Leukaemia

Janet Husband

INTRODUCTION

The leukaemias are a group of diverse neoplasms which are derived from the arrested, or aberrant, development of a clone of normal haemopoietic cells. These immature cells proliferate progressively within the bone marrow replacing normal haemopoietic tissue and circulate within the peripheral blood becoming deposited in various organs and tissues. Leukaemic cells are incapable of normal function and many of the clinical features and complications of leukaemia are a direct result of the failure of normal haemopoietic activity.

There are four major groups of leukaemia which are categorized according to the predominant type of proliferating cell:

- Acute myelogenous leukaemia (AML)
- Acute lymphoblastic leukaemia (ALL)
- Chronic myelocytic leukaemia (CML)
- Chronic lymphocytic leukaemia (CLL)

Full classification of the leukaemias has become increasingly complex as methods of discriminating dif-ferent subtypes, such as immunophenotyping and cytogenetic studies, have been developed. Thus the subclassification and characterization of the leukaemias continues to evolve.[1,2] The classification shown in Table 30.1 illustrates the wide ranging heterogeneity of these diseases.

While the radiologist working in oncological practice does not need to have a full knowledge of the different subtypes of leukaemia, the above classification is useful for reference and indeed some subtypes manifest different radiological appearances.

There is some overlap between the leukaemias and the lymphomas but in general the acute lymphoblastic leukaemias (ALL) are distinguished from lymphomas on the basis of cellular maturity and by the fact that lymphomas mainly involve extramedullary sites, at least initially. The lymphoblastic lymphomas and Burkitt's lymphoma have features of both leukaemia and lymphoma. Adult T-cell leukaemia/lymphoma (ATLL) is a distinct variety of leukaemia/lymphoma which is characterized by lymphadenopathy and hepatosplenomegaly and is endemic in certain parts of the world including Japan and the Caribbean basin.

Table 30.1. *Classification of leukaemia*

Acute
Acute myelogenous leukaemia (AML)
Acute myeloblastic leukaemia
Acute promyelocytic leukaemia
Acute myelomonocytic leukaemia
Acute monoblastic leukaemia
Acute erythroleukaemia
Acute megakaryoblastic leukaemia
Acute lymphoblastic leukaemia (ALL)
Pre-B cell acute lymphoblastic leukaemia
Common acute lymphoblastic leukaemia
Cytoplasmic immunoglobulin (+) ALL
Philadelphia chromosome (+) ALL
T cell
B cell
Acute unclassifiable leukaemia (AUL)
Chronic
Chronic myelocytic leukaemia (CML)
Chronic phase of CML
Metamorphosis of CML
Accelerated ± myelofibrosis
Lymphoblastic transformation
Myeloblastic transformation
Megakaryoblastic transformation
Juvenile chronic granulocytic leukaemia
Chronic eosinophilic leukaemia
Chronic lymphocytic leukaemia (CLL)
B cell
T cell
Hairy cell leukaemia
Polymorphocytic leukaemia
Plasma cell leukaemia
Sézary syndrome*
Adult T-cell leukaemia/lymphoma

*Leukaemic phase of mycosis fungoides.

Myelodysplasia is a syndrome characterized by pancyto-penia or chronic anaemia which results from dysfunction of the bone marrow. Transformation into acute leukaemia may develop during the course of disease.

INCIDENCE AND AETIOLOGY

The acute leukaemias account for less than 3% of all cancers in the USA but are a leading cause of cancer death in patients under the age of 35 years. In total it is estimated that there will be a total of 28,300 new cases of leukaemia diagnosed in the USA in 1997 of which about half will be acute leukaemias and half will be chronic subtypes. The total number of deaths are estimated at over 21,000.[3] Acute myelogenous leukaemia is more common than acute lymphoblastic leukaemia in adults, but acute lymphoblastic leukaemia is the most common subtype seen in childhood. In adults the most common subtypes of leukaemia are:

- Acute myelogenous leukaemia with an estimated 9,200 new cases in 1997
- Chronic lymphocytic leukaemia with an estimated 7,400 new cases in 1997

Over recent years enormous strides have been made in understanding the molecular biology and cytogenetics of leukaemia. Various chromosomal abnormalities have been identified which have helped to define subsets of AML and ALL which are listed in the classification (e.g. Philadelphia chromosome positive). These subsets of leukaemia have various clinical features and different patterns of response to therapy. Such information is used to direct patients to particular therapeutic regimes and in the longer term may allow appropriate targeting of new therapies.

While the importance of genetic changes in the development of the leukaemias is well-recognized, the underlying causes initiating these changes are largely unknown. Down's syndrome and certain other genetic syndromes are linked with leukaemia and excessive exposure to ionizing radiation is now established as an important cause,[4] as are chronic exposure to low-dose radiation in the environment, chemicals and smoking.[5]

Secondary AML may develop after treatment of childhood acute leukaemia and following therapy for other cancers such as tumours of the breast and ovary, and Hodgkin's disease.[6–9]

A human retrovirus (HTLV-1) has been identified as a cause of human T-cell leukaemia/lymphoma (ATLL).[10,11] The cumulative risk of an infected individual developing ATLL is estimated to be between 0.5 and 5%.[12,13]

Key points: general features

- The leukaemias are derived from the arrested, or aberrant, development of a clone of normal haemopoietic cells

- Various subtypes are recognized which have different clinical features, radiological features, prognosis and therapeutic implications

- ALL is the most common subtype in childhood

- AML and CLL are the most common subtypes in adults

- Various chromosomal abnormalities have been identified in the leukaemias

- Down's syndrome is strongly linked with acute leukaemia

- Ionizing radiation, chemicals and smoking have a causal relationship with leukaemia

- The human retrovirus (HTLV-1) infection is a known cause of human T-cell leukaemia/lymphoma

CLINICAL FEATURES

The replacement of normal haemopoietic cells within the bone marrow by an excessive number of abnormal functionless cells is responsible for the major clinical features of the leukaemias:

- Anaemia
- Infection
- Haemorrhage

In acute leukaemia patients usually present with a 1–3-month history of weight loss, fatigue, bruising or signs of infection such as fever. In the chronic leukaemias the onset of disease is more insidious but fever may be observed without an obvious infective cause. Occasionally, the diagnosis of chronic leukaemia is made on routine examination of the peripheral blood in an otherwise asymptomatic patient.

In all patients the diagnosis is confirmed by examination of the peripheral blood and bone marrow biopsy. Immunophenotyping and cytogenetic studies are performed to discriminate between the different subsets of the disease. In the majority of patients anaemia and thrombocytopenia are present. The peripheral white cell blood count may be normal, raised or reduced but blast cells are seen in the peripheral blood in practically all patients.

There are certain clinical features of leukaemia which are more prevalent in one subtype than another and the frequency of involvement of different organs and sites also varies (Table 30.2).[14]

Table 30.2. *Organ involvement by leukaemia cell type (1958–1982). Adapted from ref. 14*

Organ/Sites	AML (%)	CML (%)	ALL (%)	CLL§ (%)
CNS (sanctuary sites)				
Brain	9	11	14	7
Dura mater	14	14	26	21
Leptomeninges	12	10	34	8
Lymphoreticular sites				
Liver	41	55	63	83
Lymph nodes	45	59	55	76
Spleen	58	68	70	76
Cardiopulmonary				
Pericardium	8	6	11	14
Heart	15	11	21	22
Pleura	8	5	11	16
Lungs	28	29	41	41
Gastro-intestinal				
Oesophagus	17	9	16	19
Stomach	11	11	17	11
Large bowel	15	9	20	15
Pancreas	8	6	18	12
Endocrine				
Pituitary	9	10	15	20
Thyroid	6	3	5	7
Adrenals	15	22	21	33
Genito-urinary				
Kidneys	33	38	53	63
Bladder	7	6	9	8
Prostate	9	5	12	22
Uterus	11	4	25	14
Gonads (sanctuary sites)				
Testes	20	16	40	15
Ovaries	11	9	21	22
Total number of cases	585	204	308	109

§ = Percentage of all cases examined

In the acute leukaemias, central nervous system (CNS) involvement is more common in ALL than AML but is also seen in the chronic leukaemias. The CNS is resistant to chemotherapy and is therefore termed a sanctuary site of disease.

Hepatosplenomegaly due to leukaemia infiltration is seen in practically all cases of leukaemia but in the chronic forms of the disease the degree of enlargement is greater than in the acute leukaemias (Fig. 30.1).

Lymphadenopathy is most frequently seen in CLL and in juvenile CML (Fig. 30.2). It is rare in adult Philadelphia chromosome-positive CML. The incidence of enlarged lymph nodes at presentation in the acute leukaemias is as follows:

- Acute lymphoblastic leukaemia (50%) (usually T-cell or B-cell)
- Acute monoblastic leukaemia (15–20%)
- Other subtypes of acute myelogenous leukaemia (8%)[15]

Fever is a common feature of all the leukaemias whether due to infection or not. In those without documented infection, fever may arise as a result of increased metabolism due to the leukaemic process.

Anaemia is present in the majority of patients and is caused by inadequate erythrocyte production, bleeding, hypersplenism or haemolysis.

Bleeding is more common in the acute leukaemias than in the chronic subtypes and usually takes the form of small petechial haemorrhages. Occasionally, a patient may present with a catastrophic intracranial haemorrhage.

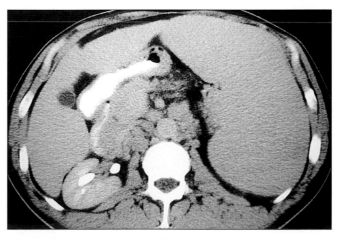

Figure 30.1. *A postcontrast CT scan in a 62-year-old male patient with CLL showing a huge spleen and multiple enlarged retroperitoneal lymph nodes.*

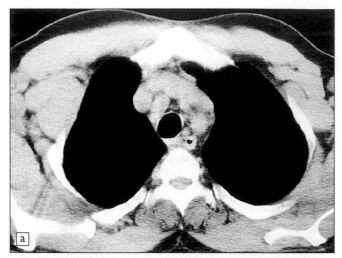

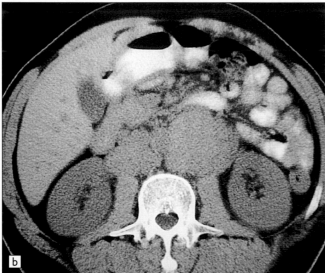

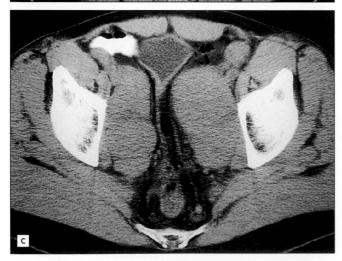

Figure 30.2. *A male patient with CLL showing multiple enlarged lymph nodes on CT: (a) in the mediastinum and axillae; (b) in the retroperitoneum; (c) in the pelvis.*

In the acute leukaemias, haemorrhage is a major cause of death and morbidity. Haemorrhage results from coagulation defects associated with the disease, thrombocytopenia and the effects of chemotherapy. The acute promyelocytic form of leukaemia is particularly prone to haemorrhage and in one study intracranial haemorrhage was the cause of death in 60% of patients.[16] Another group of patients at particularly high risk of intracranial haemorrhage are those with acute leukaemia in 'blast' crisis. In such patients the excessive numbers of leucocytes form tiny foci which plug small arterioles and destroy the vascular walls leading to haemorrhage.[17]

Patients with intracranial haemorrhage present acutely with headaches, seizures and deterioration of neurological function. Rarely, intracranial haemorrhage may herald the diagnosis of acute leukaemia.

Bone pain is a common presenting feature in children with ALL occurring in 25–30% of cases, whereas in adults it is only seen in approximately 5% of patients.[18,19] Bone pain is characteristically migratory and periarticular.[20] It is probably due to lifting of the periosteum by infiltration of leukaemic cells or from the development of bone infarction.[21] Monoarthralgia or polyarthralgia is not an uncommon presenting feature.

Abdominal pain and chest pain are also relatively common and are related to a variety of problems. For example, abdominal pain may result from stretching of the splenic capsule due to rapid enlargement or from intestinal obstruction due to leukaemic infiltration of the bowel wall. Chest pain may be caused by a large mediastinal mass compressing adjacent structures.

Granulocytic sarcoma (chloroma) is a mass composed of leukaemic cells. These tumours are usually seen in patients with AML but may also occur in CML and other myeloprolific disorders such as polycythaemia rubra vera.[22] They consist of myeloblasts, promyelocytes and myelocytes and are most frequently found in the orbits, subcutaneous tissues, paranasal sinuses, lymph nodes and bones but many other sites have also been described.[23] In a series of 728 patients with childhood myelogenous leukaemia, Pui et al. found an incidence of 4.7% of granulocytic sarcoma developing at some point during the course of disease. Others have reported an incidence ranging from 2.5 to 8%.[24,25] Rarely these tumours may be the presenting feature of leukaemia occurring before the onset of clinically overt disease.[26] They were first described by Burns in 1811[27] but it was not until 1853 that the term chloroma was coined by King to describe their typical greenish colour.[28] However, in 1966 the term chloroma was replaced by granulocytic sarcoma because less than half of them actually display the characteristic greenish colour.

Key points: clinical features

- The major clinical features of leukaemia are anaemia, infection and haemorrhage

- CNS involvement is more common in ALL than AML

- Lymphadenopathy is most frequently seen in CLL

- Bone pain is a common presenting feature in childhood leukaemia, occurring in about 25% of cases. Bone pain occurs in only 5% of adults

- Granulocytic sarcoma is a mass composed of leukaemic cells which occurs most frequently in AML. The incidence ranges from 2.5 to 8%

- The most common sites of granulocytic sarcoma are the orbits, subcutaneous tissues, paranasal sinuses and bones

TREATMENT

Treatment of acute leukaemia aims to induce a remission as quickly as possible and then to maintain remission. The success of therapy depends as much on the treatment of non-leukaemic related problems as on the eradication of leukaemia itself.

In the acute leukaemias certain features are important prognostic factors and determine the detailed approach to management. These include patient age (older patients are less likely to achieve complete remission) or previous myelodysplasia. Certain cytogenetic subtypes have a poorer prognosis (B-cell and unclassified leukaemias are rarely controlled in the long term).

Acute lymphoblastic leukaemia (common ALL) is the most sucessfully treated of all the leukaemias.[29,30,31] Complete remission is achieved in over 90% of children and in up to 80% of adults.[28] Patients with acute lymphoblastic leukaemia, other than common ALL, are not so successfully treated and relapse is common. Treatment of common ALL includes induction chemotherapy which is followed by consolidation therapy and maintenance therapy for a period of up to 2 years. Prophylactic intrathecal chemotherapy with or without cranial irradiation is used for CNS prophylaxis.[30]

The treatment of AML depends on the age of the patient at presentation. Elderly patients have a worse prognosis which is related to the high incidence of death from infection or other problems related to the disease. In young adults cure can be achieved in 20–25% of patients with induction chemotherapy using a combination of drugs[32,33] followed by intensive post-remission therapy. This is either in the form of high-dose chemotherapy supported by bone marrow transplantation or intensive short-term consolidation therapy to prevent relapse.[34–36]

The chronic leukaemias are traditionally treated with chemotherapy but recently Interferon (IFN-α) has been found to have a survival advantage in patients with chronic myeloid leukaemia.[37] Bone marrow transplantation (BMT) may be curative if preceded by destruction of all leukaemic cells. This may be achieved with total body irradiation and chemotherapy but a major problem with allogeneic BMT is graft rejection.[38]

A major cause of death in CML is transformation to an acute 'blastic' phase of the disease. In such patients BMT also offers the best chance of therapeutic response. Bone marrow transplantation may also be used elec-tively in the pretransformation (chronic) phase of the disease.

The survival of leukaemia varies according to the category of leukaemia as well as its subtype. In ALL the relative 5-year survival rates are between 50 and 80% for children and 20 and 40% for adults.[29] In AML patients under 60 years of age have a better outlook than older patients but the 5-year actuarial survival for all age groups is between 40 and 50%.[39]

In the chronic leukaemias cure is usually impossible but prolonged survival can be achieved in certain subtypes using conventional chemotherapy, BMT and new therapies such as IFN-α.[40]

Key points: treatment

- The success of therapy in leukaemia depends as much on the treatment of non-leukaemic related problems as on the eradication of leukaemia itself

- Acute lymphoblastic leukaemia (common ALL) is the most successfully treated of all the leukaemias. Complete remission is achieved in over 90% of children and in up to 80% of adults

- The 5-year survival of common ALL is 50–80% for children and 20–40% for adults

- In AML the 5-year survival for all age groups is 40–50%

- The acute leukaemias are treated with induction chemotherapy followed by consolidation therapy. Prophylactic CNS treatment is required in ALL

- The chronic leukaemias are traditionally treated with chemotherapy but recently Interferon-α has shown encouraging results

- Allogeneic bone marrow transplantation has an important role in the treatment of leukaemias. Graft rejection is a major complication

IMAGING IN LEUKAEMIA

Leukaemia is diagnosed and monitored by haematological studies of the peripheral blood and bone marrow and imaging therefore plays a lesser role in the diagnosis and staging of this disease than in the lymphomas. However, the importance of radiology in the management of leukaemia has increased over the last two decades, mainly due to the advent of cross-sectional imaging and to improvements in therapy. Imaging is used to evaluate the leukaemic process itself or to investigate its complications. Thus the imaging findings in leukaemia can be broadly categorized into two groups, those related to:

- Direct involvement of organs and tissues by leukaemic cells
- Indirect involvement of organs and tissues due to complications

In this text direct and indirect imaging findings will be discussed in relation to different anatomical sites and organ systems.

Central nervous system
Direct involvement by leukaemia

Central nervous system involvement is usually seen in acute leukaemia. It may be a manifestation of disease at diagnosis or may herald relapse in patients believed to be in remission. At diagnosis approximately 3% of children with ALL have CNS disease[41] but the number of patients who relapse with CNS involvement has been dramatically reduced by the introduction of CNS prophylactic therapy.[42]

Leukaemic spread to the CNS is presumed to be by direct infiltration from involved bone marrow of the cranium (or vertebrae) or by the haematogenous route whereby circulating leukaemia cells enter the CNS by migration through spaces in the venous endothelium.[43,44]

The leukaemic process may involve the leptomeninges, dura or both and may be diffuse or focal. Meningeal involvement occurs in up to 10% of patients with acute leukaemia and begins in the superficial arachnoid membrane, leukaemic cells then invade the cerebrospinal fluid (CSF) space and pia mater.[45,46] Extradural (parameningeal) masses (granulocytic sarcoma) may also be observed in intracranial or intraspinal sites. Involvement of the brain parenchyma is rare but when it does occur, probably results from perivascular extension of disease across the Virchow–Robin spaces through the pia-glial membrane.[47] Intracerebral granulocytic sarcomas are a rare occurrence in the myelogenous leukaemias.

Meningeal and dural disease

Symptoms of meningeal involvement of the brain include headache, nausea, vomiting and lethargy. Signs of intracranial pressure and cranial nerve palsies may be apparent on clinical examination.[42] The diagnosis of meningeal involvement is made on the finding of leukaemic cells within CSF. However, analysis of the CSF is often negative and several repeat lumbar punctures may be required to establish the diagnosis of meningeal disease. Imaging is complementary to lumbar puncture but the detection of diffuse meningeal involvement with computed tomography (CT) has been disappointing due to insufficient contrast enhancement of the abnormal meninges.[48] Computed tomography is more accurate in carcinomatous meningitis and inflammatory conditions because the contrast enhancement is usually more intense.[47]

Magnetic resonance imaging (MRI) is the method of choice for the detection of intracranial and spinal leptomeningeal disease and on occasion may demonstrate leukaemic infiltration in the presence of multiple negative cytological analyses.[42] The technique is considerably more sensitive than CT, myelography or CT myelography, and MRI has now replaced these techniques in the investigation of CNS leukaemia.[49,50] Although T2-weighted spin-echo sequences may reveal abnormal signal within the CSF space, meningeal disease is best demonstrated on gadolinium-enhanced T1-weighted images. Axial and coronal images of the head and sagittal images of the spine provide the best imaging planes to survey all the meningeal surfaces. Leukaemic infiltration is seen as abnormal nodular thickening of the meninges which enhances after injection of intravenous contrast medium (Fig. 30.3). Thickening and enhancement of nerve roots, particulary in the region of the cauda equina, is shown on MRI but may also be demonstrated on CT myelography. Diffuse dural infiltration is less common than leptomeningeal disease but is also seen as thickening and enhancement of the dural surfaces.

In patients with leukaemia, the observation of thickened enhancing meninges is not pathognomonic of leukaemic infiltration as it may also be seen in other conditions associated with leukaemia such as infectious meningitis, drug reactions and meningeal fibrosis following haemorrhage.[42]

Parameningeal disease

Intracranial and spinal parameningeal disease usually take the form of a mass of leukaemic cells known as granulocytic sarcoma (chloroma).

The majority of intracranial granulocytic sarcomas are dural-based lesions and are believed to develop by direct spread from the bone marrow. The CT and MRI appearances of granulocytic sarcomas are variable and they may mimic meningiomas, other tumours or abscesses.[51,52] On unenhanced CT, intracranial granulocytic sarcomas are isodense or slightly hyperdense compared with normal brain but frequently show intense enhancement following injection of intravenous contrast medium[53] (Fig. 30.4). On MRI these lesions may be of high signal intensity on T1-weighted images, they are bright on T2-weighting and, as with CT, show intense contrast enhancement.[51]

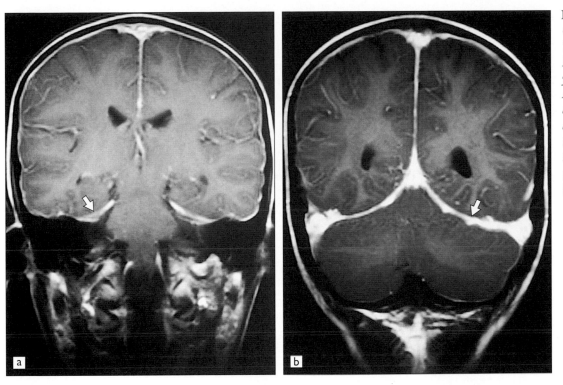

Figure 30.3. *(a, b) Contrast-enhanced T1-weighted coronal MR images in a 9-year-old boy with AML. There is extensive contrast-enhanced nodular thickening of the leptomeninges (arrows), representing leukaemic infiltration.*

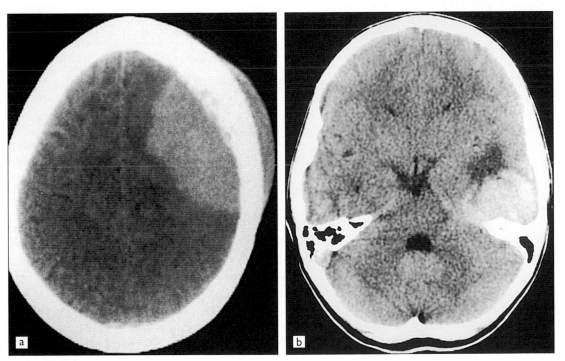

Figure 30.4. *Intracranial granulocytic sarcoma. (a) CT scan of the brain in a 14-year-old boy with relapsed ALL. The mass which probably arises from the left parietal bone extends both intracranially and into the subcutaneous soft tissues. There is homogeneous intense contrast enhancement (from ref. 54, with permission); (b) CT scan of an 8-year-old girl who relapsed following initial therapy for ALL with a large durally-based lesion in the temporal lobe. Note homogeneous enhancement and surrounding oedema.*

Spinal granulocytic sarcomas may be paraspinal or intraspinal (Fig. 30.5). Soft tissue masses in the paravertebral region extend into the spinal canal via the intervertebral foraminae[54] (Fig. 30.6). These masses invade the dura and may cause spinal cord compression, nerve root compression and bone destruction.

Although CT may show paravertebral masses and extension into the spinal canal or discrete intraspinal masses (Fig. 30.6a), MRI is now the preferred imaging technique for demonstrating these lesions because the whole spine can be examined at a single investigation (Fig. 30.6b). The multiplanar capability of MRI is also an advantage as it allows clear delineation of tumour extent. Granulocytic sarcomas have a low signal intensity on T1-weighted images and a relatively high or intermediate signal intensity on T2-weighted images.[54] They often show intense contrast enhancement.

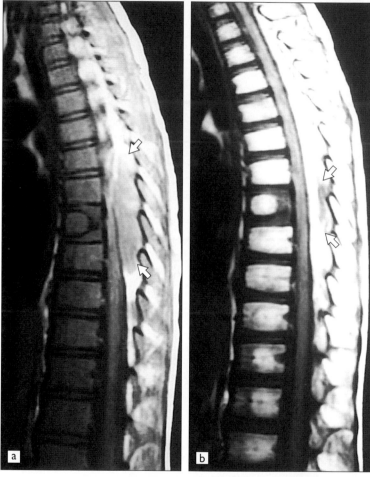

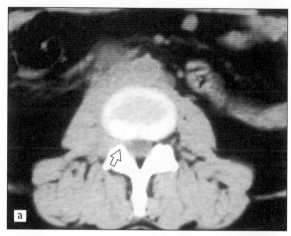

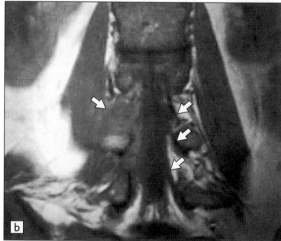

Figure 30.5. *A 9-year-old boy who presented with acute back pain and signs of spinal cord compression. (a) T1-weighted sagittal MR image showing an intraspinal extradural soft tissue mass in the midthoracic region (arrows). Note partial collapse of the vertebral body of T5. A diagnosis of AML with a granulocytic sarcoma was made on investigation. There is diffuse abnormally low signal intensity throughout the vertebral bodies indicating diffuse leukaemic infiltration; (b) repeat MR examination 6 weeks later shows an excellent response to treatment. The granulocytic sarcomatous mass has almost completely resolved (arrows) and the signal intensity of the bone marrow has increased markedly indicating reduction in bone marrow infiltration. The vertebral body of T5 still shows abnormal signal intensity posteriorly.*

Figure 30.6. *An adult male patient who presented with back pain due to a granulocytic sarcoma before clinical manifestation of AML. (a) CT scan; (b) T1-weighted coronal MR image. In (a) soft tissue mass is seen surrounding the inferior vena cava and obscuring the contour of the aorta. The mass extends posteriorly deep to the right psoas muscle and enters the spinal canal through the intervertebral foramen (arrowed); in (b) the coronal MR image shows the craniocaudal extent of the mass and clearly delineates the intraspinal component at the level of L3/L4 and L4/L5 intervertebral foraminae. Tumour surrounds the exit nerve roots. Note normal nerve roots on the left side (arrowed).*

Key points: central nervous system

- CNS involvement is usually a manifestation of acute leukaemia

- Approximately 3% of all children with ALL have CNS disease

- The leukaemic process may involve the leptomeninges, dura or extradural space

- Disease may be diffuse or focal

- Granulocytic sarcomas are usually dural based lesions

- MRI is the best imaging method for detecting intracranial meningeal and dural infiltration as well as granulocytic sarcoma

Indirect effects of leukaemia

The indirect effects of leukaemia on the CNS include vascular events, infection and toxic effects related to therapy.

Vascular complications

Haemorrhage Computed tomography or MRI is essential in patients suspected of intracranial haemorrhage. In most cases CT will be undertaken, as this is more readily available and generally quicker than MRI examinations. Unenhanced CT will show the classic features of subarachnoid and/or intracerebral haemorrhage which includes the presence of high-density material in the subarachnoid space, in the brain parenchyma and ventricular system. There may be mass effect with some surrounding oedema. On MRI, fresh blood has a high signal intensity on T1 weighting and on T2 weighting the appearances are also those of high signal intensity. Breakdown products of haemoglobin (haemosiderin) may also be present giving a low signal intensity on T2-weighting.

Computed tomography and MRI are not only valuable for demonstrating the presence of intracranial haemorrhage but also for excluding haemorrhage in patients where the diagnosis is questionable on clinical grounds. Furthermore imaging may show other associated abnormalities such as sinovenous thrombosis (*vide infra*).

Sinovenous thrombosis Sinovenous thrombosis, another vascular complication of acute leukaemia, may be related to treatment with L-asparaginase as well as to leukaemic infiltration.[48,55] Both CT and MRI are useful non-invasive methods of detecting sinovenous thrombosis. On CT, post-contrast-enhanced images may show a low density filling defect within the sinus and on precontrast images the sinus may be abnormally hyperdense. On MRI, loss of the normal signal void is apparent on T2-weighted sequences and on postcontrast images a filling defect may be observed, as on CT. Gradient-echo or other flow sensitive techniques may also demonstrate sinovenous thrombosis on MRI.[48] Leukaemic infiltration of meninges and sinus thrombosis may coexist.

Patients present with headache and signs of intracranial pressure and therefore may mimic direct involvement of the CNS by the leukaemic process.

Cerebral infarction Patients with leukaemia are at an increased risk of cerebral infarction for several reasons which include:[48]

- General risks — patient age, atherosclerosis
- Intravascular coagulation
- Sinovenous occlusion
- Tumour emboli
- Septic emboli
- Effects of therapy[16]

As in the diagnosis of intracranial haemorrhage, CT is valuable for demonstrating the presence of cerebral infarction and for distinguishing infarcts from other intracranial lesions such as haemorrhage, infection and drug related toxicity.

Infection

In leukaemic patients intracranial infection results from direct spread of infection from the paranasal sinuses or by the haematogenous route. Sinusitis is usually aggressive in immunocompromised patients and infection with organisms such as Aspergillus results in invasion of local structures and destruction of bone (Fig. 30.7), thereby giving access to the dura, meninges and underlying brain parenchyma. Other organisms including bacteria (e.g. Klebsiella pneumonii) and viruses are also associated with intracranial infection in leukaemia.[56] Abscesses may develop and whether solitary or multiple, may simulate parenchymal leukaemic deposits.[56] On CT, abscesses usually show rim enhancement with a relatively low density centre; on MRI these masses have a high signal intensity on T2 weighting and a relatively low signal intensity on T1 weighting. As on CT, rim enhancement is noted following injection of intravenous contrast medium.

Treatment-related complications

There are many neurological complications associated with the treatment of leukaemia but such complications are especially related to the treatment or prophylaxis of the CNS. Different syndromes and clinical features are associated with particular drugs or radiotherapy. In general, CNS toxicity can be divided into acute, subacute and chronic forms.

In general, the acute or subacute neurological complications are more likely to be reversible than the complications

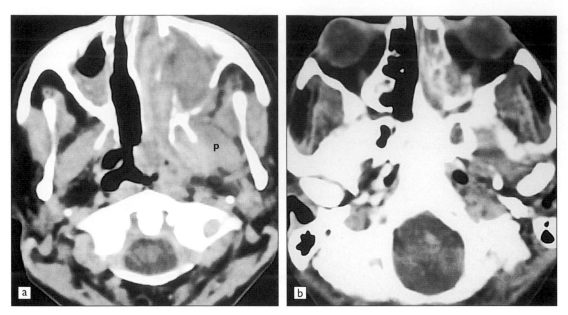

Figure 30.7. *CT scan in a 53-year-old male patient with relapsed AML showing extensive paranasal sinus infection with Aspergillus. (a) The soft tissue mass occupies the left maxillary sinus. There is almost complete destruction of the medial wall of the maxillary sinus with extension of the soft tissue mass into the nasal cavity and nasopharynx. There is also destruction of the lateral wall of the maxillary sinus with extension of disease into the pterygoid region. Note enlargement and poor definition of the lateral pterygoid muscle (p); (b) the soft tissue mass is also seen extending into the posterior aspect of the left orbit. The left ethmoid sinuses are replaced by soft tissue and there is destruction of the medial wall of the orbit.*

which develop in the longer term. Patients present with symptoms and signs of raised intracranial pressure, and on examination neurological deficit is common.[57] On clinical evaluation it may be impossible to distinguish CNS leukaemic relapse from the effects of therapy and in this situation imaging plays a key role. Delayed or chronic toxic effects are more likely to be irreversible and may develop several years after initial treatment.

Radiotherapy neurotoxicity is usually subacute, developing several weeks after treatment. It is characterized by drowsiness, nausea and malaise as well as somnolence.[42] Imaging is not usually required to reach a definitive diagnosis.

The delayed effects of radiotherapy include cerebral atrophy and even necrosis. This results in growth disturbance, intellectual impairment and neuro-endocrine problems. Magnetic resonance imaging shows abnormally high signal intensity in the white matter following cranial irradiation and may demonstrate abnormalities even in patients without clinical evidence of toxicity. Computed tomography may reveal areas of low attenuation within the white matter and calcifications. Long-term survivors of childhood ALL treated with cranial irradiation and intrathecal methotrexate frequently show abnormalities on MRI; this is more common in patients treated withboth modalities than with intrathecal methotrexate alone.[58,59]

Intrathecal methotrexate may cause acute arachnoiditis and imaging is not required in the diagnostic work-up. Subacute neurotoxicity and delayed reactions are characterized by seizures and other manifestations of motor dysfunction such as paraplegia. Imaging may be required to exclude direct involvement of the CNS by leukaemia, for example the presence of a granulocytic sarcoma. Delayed effects of methotrexate include white matter ischaemia and imaging shows intracerebral calcifications and cerebral atrophy. Both CT and MRI are useful for demonstrating the extent of these abnormalities.

Disseminated necrotizing leuco-encephalopathy is more likely to develop when CNS irradiation is combined with intrathecal methotrexate and high-dose methotrexate (Fig. 30.8).[42,57,60] This condition may be fulminating and rapidly fatal or less severe leading to chronic neurological deficit. Leuco-encephalopathy affects the white matter of the brain and is seen on CT as multifocal areas of low attenuation and on MRI as areas of high signal intensity on spin-echo T2-weighted images. Enhancement of these lesions can sometimes be seen on MRI.[61–63] Calcification may also be observed in the basal ganglia and in the subcortical white matter.

Other drugs such as cytarabine and cyclosporin A are also associated with severe neurotoxicity.[42]

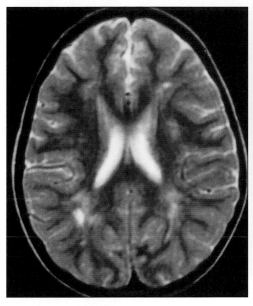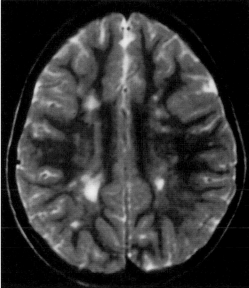

Figure 30.8. *Necrotizing leuco-encephalopathy. T2-weighted axial MR images of the brain showing abnormal high signal intensity in the white matter following cranial irradiation and methotrexate therapy.*

Key points: CNS complications

■ Haemorrhage is a major cause of death in acute leukaemia, particularly in acute promyelocytic leukaemia and patients in 'blast' crisis

■ Sinovenous thrombosis may be demonstrated by MRI and CT but may co-exist with leukaemic meningeal infiltration

■ Cerebral infarction has an increased incidence in patients with leukaemia

■ Intracranial infection usually results from spread of infection from paranasal sinuses directly by organisms such as Aspergillus

■ CNS toxicity is related to irradiation, intrathecal methotrexate and high-dose methotrexate

■ Disseminating necrotizing leuco-encephalopathy affects the white matter of the brain and is demonstrated on MRI as areas of high signal intensity with foci on T2-weighted images. Enhancement of the lesions may be seen

Head and neck
Direct involvement by leukaemia
The most important extracranial site of leukaemia of the head and neck region is the orbit. Leukaemic deposits may infiltrate around the optic nerve, often in association with meningeal disease and the choroid and retina may also be involved by diffuse infiltration. The orbit is a well-recognized

site of granulocytic sarcoma (chloroma).[52] On both CT and MRI, intra-orbital granulocytic sarcomas enhance with intravenous contrast medium and are usually seen as soft tissue masses related to the intra-ocular muscles.[23] Granulocytic sarcoma in the paranasal sinuses may spread by direct extension into the orbit.

Key point: granulocytic sarcoma

■ The orbit is a common site of granulocytic sarcoma

Indirect effects of leukaemia
Major indirect effects of leukaemia in the head and neck are haemorrhage and infection. Infection of the paranasal sinuses may be extremely aggressive, resulting in intracranial disease as described above. Imaging with CT or MRI may be required to define the extent of infection extracranially as well as the presence of meningeal or brain involvement.

Intrathoracic disease
Direct involvement by leukaemia
Mediastinal lymphadenopathy is a common feature of ALL as well as CLL (Fig. 30.9). A large anterior mediastinal mass on plain chest films is a characteristic feature of childhood T-cell leukaemia and indeed over 50% of patients with adult T-cell leukaemia have mediastinal disease.[15,64] These large masses may cause superior vena caval obstruction or tracheal compression. Hilar lymphadenopathy may also be seen.

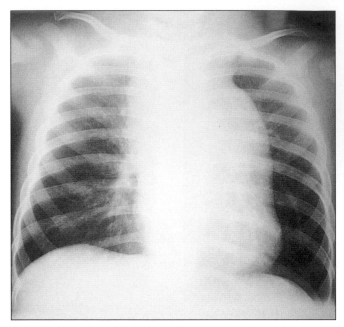

Figure 30.9. *Chest radiograph in a 4-year-old boy with ALL showing a large mediastinal mass at presentation.*

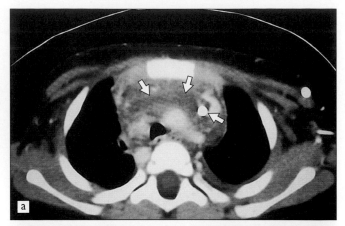

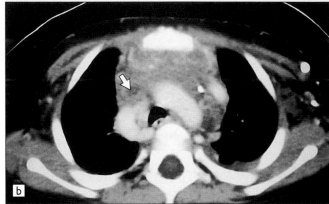

Figure 30.10. *(a, b) Contrast-enhanced CT scans in a 3-year-old child with massive mediastinal widening due to extrusion of the central line from the left innominate vein into the mediastinal soft tissues. Note thrombus in the left innominate vein shown as tubular low attenuation (arrowed). Thrombus is also present in the superior vena cava (arrowed). The mediastinum is widened and contains generalized increased soft tissue density due to mediastinitis. Note the central line.*

Pulmonary leukaemic infiltration is only rarely diagnosed on plain chest radiographs but is found more commonly at autopsy.[65] On a plain chest film, leukaemic infiltration appears as diffuse peribronchial infiltration accompanied by septal lines. The findings are usually indistinguishable from infection or pulmonary oedema and therefore the diagnosis is rarely made radiologically. In a series of 109 patients reported by Green and Nichols, 30 had autopsy evidence of pulmonary infiltration but only two of these patients showed evidence of infiltration on chest radiographs.[66]

Indirect effects of leukaemia

Mediastinal widening may be due to haemorrhage within the mediastinum, thrombus within the superior vena cava (usually as a result of central line insertion) or to mediastinitis (this may be associated with central line insertion due to an extraluminal placement of a catheter tip or infection). The cause can be detected on contrast-enhanced CT and is readily distinguished from lymphadenopathy (Fig. 30.10).

Pulmonary infection is a major cause of abnormal shadowing detected on plain chest radiographs in leukaemic patients. These infections result from immunosuppression and may be bacterial, viral or fungal. The most common organisms which have a predilection for immunosuppressed hosts include cytomegalovirus (CMV), Pneumocystis carinii and fungal infection by organisms such as Aspergillus and Cryptococcus.[67–69] On occasion, CT may be useful in the differential diagnosis of pulmonary infiltration, for example CT may demonstrate the rounded lesions of Aspergillus fumigatus not visualized on plain chest films. Oropharyngeal and oesophageal infection with Candida albicans is common and results from antibiotic therapy as well as the impaired immune response.[67] These complications of treatment are discussed further in Chapter 46.

Pulmonary haemorrhage should be considered in the differential diagnosis of abnormal air space pulmonary shadowing on plain chest films, particularly if accompanied by haemoptysis. Pulmonary oedema may mimic infection and indeed may coexist with an inflammatory process.

Treatment-related pulmonary damage is important in the differential diagnosis of abnormal pulmonary shadowing and chest symptoms in the leukaemic patient.

Drugs cause pulmonary oedema and vasculitis. In the early stages of lung toxicity, plain chest radiographs are usually normal. Alveolar damage is usually a generalized process at the lung bases and in moderate to severe cases is seen as bilateral abnormal non-specific shadowing both on plain films and on CT. Such injury may be caused by busulphan, carmustine (BCNU) and methotrexate. Pulmonary vasculitis leads to infarction and in some cases cavitation may result. Pulmonary vascular damage may occur with busulphan therapy.[70]

Chronic graft versus host disease is characterized by lymphocytic infiltration of the interstitial tissues and bronchial walls. Bronchiolitis obliterans is also seen.[71] Plain chest radiographs may be normal but on CT abnormal shadowing around peripheral bronchi may be observed.[72]

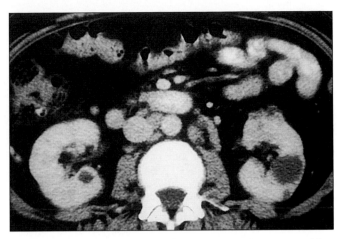

Figure 30.11. *CT scan in a 47-year-old female patient with CLL showing bilateral renal masses. The anterior aspect of the left kidney shows an area of diminished attenuation with an irregular poorly defined outer edge. This probably represents leukaemic infiltration. Note enlarged retroperitoneal lymph nodes.*

Key points: thoracic manifestations

- Mediastinal lymphadenopathy is a common feature of ALL and CLL

- Mediastinal lymphadenopathy is also seen in T-cell childhood leukaemia and in adult T-cell leukaemia/lymphoma

- Leukaemic infiltration of the lungs is rarely diagnosed during life. The appearances are often indistinguishable from infection or pulmonary oedema

- Mediastinal widening may be due to mediastinitis, haemorrhage or superior vena caval thrombosis as well as lymphadenopathy

- Pulmonary infection is a major cause of morbidity in leukaemic patients. Organisms include CMV, Pneumocystis carinii and fungal infections such as invasive pulmonary aspergillosis

Abdomen and pelvis
Direct involvement
Hepatosplenomegaly due to diffuse involvement of the liver and spleen is a frequent manifestation of leukaemia (Fig. 30.1). Imaging is not usually undertaken to evaluate these organs but both CT and ultrasound will demonstrate hepatosplenomegaly. Focal lesions within the liver and spleen due to leukaemia are rarely seen. Splenic infarction may be associated with gross splenomegaly and on CT these lesions appear as an irregular relatively low-density area within a massively enlarged spleen and as hypoechoic lesions on ultrasound.

Renal involvement in leukaemia is common, occurring in approximately 50% of cases at autopsy.[15] As in patients with lymphoma, leukaemia may involve the kidneys by:

- Diffuse parenchymal infiltration (bilateral or unilateral)
- Discrete renal mass or masses
- Obstruction due to lymphadenopathy at the hilum

Ultrasound is a useful technique for detecting leukaemic infiltration. The kidneys are diffusely enlarged and show patchy areas of low echogenicity. On contrast-enhanced CT the parenchyma shows an inhomogeneous pattern with areas of diminished density interspersed with areas of enhancement, findings which are similar to those seen in lymphoma.[73] Solid renal masses may also be observed on CT (Fig. 30.11).

The gastro-intestinal tract is involved in leukaemia in about 25% of cases.[74] Leukaemic infiltrates spread through the lamina propria or submucosa of the bowel wall producing localized areas of bowel wall thickening. Imaging is seldom required as it is unusual for such lesions to become clinically manifest. Occasionally, a granulocytic sarcoma may develop within the bowel wall and may present as abdominal pain or intestinal obstruction.

As in other anatomical sites, abdominal lymph node involvement is more commonly seen in the acute lymphoblastic and chronic lymphocytic leukaemias than in the myelogenous leukaemias. Multiple enlarged nodes may be seen within the retroperitoneum, mesentery, splenic hilum, porta hepatis and other intra-abdominal and pelvic sites (Figs. 30.2 and 30.11). Nodes are usually discretely enlarged and on imaging the appearances are indistinguishable from those of non-Hodgkin's lymphoma.

Other sites of involvement in the abdomen and pelvis include the prostate gland, uterus and adrenal glands. The testis and ovary are sanctuary sites and are therefore relatively resistant to chemotherapy[14] (See Table 30.2).

Key points: abdominal/pelvic manifestations

- Hepatosplenomegaly is a common feature of all the leukaemias

- Splenic infarcts may be demonstrated on imaging

- Renal involvement is seen in 50% of cases at autopsy

- Renal involvement may be diffuse or focal

- Enlarged lymph nodes in the abdomen and pelvis occur in multiple sites in ALL and CLL

- The gastro-intestinal tract is involved in approximately 25% of cases. In the majority of patients the disease is silent

Indirect effects of leukaemia

The most important indirect effects of leukaemia within the abdomen and pelvis are graft versus host disease, haemorrhage and infection.

Graft versus host disease

Graft versus host disease (GVHD) most commonly affects the skin, gastro-intestinal tract and liver. This disease is a major complication of allogeneic bone marrow transplantation, occurring in about 50% of patients. The phenomenon is a manifestation of graft rejection in which the immunocompetent donor lymphoid cells react against host antigens. The principal bowel abnormalities are those of lymphocytic infiltration of the lamina propria, crypt dilatation and necrosis and focal micro-abscess formation.[75,76]

Involvement of the bowel can be demonstrated on conventional plain abdominal radiographs, barium studies and on CT.

On plain radiography air fluid levels, bowel wall and mucosal fold thickening and ascites may be seen.[77] On barium studies the small bowel shows thickening and flattening of the mucosal folds, a rapid transit time and air/fluid levels.[78] Pneumotosis intestinalis may be observed in severe cases.[79] Graft versus host disease may resolve completely in which case the abnormal plain film and barium findings return to normal. Computed tomography findings of GVHD include bowel wall thickening, stenosis of small bowel loops and oedema of the bowel wall. Oedema is typically seen as a 'target sign' with decreased attenuation centrally bounded by high attenuation on both the serosal and mucosal surfaces of the bowel. In addition, there is usually generalized increased density within the mesenteric fat.[80] These findings are non-specific and may be seen in other benign and malignant conditions.

Haemorrhage

Occasionally, imaging is required to investigate clinical features suggestive of intra-abdominal haemorrhage in leukaemic patients. This is usually manifested by acute abdominal pain together with clinical features of blood loss. Retroperitoneal haemorrhage may present as acute back pain and in such patients CT is the ideal imaging modality to demonstrate the presence of fresh blood and the extent of haemorrhage (Fig. 30.12).

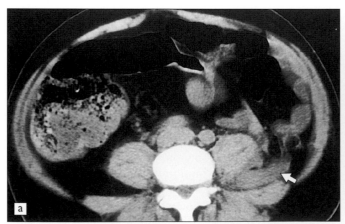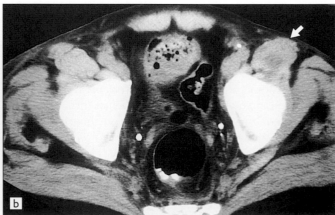

Figure 30.12. *(a and b) CT scans showing retroperitoneal haemorrhage in a 33-year-old male patient with ALL. There is an infected haematoma in the left psoas muscle which extends caudally, representing as a high attenuation mass in the left groin (arrows).*

Infection

Intra-abdominal infection is an important cause of abdominal pain in leukaemic patients. Infectious caecitis (typhlitis), perirectal abscesses and appendicitis may all complicate the clinical picture of leukaemia. Computed tomography may be helpful in the management of these patients since haemorrhage may be distinguished from infection and the site of infection localized.

Key points: abdominal/pelvic complications

■ Graft versus host disease is a major complication of allogeneic bone marrow transplantation

■ Acute GVHD most commonly affects the skin, liver and gastro-intestinal tract

■ Plain radiographs, barium studies and CT may all show dilatation, stenosis and thickening of small bowel loops with air fluid levels

■ Ascites and pneumotosis intestinalis are seen in severe cases

■ Intra-abdominal/retroperitoneal haemorrhage may account for the onset of abdominal pain in leukaemic patients

■ Intra-abdominal infection such as caecitis (typhlitis) may complicate acute leukaemia

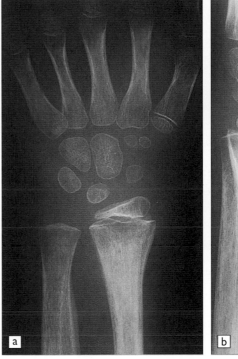
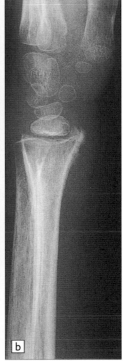

Figure 30.13. *Plain radiographs of the wrist in a 4-year-old boy with ALL. (a) Anterior/posterior view; (b) lateral view, showing diffuse osteoporosis throughout the radius and ulna as well as the bones of the wrist. Transverse metaphyseal bands of diminished density are noted. There is an extensive periosteal reaction on the distal surfaces of the radius and ulna.*

Skeletal system
Direct effects of leukaemia

The incidence and radiographic manifestations of skeletal involvement in leukaemia vary with patient age and subtype of the disease.

Radiographic findings

In children, leukaemic infiltration of the long bones produces characteristic appearances on plain radiographs (Fig. 30.13), which include:

- Diffuse osteoporosis
- Transverse metaphyseal bands of diminished density
- Dense transverse metaphyseal lines of arrested growth
- Subperiosteal new bone formation
- Osteolytic lesions
- Osteosclerotic lesions in less than 2% of patients[81]

Diffuse osteoporosis is the most common skeletal abnormality in childhood ALL, occurring in up to 60% of cases, and is most obvious in the spine.

In adults osteoporosis and cortical thinning of long bones due to expansion of the marrow space are common. Other features such as metaphyseal bands, so characteristic of childhood leukaemia, are not seen in adults. In adult T-cell leukaemia/lymphoma lytic bone lesions are common.[64] Subperiosteal bone resorption may be seen in this subtype of leukaemia and probably results from hypercalcaemia.[64]

In children with acute leukaemia presenting with back ache, plain radiographs may show collapse of one or several vertebral bodies (Fig. 30.14a). This is either due to vertebral compression fractures as a result of osteoporosis or from destruction of bone trabeculae by leukaemic infiltration. With treatment, remodelling of the vertebral body with reconstitution of the vertebral height may be observed (Fig. 30.14b). A characteristic but unusual feature is that of a 'bone' within a bone.[82]

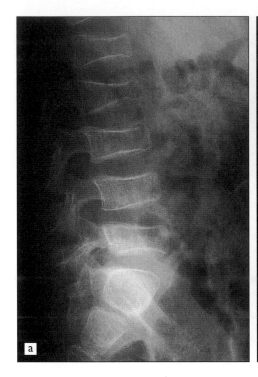

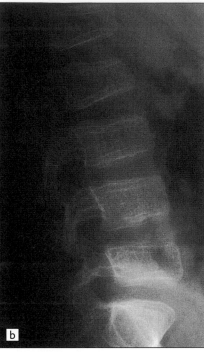

Figure 30.14. *Lateral plain radiographs in a 4-year-old boy who presented with back pain due to ALL. (a) At presentation partial collapse of the lumbar vertebral bodies is noted. The most severely affected vertebra is L2; (b) 2 years later following treatment, there has been remodelling of the bone. Note the thin dense lines adjacent to the vertebral end-plates giving the appearance of a bone within a bone. There is still extensive osteoporosis.*

Submetaphyseal bands are seen in approximately 40% of children and probably represent osteoporosis in the rapidly growing region of the long bone. They are seen most frequently in the distal femur, proximal tibia, proximal humerus and vertebral bodies.

Focal lytic lesions are less common in AML than in ALL but may develop in CML during the accelerated growth phase and in this group of patients, hypercalcaemia may also be evident.[83] Focal lesions are usually permeative and may show cortical destruction with pathological fracture. In the skull, lucent areas with a 'moth-eaten' appearance may be identified due to leukaemic infiltration and in children, widening of the sutures is associated with underlying meningeal disease. This has been less commonly observed since the introduction of CNS prophylaxis.

Bone is one of the most frequent sites for development of granulocytic sarcoma. An area of bone destruction is seen on plain radiographs which may be accompanied by a soft tissue mass. The lesions are most commonly found in the skull, spine, ribs and sternum.[84]

Computed tomography is indicated for the evaluation of leukaemic masses (granulocytic sarcoma) in various sites, as the technique can define the soft tissue disease as well as the extent of bone destruction.

Radionuclide bone scanning either with technetium-99m-diphosphonate or bone marrow imaging with colloid is not required in the routine management of leukaemia[85,86] but bone scans may be helpful in patients suspected of harbouring occult bone infection.

When MRI was first introduced into clinical practice over a decade ago there was considerable enthusiasm regarding its potential to evaluate diffuse bone marrow disease. Certainly diffuse infiltration of the bone marrow can be elegantly demonstrated on spin-echo imaging as diffuse abnormally low signal intensity on T1-weighted images accompanied by an intermediate signal intensity on T2-weighted images. In leukaemia the axial skeleton is mainly involved (Fig. 30.15). However, MRI is non-specific and benign and malignant disorders give similar appearances (Fig. 30.16).[87,88] Clear advantages of MRI are the ability to survey large volumes of the bone marrow at a single investigation and the high sensitivity of the technique in detecting bone marrow pathology. However, the current role of MRI in the evaluation of leukaemia is limited since clinical and haematological investigations usually direct patient management.

Magnetic resonance imaging may demonstrate changes within the bone marrow in leukaemic patients in response to treatment (Fig. 30.17) and some authors have used quantitative measurements of T1-relaxation times to evaluate therapeutic response.[89,90] In a recent study Vande Berg et al. showed that sequential quantitative MR imaging during therapy for ALL and AML revealed significant differences in the initial bulk values of T1 relaxation between these sub-types of leukaemia and also in the changes observed in T1 between the two groups during therapy. As a result these authors suggest that bone marrow imaging with MRI may be a useful method of predicting response in ALL.[91]

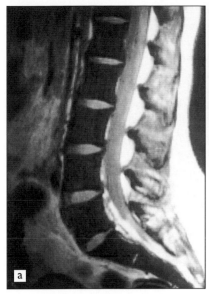

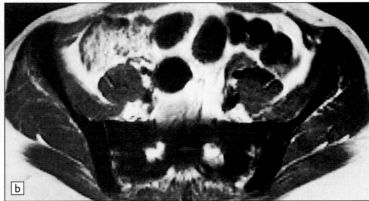

Figure 30.15. *T1-weighted spin-echo MR images in a 21-year-old female with ALL. (a) Sagittal image of the spine; (b) axial image through the pelvis. The MR examination shows widespread diffuse abnormal low signal intensity throughout the vertebral bodies and pelvis, indicating extensive bone marrow infiltration.*

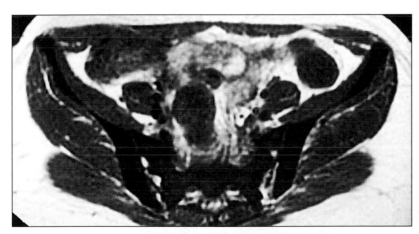

Figure 30.16. *A 50-year-old female patient with myelofibrosis. The spin-echo T1-weighted axial MR image of the pelvis shows diffuse abnormal low signal intensity throughout the iliac bones and sacrum. The appearances are identical to those of leukaemic infiltration.*

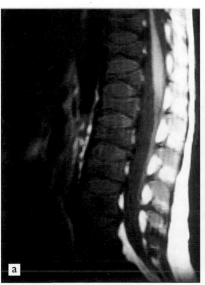

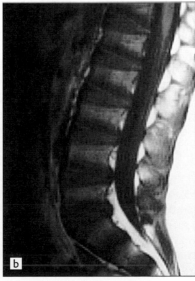

Figure 30.17. *MR images in a 4-year-old boy with ALL. This is the same patient as shown in Figure 30.13. T1-weighted sagittal images through the thoracic and lumbar spine: (a) before treatment; (b) 2 years after treatment. The MR image at presentation shows diffuse abnormal low signal intensity throughout the vertebral bodies indicating leukaemic infiltration. Note that the signal intensity of the bone marrow is lower than that of the adjacent intervertebral discs. There is partial collapse of multiple vertebrae. Two years later the signal intensity of the vertebral bodies is higher than the adjacent intervertebral discs. This represents response to treatment.*

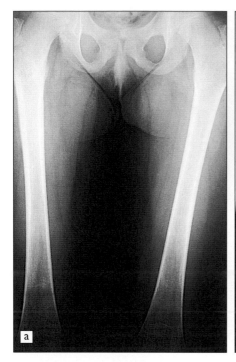

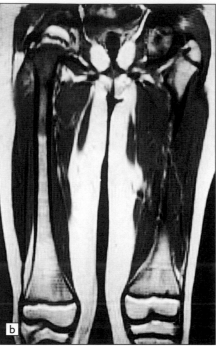

Figure 30.18. *A 10-year-old boy treated 3 years previously for ALL with CNS relapse. He re-presented with right leg pain: (a) plain radiograph of the femora did not reveal any abnormality; (b) coronal T1-weighted MR image of the femora showing extensive abnormal low signal intensity throughout the metaphyseal region and upper diaphysis of the right femur. This represented leukaemic relapse.*

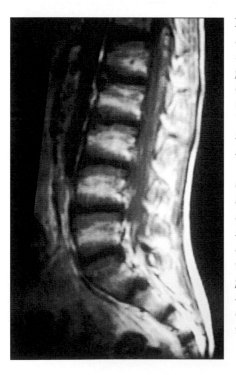

Figure 30.19. *MR image in a 21-year-old male patient following bone marrow transplantation. T1-weighted sagittal image showing typical 'bandlike' pattern of repopulation of bone marrow with areas of low signal intensity adjacent to the vertebral end-plates. Higher signal intensity centrally represents fat.*

Key points: skeletal involvement

■ In childhood ALL, osteoporosis occurs in up to 60% of cases

■ Metaphyseal translucencies are seen in the long bones in approximately 40% of children with ALL

■ Focal bone lesions are more common in ALL than AML

■ Granulocytic sarcoma in AML occurs most frequently in the skull, ribs and sternum

■ MRI shows diffuse bone marrow abnormality in acute leukaemia but the appearances are non-specific

■ MRI has a valuable role in the detection of leukaemic relapse in patients with bone pain

Indirect effects of leukaemia

Following therapy with bone marrow transplantation repopulation of the bone marrow gives rise to striking appearances with bands of low signal intensity adjacent to the vertebral end-plates with higher signal intensity centrally on MRI (Fig. 30.19). These appearances are related to repopulation of the marrow in the region of the capillary network which lies adjacent to the vertebral end-plates.[92,93] Treatment with steroids may lead to avascular necrosis of the femoral head (Fig. 30.20). Magnetic resonance imaging is well established as the best imaging technique for detecting avascular necrosis and is indicated in all symptomatic

Although MRI seems to have little role in the routine evaluation of the bone marrow in leukaemia, it is useful in patients suspected of relapse, for example in patients believed to be in remission who re-present with bone pain (Fig. 30.18) or in patients at high risk of relapse in whom serial bone marrow biopsies are negative.

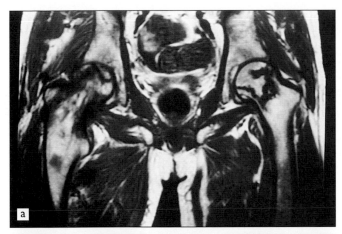

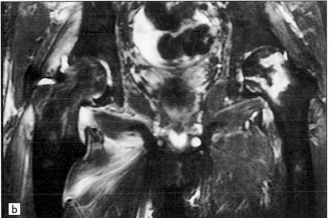

Figure 30.20. *An adult male patient with ALL with bilateral avascular necrosis of the femoral heads. (a) Coronal T1-weighted MR image, (b) turbo STIR image. The T1-weighted image shows classic signs of avascular necrosis with irregular areas of low signal intensity within the femoral heads bilaterally. The STIR image shows abnormal high signal intensity areas within the femoral heads and also in the femoral neck on the right, indicating associated oedema.*

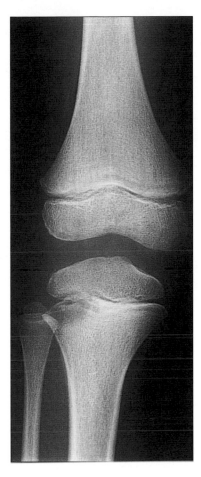

Figure 30.21. *Plain film of the right knee in a 5-year-old boy with ALL complaining of severe bone pain around the knee joint. There is a destructive lytic lesion in the lateral aspect of the tibial metaphysis. This was due to osteomyelitis and was surgically drained.*

patients with normal plain films. As in other areas of the body, infection is a major hazard in the acute leukaemias and bone pain may represent osteomyelitis as well as leukaemic relapse (Fig. 30.21).

CONCLUSION

Leukaemia comprises a heterogeneous group of neoplasms for which the investigation and treatment has changed markedly over recent years. Cross-sectional imaging, as well as conventional radiology, has an important place in the management of this disease. However, it is impossible to define strict algorithms for the use of imaging because the disease is manifested in many different organs and organ systems and the complications of leukaemia are common and diverse. As in other malignant tumours, close liaison between clinician and radiologist is essential to determine the most appropriate use of imaging for individual patient care.

Summary

- There are four major groups of leukaemia which are categorized according to the predominant type of proliferating cell — ALL, AML, CML, CLL.

- Acute lymphoblastic leukaemia (ALL) is the most common subtype in childhood.

- Acute myelogenous leukaemia (AML) and chronic lymphocytic leukaemia (CLL) are the most common subtypes in adults.

- Chromosomal abnormalities have been identified in many of the subtypes of leukaemia.

- The major clinical features of leukaemia relate to anaemia, infection and haemorrhage.

- Bone pain is a common presenting feature in children with ALL but is uncommon in adults.

- Granulocytic sarcoma (chloroma) is a mass composed of precursors of myelocytes. It occurs in AML disorders but also occurs in other myeloprolific disorders.

- Granulocytic sarcoma most commonly involves the orbits, subcutaneous tissues, paranasal sinuses and bones.

- Leukaemia is primarily treated with combination chemotherapy. Bone marrow transplantation, craniospinal irradiation and Interferon-α (IFN-α) all have a place in patient management.

- The 5-year survival rate of ALL in children is 50–80% and in adults it is 20–40%.

- The 5-year survival in AML is 40–50%.

- Imaging findings in leukaemia are related to direct involvement of organs and tissues by the disease and to indirect involvement of organs due to complications.

- In the CNS leukaemia involves the leptomeninges, dura and rarely the brain parenchyma. It may be diffuse or focal.

- Haemorrhage, sinovenous thrombosis and cerebral infarction, as well as infection, are all indirect effects of leukaemia on the CNS.

- Intrathoracic leukaemia usually involves mediastinal and hilar lymph nodes. Pulmonary complications include infection, haemorrhage, oedema and graft versus host disease (GVHD).

- Diffuse involvement of intra-abdominal organs is common (liver, spleen, kidneys, gastro-intestinal tract, intra-abdominal lymph nodes).

- Graft versus host disease (GVHD) is an important intra-abdominal complication.

- Skeletal manifestations of childhood leukaemia are seen in up to 60% of patients and include osteoporosis, trans-metaphyseal bands and subperiosteal new bone formation.

- Focal lytic lesions in the bone are more common in AML than ALL.

- MRI may demonstrate diffuse bone marrow abnormalities, both in acute and chronic leukaemia, but is not widely used for routine evaluation.

- MRI is useful in the investigation of pain in patients suspected of relapse with bone pain.

REFERENCES

1. Caligiuri M A. Ritz J. Immunology. In: Henderson E S, Lister T A (eds). Leukaemia (5th ed). Philadelphia: W B Saunders, 1990: 105–130

2. Garson C M. Cytogenetics of leukemic cells. In: Henderson E S, Lister T A (eds). Leukaemia (5th ed). Philadelphia: W B Saunders 1990: 131–152

3. Cancer Facts and Figures, 1997. Atlanta: American Cancer Society, Inc., 1997

4. Preston D L, Kusumi S, Tomonaga M et al. Cancer incidence in atomic bomb survivors. III. Leukaemia, lymphoma and multiple myeloma 1950–1987. Radiat Res 1994; 137: S68

5. Sandler D P. Recent studies in leukaemia epidemiology. Curr Opin Oncol 1995; 7: 12–18

6. Arseneau J C, Sponzo R W, Levin D L et al. Non-lymphomatous malignant tumours complicating Hodgkin's disease. Possible association with intensive therapy. N Engl J Med 1972; 287: 1119

7. Aisenberg A C. Acute nonlymphocytic leukaemia after treatment for Hodgkin's disease. Am J Med 1983; 75: 449–454

8. Curtis R E, Boice Jr, Stovall M et al. Risk of leukaemia after chemotherapy and radiation treatment for breast cancer. N Engl J Med 1992; 326: 1745–51

9. Kaldor J M, Day N E, Pettersson F et al. Leukaemia following chemotherapy for ovarian cancer. N Engl J Med 1990; 322: 1–6

10. Robert-Guroff M, Reitz M S, Robcy W G et al. In vitro generation of an HTLV-III variant by neutralizing antibody. J Immunol 1986; 137: 3306–3309

11. Kalyanaraman V S, Sarngadharan M G, Nakao Y et al. Natural antibodies to the structural core protein (p24) of the human T-cell leukemia (lymphoma) retrovirus found in sera of leukemia patients in Japan. Proc Natl Acad Sci USA 1982; 79: 1653

12. Weber J. HTLV-1 infection in Britain (Editorial). BMJ 1990; 301: 71–72

13. HTLV-1 comes of age (Editorial). Lancet 1988; I: 217–219

14. Barcos M, Lane W, Gomez G A et al. An autopsy study of 1206 acute and chronic leukemias (1958–1982). Cancer 1987; 60: 827–837

15. Henderson E S, Afshani E. Clinical manifestation and diagnosis. In: Henderson E S, Lister T A, (eds). Leukaemia 5th ed. Philadelphia: W B Saunders, 1990; 291–359

16. Graus F, Rogers L R, Posner J B. Cerebrovascular complications in patients with cancer. Medicine 1985; 64: 16–35

17. Freireich E J, Thomas L B, Frei E III et al. A distinctive type of intracerebral haemorrhage associated with blastic crisis in patients with leukaemia. Cancer 1960; 13: 146–154

18. Fernbach D J. Natural history of acute leukemia. In: Sutow W W, Vietti T J, Fernbach D J (eds). Pediatric Oncology (2nd ed). St. Louis: Mosby, 1977: 291–333

19. Thomas L B, Forkner C E, Frei E et al. The skeletal lesions of acute leukemia. Cancer 1961; 14: 608–621

20. Hann I M, Gupta S, Palmer M K et al. The prognostic significance of radiological and symptomatic bone involvement in childhood acute lymphoblastic leukemia. Med Pediat Oncol 1979; 6: 51–55

21. Nies B A, Kundel D W, Thomas L B et al. Leucopenia, bone pain, and bone necrosis in patients with acute leukemia. A clinicopathological complex. Ann Intern Med 1965; 62: 698

22. Neiman R S, Barcos M, Berard C et al. Granulocytic sarcoma: a clinicopathologic study of 61 biopsied cases. Cancer 1981; 48: 1426–1437

23. Pui M H, Fletcher B D, Langston J W. Granulocytic sarcoma in childhood leukemia: imaging features. Radiology 1994; 190: 698–702

24. Muss H B, Moloney W C. Chloroma and other myeloblastic tumors. Blood 1973; 42: 721–728

25. Liu P I, Ishimaru T, McGregor D H et al. Autopsy study of granulocytic sarcoma (chloroma) in patients with myelogenous leukemia, Hiroshima–Nagasaki 1949–1969. Cancer 1973; 31: 948–955

26. Krause J R. Granulocytic sarcoma preceding acute leukemia. A report of six cases. Cancer 1979; 44: 1017–1021

27. Burns A. Observation on the surgical anatomy of the head and neck. Edinburgh, Scotland: Thomas Bryce, 1811: 364–366

28. King A. A case of chloroma. Monthly J Med Soc 1853; 17: 97

29. Henderson E S, Hoelzer D, Freeman A I. The treatment of acute lymphoblastic leukaemia. In: Henderson E S, Lister T A (eds). Leukaemia (5th ed). Philadelphia: W B Saunders, 1990: 443–484

30. Ortega J A, Nesbit M E, Sather H N et al. Long-term evaluation of a CNS prophylaxis trial — treatment comparisons and outcome after CNS relapse in childhood ALL: a report from the Children's Cancer Study Group. J Clin Oncol 1978; 5: 1646

31. DeVries E G E, Mulder N H, Houwen B et al. Combination chemotherapy for acute lymphocytic leukaemia in 25 adults. Blut 1982; 44: 151–158

32. Lister T A, Whitehouse J M A, Oliver R T D et al. Chemotherapy and immunotherapy for acute myelogenous leukemia. Cancer 1980; 46: 2142–2148

33. Weinstein H J, Mayer R J, Rosenthal D S et al. Chemotherapy for acute myelogenous leukemia in children and adults: VAPA update. Blood 1983; 62: 315–319

34. Gale R P, Champlin R E. Bone marrow transplantation in acute leukemia. Clin Hematol 1986; 15: 851–872

35. Gale R P, Foon K A, Cline M J et al. Intensive chemotherapy for acute myelogenous leukemia. Ann Intern Med 1981; 94: 753–757

36. Tricot G, Boogaerts M A, Vlietinek R et al. The role of intensive remission induction and consolidation therapy in patients with acute myeloid leukaemia. Br J Haematol 1987; 66: 37–44

37. Kantarjian H M, Smith T L, O'Brien S et al. Prolonged survival in chronic myelogenous leukaemia after cytogenetic response to IFN-α therapy. Ann Intern Med 1995; 122: 254–261

38. Thomas E D, Clift R A, Fefer A et al. Marrow transplantation for the treatment of chronic myelogenous leukemia. Ann Intern Med 1986; 104: 155–163

39. Goldman J M. Leukaemia. In: Price P, Sikora K (eds). Treatment of Cancer (3rd edition). London: Chapman and Hall, 1995; 825–839

40. Kantarjian H M, Talpaz M, Keating M J et al. Intensive chemotherapy induction followed by interferon-alpha maintenance in patients with Philadelphia chromosome-positive chronic myelogenous leukaemia. Cancer 1991; 68: 1201–1207

41. Coccia P F, Bleyer W A, Siegel S E et al. Development and preliminary findings of Children's Cancer Study Group Protocols (#161,162,163) for low, average and high risk acute lymphoblastic leukemia in children. In: Murphy S, Gilbert J R (eds). Leukemia Research — Advances in Cell Biology and Treatment. Amsterdam: Elsevier/North Holland, 1983: 241

42. Bleyer W A. Central nervous system leukemia. In: Henderson E S, Lister T A (eds). Leukaemia (5th ed). Philadelphia: W B Saunders, 1990: 733–768

43. Price R A, Johnson W W. The central nervous system and childhood leukaemia. I. The arachnoid. Cancer 1973; 31: 520–533

44. Azzarelli B, Roessman U. Pathogenesis of central nervous system infiltration in acute leukemia. Arch Pathol Lab Med 1977; 191: 203–205

45. Zawadzki M B, Enzmann D R. Computed tomographic brain scanning in patients with lymphoma. Radiology 1978; 129: 67–71

46. Enzmann D R, Krikorian J, Yorke C. et al. Computed tomography in leptomeningeal spread of tumour. J Comput Assist Tomogr 1978; 2: 448–455

47. Pagani, J J, Libshitz H I, Wallace S et al. Central nervous system leukemia and lymphoma: computed tomographic manifestations. Am J Roentgenol 1981; 137: 1195–1201

48. Ginsberg L E, Leeds N E. Neuroradiology of leukemia. Am J Roentgenol 1995; 165: 525–534

49. Paako E, Patronas N J, Schellinger D. Meningeal Gd-DTPA enhancement in patients with malignancies. J Comput Assist Tomogr 1990; 14: 542–546

50. Sze G, Abramson A, Krol G et al. Gadolinium-DTPA in the evaluation of intradural extramedullary spinal disease. Am J Neuroradiol 1988; 9: 153–163

51. Kao S C S, Yuh R C, Sato Y et al. Intracranial granulocytic sarcoma (chloroma): MR findings. J Comput Assist Tomogr 1987; 11: 938–941

52. Pomeranz S J, Hawkins J J, Towbin R et al. Granulocytic sarcoma (chloroma): CT manifestations. Radiology 1985; 155: 167–170

53. Barnett M J, Zussmann W V. Granulocytic sarcoma of the brain: a case report and review of the literature. Radiology 1986; 160: 223–225

54. Williams M P, Olliff J F C, Rowley M R. CT and MR findings in parameningeal leukaemic masses. J Comput Assist Tomogr 1990; 14: 736–742

55. Lockman L A, Masatri A, Priest J R et al. Dural venous sinus thrombosis in acute lymphoblastic leukemia. Pediatrics 1980; 66: 943–947

56. Henderson E S. Complications of leukaemia: a selective overview. In: Henderson E S, Lister T A (eds). Leukaemia (5th ed). Philadelphia: W B Saunders, 1990: 671–685

57. Bleyer W A. Neurologic sequelae of methotrexate and ionizing radiation: a new classification. Cancer Treat Rep 1981; 65: 89–98

58. Packer R J, Zimmermann R A, Bilaniuk L T. Magnetic resonance imaging in the evaluation of treatment-related central nervous system damage. Cancer 1986; 58: 635

59. Duffner P D, Cohen M E, Brecher M L et al. CT abnormalities and altered methotrexate clearance in children with CNS leukaemia. Neurology 1984; 34: 229

60. Rubenstein L J, Herman M M, Long T F et al. Disseminated necrotizing leukoencephalopathy: a complication of treated central nervous system leukemia and lymphoma. Cancer 1975; 35: 291–305

61. Price R A, Birdwell D A. The central nervous system in childhood leukaemia: III. Mineralising microangiography and dystrophic calcification. Cancer 1978; 42: 717–728

62. Ito M, Akiyama Y, Asato R et al. Early diagnosis of leukoencephalopathy of acute lymphocytic leukaemia by MRI. Pediatr Neurol 1991; 7: 436–439

63. Bjorgen J E, Gold L H A. Computed tomographic appearance of methotrexate-induced necrotising leuko-encephalopathy. Radiology 1977; 122: 377–378

64. George C D, Wilson A G, Philpott N J et al. The radiological features of adult T-cell leukaemia/lymphoma. Clin Radiol 1994; 49: 83–88

65. Armstrong P, Dyer R, Alford A B et al. Leukemic pulmonary infiltrates: rapid development mimic-king pulmonary oedema. Am J Roentgenol 1980; 135: 373–374

66. Green R A, Nichols N J. Pulmonary involvement in leukemia. Am Rev Resp Dis 1959; 80: 833–844

67. Schimpff S C. Infection in the leukaemia patient: Diagnosis, therapy and prevention. In: Henderson S A, Lister T A (eds). Leukaemia (5th ed). Philadelphia: W B Saunders, 1990; 687–709

68. Degregorio M W, Lee W M F, Linker C A et al. Fungal infections in patients with acute leukaemia. Am J Med 1982; 73: 543–548

69. Olliff J F C, Williams M P. Appearances of cyto-megalovirus infections. Clin Radiol 1989; 40: 463–467

70. Dee P. Drug- and radiation-induced lung disease. In: Armstrong P, Wilson A G, Dee P Hansell D M (eds). Imaging Diseases of the Chest (2nd ed). St. Louis: Mosby, 1995: 461–484

71. Chaan C, Hyland R H, Hutcheon M A at al. Small airways disease in recipients of allogeneic bone marrow transplantations. Medicine 1987; 66: 327–340

72. Graham J, Muller N L, Miller R R et al. Intrathoracic complications following allogeneic bone marrow transplant: CT findings. Radiology 1991; 181: 153–156

73. Gore R M, Skolnik A. Abdominal manifestations of pediatric leukemias: sonographic assessment. Radiology 1982; 143: 207–210

74. Boggs D A, Wintrobe M M, Cartwright G E. The acute leukaemias. Analysis of 322 cases and review of the literature. Medicine 1962; 41: 163

75. Epstein R J, McDonald G B, Sale G E et al. The diagnostic accuracy of the rectal biopsy in acute graft-versus-host disease: a prospective study of thirteen patients. Gastroenterology 1980; 78: 764–771

76. Slavin R E, Woodruff J M. The pathology of bone marrow transplantation. In: Somers S C (ed). Pathology Annual. New York: Appleton-Century Crofts, 1974: 291

77. Belli A-M, Williams M P. Graft versus host disease: findings on plain abdominal radiography. Clin Radiol 1988; 39: 262–264

78. Fisk J D, Shulman H M, Greening R R et al. Gastrointestinal radiographic features of human graft versus host disease. Am J Roentgenol 1981; 136: 329–336

79. Maile C W, Frick M P, Crass J R et al. The plain abdominal radiograph in acute gastro-intestinal graft versus host disease. Am J Roentgenol 1985; 145: 289–292

80. Jones B, Fishman E K, Kramer S S et al. Com-puted tomography of gastro-intestinal inflammation after bone marrow transplantation. Am J Roentgenol 1986; 146: 691–695

81. Thomas L G, Forkner C E Jr, Frei E III et al. The skeletal lesions of acute leukemia. Cancer 1961; 14: 608

82. DeCastro L A, Kuhn J P, Freeman A E et al. Complete remodeling of the vertebrae in a child successfully treated for acute lymphocytic leukemia (ALL). Cancer 1977; 40: 398–401

83. Tricot G, Boogaerts M A, Broeckaert-Van Orshoven A et al. Hypercalcemia and diffuse osteolytic lesions in the acute phase of chronic myelogenous leukemia. A possible relation between lymphoid transformation and hypercalcemia. Cancer 1983; 52: 841–845

84. Van Slyck E J. The bony changes in malignant hematologic disease. Orthop Clin North Am 1972; 3: 733–744

85. Georgen T G, Alazrake N P, Halpern S E et al. 'Cold' bone lesions: a newly recognised phenomenon of bone imaging. J Nucl Med 1974; 15: 1120–1124

86. Parker B R, Marglin S, Castellino R A. Skeletal manifestations of leukemia. Hodgkin's disease, and non-Hodgkin's lymphoma. Semin Roentgenol 1980; 15: 302–315

87. Porter B A, Shields A F, Olson D O. Magnetic resonance imaging of bone marrow disorders. Radiol Clin North Am 1986; 24: 269–289

88. Jones R J. The role of bone marrow imaging. Radiology 1992; 183: 321–322

89. Moore S G, Gooding C A, Brasch R C et al. Bone marrow in children with acute lymphocytic leukemia: MR relaxation times. Radiology 1986; 160: 237–240

90. McKinstry C S, Steiner R E, Young A T et al. Bone marrow in leukaemia and aplastic anaemia: MR imaging before, during and after treatment. Radiology 1987; 162: 701–707

91. Vande Berg B C, Michaux L, Scheiff J-M et al. Sequential quantitative MR analysis of bone marrow: differences during treatment of lymphoid versus myeloid leukaemia. Radiology 1996; 201: 519–523

92. Stevens S K, Moore S G, Amylon M D. Repopulation of marrow after transplantation: MR imaging with pathologic correlation. Radiology 1990, 175: 213–218

93. Tanner S F, Clarke J, Leach M O, et al. MRI in the evaluation of late bone marrow changes following bone marrow transplantation. Br J Radiol 1996; 69: 1145–1151

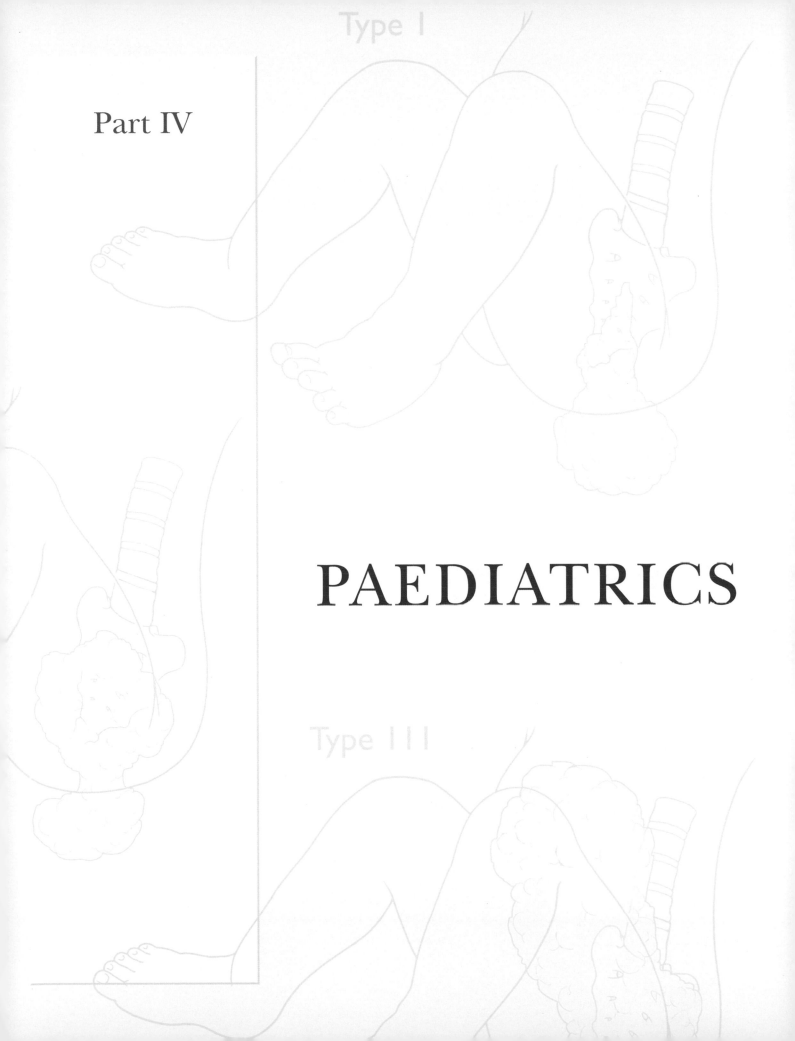

Part IV

PAEDIATRICS

Chapter 31

General principles in paediatric oncology

Helen Carty

INTRODUCTION

Children with cancer place significant demands on a department of paediatric radiology. The children are often ill. There is considerable parental and family anxiety while awaiting the outcome of the radiological investigations. There is an urgency of response required by the oncologist, anxious to reach a diagnosis and plan the treatment for the patient. In providing this service, the radiologist should be objective, decisive, sensitive and diagnostically accurate.

For the complete assessment of children with cancer the radiology department must have on-site access to or easy availability of all five main imaging modalities — plain radiography, ultrasound, nuclear medicine, computed tomography (CT) and magnetic resonance imaging (MRI).

THE DEPARTMENT

General points

In this section, points are highlighted which are often overlooked in non-specialized paediatric departments. Children are best managed in departments of paediatric radiology where the ambient environment is designed for children, where staff are familiar with the handling of children and can easily communicate with the child. Successful examinations are more readily achieved if the child's full cooperation is obtained. There should be explanatory books and leaflets available, written with the child in mind. The procedures should be explained in a language that the child can understand, and explained to the child and not just the parent. Knowledge allays anxiety and fear.

Heat loss

Much modern computer-controlled equipment requires an air-conditioned, stable, environmental temperature for its operation. Heat loss in children in relation to body surface area is greater than in adults. Children who are cold become restless. In small infants, hypothermia can be dangerous but heat loss can be combated by covering the child with blankets and other heat-retaining devices.

Injections

Most children fear pain and are aware that they need intravenous injections for many of their examinations. The discomfort of an injection can be minimized by a combination of prior application of a local anaesthetic cream to a suitable vein and ensuring that children's injections are done by a radiographer or doctor skilled in obtaining intravenous access in children. In most departments, even within paediatric departments, needle skills are variable and it is only fair that the most skilled should undertake the difficult patient. Intravenous injection of any contrast medium can be satisfactorily achieved with 23 and 25 French guage needles, although in difficult veins, 27 guage needles may be required. A butterfly system should be used because needle stability is better controlled.

Once a cancer is diagnosed and the child is on treatment, intravenous access via a long line such as a Hickman or Broviac catheter is almost invariably established. When these are used for intravenous access there must be clear protocols in place, agreed with the oncology ward, to avoid cross infection. In general the parents are fully versed with the management of central lines and can be consulted if in doubt.

Before embarking on an intravenous puncture, the radiologist should always check that there is no requirement for blood samples or subsequent chemotherapy that day. The insertion of an IV cannula instead of a simple butterfly system may avert a second venepuncture.

There are a group of children who require regular scanning with the use of intravenous contrast but do not have long lines, who are absolutely terrified at the prospect of the venepuncture in spite of all the best care. Consideration should be given to referring these children for psychological support and play-therapy in an effort to help them overcome their fears. This type of service is increasingly available in children's hospitals.

Equipment

The equipment used for imaging children with oncological problems has by definition to be that which is commercially available and is designed mainly for the adult population. When choosing equipment for mixed adult and childhood use, the requirements of the child should be considered.

Ultrasound

It is essential that a full range of probes is available, including a high frequency linear-array probe. Colour Doppler is essential. There should be high quality mobile ultrasound facilities available as well as the departmental machines.

Nuclear medicine

Nuclear medicine facilities are required as an integral part of imaging children with cancer. The camera head should not be placed over the child — it frightens them. Anterior views can be obtained by placing the child prone. High resolution collimation must be available for bone imaging. A liberal supply of cassettes and tapes played during the examination help to allay boredom.[1] This type of distraction therapy also works with CT and MRI.

Computed tomography scanner

The choice of a CT scanner should be influenced by the availability of fast scan times which reduce sedation and general anaesthetic requirements, and detector systems, which minimize radiation dose. Scan planes should be chosen to minimize the number of slices consistent with obtaining accurate information. For example, angling the gantry away from the orbitomeatal line during head scanning reduces the lens dose and reduces the number of slices for a head scan when compared with scanning in the orbitomeatal plane. The question requiring an answer needs to be defined and the scan protocol designed to obtain the correct answer.

Magnetic resonance imaging equipment

The main MRI equipment requirements are that the system should be as non-intimidating as possible, with maximum tunnel width and openness, good air flow within the tube, and the ability to leave several coils *in situ* at the same time, so that moving a child to change a coil is avoided. For example, routine scanning of the head and spine may be required in the follow-up of a child with a medulloblastoma. Moving a sedated child to change from a head to spinal coil may awaken him/her. Prior play-therapy with mock ups of the scanner and familiarization with the noise by playing audio tapes will improve the success rate of non-sedated scanning. Ease and reliability in achieving cardiac and respiratory gating must also be ensured.

Radiographers

Radiographers at ease with children and with good communication skills will achieve a higher success rate in scanning children without sedation than those who only occasionally examine children. In mixed adult and children's units, children should be scanned by a small number of specially trained radiographers.

PRINCIPLES OF IMAGING

Certain principles underpin diagnostic imaging of children with cancer:

- Diagnosis
- Staging
- Tissue diagnosis
- Communication
- Research

Diagnosis

The ultimate diagnosis of a tumour depends on tissue histology, but while awaiting this, patterns of imaging are sufficiently diagnostic in most childhood cancers that a working diagnosis can be established by imaging, and initial patient management planned on this basis. In arranging imaging for a child with a suspected cancer, tests should be arranged using the most appropriate, least invasive, first. In general, the initial imaging of such a child needs plain films of the suspect area, ultrasound of any palpable mass lesion, and a chest radiograph. When planning crosssectional imaging, if a general anaesthetic is required, arrangements should be made following discussion between the radiologist and oncologist. Thus, where appropriate, bone marrow aspiration, lumbar puncture, insertion of a long line and biopsy, should all be done at the same time, thereby maximizing the scope of investigation under general anaesthesia and avoiding the need to repeat it.

Imaging protocols must be designed to yield maximum information with minimum invasiveness and discomfort for the patient.

Once a decision to image is made, it should be done once, properly. In general, this is best done in the centre in which the child is to be treated. Tempting though it may be for a peripheral unit to image an 'interesting' case, it could be argued that it is a waste of resources to use a slot on a hard-pressed CT or MRI schedule when the examination done outside the specialist centre is often inadequate, does not answer the specific diagnostic questions, and may have to be repeated.

Staging

Imaging is required to stage a tumour. The pattern of this imaging should be designed with full knowledge of the pattern of spread of the disease. For example, children with neuroblastoma do not require routine chest CT as the tumour rarely metastasizes to the lungs. The choice of CT or MRI for cross-sectional imaging and staging depends on ease of local availability, tumour type and the requirement to obtain lung parenchymal images for identification of metastases. In a child with a Wilms' tumour, staging by CT alone is satisfactory, as both abdominal and chest imaging is required. However, staging of a child with osteosarcoma will require both CT and

MRI; CT is needed for identification of lung metastases, MRI for staging of the primary bone lesion.

Tumours in which it is currently considered that MRI is mandatory include tumours of the:

- Brain
- Spine
- Liver
- Bone
- Soft tissue

MRI is the preferred technique for staging:

- All pelvic tumours
- Neuroblastomas
- Lymphoma

CT is still considered satisfactory for Wilms' tumour, ovarian tumours and lymphoma if MRI is not easily available.

Tissue diagnosis

Where technically feasible and medically appropriate, tissue diagnosis by excision of the primary tumour or an accessible lymph node is the primary choice. In many tumours, the appropriate management of the primary tumour is by neo-adjuvant chemotherapy with excision of residual tumour later. A biopsy is required for tissue diagnosis. The basic principles underlying tumour biopsy are:

- The choice of biopsy route, open or closed, is dictated by safety with avoidance of complications
- In general, today open surgical biopsy by laparotomy should be avoided. Adequate tissue can be obtained by image guided biopsies or by laparoscopy or thoracoscopy
- Prior to biopsy the child should have a clotting screen, and any identified deficiency corrected by the haematologist
- Imaging is required to establish the safest biopsy route. For example, if a child has chest lymphoma, no palpable nodal disease but splenic or renal involvement, it may be preferable to biopsy the spleen or kidney instead of the mediastinum to obtain tissue
- Biopsy tissue must be obtained from viable and not necrotic tumour
- Tissue samples must be sufficiently large to enable the pathologist to undertake all the required stains, immunohistochemistry and cytogenetic studies required for diagnosis. Also ideally there should be enough tumour tissue to store in a tissue bank for further research. Primary diagnosis takes precedence if tissue is sparse

- The handling of the tissue must be agreed in advance by radiologist and pathologist. Placing tissue in formalin will destroy it for cytogenetic studies
- When carrying out the biopsy the radiologist must be familiar with the subsequent surgical requirements, such as excision of the biopsy track if this is appropriate

Communication

Reference has already been made to the importance of good communication between the radiographer and the child when carrying out the technical aspects of scanning. Just as important are clear lines of communication between the radiologist and oncologist as to the information the parent is given at the end of an examination.

Research

Much of the improvement in survival and cure of children with cancer is attributable to collaborative research and multicentre therapy trials. Imaging to monitor progress of disease is important in this research, and will on occasion entail imaging for research purposes alone. This is acceptable but in designing these trials, the tolerance of the child and their family in coping with these tests, in addition to cost effectiveness, must be borne in mind. Families, though grateful for the success of the treatment and cure, have a finite tolerance for being part of research programmes and require great sensitivity in their handling.

Key points: general considerations

- Precautions should be taken to prevent heat loss, particularly in small infants and babies

- Clear protocols should be in place for the use of intravenous central lines for the administration of contrast medium

- Imaging and other tests such as bone marrow biopsy should all be performed as a single procedure under the same sedation or general anaesthesia

- Percutaneous biopsy under imaging control should obviate the need for surgical open biopsy or laparotomy in a high proportion of patients

- Even in mixed adult and children scanning units, radiographers should be specially trained for paediatric scanning

ACUTE COMPLICATIONS

There are certain acute complications of cancer treatment in children common to many types of cancer. Many of these are either directly related to the toxic effects of the drugs used in treatment or the neutropenia and immunosuppression associated with the drug treatment. These include:

- Intravenous access complications
- Abdominal complications
- Chest infection
- Haemorrhagic complications

Intravenous access complications

Most children will have some form of long line inserted for chemotherapy and on occasion parenteral nutrition. Fracture of the line will lead to extravasation of infused substances and may cause pain during infusion with or without visible soft tissue swelling. Fluoroscopy during infusion of radio-opaque contrast medium is the best method of identifying the site of the fracture, or line blockage. All such studies must be performed with a rigorous aseptic technique and non-ionic contrast media.

Venous thrombosis distal to the catheter tip is clinically manifest by pain on infusion, difficulty in aspirating blood and frequent stoppage of the infusion pump. More rarely there are signs of obstruction with limb oedema or superior vena caval compression symptoms. Initial assessment of such a problem should be by Doppler ultrasound but venous angiography either by digital subtraction angiography or magnetic resonance angiography may be needed for complete assessment. Doppler ultrasound is very helpful in identifying venous anatomy and patency for the resiting of a new IV line.

Line infection

This is a frequent cause of pyrexia in neutropenic children. Bacterial thrombi can form on the line and lead to bacterial endocarditis and septic emboli. Echocardiography is the method of choice for the identification of bacterial thrombi on the line tip or the heart valves. Septic emboli to the brain are best imaged by MRI or CT depending on what is easily locally available. Suspect septic emboli to the lung leading to perfusion defects are best imaged by a perfusion lung scan. Computed tomography may be needed to assess any abscess formation. A potential pitfall of CT is that such lesions may in theory be multiple and can, of course, resemble metastases. If the tumour undergoing treatment is not one that metastasizes to the lungs, caution in interpretation should be exercised. Review of the current scan with previous imaging and correlating the scan and clinical details should avoid confusion. This complication is more a theoretical than a practical reality.

Abdominal complications

A full review of these conditions is outside the scope of this chapter but they are discussed in more detail in Chapter 46. There are also several articles in the literature which review the problem.[2] The imaging approach to the common lesions is described which include:

- Neutropenic colitis
- Pseudomembranous colitis
- Graft versus host disease

Neutropenic colitis

Any child who is immunosuppressed on chemotherapy is potentially at risk for the development of neutropenic colitis (or typhlitis) but it is most commonly seen in children with leukaemia.[3,4,5,6] Clinical presentation is with abdominal pain and fever. There may be associated diarrhoea which may be bloody. The pain, though often generalized, may be localized to the right lower quadrant and simulate appendicitis. The abdomen is tender on palpation and there is often ileus and peritonism. Bowel sounds are diminished. Initial imaging is by plain abdominal radiography. On plain abdominal radiographs the appearances are variable. Thickened bowel may be visible but this is unusual. More commonly there is distended bowel with a pattern of ileus. A distended abdomen, with displacement of bowel gas centrally and distension of the flank stripes will be present if there is sufficient ascites. Perforation, although unusual, is manifest by free intra-abdominal air. The best further method of investigation is abdominal ultrasound. Ultrasonic findings mirror the combination of the clinical features and plain radiographs. The bowel wall is thickened, the right colon and caecum being most affected (Fig. 31.1). These features are also seen on CT but this is usually not necessary.[5] Free fluid, which is usually clear and not turbulent, is present in variable quantity. Ileus of the bowel is noted. This thickened bowel may act as the lead point of an intussusception. The ultrasonic findings will then be those of intussusception, with the intussuscipiens lying in the thickened bowel (Fig. 31.2). Unless there is perforation, hydrostatic reduction of the intussusception should be undertaken. As the bowel is already compromised, the reduction should be done using water soluble contrast medium to avoid barium contamination of the peritoneum if a perforation should occur (Fig. 31.3). In general the child will require analgesia for the reduction. This is one occasion in which reduction under general anaesthetic may be indicated with a view to proceeding to surgery if the reduction fails.

Monitoring of the progress of neutropenic colitis is by ultrasound and plain films, as clinically indicated. Abscess formation is most easily detected by ultrasound or CT, perforation by plain radiographs.

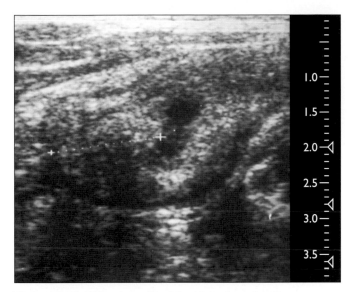

Figure 31.1. *Nine-year old girl with leukaemic relapse. Ultrasound of the caecum. Note thickened wall between crosses. The bowel wall measured 2.0 cm.*

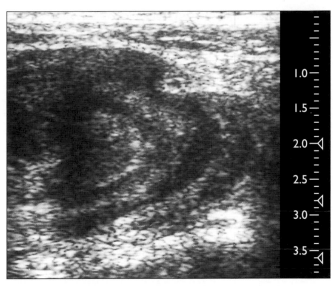

Figure 31.2. *Same child as Figure 31.1. 2 days later. Classical appearances of ileo-ileo-colic intussusception. Note multiple layers of bowel wall.*

Children who are immunocompromised are, in theory, at risk from many other abdominal inflam-matory conditions, but in practice these are quite rare. Neutropenic colitis is the most frequent.

Pseudomembranous colitis

Pseudomembranous colitis due to overgrowth with Clostridium difficile and its toxin is caused by antibiotic therapy. There is diffuse thickening of the colonic wall which may be seen on ultrasound or CT and may also be visible on plain radiographs as thumbprinting.[6–8] A barium enema will show marked coarse mucosal irregularity.

Graft versus host disease

Graft versus host disease (GVHD) is unique to children who have had a bone marrow transplant. On CT examination there is mucosal enhancement, a fluid filled bowel due to ileus with murkiness and oedema of the mesenteric fat.[9] On the plain abdominal radiograph, bowel wall thickening and non-specific dilatation may be seen. Pneumatosis intestinalis is a recognized feature.[2,10] Infectious enteritis may occur due to a whole host of organisms. The imaging features are non-specific and include mild bowel wall thickening, ileus and variable amounts of free intra-abdominal fluid.

As for neutropenic colitis, primary imaging should be with plain radiographs and abdominal and bowel ultrasound, supplemented by CT if the information is inadequate or conflicts with clinical assessment.

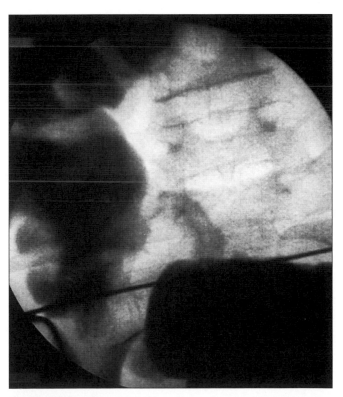

Figure 31.3. *Water soluble enema under general anaesthetic. Same child as Figures 31.1. and 31.2. The intussusception was reduced. There is a little caecal oedema but marked oedema of the terminal ileum.*

In all these children, management is conservative, surgery being reserved for perforation, obstruction or abscess drainage if the latter cannot be drained percutaneously.

GVHD is also discussed in relation to leukaemia in Chapter 30.

Chest infection

Children undergoing chemotherapy are neutropenic and therefore prone to developing infection. The infection may be a simple common viral or bacterial infection. The radiological appearance of these does not differ from patterns seen in the non-compromised child. The dilemma for the clinician is to diagnose opportunistic infections such as Pneumocystis carinii pneumonia (Fig. 31.4), fungal and viral infection, tuberculosis or aspergillosis, and to institute appropriate antimicrobial treatment as early as possible. Many of these infections have characteristic radiographic patterns, well described in standard texts[9,11,12,13] and will not be repeated here. The patterns in immunocompromised children on chemotherapy are similar to those in children with auto-immune deficiency syndrome (AIDS) or other immune deficiency syndromes. Most of these radiographic patterns are only seen when infection is well established. Early diagnosis is best achieved by bronchial lavage and, once a diagnosis of opportunistic infection is suspected, this is indicated.

If there is doubt about the presence of pulmonary infiltration on a chest radiograph, high-resolution CT (HRCT) is valuable. CT is also excellent for showing the extent of mycetoma in cavities and assessment of mediastinal nodal disease.[9]

Graft versus host disease is a recognized complication of bone marrow transplantation and may be acute or chronic. Symptoms include cough and bronchospasm. There is an obstructive pattern to pulmonary function. Radiographic findings are variable and range from a normal appearance to mild hyperinflation (Fig. 31.5). There may be patchy perihilar infiltrates which in severe cases, progress to a diffuse infiltrative pattern.[11,12] The underlying pathology is that of lymphocytic infiltrates with the development of bronchiolitis obliterans in severe cases. Once suspected, the child requires HRCT, but the diagnosis is confirmed by biopsy.

Haemorrhagic complications

These are relatively infrequent in spite of the low platelet counts that accompany chemotherapy. Imaging will depend on the location. In the brain, non-contrast enhanced CT is the method of choice. Elsewhere in the body, initial investigation is with plain radiographs, ultrasound and CT, with MRI being the imaging technique of choice for suspected intramuscular haemorrhage.

LONG-TERM EFFECTS OF TREATMENT OF CHILDREN WITH CANCER

As children survive their primary oncological disease, there are a number of important effects of treatment that may affect almost any body organ.[14] These complications may be due to radiation therapy or the potent anticancer drugs. Imaging of these effects will depend on the nature and location of the clinical problem and, as for the imaging of the primary disease, full diagnostic facilities are required. A multidisciplinary approach to the management of the problem is also frequently essential.

Routine imaging surveillance for most of these long-term complications is not indicated. Each is imaged as it clinically presents. The radiologist must be familiar with these known complications so that he/she can advise the most appropriate investigations. When a child with a previous history of cancer treatment is referred for imaging, a proper history of the drugs and the radiation field used must be available to the radiologist so that a correct interpretation of

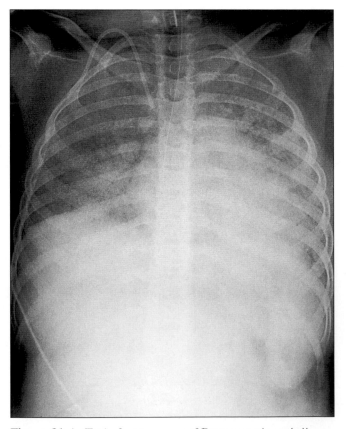

Figure 31.4. *Typical appearance of Pneumocystis carinii pneumonia.*

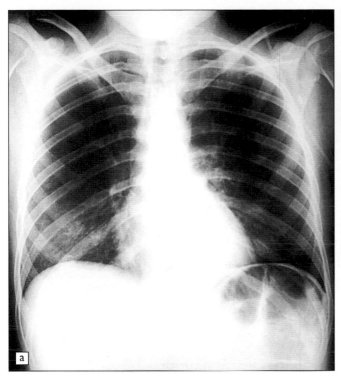

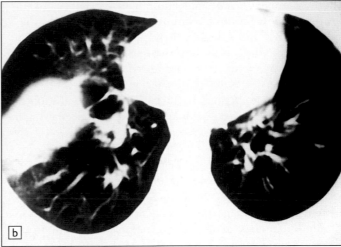

Figure 31.5. *Graft versus host disease. Biopsy proven. (a) Plain radiograph. There is non-specific right middle lobe infiltrate; (b) CT scan. There is a paucity of vessel markings on the left due to bronchiolitis obliterans but without hyperinflation. On the right there is segmental consolidation of the right middle lobe and patchy infiltration in the right lower lobe. The appearances of both the radiograph and the CT scan are non-specific.*

imaging findings is made. Great confusion can be caused by the incorrect interpretation of imaging findings which, if interpreted out of context, may be misconstrued and mistakenly diagnosed as other diseases. Conversely, the radiologist must always be careful not to miss a new disease if imaging findings are not compatible with the late effect of cancer therapy. An increasingly important late effect of cancer treatment is the development of second primary cancers. This topic is discussed in detail in Chapter 47.

The main regions affected by therapy which will be considered are:

- Central nervous system
- Musculoskeletal system
- Cardiopulmonary system
- Gonads
- Thyroid
- Kidneys

Central nervous system (CNS) effects

Effects of treatment on the central nervous system can be divided into general effects on brain function and specific injury to the special senses and neuro-endocrine function. The main effect of radiation and chemotherapy on general brain function is a resultant deterioration in intellectual ability. Imaging studies may show varying degrees of generalized cerebral atrophy associated with ventricular dilatation. There may be further focal damage at the site of the primary brain tumour. Cerebral atrophy may also occur in children with leukaemia who have central nervous system irradiation even though there is no focal primary tumour. Cerebral calcification may develop in either group. The best imaging technique for the demonstration of the late effects of treatment is MRI.

Damage to the hypothalamus or pituitary gland may occur from radiation, not just to primary central brain tumours but also in those children with tumour of the orbit or nasopharynx. The damage is usually functional, rather than physical, but if imaging of the hypothalamus or pituitary gland is indicated, MRI is the technique of choice. Suspected damage to the auditory or optic nerves is also best imaged by MRI. Radiation-induced cataracts are best imaged by ultrasound.

Radiation-induced musculoskeletal disease

Radiation to the growing skeleton may damage growth of both bones and soft tissues. This can lead to complications such as scoliosis, limb shortening and asymmetry of development of the structures in the irradiated field. Imaging of these complications is similar to imaging primary growth abnormalities. Scoliosis monitoring is by plain posterior–anterior (PA) full spinal radiographs with special lateral bending and traction views preoperatively if surgery is planned. Leg asymmetry is monitored by leg length monitoring. Scout view on CT is the most efficient method.

Facial asymmetry may result from irradiation. If surgical correction of this is contemplated, 3D craniofacial CT will be required.

Late cardiopulmonary effects

Mediastinal radiation may rarely result in radiation induced constrictive pericarditis.[14] This is increasingly rare as mediastinal radiation is used less frequently since the advent of chemotherapeutic drugs for the treatment of mediastinal tumours, notably Hodgkin's disease.

The main long-term cardiac effects of cancer treatment use relate to drug treatment, especially the anthracyclines.[15] Left ventricular function is impaired. Monitoring of cardiac function is predominantly by echocardiography but nuclear medicine studies have a part to play, especially if there is difficulty in obtaining good echo studies due to the patient's habitus or the results are equivocal. Radiation pneumonitis and fibrosis has long been recognized and is best imaged by HRCT. Pulmonary toxicity with infiltration as well as basal fibrosis may also result from chemotherapeutic drugs such as methotrexate, bischloroethyl nitrosourea (BCNU), busulphan and bleomycin. If suspected, high-resolution CT is indicated, but once a diagnosis is made should only be repeated if there is clinical deterioration. Ventilation/perfusion (V/Q) nuclear medicine studies will also show the functional distribution of the disease.

Gonadal dysfunction

This is a well recognized complication of both radiation and chemotherapy. In general, no radiological imaging of the affected gonad is required. Gonadal dysfunction may be associated with growth failure and delayed bone maturation. Bone maturation is assessed by hand and wrist radiography. The most sensitive and widely accepted method of assessment for height prediction is the Tanner–Whitehouse System 2 (TW2) method.[16] This, where necessary, can be repeated at yearly intervals until skeletal maturity.

Thyroid dysfunction

Thyroid dysfunction may result from radiation to the neck. Monitoring is by biochemical studies but, if required, these can be correlated with imaging of the thyroid by nuclear medicine studies. The latter are indicated if there is any palpable nodularity of the gland to show whether the nodules are functional or not. Ultrasound of the thyroid gland will identify cystic nodules. Both are only indicated in symptomatic patients.

Nephrotoxicity

Radiation nephritis has long been recognized to cause hypertension. Monitoring general renal function is mainly by biochemistry. If there is any reason to suspect unilateral disease then nuclear medicine studies are indicated for divided renal function. Radiation-induced renal artery stenosis has been described. Duplex Doppler ultrasound should be the initial investigation, followed by captopril renography and MR angiography. The gold standard for the detection of renal artery stenosis is by contrast angiography. Angioplasty of the stenosed segment may result in the relief of hypertension.

Chemotherapy with cis-platinum, BCNU, ifosfamide and methotrexate may cause acute nephrotoxicity. Long-term effects may persist but as both kidneys are af-fected, monitoring of renal function is in general non-radiological.

Cyclophosphenol and ifosfamide may both cause damage to the bladder wall with telangiectatic lesions. These may cause haematuria. The lesions are seen at cystoscopy. Radiation cystitis will cause thickening of the bladder wall and a small volume bladder. The thickening is well demonstrated by ultrasound. Bladder volume pre- and post-micturition may be measured by ultrasound.

Summary

- Children are most appropriately imaged in paediatric centres where treatment will be given.

- Techniques and protocols of examination should be defined according to pattern of tumour spread.

- A multidisciplinary approach to obtain all the information at a single investigation is essential if general anaesthesia or sedation is used — e.g. imaging, bone marrow biopsy, etc.

- Acute complications of therapy include intravenous access blockage, abdominal infections, graft versus host disease, chest infections and haemorrhage.

- Long-term complications include cerebral atrophy, musculoskeletal growth problems, cardiopulmonary effects, thyroid and gonadal dysfunction and nephrotoxicity. The development of second primary tumours is becoming increasingly important.

REFERENCES

1. Sherazi Z, Gordon I. Quality of care: identification and quantification of the process of care among children undergoing nuclear medicine studies. Nucl Med Comm 1996; 17: 363–366

2. Jones B, Wall S D. Gastrointestinal disease in the immunocompromised host. Radiol Clin North Am 1992; 30(3): 555–577

3. Wall S D, Jones B. Gastrointestinal tract in the immunocompromised host: opportunistic infection and other complications. Radiology 1992; 185: 327–335

4. Alexander J E, Williamson S L, Seibert J J, Golladay E S, Jimenez J F. The ultrasonographic diagnosis of typhlitis — neutropenic colitis. Pediatr Radiol 1988; 18: 200–204

5. Suarez B, Kalifa G, Adamsbaum C et al. Sonographic diagnosis and follow-up of diffuse neutropenic colitis: case report of a child treated for osteogenic sarcoma. Pediatr Radiol 1995; 25: 373–374

6. Donnelly L F. CT Imaging of immunocompromised children with acute abdominal symptoms. Am J Roentgenol 1996; 167: 909–913

7. Ros P R, Buetow P C, Pantograg-Brown L et al. Pseudomembranous colitis. Radiology 1996; 198: 1–9

8. Benya E C, Sivit C J, Quinones R R. Abdominal complications after bone marrow transplantation in children: sonographic and CT findings. Am J Roentgenol 1993; 161: 1023–1027

9. Donnelly L F, Morris C L. Acute graft-versus-host disease in children: abdominal CT findings. Radiology 1996; 199: 265–268

10. Yeager A M, Kanof M E, Kramer S S et al. Pneumatosis intestinalis in children after allogeneic bone marrow transplantation. Pediatr Radiol 1987; 17: 18–22

11. Pagani J J, Kangarloo H, Gyepes M T et al. Radiographic manifestations of bone marrow trans-plantation in children. Am J Roentgenol 1979; 132: 883–890

12. Shaw D. The chest. In: Carty H, Brunelle B, Shaw D, Kendall B (eds). Imaging in Children. Edinburgh: Churchill Livingstone 1994: 118

13. McLoud T C, Naidich D P. Thoracic disease in the immunocompromised patient. Radiologic Clin North Am 1992; 30(3): 525–554

14. Malpas J S. Clinical Review. Long-term effects of treatment of childhood malignancy. Clin Radiol 1996; 51: 466–474

15. Lipschultz S E, Colon S D, Gelber R D et al. Late cardiac effects of doxorubicin therapy. N Engl J Med 1991; 324: 808–815

16. Tanner J M, Whitehouse R H, Marshall W A et al. In: Assessment of Skeletal Maturity and Prediction of Adult Height (TW2 Method). London: Academic Press, 1975

Chapter 32

Wilms' tumour and associated neoplasms of the kidney

Helen Carty

WILMS' TUMOUR

Incidence and epidemiology

Wilms' tumour or nephroblastoma is the most frequent renal tumour in childhood, with an incidence of 1 per 10,000 live births per year[1,2] and 6% of all childhood malignancies.[3] It typically occurs in the first 6 years of life, most children presenting between 6 months and 4 years, with an average age of 36 months, but it can occasionally present in older children. The sex incidence is equal. The tumour is mainly unilateral, but in 5–10% of cases is bilateral.[2,4] Children with bilateral tumours tend to present at a slightly earlier age than those with unilateral disease. Population studies have shown a relatively increased incidence of Wilms' tumour in the black population relative to Asian or Caucasian races.[5,6]

Predisposing factors

It is now generally accepted that there are two gene mutations that lead to the development of Wilms' tumour. One mutation occurs either before or after the formation of the zygote, the other always after zygote formation.[7] Tumours due to mutation in a prezygote germ cell are likely to be hereditary, occur in younger patients, be multicentric and bilateral, while those occurring in somatic cells, requiring two mutations, are more likely to be sporadic and unilateral, and occur in the slightly older child.[7] Children with bilateral tumours have a median age of presentation of 23–30 months, while those with unilateral tumours have a median age of 36–42 months.[7] The hereditary form tends to occur in those in whom the mutation took place at germ cell level.[8] The true incidence of hereditary Wilms' is said to be around 20%.[9] Chromosomal deletion at locus 11p13 is present in many patients with Wilms' tumour, especially the hereditary forms associated with aniridia, Denys–Drash and WAGR (Wilms' tumour, aniridia, genito-urinary malformations and mental retardation) syndromes.[6,9,10] Chromosome locus 11p15 is implicated in the association of Wilms' tumour and Beckwith–Wiedemann syndrome,[6,9] the genetic change being duplication of paternal allele. Loss of heterozygosity for chromosome 16q has been shown to have a relapse rate three times higher and a mortality rate 12 times higher than in patients without this,[6] but this chromosomal abnormality is said to affect tumour regression and prognosis rather than tumour incidence.[6] The loss of heterozygosity for chromosome 11p affects tumour incidence but not outcome.[6]

Associations of Wilms' tumour

For years it has been recognized that there are many syndromes associated with Wilms' tumour:

- WAGR syndrome
- Denys–Drash Syndrome
- Beckwith–Wiedemann syndrome
- Perlman syndrome
- Hemihyperplasia

WAGR syndrome

Sporadic aniridia has long been recognized to be associated with Wilms' tumour.[1] The WAGR syndrome — Wilms' tumour, aniridia, genito-urinary malformation and mental retardation — is another recognized association of abnormalities. There is a deletion at the 11p13 chromosome. The incidence of Wilms' tumour is greater than 30%.[6] There is no increased incidence of Wilms' in other forms of aniridia.

Denys–Drash syndrome

The association of XX/XY gonadal dysgenesis with ambiguous genitalia, glomerulonephropathy and Wilms' tumour was first reported in 1967.[10] Since then there have been several more reports of both the complete and incomplete syndrome. When two components are present the syndrome is regarded as being incomplete.[11,12] The chromosomal abnormality is at 11p13 with an incidence of over 90% of Wilms' tumours,[6] but clear cell sarcoma has also been described.[11]

Beckwith–Wiedemann syndrome

The main characteristics of this syndrome are macroglossia, omphalocoele, umbilical hernia, visceromegaly, gigantism and hemihypertrophy. All features are not present in every patient. The incidence of Wilms' tumour is said to be less than 5%[6] but patients with hemihypertrophy as part of the syndrome have a threefold increase in neoplasms. Other neoplasms associated with Beckwith–Wiedemann syndrome include rhabdomyosarcoma, hepatoblastoma and adrenal carcinoma.[13] Renal cell carcinoma has been reported.[13] The chromosomal locus associated with the syndrome is 11p15.[6,13]

Perlman syndrome

This syndrome which is autosomal recessive has many features in common with Beckwith–Wiedemann syndrome; macrosomia, organomegaly but not macroglossia, ear pits or creases and umbilical abnormalities.[14] Children with Perlman syndrome have a characteristic facial appearance, high neonatal mortality and a high incidence of mental retardation rates as well as a high frequency of Wilms' tumour — 45% in the published cases,[14] but there is no apparent increase in other neoplasms. No chromosomal abnormality is yet identified in Perlman syndrome.

Hemihyperplasia

There is a long recognized association between hemihyperplasia and neoplasms in childhood, Wilms' tumour being the most frequent of these.[11] The true incidence of Wilms' tumour associated with hemihyperplasia is 3–4%.[15,16] In a series of 30 patients with hemihypertrophy and a childhood neoplasm — 19 patients had Wilms' tumour and 1 nephroblastomatosis[15] but this report does not reflect the true incidence of the association as it does not include those children with hemihypertrophy without tumour. Children with solid tumours usually have the mass on the same side as the hemihypertrophy.

Clinical presentation

Most children with Wilms' tumour present as a result of the incidental palpation of an abdominal mass, usually by a parent. The mass grows rapidly — parents often commenting that they 'are sure the "tummy" was normal the previous week'. The child is usually asymptomatic. Other presenting features include an increasing abdominal girth, abdominal pain and frank haematuria. The latter is a rare primary presentation but is a relatively common presentation in a child sustaining minor abdominal trauma which causes rupture of or bleeding within a Wilms' tumour (Fig. 32.1).

Microscopic haematuria is present in about one-third of children with Wilms' tumour. Hypertension or polycythemia may also be present. Tumour invasion of the renal vein and inferior vena cava (IVC) is usually asymptomatic

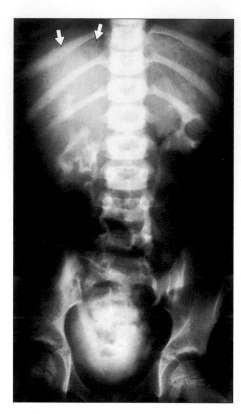

Figure 32.1.
Five-year old girl who fell from her bicycle and then had profound haematuria. Ten minute intravenous urogram film shows clot in the right renal pelvis, an enlarged right kidney, distorted upper pole calyx due to tumour and dilatation of the lower end of the ureter due to partial obstruction from the blood clot (arrowed).

but is an important cause of operative morbidity and mortality due to tumour thrombus embolism if not diagnosed preoperatively. A rare presentation is left-sided varicocoele due to tumour compression of the left renal vein.[17] Symptomatic presentation of vascular invasion is rare but has been reported with clinical presentation of a non-reducible varicocoele[18] and Budd–Chiari syndrome.[19] Complete IVC obstruction may lead to ascites and distal limb oedema.[20] Inferior vena cava tumour thrombus may extend into the right atrium. Primary presentation with metastatic disease is rare.

Staging

The prognosis for and treatment of children with Wilms' tumour depends on staging and histological type. Preoperative staging is clinical and radiological with further assessment being visually carried out during surgery. The internationally accepted staging system for Wilms' tumour is the NWTS system (National Wilms' Tumour Study) (Table 32.1).

An attempt should be made to stage each side according to the above criteria on the basis of extent of disease before biopsy.

A staging system of intracaval thrombus has been proposed which influences surgical management.[21]

Table 32.1. *Wilms' tumour staging (N.W.T.S.)*

Stage I	Tumour limited to kidney and completely excised. The surface of the renal capsule is intact. Tumour was not ruptured before or during removal. There is no residual tumour apparent beyond the margins of resection
Stage II	Tumour extends beyond the kidney but is completely removed. There is regional extension of the tumour (i.e. penetration through the outer surface of the renal capsule into perirenal soft tissues). Vessels outside the kidney substance are infiltrated or contain tumour thrombus. The tumour may have been biopsied or there has been local spillage of tumour confined to the flank. There is no residual tumour apparent at or beyond the margins of excision
Stage III	Residual non-haematogenous tumour confined to abdomen. Any one or more of the following occur: • Lymph nodes on biopsy are found to be involved in the hilum, the periaortic chains, or beyond • There has been diffuse peritoneal contamination by tumour such as by spillage of tumour beyond the flank before or during surgery, or by tumour growth that has penetrated through the peritoneal surface • Implants are found on the peritoneal surfaces • The tumour extends beyond the surgical margins either microscopically or grossly • The tumour is not completely resectable because of local infiltration into vital structures
Stage IV	Haematogenous metastases
	Deposits beyond Stage III (i.e. lung, liver, bone, and brain)
Stage V	Bilateral renal involvement at diagnosis

Table 32.2. *Staging for intracaval thrombus*

Stage Ia	Small intracaval thrombus
Stage Ib	Subintimal attached small intracaval thrombus
Stage II	Large thrombus under the liver veins level
Stage III	Thrombus extending to the liver veins junction
Stage IV	Thrombus extending to the right atrium

Diagnostic imaging techniques

The principles of imaging the child presenting with an abdominal mass are:

- Identification of the organ of origin of the lesion
- Characterization of the mass
- Assessment of extent
- Suitability for primary excisional surgery
- Detection of metastatic disease

The accepted initial investigation of the child is a plain radiograph of the chest and abdomen followed by ultrasonic examination.

Plain abdominal radiograph

On abdominal radiography, the tumour will be seen to lie predominantly in a flank displacing the bowel gas laterally or medially and inferiorly (Fig. 32.2). Very large tumours may displace the diaphragm upwards and occasionally lead to respiratory embarrassment. Calcification is rarely seen on the plain radiographs. If the tumour has ruptured into the peritoneum, there may be evidence of ascites. Other than showing the mass, the radiographic appearance is non-specific.

Intravenous urography

Prior to the availability of ultrasound and cross sectional imaging, intravenous urography (IVU) was the primary investigation for abdominal mass lesions. The appearance of a Wilms' tumour at urography is that of an intrarenal mass lesion with displacement of the collecting system by the mass (Fig. 32.3). In between 3–18% of patients[22] the kidney with the tumour is non-functional at urography due to renal vein invasion, obstructive uropathy or, rarely, complete replacement of the kidney by tumour (Fig. 32.4). Bleeding from the tumour may appear as filling defects in the calyces and renal pelvis due to clot (Fig. 32.1). The child may present with renal colic due to clot as well as haematuria. In the context of the appropriate clinical presentation the IVU appearances are characteristic. The main differential diagnosis is a renal abscess or benign cyst.

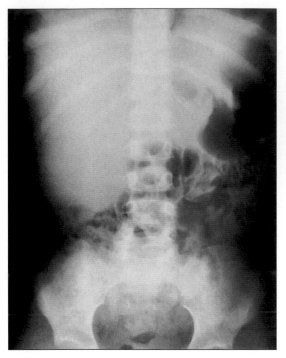

Figure 32.2. *Plain abdomen radiograph of a child with a right-sided Wilms' tumour. Clinical presentation was with an abdominal mass. Note displacement of the hepatic flexure downwards.*

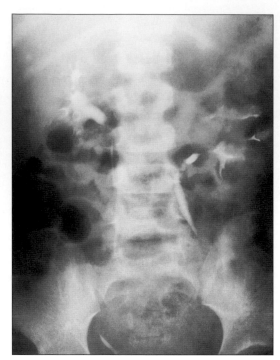

Figure 32.3. *Ten minute film of intravenous urogram. Left Wilms' tumour. Note distortion of the collecting systems mainly in the upper pole with displacement downwards of the renal pelvis and lower pole calyces which are not involved by the tumour.*

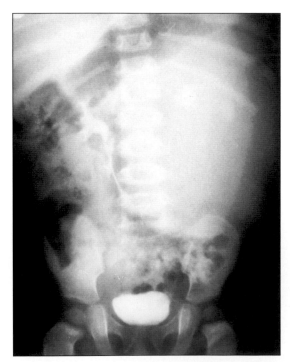

Figure 32.4. *Left Wilms' tumour. Fifteen minute intravenous urogram film. Normal right kidney. The left kidney is virtually non-functioning but is obviously enlarged.*

Ultrasound

The examination should include examination of the whole abdomen, with careful assessment of the contralateral kidney to ensure that the tumour is unilateral. Most Wilms' tumours are predominantly solid and intrarenal (Fig. 32.5) though tumour bulk will usually cause an exophytic component. Tumour necrosis and haemorrhage alter the appearance, these areas appearing either as areas of low reflectivity or increased reflectivity dependent upon the degree of haemorrhage (Fig. 32.6). The tumour usually arises intrarenally, thus distinguishing it from neuroblastoma which displaces the kidney. Careful examination will usually show a rim of more normal renal tissue around the main body of the tumour (Fig. 32.7). This compression of normal tissue may give the impression of a pseudocapsule. Calcification, seen at ultrasound in approximately 5% of patients, is usually minimal.[22] Note should be made of nodal disease which when present usually affects the periaortic region and is contiguous with the lesion. Examination of the inferior vena cava (IVC) and renal vein should be undertaken to ensure that there is no macroscopic tumour extension into them, which occurs in between 4–10% of cases (Fig. 32.8).[23] These are best examined by a combination of real time and colour Doppler modes. The tumour may be so large that it compresses the IVC, rendering it impossible to fully visualize. However, it is usually possible to see the proximal portion of the IVC where it enters the right atrium, thus ensuring that tumour thrombosis does not reach this level. Patency of a compressed IVC can be assessed using Doppler and leg vein compression but small amounts of tumour thrombosis may not be visible in a compressed renal vein or IVC.

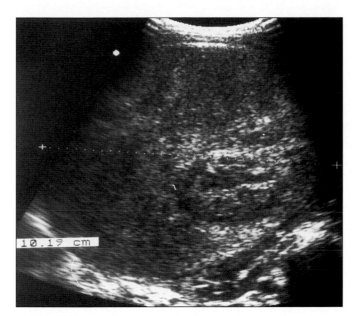

Figure 32.5. *Large left Wilms' tumour which on this ultrasound section is well encapsulated. The tumour is mainly solid. The bright echoes may represent haemorrhage or microcalcification. CT will show necrosis better.*

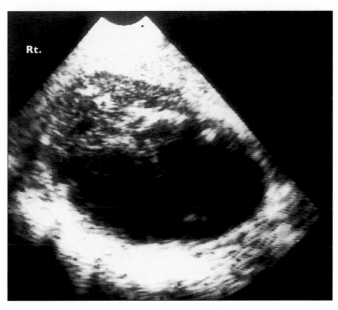

Figure 32.6. *Ultrasound scan showing large necrotic area within a Wilms' tumour at the lower pole.*

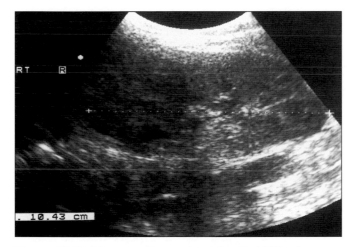

Figure 32.7. *Ultrasound scan of a right-sided Wilms' tumour involving the upper pole. Note normal lower pole architecture.*

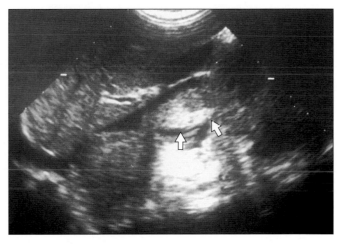

Figure 32.8. *Ultrasound scan of IVC. Note tumour thrombus in IVC (arrows).*

Liver metastases are rarely found with Wilms' tumour and are mainly associated with rhabdoid and anaplastic lesions. Wilms' tumours occasionally rupture into the peritoneum and cause ascites.

While some cystic areas, mainly due to tumour necrosis, are common in Wilms' tumour, there are rare cases of predominantly cystic Wilms' tumour (Fig. 32.9) which are ultrasonically indistinguishable from multilocular cystic

nephroma — a benign tumour. The identification of cysts within the septae is a useful feature in distinguishing neoplastic from benign renal lesions.[24]

Computed tomography

This is the usual primary cross sectional imaging technique to establish tumour extent in a format that is more easily understood by paediatricians and surgeons than ultrasound.

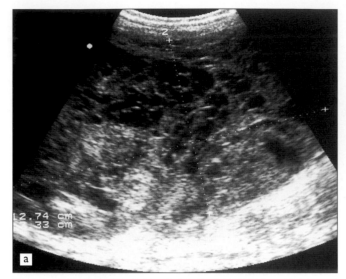

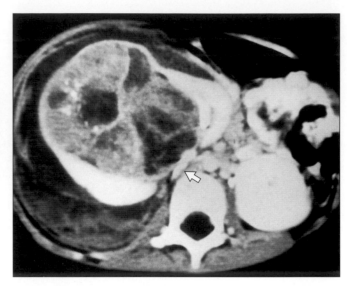

Figure 32.10. *Right-sided Wilms' tumour shown on CT scan. Note opacification of normal renal tissue medially and inferiorly following intravenous contrast medium injection. There is a perirenal collection due to rupture of the tumour capsule. The tumour solid areas are seen laterally. Medially the areas of low attenuation are due to tumour necrosis. The IVC (arrow) is patent but compressed.*

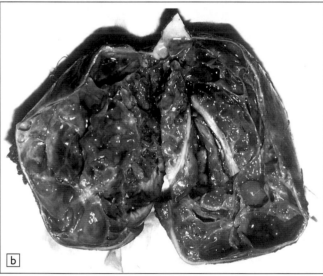

Figure 32.9. *(a) Ultrasound scan showing a large left-sided Wilms' tumour which has multiple small cysts; (b) excised specimen.*

At contrast-enhanced CT the tumour is of lower density than the normal kidney tissue (Fig. 32.10) Tumour necrosis, which may be hyperechoic due to haemorrhage and therefore mistaken as solid tumour at ultrasound, shows non-enhancement with contrast medium and is easier to appreciate than on ultrasound (Fig. 32.11). Contrast-enhanced CT should be performed using dynamic scanning commencing following injection of half the bolus. Contiguous maximum thickness slices from diaphragm to the bottom of the tumour to include both kidneys should be performed. Opacification of aorta and IVC makes it easier to appreciate nodal disease and tumour invasion of the IVC, although the latter is better demonstrated with ultrasound.

CT may give a false impression of tumour invasion of the liver due to a partial-volume effect. The dynamic movement of a right Wilms' tumour relative to the liver and therefore lack of invasion is easier to appreciate with ultrasound.

Both kidneys must be completely examined to:

- Ensure function of contralateral kidney
- To exclude nephroblastoma rests in the contralateral kidney

Magnetic resonance imaging

There are no large series reporting on the relative merits of CT versus magnetic resonance imaging (MRI) in the staging of Wilms' tumour, as both techniques are satisfactory. The known advantages of MR with direct multiplanar imaging, non-ionising radiation and excellent soft tissue contrast have little practical advantage over CT. Computed tomography is quicker, readily accessible and can frequently be carried out without sedation. Disadvantages of MRI include a longer examination time, greater cost, limited availability, increased sedation requirements and more susceptibility to degradation of images by bowel or body movement.

If MRI is undertaken, T1- and T2-weighted spin-echo sequences in axial and coronal planes, together with STIR sequences should be obtained. Contrast-enhanced images are also required. The tumour has low to intermediate

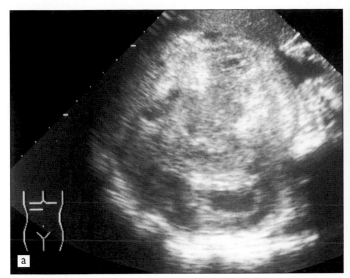

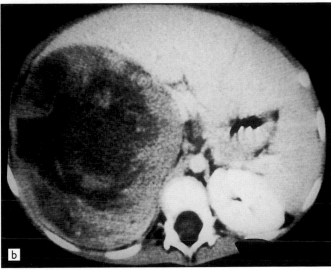

Figure 32.11. *(a) Ultrasound; (b) contrast-enhanced CT scan. Large right-sided tumour. Both examinations show an intact capsule around the tumour. At ultrasound the tumour looks* *mainly solid but is obviously necrotic on CT. The solid appearance at ultrasound is due to reflectivity from haemorrhage and necrosis.*

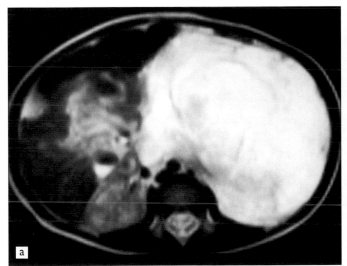

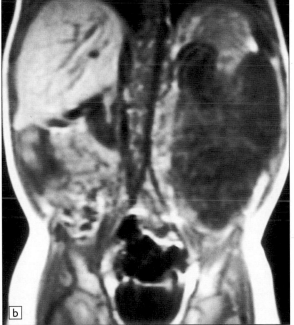

Figure 32.12. *MR images of a left Wilms' tumour. (a) Axial T2-weighted image; (b) coronal T1-weighted image. Note the heterogeneity within the mass due to areas of necrosis. The aorta and IVC are very well displayed by MRI.*

intensity on T1-weighted images with high signal intensity on T2-weighted (Fig. 32.12).[25] There is usually heterogeneity within the tumour due to areas of haemorrhage and necrosis. Fresh haemorrhage will appear as high signal intensity on T1-weighting. Tumour enhancement with Gadolinium-DTPA is inhomogeneous[26] and reflects the heterogeneity of composition of the mass.

Angiography

There is no role for preoperative angiography in the routine assessment of children with Wilms' tumour. If partial nephrectomy is being considered, especially in children with bilateral tumours, or in the case of a tumour arising in a horseshoe kidney, then vascular mapping may be indicated. A decision is made for each individual patient.

Magnetic resonance angiography (MRA) provides a potentially attractive alternative to invasive arteriography but there is still insufficient experience[27] to determine categorically whether MRA is accurate. The quality of MR angiography is now such that it is probably appropriate to carry this out initially and proceed to invasive arteriography if the information is deemed inadequate.

Magnetic resonance venography (MRV) is an alternative to ultrasound for detecting thrombus in the IVC and should be attempted if ultrasound is equivocal or inconclusive. It has been claimed that MRV is the best non-invasive method of demonstrating IVC tumour thrombus in a limited series of patients with Wilms' tumour.[28]

Radionuclide studies

There is no indication for either renal or bone studies in the routine preoperative assessment of children with Wilms' tumour. Bone scanning should only be performed if the child presents with bone pain.

Radionuclide studies are useful in establishing preoperative differential renal function in children in whom the Wilms' tumour arises in an otherwise normal kidney but also have an abnormal contralateral kidney. This provides a guide to prognosis for long-term renal function and potential need for renal dialysis or transplant.

The role of imaging: special aspects
Chest radiography and computed tomography

At diagnosis a routine chest radiograph is indicated. Metastatic disease in the lungs appears as round lesions and are present in about 10% of patients at diagnosis (Fig. 32.13). Although there is debate about the role of a staging chest CT, both in patients who have obvious metastatic disease on the radiograph and those with a normal radiograph, most radiologists would agree that chest CT should be carried out at presentation. Contiguous maximum thickness slices should be done in full inspiration to avoid small areas of basal atelectasis mimicking metastases. Many studies have found that between 7–29% of children at presentation will be plain chest film negative but CT positive.[22] Most of these will have small subpleural lesions. Debate has arisen over the staging of a patient with lung metastases seen only on CT. Distant metastases would normally upgrade staging to Stage IV and warrant more aggressive treatment, but there is inconsistency as to how CT positive/plain film negative patients are staged making comparative studies of outcome difficult to interpret.[29] The evidence appears to be that if patients are downstaged by ignoring metastatic lesions visible only on CT, there is a higher relapse rate.[29,30,31] The debate continues, and one recent study[32] suggests that neither preoperative CT of the chest or abdomen is cost effective. The authors place reliance on surgical exploration and histological proof of disease as the only truly accurate method of staging Wilms' tumour. This policy is not advocated by the author.

Caution as to the interpretation of the significance of pulmonary nodules seen on CT must be exercised in children coming from parts of the world in which other causes of pulmonary nodules are endemic, for example histoplasmosis. These difficulties usually arise in the slightly older child and not those under 3 years of age. The interpretation of the significance of a solitary non-calcified nodule in a child with Wilms' tumour also poses difficulty. If the nodule is easily accessible to percutaneous biopsy, then this should be performed. If not, there are two possible courses of action. One is thoracotomy with excision of the lesion

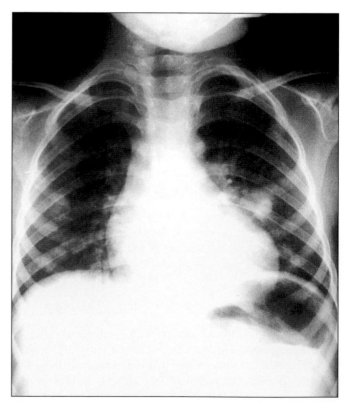

Figure 32.13. *Chest radiograph of a child with a Wilms' tumour. Note the bilateral pulmonary metastases.*

and histological examination, but with this approach there is an increased morbidity for the child. The other is to assume that the lesion is metastatic and treat accordingly with monitoring of the response of the lesion as a means of diagnosis, on the presumption that only metastatic disease will respond to chemotherapy. This is the path most frequently followed.

Percutaneous biopsy

Most children presenting with tumours which are localized to the abdomen and which are unilateral, do not have liver metastases and in whom primary surgical excision is deemed appropriate, do not require preoperative biopsy. If it is decided clinically that primary excisional surgery is not appropriate and initial treatment should be with chemotherapy, then it is desirable to have histological tumour typing before treatment.

Percutaneous biopsy has some advantages over open biopsy:

- It is relatively non-invasive
- Direct imaging control can ensure that the biopsy is made through viable and non-necrotic tissue
- The procedure can be combined with other surgical procedures, e.g. the insertion of a long line for chemotherapy

A disadvantage of percutaneous biopsy is that the tissue sample is likely to be smaller than any obtained by open biopsy. There are also rare reports of tumour seeding in the biopsy track. A decision should be agreed locally as to the most appropriate method of obtaining tissue. If the biopsy is to be percutaneous, before the procedure the radiologist must ensure that clotting studies are normal or, if abnormal, appropriate correction has taken place before the biopsy.

Key points: pulmonary metastases

- 7–29% of patients will be plain chest film negative and CT positive for subpleural/pulmonary nodules

- Downstaging by ignoring small nodules in the lungs leads to a higher relapse rate

- A solitary nodule may be benign. This should be biopsied or assumed to be metastatic and treated

---

Follow-up radiology

Following excision of the tumour, monitoring of the child during treatment for evidence of metastatic disease is by chest radiographs every 2 months while on treatment and for the first year off treatment, the intervals increasing to every 3 months for a further 1 year, and then 6 monthly and annually for a further 2 years.

Chest CT and abdominal ultrasound should be repeated on the completion of chemotherapy. Abdominal ultrasound should be performed routinely every 6 months for 2 years and further investigation by CT or MRI should be conducted if there are symptoms of:

- Abdominal pain
- Loin discomfort
- Haematuria
- Recurrent mass

Routine post-treatment CT in the asymptomatic child is not indicated.

In the child presenting with lung metastases, CT of the chest should be repeated following two courses of treatment and again on completion of treatment.

Abdominal CT during treatment to monitor response is indicated in the child in whom management of the primary tumour is by chemotherapy or in the child with bilateral disease, and should be repeated immediately before planned surgery.

Ultrasonic monitoring of the child at risk for Wilms' tumour

The question is often asked, for how long and how frequently, should the child with risk factors for developing a Wilms' tumour be monitored? There are no reliable long-term prospective trials which answer this question and most advice is based on anecdotal statements. It is well recognized that as the mass of a Wilms' tumour appears rapidly — an interval of even 6 months between sonograms will not detect lesions at a time when they are clinically silent. Ninety-five percent of children[33,34,35] with Wilms' tumour associated with hemihypertrophy syndromes will develop the tumour before his/her eighth birthday and 92% of children with aniridia develop his/her tumour under the age of 5.[33]

Most would accept that sonography at 3 monthly intervals up to the age of 5 years in children with aniridia, and 8 in children with hemihypertrophy is the best counsel if monitoring is to be undertaken. This policy has to be reviewed in the light of the likely incidence of developing a tumour and set against the expense and anxiety and inconvenience of such regular attendance at hospital. The prognosis for cure is related more to histological type than stage at presentation, those with unfavourable histology having a significantly worse prognosis. However, there is some deterioration in outlook with more advanced disease — 97% survival at 4 years with Stage I versus 82% with Stage IV.[32]

- Regular chest radiographs are essential as a survey for the detection of lung metastases up to 2 years after diagnosis

- Chest CT and ultrasound should be repeated after chemotherapy

- Abdominal ultrasound should be performed at 6 monthly intervals for 2 years

- Abdominal ultrasound should be used at 3-monthly intervals to monitor children at risk

OTHER TUMOURS OF CHILDHOOD

- Nephroblastomatosis
- Bilateral Wilms' tumour
- Wilms' tumour with unfavourable histology
- Clear cell sarcoma of the kidney (CCSK)
- Rhabdoid tumour of the kidney (RTK)
- Anaplastic Wilms' tumour
- Wilms' tumour variants
- Cystic partially differentiated nephroblastoma (CPDN)
- Renal cell carcinoma
- Renal lymphoma
- Congenital mesoblastic nephroma (CMN)

Nephroblastomatosis

Nephroblastomatosis is defined as the presence within the kidneys of nephrogenic rests which may be multifocal or diffuse. There is failure of complete maturation of the primitive nephrogenic cells.[36,37] These foci are recognized as a precursor of Wilms' tumour but the foci are themselves not necessarily malignant. Microscopic foci cannot be detected by imaging. Macroscopic foci act as space-occupying lesions within the kidney, are usually hypoechoic on ultrasound examination, but may be iso- or even hyperechoic compared with normal renal parenchyma.[36] On contrast-enhanced CT, the rests appear as foci of low attenuation within the kidney (Fig. 32.14). The kidney may be enlarged by these foci and at IVU they have an appearance similar to autosomal dominant polycystic disease or infiltration of the kidney by lymphoma, especially if they are bilateral (Fig. 32.15).[38] Ultrasound will demonstrate the non-cystic structure of the lesions. Children with bilateral Wilm's tumours have almost 100% incidence of nephroblastomatosis.[37] The tumour staging equates to that for a Wilm's without nephroblastomatosis.[37] Minor degrees are present in many children within the affected kidney with unilateral Wilms' tumour, but do not affect the staging.

Palpation of the contralateral kidney at surgery in the child with a unilateral Wilms' tumour has been the traditional way to detect nephroblastomatosis rests prior to CT, but clinical palpation will miss deep-seated intralobar rests and CT is now recognized as the most sensitive method to detect them.

There are no imaging criteria to determine whether the rests are benign or malignant. This distinction is made only by histology but it may be impossible or impractical to biopsy all the lesions. Nephroblastomatosis is usually diagnosed when the child is under investigation for a clinically apparent Wilms' tumour and is seldom discovered by serendipity. The usual management of a patient is to treat the clinically presenting Wilms' as per protocol and to biopsy accessible contralateral lesions and then to monitor the kidney by imaging surveillance. Once detected, nephroblastomatosis rests must be monitored regularly for growth, as increase in size is recognized as demonstrating malignant transformation. A suggested monitoring scheme is:

- Three monthly sonography for 1 year after diagnosis, increasing to 4-monthly intervals for a second year, then 6 monthly until the child reaches his/her 10th birthday
- Computed tomography at 6-monthly intervals for 2 years, increasing to yearly until the age of 10 years

Any change in appearance on ultrasound or change in symptoms during that period will require more intensive investigation to exclude the development of a Wilms' tumour.

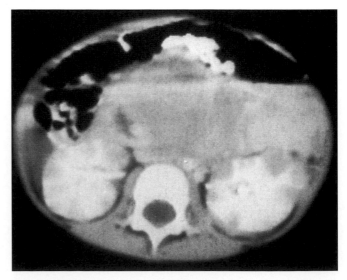

Figure 32.14. *Nephroblastoma rests appearing as focal areas of low attenuation in both kidneys on a CT scan.*

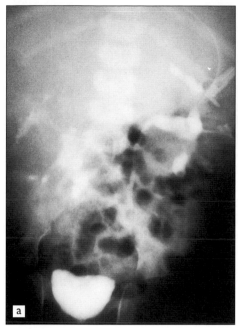

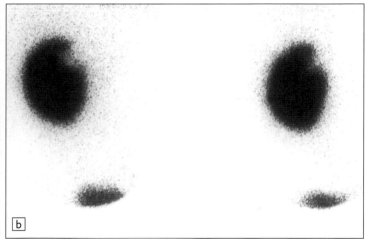

Figure 32.15. *(a) Child of 6 months with nephroblastomatosis. Note distortion of both collecting systems on the intravenous urogram. The right tumour was excised. (b) Dimercaptosuccinic acid scan after chemotherapy showing residual rest in left kidney as a photopenic area.*

Bilateral Wilms' tumour

Synchronous bilateral Wilms' tumour occurs in about 5% of all patients presenting with Wilms' tumour (Fig. 32.16).[39,40] There is a higher incidence of associated abnormalities than in the children presenting with unilateral disease. As already stated, there is an almost 100% incidence of nephroblastomatosis compared with unilateral tumours. There is a higher incidence of:

- Aniridia
- Beckwith–Wiedemann syndrome
- Genito-urinary malformation
- Hemihypertrophy[39,40]

The average age of presentation is approximately 27 months[39] almost 1 year younger than children presenting with unilateral disease. There is a reported increased incidence of bilateral Wilms' tumour in girls compared with boys.[40]

Metachronous bilateral disease, that is either a new tumour or relapse presenting in the contralateral kidney is rarer than synchronous bilateral tumours with an incidence of about 1%. Children with metachronous lesions tend to have their first presentation at about 1 year of age, much younger than the average age of presentation.[40] The disease-free interval is variable with a median time of diagnosis of the second tumour being 5 months in one series.[39] The incidence of intralobar nephroblastomatosis rests in metachronous tumours is higher than perilobar rests.[40] The imaging of bilateral tumours is similar to that for unilateral disease, but radionuclide studies which provide information about individual renal function may be useful in planning salvage surgery following initial chemotherapy. The aim of treatment is to avoid bilateral nephrectomy with the subsequent requirement for dialysis and possible transplant. The overall survival of children with bilateral tumours is high, at about 70% at 10 years[41] and 82% at 2 years.[40] As with unilateral tumours, survival is dependent on stage at presentation and histological type.

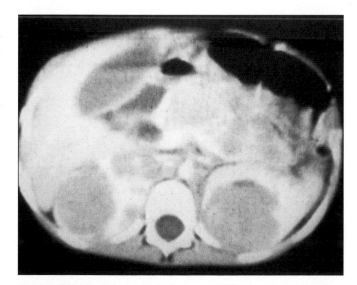

Figure 32.16. *Bilateral synchronous Wilms' tumour in a boy of 6 months shown on CT.*

Wilms' tumour with unfavourable histology

There are three types of tumour with unfavourable histology and a poor outcome which are indistinguishable from a Wilms' tumour with favourable histology on the basis of imaging the primary tumour. These are:

- Clear cell sarcoma of the kidney (bone metastasizing Wilms' tumour)
- Rhabdoid tumour of the kidney
- Anaplastic Wilms' tumour

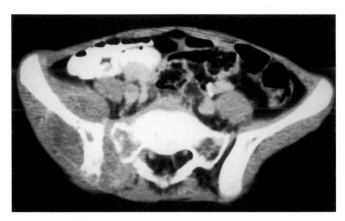

Figure 32.17. *Metastasis from a clear cell sarcoma of the kidney. Note destruction of the right hemisacrum and iliac blade with a large soft tissue mass.*

Clear cell sarcoma of the kidney

Clear cell sarcoma of the kidney (CCSK) comprise 4–6% of renal tumours in children.[37] This tumour has a high incidence of haematogenous spread with bone metastases in 60–70% of patients (Fig. 32.17).[42,43] The incidence of bone metastases in true Wilms' tumour is 2%.[42] When metastases occur they present clinically with pain. They are usually multiple, affecting the spine, pelvis and long bones, but any bone may be involved. The lesions as seen on plain radiographs are mainly destructive but sclerotic lesions have also been described.[43] The lesions are detectable by bone scintigraphy, which is indicated in any patient in whom histological examination reveals a CCSK. The prognosis for children with this type of tumour is generally poor compared with a typical Wilms' tumour with survival rates of about 40% at 2 years, but Wood et al.[42] have reported a 93% survival at 2 years using aggressive chemotherapy regimes.

Rhabdoid tumour of the kidney

This variant is regarded as the most malignant of the three tumour types with unfavourable histology.[37] Its overall incidence within the Wilms' tumour group is 2–3%.[37,42] There is a 2:1 male to female ratio. Approximately 50% of the patients present in the first 12 months of life. There is an association with midline posterior fossa primary central nervous system tumours which may present prior to the renal tumour. The tumour metastasizes via lymphatic and haematogenous spread and by direct extension. Metastases may occur in the lungs, liver, brain, bone and other sites (Fig. 32.18).

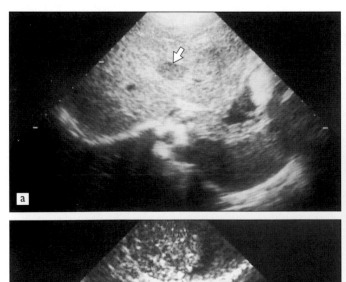

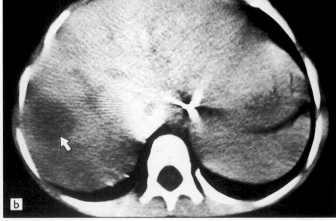

Figure 32.18. *A boy with a rhabdoid tumour of the kidney. (a) Ultrasound scan of liver; (b) CT scan of the liver showing liver metastases (arrows); (c) ultrasound scan showing a testicular metastasis in the same boy. The primary tumour was in the left kidney. It is presumed that the testicular metastasis was due to seeding down the testicular vein.*

Anaplastic Wilms' tumour

This is an histological variant of a Wilms' tumour and has no specific radiological features. It represents less than 1% of all Wilms' tumours. Metastases are predominantly to the lungs.

None of these tumours can be distinguished from a Wilms' with favourable histology on imaging criteria.

Wilms' tumour variants

Intrapelvic Wilms' tumour

Wilms' tumour most commonly arises in the renal parenchyma, but there are several reports, mainly of isolated cases, where the tumour arises mainly within the renal pelvis.[44–47] Clinical presentation is similar to a classical Wilms', with haematuria and pain being frequent. A mass may or may not be present. At imaging, there is a space-occupying lesion in the renal pelvis. The kidney may be non-functioning. The renal parenchyma is normal. Because the lesion is mainly within the collecting system and can extend down the ureter, the tumour may mimic pus and simulate xanthogranulomatosis pyelonephritis or pyonephrosis.[47]

Cystic partially differentiated nephroblastoma

Cystic partially differentiated nephroblastoma and a multilocular cystic nephroma (MCN) are difficult to distinguish on imaging grounds, the distinction being mainly made by histological examination when blastemal elements are found within the septae. Multilocular cystic nephroma is a benign lesion but CPDN may recur locally.[48] In MCN the septae are thin walled on sonography[49] and not thickened (Fig. 32.19). The following features suggest CPDN, but are not found in MCN:[20,27]

- Thickened septae
- Cysts within the septae
- Nodules

At IVU the tumour has an appearance similar to a Wilms' tumour with stretched calyces indicating an intrarenal lesion. One report of MRI in a CPDN has demonstrated the septal nature of the lesion with heterogeneity in the signal intensity from different components of the mass,[50] but as yet it is not possible to ascertain whether this is a reliable diagnostic feature. Two incidence peaks of multiloculated cystic renal tumours occur. The first is in children between 3 and 24 months of age. In this group there is a 2:1 male sex preponderance. Fifty percent of these tumours will contain blastoma and should be classified as CPDN.[48] A further group of patients with these tumours presents over the age of 30 years with an 8:1 female preponderance. The prognosis for children with CPDN is excellent.

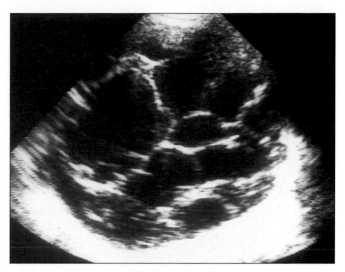

Figure 32.19. *Typical ultrasound appearance of multiloculated cystic nephroma on ultrasound.*

Renal cell carcinoma

Renal cell carcinoma is a tumour of adults with rare reports of occurrence in childhood. When this tumour does occur in children, it behaves in a similar fashion to the adult tumour.[51] The average age of presentation is 11 years but renal cell carcinoma has been described across the whole paediatric age range. On imaging criteria, the tumour cannot be distinguished from Wilms' tumour. Rarely within a Wilms' tumour rests of renal cell carcinoma may be found histologically. There are also rare reports of renal cell carcinoma arising as a recurrence following treatment of a Wilms' tumour which then carry a poor prognosis.[52]

Renal lymphoma

The kidney is a common extranodal site for lymphoma. When kidney involvement is present together with typical nodal disease, the diagnosis is obvious. Most commonly the disease is bilateral. The kidneys are enlarged and have multiple tumour deposits. At IVU, the calyces are stretched around the deposits and have an appearance resembling adult polycystic disease (Fig. 32.20). At sonography, the lesions are solid but of low echogenicity compared with the normal renal parenchyma. They are of low signal intensity on T1-weighted MR images (Fig. 32.21). Rarely lymphoma may occur unilaterally as a manifestation of relapsed disease, or as a primary presentation of the lymphoma. The appearance is that of a space-occupying lesion within the kidney. Inevitably the presumptive initial diagnosis is Wilms' tumour, especially if it occurs in the appropriate age group. The diagnosis is made by histological examination.[51,53] Renal lymphoma presenting as a solitary lesion with bony metastases may be misdiagnosed as a clear cell sarcoma of the kidney.[53]

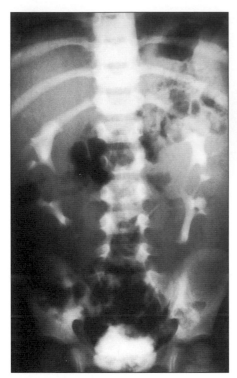

Figure 32.20. *Intravenous urogram showing lymphomatous infiltration of the kidneys. Note enlarged kidneys with marked stretching of the calyces.*

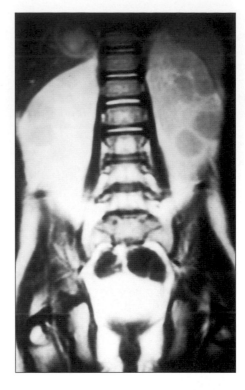

Figure 32.21. *T1-weighted MR image showing lymphoma deposits in the left kidney.*

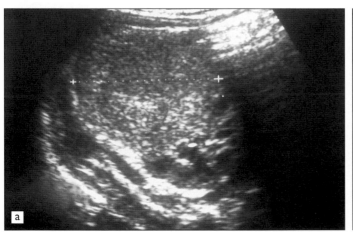

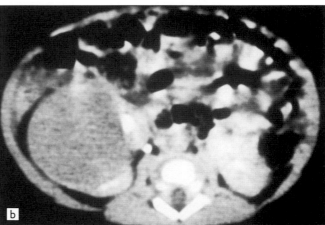

Figure 32.22. *Mesoblastic nephroma: (a) ultrasound scan; (b) CT scan. The tumour involves the upper pole of the right kidney and is solid.*

Congenital mesoblastic nephroma

Congenital mesoblastic nephroma (CMN) is the most frequent solid renal tumour in the newborn period. It is now often diagnosed antenatally when it is discovered as an incidental finding on routine fetal sonography, or when it becomes symptomatic due to its size causing obstruction to the foetal intestine with consequent polyhydramnios.[54] Post-birth, the tumour is most commonly identified by the incidental palpation of a loin mass. The child may be hypertensive and hypercalcaemia is a well recognized association.

Most CMNs are diagnosed by the age of 6 months.[54] The tumour is usually unilateral but may affect only part of the kidney. In general, it carries a very favourable prognosis and treatment is by nephrectomy alone, without adjunctive chemotherapy. Management is complicated should the tumour occur in a solitary kidney.[55]

Initial imaging is by sonography. The tumour is usually solid and well encapsulated (Fig. 32.22). Calcified and cystic components have been described but these are unusual.[54] The examination must include a survey of the contralateral kidney and the IVC and renal vein. If tumour extension into the IVC is discovered, this suggests that the lesion is not a mesoblastic nephroma but is a Wilms' or other renal tumour. On CT the mass is seen as an intrarenal space-occupying lesion indistinguishable from a Wilms' tumour. The age of the child suggests the correct diagnosis.

While the tumour is most commonly a benign lesion, aggressive forms have been reported with metastases to the brain, liver, heart and bone,[56] with many of the reported patients having atypical histology. Children with typical CMN have a mean age of presentation of 5 days while those with atypical CMN, have a mean age at diagnosis of 5 months.[57]

COMPLICATIONS OF TREATMENT OF WILMS' TUMOUR

The complications may be regarded as those that occur acutely during chemotherapy and are in the main related to the effects of immunosuppression or late complications. The former are discussed in Chapter 31 on the general principles of oncological imaging in children. In this section the late complications will be discussed.

Hepatotoxicity and radiation hepatitis

The development of hepatotoxicity due to radiation hepatitis or radiation-induced veno-occlusive disease in children who undergo abdominal irradiation during chemotherapy especially with adriamycin and actinomycin D is a rare acute complication of treatment of children with Wilms' tumour. This has become rarer since the current management of children with Wilms' infrequently involves combined radiotherapy and chemotherapy.

Radiation hepatitis is dose related and is more frequently seen with right-sided tumours than left, due to the likelihood of increased liver volume being injured.[58] The children present clinically with hepatomegaly, icterus and ascites. The median time of onset of liver toxicity is 6.5 weeks.[58] On ultrasound examination, the liver is initially enlarged, and has an altered echotexture. Ascites is present. As portal hypertension develops, splenic enlargement occurs. There is alteration in portal venous flow, as seen on Doppler studies. Sulphur colloid radionuclide studies demonstrate partial or complete photopenia of the liver with splenic enlargement due to portal hypertension. The outcome is generally good, with recovery of hepatic function, but portal hypertension with all its consequences may persist.

This author has seen one patient who presented 18 years after nephrectomy and liver radiation with sclerosing cholangitis, presumably a result of the radiotherapy. Liver toxicity may also occur from chemotherapy, in particular, dactinomycin and doxorubicin, with changes in liver enzymes and thrombocytopenia.[59]

Lungs

Pulmonary irradiation for metastatic disease can result in lung damage with reduced vital capacity, and was reported by Wohl et al. to be 72% of predicted values.[60] Lung function can be further reduced by thoracotomy for excision of metastases. Serial evaluation of patients showed progression up to 48 months following treatment.[61]

Kidney

Compensatory hypertrophy of the contralateral kidney occurs following unilateral nephrectomy. Abdominal irradiation which includes the contralateral renal parenchyma or the renal artery may result in impaired renal function or renal artery stenosis.[59] Renal artery stenosis can lead to hypertension. The stenosis may require angioplasty. Nephrotoxic chemotherapeutic agents may also result in impaired renal function with reduced creatinine clearance.

There have been reports[62,63] of patients with Wilms' tumours and unilateral nephrectomy, chemotherapy and local irradiation developing proteinuria and hypertension 10–20 years later. Hypertension, although it can occur following radiation-induced renal artery stenosis, is not found more frequently in survivors of Wilms' tumour than in the normal population. Patients who have bilateral tumours who have significantly diminished residual renal parenchyma may progress to chronic renal failure but usually not until late childhood or adulthood.[64]

Skeletal system

- Rickets
- Scoliosis
- Osteochondroma

Rickets

Treatment with ifosfamide may result in tubular defects of sufficient severity to result in rickets (Fig. 32.23). The kidneys usually recover but any persisting skeletal deformity of rickets may require corrective orthopaedic surgery.[65,66]

Scoliosis

A well-recognized complication of nephrectomy with associated radiotherapy is scoliosis which may be severe enough to require corrective surgery.[67] This is often accompanied by hemiatrophy (Fig. 32.24). The investigation of such a scoliosis is by radiographic surveillance with plain radiographs.

Osteochondroma

Osteochondromas may develop in the radiation field and therefore in children may be found on the ribs or lower scapular blade.

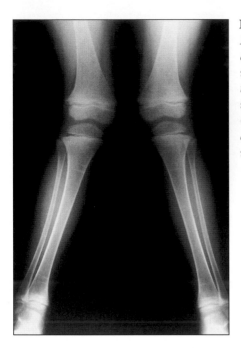

Figure 32.23. *Bowing of the legs as a result of rickets secondary to treatment with ifosfamide. Corrective osteotomies were required.*

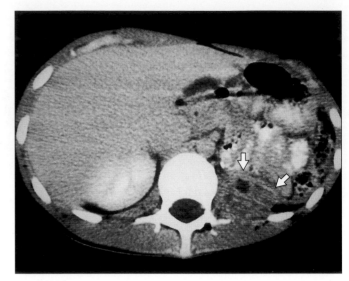

Figure 32.24. *CT scan showing postirradiation hemiatrophy of the left side of the abdomen. Left nephrectomy. There is a recurrent tumour (arrows) in the left psoas muscle.*

Reproductive organs

Whole abdominal irradiation in childhood may result in ovarian failure and amenorrhoea. Pregnancy outcome in those who conceive is less successful following childhood irradiation, with low birth weights and an increase in perinatal deaths.[68,69] There is no increase in congenital abnormalities and there is not an increased incidence of Wilms' tumour in the offspring of survivors.[70]

Testicular function is also adversely affected by irradiation even in those patients in whom the scrotum is excluded from the radiation field or covered by 3 mm lead.[71]

Second malignant neoplasm

A recent study[72] has calculated that the cumulative risk for a second malignant neoplasm following treatment for Wilms' tumour was 1.6% at 15 years, this risk being increased by adjunctive therapy with abdominal irradiation and potentiated by doxorubicin. The neoplasms reported can be divided into those which occurred directly in the radiation field and those distant from this. The solid tumours in the radiation field included:

- Breast
- Hepatocellular carcinoma
- Thyroid cancer
- Skin neoplasms
- Colonic adenocarcinoma
- Osteosarcoma
- Chondrosarcoma

Most of the lesions not directly in the radiation field were either lymphoma or myeloid leukaemia. The radiology of these lesions is identical to that of these tumours arising *de novo*. The topic is discussed in more detail in Chapter 47.

Key points: complications

- Radiation hepatitis is rare now that chemotherapy is the preferred treatment

- Liver toxicity may occur with chemotherapy, particularly dactinomycin and doxorubicin

- Pulmonary irradiation and metastectomy reduce lung function

- Compensatory hypertrophy of a contralateral kidney follows unilateral nephrectomy. Irradiation may impair renal function or induce renal artery stenosis. Chemotherapy may also impair renal function

- Patients with bilateral tumours may progress to chronic renal failure due to significantly diminished ring parenchyma

- Rickets may result from treatment with ifosfamide and scoliosis is seen following radiotherapy. Osteochondromas may develop in the irradiation field

- Abdominal radiation may result in ovarian and testicular dysfunction

- The cumulative risk for a second malignancy is 1.6% at 15 years

Summary

- Wilms' tumour is the most common renal tumour of childhood with a peak incidence between 6 months and 4 years.

- Bilateral tumours are seen in 5–10% of children.

- Two gene mutations lead to the development of Wilms' tumour and several distinct syndromes are also associated with it.

- Contrast-enhanced CT is the primary imaging technique for staging the primary tumour.

- Ultrasound is the best technique for detecting inferior vena caval and renal vein involvement.

- MR angiography has a potential role in determining vascular anatomy and MR venography for detecting inferior vena caval tumour.

- Metastases are predominantly to the lungs and routine CT of the chest is recommended.

- Routine follow-up with chest radiographs and ultrasound should be performed for at least 4 years following primary tumour resection.

- Nephroblastomatosis represents nephrogenic rests which may be focal or diffuse and are the precursors of Wilms' tumour.

- Wilms' tumour with unfavourable histology is indistinguishable from Wilms' tumour with favourable histology on imaging.

- Congenital mesoblastic nephroma is the most frequent solid renal tumour in the newborn. Malignancy is uncommon but occasionally it metastasizes to a distant site.

- Late complications of treatment include hepatotoxicity, pulmonary damage, renal impairment and musculo-skeletal growth abnormalities.

REFERENCES

1. Coppes M J, Williams B R G. The molecular genetics of Wilms' tumour. Cancer Invest 1994; 12: 57–65
2. Webber B L, Parham D M, Drake L G et al. Renal tumours in childhood. Pathol Annual 1992; 27: 191–232
3. Marina N M, Krance R, Ribeiro R C et al. Diagnosis and treatment of the most common solid tumours in childhood. Primary Care Diag Treatment 1992; 19: 871–889
4. Coppes M J, De Kraker J, Van Dijken P J et al. Bilateral Wilms' tumour — long term survival and some epidemiological features. J Clin Oncol 1989; 7: 310–315
5. Stiller C A, McKinney P A, Bunch K J et al. Childhood cancer and ethnic group in Britain: a United Kingdom Children's Cancer Study Group (UKCCSG) study. Br J Cancer 1991; 64: 543–548
6. Julian J C, Merguerian P A, Shortliffe L M D. Pediatric genitourinary tumours. Curr Op Oncol 1995; 7: 265–274
7. Smyth T B, Shortliffe L M D. Pediatric genitourinary tumours. Curr Opin Oncol 1990; 2: 507–513
8. Knudson A G, Strong L C. Mutation and cancer: a model for Wilms' tumour of the kidney. J Natl Cancer Instit 1972; 48: 313–324
9. Shochat S J. Wilms' tumour: diagnosis and treatment in the 1990s. Semin Pediatr Surg 1993; 2(1): 59–68
10. Denys P, Malvaux P, van den Berghe H et al. Association d'un syndrome au anatompathologique de pseudohermaphroditisme masculin, d'une tumeur de Wilms' d'une nephropathie parenchymateuse et d'un mosaicism xx/xy. Arch Francaises Pediatr 1967; 24: 729–739
11. Buyukpamukcu M, Kutluk T, Buyukpamukcu N et al. Renal tumours with pseudohermaphroditism and glomerular disease. Acta Oncol 1992; 31: 745–748
12. Schmitt K, Zabel B, Tulzer G et al. Nephropathy with Wilms' tumours or gonadal dysgenesis: incomplete Denys–Drash syndrome or separate diseases? Eur J Pediatr 1995; 154: 577–581
13. Yamaguchi T, Fukuda T, Uetani M et al. Renal cell carcinoma in a patient with Beckwith–Wiedemann syndrome. Pediatr Radiol 1996; 26: 312–314
14. Grundy R G, Pritchard J, Baraitser M et al. Perlam and Wiedemann–Beckwith syndromes: two distinct conditions associated with Wilms' tumour. Eur J Pediatr 1992; 151: 895–898

15. Smith P J, Sullivan M, Algar E et al. Analysis of paediatric tumour types associated with hemihyperplasia in childhood. Paediatr Child Health 1994; 30: 515–517

16. Cohen M D. Biological approach to tumour imaging. Semin Paediatr Surg 1992; 1: 308–313

17. Caty M G, Shamberger R C. Abdominal tumours in infancy and childhood. Pediatr Clin North Am 1993; 40: 1253–1271

18. Navoy J F, Royal S A, Vaid Y N et al. Wilms' tumour: unusual manifestations. Pediatr Radiol 1995; 25: 76–86

19. Jose B, Nakayan P L, Pietsch J B et al. Budd–Chiari syndrome secondary to hepatic vein thrombus from Wilms' tumour: case report and literature review. J Kentucky Med Assoc 1989; 87: 174–176

20. Arens R, Frand M, Rechavi G et al. Radiological cases of the month. Am J Dis Child 1992; 146: 1091–1092

21. Daum R, Roth H, Zachariou Z. Tumour infiltration of the vena cava in nephroblastoma. Eur J Pediatr Surg 1994; 4: 16–20

22. Babyn P, Owens C, Gyepes M et al. Imaging patients with Wilms' tumour. Hematol Oncol Clin North Am 1995; 9: 1217–1252

23. Federici S, Galli G, Ceccarelli P L et al. Wilms' tumour involving the inferior vena cava: preoperative evaluation and management. Med Pediatr Oncol 1994; 22: 39–44

24. Duncan A W, Charles A K, Berry P J. Cysts within septa: an ultrasound feature distinguishing neoplastic from non-neoplastic renal lesions in children? Pediatr Radiol 1996; 26: 315–317

25. Lubat E, Weinreb J C. Magnetic resonance imaging of the kidneys and adrenals. Topics Magnet Reson Imag 1990; 2: 17–36

26. Gylys-Morin V, Hoffer F A, Kozakewich H et al. Wilms' tumour and nephroblastomatosis: imaging characteristics at gadolinium-enhanced MR imaging. Radiology 1993; 188: 517–521

27. Ferrer F A, Mckenna P H, Donnal J F. Non-invasive angiography in preoperative evaluation of complicated pediatric renal masses using phase contrast magnetic resonance angiography. Urology 1994; 44(2): 254–259

28. Weese D L, Applebaum H, Taber P. Mapping intra-vascular extension of Wilms' tumor with magnetic resonance imaging. J Pediatr Surg 1991; 26: 64–67

29. Cohen M D. Commentary. Imaging and staging of Wilms' tumours: problems and controversies. Pediatr Radiol 1996; 26: 307–311

30. Williams J A, Douglass E C, Magill H L et al. Significance of pulmonary computed tomography at diagnosis of Wilms' tumour. J Clin Oncol 1988; 6: 1144–1146

31. Cohen MD. Review: staging of Wilms' Tumour. Clin Radiol 1993; 47: 77–81

32. Ditchfield M R, De Campo J F, Waters K D et al. Wilms' Tumour: a rational use of preoperative imaging. Med Pediatr Oncol 1995; 24: 93–96

33. Beckwith J B. In: Questions and answers. Am J Roentgenol 1995; 164: 1291–1295

34. Green D M, Breslow N E, Beckwith J B et al. Screening of children with hemihypertrophy, aniridia, and Beckwith–Wiedemann syndrome in patients with Wilms' tumour: a report from the National Wilms' Tumour Study. Med Pediatr Oncol 1993; 21: 188–192

35. Garber J E, Diller L. Screening children at genetic risk of cancer. Curr Opin Pediatr 1993; 5: 712–715

36. White K S, Kirks D R, Bove K E. Imaging of nephro-blastomatosis: an overview. Radiology 1992; 182: 1–5

37. White K S, Grossman H. Wilms' and associated renal tumours of childhood. Pediatr Radiol 1991; 21: 81–88

38. Papadopoulou F, Efremidis S C, Gombakis N et al. Nephroblastomatosis: the whole spectrum of abnormalities in one case. Pediatr Radiol 1992; 22: 598–599

39. Shearer P, Parham D M, Fontanese J et al. Bilateral Wilms' tumour. Review of outcome, associated abnormal-ities, and late effects in 36 pediatric patients treated at a single institution. Cancer 1993; 72: 1422–1426

40. Ritchey M L, Coppes M J P. The management of synchronous bilateral Wilms' tumour. Hematol Oncol Clin North Am 1995; 9: 1303–1315

41. Coppes M J, de Kraker J, van Dijken P L et al. Bilateral Wilms' tumor: Long term survival and some epidemio-logical features. J Clin Oncol 1989; 7: 310–315

42. Wood D P, Kay R, Norris D. Renal sarcomas of childhood. Urology 1990; 36: 73–78

43. Gururangan S, Wilimas J A, Fletcher B D. Bone metastases in Wilms' tumour — report of three cases and review of literature. Pediatr Radiol 1994; 24: 85–87

44. Engel R M. Unusual presentation of Wilms' tumour. Urology 1976; 8: 288–289

45. Chen-Kuang N, Wei Fen C, Jiin-Haur C et al. Intrapelvic Wilms tumour: report of 2 cases and review of the literature. J Urol 1993; 150: 936–939

46. Weinberg A G, Currarino G, Hurt G E. Botryoid Wilms' tumour of the renal pelvis. Arch Pathol Lab Med 1984; 108: 147–148

47. Groeneveld D, Robben S G F, Meradji M et al. Intra-pelvic Wilms' tumour simulating xanthogranulomatous pyelonephritis. Pediatr Radiol 1995; 25: 68–69

48. Agrons G A, Wagner B J, Davidson A J et al. Multilocular cystic renal tumour in children: radiologic–pathologic correlation. RadioGraphics 1995; 15: 653–669

49. Garrett A, Carty H, Pilling D W. Multilocular cystic nephroma: report of three cases. Clin Radiol 1987; 38: 55–57

50. Abara O E, Liu P, Churchill B M et al. Magnetic resonance imaging of cystic partially differentiated nephroblastoma. Urology 1990; 36: 424–427

51. Levine C, Levine E. Small pediatric renal neo-plasms detected by CT. J Comput Assist Tomogr 1990; 14: 615–618

52. Allsbrook W C, Boswell W C, Takahashi H et al. Re-current renal cell carcinoma arising in Wilms' tumour. Cancer 1991; 67: 690–695

53. Capps G W, Das Narla L. Renal lymphoma mimicking clear cell sarcoma in a pediatric patient. Pediatr Radiol 1995; 25: 87–89

54. Fernbach S K, Feinstein K A. Renal tumours in children. Semin Roentgenol 1995; 333: 200–217

55. Nicholson D A, Gupta S C. Case report: congenital mesoblastic nephroma occurring in a solitary kidney. Clin Radiol 1990; 41: 211–218

56. Schlesinger A E, Rosenfield N S, Castle V P et al. Congenital mesoblastic nephroma metastatic to the brain: a report of two cases. Pediatr Radiol 1995; 25: 73–75

57. Chan H S, Mancer K, Weitzman S S et al. Congenital mesoblastic nephroma: a clinico-radiologic study of 17 cases representing the pathologic spectrum of the disease. J Pediatr 1987; 111: 64–70

58. Flentje M, Weirich A, Optter R et al. Hepatotoxicity in irradiated nephroblastoma patients during postoperative treatment according to SIOP9/GPOH. Radiother Oncol 1994; 31: 222–228

59. Green D M, Donckerwolcke R, Evans A E et al. Late effects of treatment for Wilms' tumour. Hematol Oncol Clin North Am 1995; 9: 1317–1337

60. Wohl M E, Griscom N T, Traggis D G et al. Effects of therapeutic irradiation delivered in early childhood upon subsequent lung function. Pediatrics 1975; 55: 507–516

61. Benoist M R, Lemerle J, Jean R et al. Effects on pulmonary function of whole lung irradiation for Wilms' tumour in children. Thorax 1982; 37: 175–180

62. Inglefinger J R, Colvin R B. Case records of the Massachusetts General Hospital (Case 17–1985). N Engl J Med 1985; 312: 1111

63. Welch T R, McAdams A J. Focal glomerulosclerosis as a late sequela of Wilms' tumour. J Pediatr 1986; 108: 105–109

64. Ritchey M L, Green D M, Thomas P et al. Renal failure in Wilms tumor patients: a report from the National Wilms' Tumor Study Group. Med Pediatr Oncol 1996; 26: 75–80

65. Skinner R, Pearson A D J, Price L et al. Nephrotoxicity after ifosfamide. Arch Dis Child 1990; 65: 732–738

66. Sweeney L E. Hypophosphataemic rickets after ifosfamide treatment in children. Clin Radiol 1993; 47: 345–347

67. Evans A E, Norkool P, Evans I et al. Late effects of treatment for Wilms' tumour. A report from the National Wilms' Tumour Study Group. Cancer 1991; 67: 331–336

68. Hawkins M M, Smith R A. Pregnancy outcomes in childhood cancer survivors: probable effects of abdominal irradiation. Int J Cancer 1989; 43: 399–402

69. Li F P, Gimbrere K, Gelber R D et al. Outcome of pregnancy in survivors of Wilms' tumour. J Am Med Assoc 1987; 257: 216–219

70. Byrne J, Mulvihill J J Connelly R R et al. Reproduc-tive problems and birth defects in survivors of Wilms' tumour and their relatives. Med Pediatr Oncol 1988; 16: 233–240

71. Shalet S M, Beardwell C G, Jacobs H S et al. Testicular function following irradiation of the human prepubertal testis. Clin Endocrinol (Oxford) 1978; 9: 483–490

72. Breslow N E, Takashima J R, Whitton J A. Second malignant neoplasms following treatment for Wilms' tumour: a report from the National Wilms' Tumour Study Group. J Clin Oncol 1995; 13: 1851–1859

Chapter 33

Neuroblastoma

Claire Dicks-Mireaux

INTRODUCTION

Neuroblastomas are tumours of sympathetic nervous tissue of unknown aetiology and, with the exception of infants under the age of 1 year, the prognosis is poor. Imaging plays a crucial role in the determination of stage and is extremely important as, the stage of the disease, the site of the tumour and the age of the patient at the time of diagnosis are all important predictors of response.[1] Despite its poor prognosis, neuroblastoma has the ability to regress spontaneously and also to mature to benign ganglioneuroma.[2] It therefore remains an intriguing and enigmatic tumour which poses many challenges to scientists, oncologists, pathologists and radiologists.

INCIDENCE

Neuroblastoma is the most common extracranial malignant tumour of childhood. It accounts for 8–10% of all childhood cancers. The incidence is about one case per 8000 live births and there are about 515 newly diagnosed cases of neuroblastoma in the US annually.[3,4] The median age at diagnosis of children with neuroblastoma is 22 months. About 35% of patients are under 1 year of age; 80% are under 4 years and 95% are under 10 years of age.

PATHOLOGY AND PROGNOSIS

Neuroblastoma arises from primitive sympathetic neuroblasts of the embryonic neural crest and consists of small round cells with scanty cytoplasm, often arranged in clusters resembling rosettes. Macroscopically, neuroblastomas average 6–8 cm in size, are lobulated and often haemorrhagic. Microscopically, the tumour may be difficult to differentiate from other tumours made up of small round cells, such as Ewing's sarcoma, primitive neuro-ectodermal tumour, rhabdomyosarcoma, leukaemia and lymphoma.

Half the tumours arise in the adrenal medulla, about 30% in the pelvis or visceral ganglia, paraganglia or in the organ of Zuckerkandl, and about 20% in the thorax or neck.[4]

There is a spectrum of disease from malignant undifferentiated neuroblastoma to well differentiated ganglioneuroma with a high degree of maturation. Tumours may consist of both mature and undifferentiated elements and are then called ganglioneuroblastoma.

Shimada et al. in 1984[5] produced a scheme whereby histological criteria are used to define tumour as stroma-poor or stroma-rich on the basis of neuritic or neuromatous content. The stroma-poor group is further classified on the basis of age at diagnosis, degree of maturation and frequency of mitosis, and the stroma-rich group into well-differentiated, mixed and nodular. The stroma-poor group is associated with a worse prognosis than the stroma-rich group.

Genetic features of the tumour cells may also have prognostic significance. Expression of the *N-myc* oncogene and amplification of the *N-myc* region on the chromosome indicate a poor prognosis and more advanced stage of disease.[6] Other genetic features such as chromosome number, chromosome 1p deletion, the DNA index, and expression of the nerve growth receptor TRK-A may have prognostic significance. Certain characteristic serum and urinary tumour markers occur in neuroblastoma which have diagnostic significance. Approximately 90% of children with neuroblastoma will have elevated levels of urine or serum catecholamine metabolites (vanillylmandelic acid VMA, homovanillic acid HVA, and dopamine).[7] Other serum markers are less specific but also have prognostic significance. These include serum ferritin, lactic dehydrogenase and neuron-specific enolase.

DIAGNOSIS

In most cases, tissue diagnosis is based on conventional staining with haematoxylin and eosin using light microscopy. Electron microscopy or immunohistological examination can also establish the diagnosis.

The diagnosis may also be made on the basis of bone marrow involvement (detected by bone marrow biopsy or trephine) combined with significantly raised serum or urinary catecholamines or metabolites (VMA and HVA). True-cut core

Table 33.1. *The three major staging systems for neuroblastoma in use until 1988*

Evans[9]	
Stage I	Tumour confined to the organ or structure of origin
Stage II	Tumour extending in continuity beyond the organ or structure or origin but not crossing the midline. Regional lymph nodes on the homolateral side may be involved
Stage III	Tumours extending in continuity beyond the midline. Regional lymph nodes bilaterally may be involved
Stage IV	Remote disease involving bone, parenchymatous organs, soft tissues or distant lymph node groups, or bone marrow
Stage IV–S	Patients who would otherwise be Stage I or II but who have remote disease confined to one or more of the following sites: liver, skin or bone marrow (without evidence of bone metastases)

Hayes[10]	
Stage A	Complete gross excision of primary tumour, margins histologically negative or positive. Intracavitary lymph nodes not intimately adhered to and removed with resected tumour are histologically free of tumour. If primary is in abdomen (including pelvis), liver is histologically free of tumour
Stage B	Incomplete gross resection of primary. Lymph nodes and liver histologically free of tumour as in Stage A
Stage C	Complete or incomplete gross resection of primary. Intracavitary nodes histologically positive for tumour. Liver histologically free of tumour
Stage D	Disseminated disease beyond intracavitary nodes (i.e. bone marrow, bone, liver, skin or lymph nodes beyond cavity containing primary tumour)

TNM[11]		
Stage I	T1	Single tumour, <5 cm in diameter
	N0	No evidence of lymph node involvement
	M0	No evidence of distant metastases
Stage II	T2	Single tumour, >5 cm but <10 cm
	N0	No evidence of lymph node involvement
	M0	No evidence of distant metastases
Stage III	T1/2	As above
	N1	Regional lymph node involvement
	M0	No evidence of distant metastases
	T3	Single tumour, >10 cm
	Any N	Regional lymph nodes involved/not involved/cannot be assessed
	M0	No evidence of distant metastases
Stage IVA	T1/2/3	As above
	Any N	As above
	M1	Evidence of distant metastases
Stage IVB	T4	Multiple simultaneous tumours
	Any N	As above
	Any M	Distant metastases evident/not evident/cannot be assessed

T, primary tumour; N, regional lymph nodes; M, metastases.

needle biopsies performed as an open or closed procedure with imaging guidance are acceptable for diagnosis,[8] but fine-needle aspiration is thought to be suboptimal.

CLINICAL PRESENTATION

The clinical presentation varies depending on the site of tumour and extent of disease. Non-specific signs and symptoms may include fever, irritability, weight loss and anaemia. Patients, not uncommonly, present with abdominal distension due to a large abdominal mass. Additional presenting complaints include anorexia, vomiting, back pain and paraplegia. Localized tumours in the thorax may be asymptomatic and discovered incidentally on a chest radiograph. Paraspinal tumours in the chest or abdomen may present with acute neurological symptoms, such as increasing limb weakness with eventual paralysis, due to spinal cord compression, following extension of the tumour into the spinal canal.

Cervical neuroblastoma presents as a neck mass, occasionally resulting in dysphagia, airway compromise, Horner's syndrome or heterochromia of the iris. Primary cerebral neuroblastoma is rare and, similar to other intracranial malignancies, presents with signs and symptoms of raised intracranial pressure.

At least 70% of patients will have disseminated disease at the time of diagnosis and may present with symptoms and signs secondary to metastatic spread to bone, bone marrow, skin and liver, such as pathological fractures or skin nodules. Metastatic disease affecting the orbits results in proptosis and periorbital bruising giving a characteristic racoon-like appearance. Other more unusual clinical presentations include intractable diarrhoea, sweating, hypertension and cerebellar encephalopathy, typically opsomyoclonus (dancing eyes), all attributable to metabolic and immunological disturbances associated with the tumour.

In infants presenting under the age of 12 months, massive hepatomegaly and raised bluish skin nodules may be seen. These patients, despite the presence of metastatic disease, are not particularly unwell, unless the hepatomegaly causes respiratory distress, and have a relatively good prognosis requiring little or no treatment.

STAGING AND PROGNOSIS

Up until 1988, three major staging systems were in use. (summarized in Table 33.1). The two most important criteria used in staging by the Evans' system[9] are tumour extension across the midline and the presence of metastases. In the Hayes' system,[10] regional lymph node involvement replaces extension across the midline as a criterion for

Stage-III disease. The UICC-TNM system[11] stages according to size of the primary tumour, presence of lymph node involvement and distant metastases. Staging by the Hayes' and TNM systems requires biopsy or excision of macroscopically abnormal lymph nodes at surgery.

In an attempt to combine these different factors and provide a uniform system for the organization and interpretation of clinical studies, the International Neuroblastoma Staging System (INSS)[12,13] has recently been formulated (Table 33.2). All of these staging systems include the surgical findings at initial presentation.

The INSS distinguishes between ipsilateral and contralateral lymph node involvement, the latter being a criterion for Stage-3 disease, and categorizes a midline tumour as Stage 3.

Table 33.2. *The International Neuroblastoma Staging System (INSS)*

Stage 1	Localized tumour with complete gross excision, with or without microscopic residual disease; representative ipsilateral lymph nodes negative microscopically
Stage 2a	Localized tumour with incomplete gross excision; representative ipsilateral non-adherent lymph nodes negative for tumour microscopically
Stage 2b	Localized tumour with or without complete gross excision, with ipsilateral non-adherent lymph nodes positive for tumour. Enlarged contralateral lymph nodes must be negative microscopically
Stage 3	Unresectable unilateral tumour infiltrating across the midline, with or without regional lymph node involvement; or localized unilateral tumour with contralateral regional lymph node involvement; or midline tumour with bilateral extension by infiltration (unresectable) or by lymph node involvement
Stage 4	Any primary tumour with dissemination to distant lymph nodes, bone, bone marrow, liver, skin and/or other organs (except as defined for Stage 4S — see below)
Stage 4S	Localized primary tumour (as defined for Stage 1, 2a or 2b), with dissemination limited to skin, liver, and/or bone marrow (limited to infants less than 1 year of age)
Stages 1, 2a and 2b	Defined by the surgical and pathological findings at diagnosis. Imaging has a crucial role in the assessment of Stages 3 and 4, as surgery, if possible, is delayed and follows treatment with chemotherapy

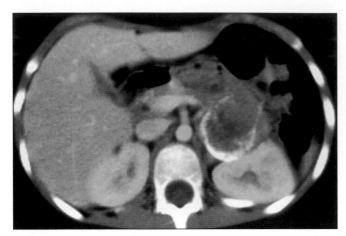

Figure 33.1. *Partially calcified Stage-1 abdominal neuroblastoma extending up to, but not beyond, the midline.*

The definition of the *midline* in Stage 3 merits clarification. The vertebral column is considered as the midline; only tumours which extend by continuous invasion to, or beyond, the opposite side of the vertebral body are classified as Stage 3 (Fig. 33.1). The absence of bony metastases as demonstrated by a negative isotope bone scan is essential for the diagnosis of Stage 4S.

PROGNOSIS

Prognosis is correlated with pathological and clinical features. Pathological features include: the degree of differentiation of the tumour,[5] stromal content,[14] degree of mitosis and *N-myc* oncogene amplification.[6,15] Clinical factors affecting survival include the patient's age, site of tumour and stage of disease. Currently, 5-year survival of patients is as follows:

- Stage 1 — 94%
- Stage 2 — 90%
- Stage 3 — 64%
- Stage 4 — 24%, with only modest improvement in the last three decades
- Stage 4S — 75%

Younger people have a better prognosis. When all stages are combined, 75% of children under 1 year of age survive compared with 20% of children over 1 year of age.[3,4]

TREATMENT

The treatment of neuroblastoma is determined by the stage of the tumour at diagnosis. Patients with Stage 1 and 2 tumours are candidates for primary surgical resection. If the tumour is very large, encases vessels and is thought to be unresectable, and if metastatic disease is present, treatment is with chemotherapy, initially, to shrink the tumour and eradicate metastatic deposits. Surgery may be necessary if the tumour requires debulking and is compressing a vital organ.[16] Once unresectable tumours decrease sufficiently in volume, and all metastatic disease is cleared, delayed surgical resection is performed. Following this, any residual tumour is treated with one or a combination of the following: chemotherapy, radiation therapy and total body irradiation followed by autologous bone marrow transplantation. Treatment with radiolabelled metaiodobenzylguanidine (MIBG) has been assessed and responses to localized bulky disease have been documented.

Key points: incidence, prognosis, staging

- Neuroblastoma is the most common extracranial malignant tumour of childhood

- 80% of tumours occur under 4 years of age

- Approximately 80% of tumours occur in the abdomen, 50% in the adrenal medulla

- Approximately 90% of tumours result in elevated VMA, HVA and dopamine

- At least 70% of patients have disseminated disease at the time of diagnosis

- The International Neuroblastoma Staging System (INSS) is now the most widely used staging classification

- Prognosis depends not only on stage but also on differentiation, stromal content, *N-myc* oncogene amplification, patient's age and the site of the tumour

IMAGING

Imaging is used to identify the primary tumour, to demonstrate its extent and to detect metastatic disease. Subsequently, imaging has an important role in assessing response to treatment, the detection of recurrent disease and late sequelae of treatment.

Imaging in detection
The imaging examination used to detect neuroblastoma varies with its location.

Abdominal neuroblastoma
Any child with an abdominal mass should have an ultrasound scan initially to confirm the presence of a solid mass and to

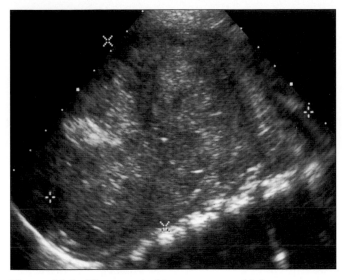

Figure 33.2. *Ultrasound of large tumour with heterogeneous echo pattern and calcification.*

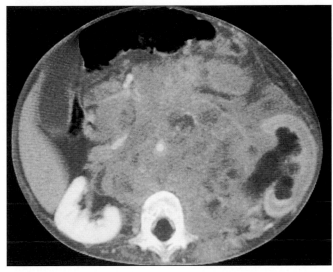

Figure 33.3. *Extensive NBL with encasement and displacement of aorta, inferior vena cava and left kidney.*

exclude a cystic lesion. This should be followed by computed tomography (CT) or magnetic resonance imaging (MRI).

Ultrasound

Ultrasound will demonstrate a large, poorly defined, central abdominal or suprarenal mass with a heterogeneous echo pattern (Fig. 33.2). The heterogeneity apparently reflects the frequent foci of microcalcification, haemorrhage and necrosis. Calcific deposits with acoustic shadows may be present. The kidney is displaced laterally and inferiorly and is separate from the mass, distinguishing between neuroblastoma and the other important abdominal tumour in this age group — Wilms' tumour.

In the new-born, neuroblastomas may be predominantly cystic or anechoic.[17] This appearance reflects either degenerative change in the tumour or, in some cases, clusters of microcysts in the tumour cells on pathological section. Unfortunately, this appearance is non-specific and can mimic adrenal haematoma, another common lesion of the neonate. Differentiation requires demonstration of metastatic disease or positive laboratory studies, i.e. VMA analysis, or serial sonographic examination.

Computed tomography

The role of ultrasound in the diagnosis of neuroblastoma is primarily confirmation of the presence of a mass lesion. Other studies are needed to determine the extent of disease. Either CT or MRI can validate the plain radiographic or sonographic findings. Both studies are comparable in determining the presence of tumour. On CT, neuroblas-

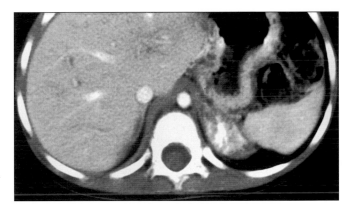

Figure 33.4. *Small calcified abdominal tumour.*

toma appears as a homogeneous or heterogeneous, pararenal, soft tissue mass with lobulated margins[18–22] The tumour enhances less than that of surrounding tissues after intravenous administration of contrast material. Calcifications within the tumour, which may be coarse, mottled, solid or ring-shaped, are observed in approximately 85% of abdominal neuroblastomas and in 50% of thoracic tumours on CT. Computed tomography with intravenous injection of contrast medium will demonstrate the full extent of the tumour more clearly than ultrasound and confirm the characteristic displacement and encasement of vessels (Fig. 33.3). Smaller Stage-1 and -2 tumours are clearly delineated and calcification is also demonstrated (Fig. 33.4).

Magnetic resonance imaging

On T1-weighted MR images, neuroblastoma appears either hypointense or isointense relative to the liver.[23,24] On T2-weighted sequences, it appears slightly to markedly hyperintense relative to liver (Fig. 33.5). The centre of the tumour may be heterogeneous, reflecting calcification, haemorrhage or necrosis.[25–27] Prevertebral extension across the midline with vascular encasement is characteristic, and hepatic metastases, intraspinal extension, and renal invasion or infarction may also be seen.[28] Following surgery or chemotherapy, CT or MRI can be used to monitor treatment response and detect recurrent disease.

Imaging in staging

The staging of neuroblastoma requires radiological studies and marrow aspiration to determine the extent of local disease and distant spread. The choice of the most appropriate treatment protocol for an individual patient with neuroblastoma depends on non-operative, radiological methods for provision of staging information. The same principles that apply to staging can be used for follow-up examinations. The principal morphological parameters that influence disease control and patient survival are: the site of tumour: encasement of vascular structures; lymph node involvement; and haematogenous dissemination (chiefly to bone or to bone marrow and occasionally to liver).

Both local and distant extent of tumour need to be determined. With respect to local disease, the diagnostic questions that need to be answered are:

- Is there midline extension
- Vascular encasement
- Regional lymph node enlargement
- Intraspinal extension?

Midline extension and lymphnode enlargement are important because they change stage. Vessel encasement is of significance because it is a contraindication to primary surgical resection. Intraspinal extension will require urgent preoperative chemotherapy and sometimes decompressive laminectomy if clinical signs of cord compression are present.

Choice of technique

Plain radiographs and intravenous urography are now rarely used to diagnose and stage abdominal neuroblastoma. A plain film of the abdomen may show some helpful features, such as stippled or mottled calcification in up to 55% of patients (Fig. 33.6), displacement of bowel gas, paravertebral widening, bone destruction, and widened interpedicular distances indicating extension of tumour into the spinal canal. Intravenous urography will demonstrate displacement of the kidney, laterally and inferiorly, without distor-

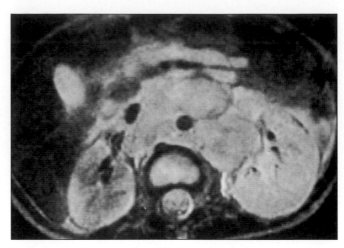

Figure 33.5. *Axial T2-weighted MR image of abdominal NBL with encasement and displacement of aorta and inferior vena cava.*

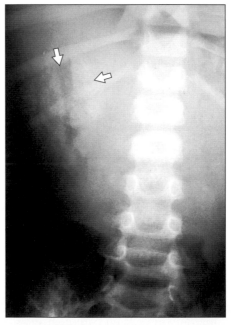

Figure 33.6.
Plain radiograph of calcified right suprarenal neuroblastoma (arrowed) with retrocrural nodes and metastases in right iliac wing.

tion of the calyces or renal pelvis. Only approximately two-thirds of neuroblastomas are demonstrated with intravenous urography and additional disadvantages are an inability to measure the size of the mass, difficulty in demonstrating vessel encasement and extension across the midline, and an inability to demonstrate lymph node or liver involvement.

Ultrasound is seldom able to demonstrate the full extent of a very large tumour. It has limited value in demonstrating involvement of retroperitoneal and retrocrural nodes and is unable to detect extension into the spinal canal.[18]

The appropriate choice of CT or MRI has been the subject of continuing debate. Unfortunately, there are no large prospective series that compare MR and CT in neuroblastoma for staging accuracy. CT with contrast enhancement can reliably demonstrate the primary tumour and it is superior to MRI in demonstrating calcification. However, based on small series in the literature, MRI appears to be superior to CT in determining the full extent of local disease. These advantages relate to its multiplanar imaging capability and superb contrast resolution (Fig. 33.7).

In 20 patients at Great Ormond Street Hospital, who had both CT and MR at diagnosis, staging of local disease was more accurate with MRI due to more accurate demonstration of nodal disease and the ability to show vertebral marrow abnormalities not seen on CT. With MRI findings alone, disease was correctly staged in 75% of patients fully-staged at diagnosis. The choice of technique is therefore often governed by the availability of equipment and need for anaesthesia.

Local disease: imaging characteristics

Midline extension or vascular encasement occurs in more than 30% of tumours. Midline extension is defined as tumour extending to or across the contralateral pedicle. Vascular encasement is defined as a mass of soft tissue attenuation or intermediate signal intensity surrounding the aorta, superior mesenteric artery and vein, inferior vena cava, or right or left renal artery and vein (Fig. 33.3). Detection of midline extension is important because it alters staging and upgrades the disease to Stage 3. Vascular encasement affects management not staging.

Adenopathy is another indicator of local spread of tumour, occurring in abut 30% of patients with neuroblas-toma. Lymph node involvement is defined as discrete masses of soft tissue attenuation or intermediate signal intensity separate from the main tumour mass. Detection of nodal disease is important because it alters stage. Ipsilateral nodes correspond to a Stage-2 disease. Contralateral tumour indicates Stage-3 tumour.

Intraspinal extension of neuroblastoma occurs in about 15% of patients and is defined as a mass of soft tissue attenuation or intermediate signal intensity within the spinal canal (with or without cord displacement) that is contiguous with the main tumour mass.[28] Detection of intraspinal extension is important as the possibility of cord compression requires urgent treatment with chemotherapy and steroids to shrink the tumour and reduce swelling of the cord. This is particularly well documented on MRI (Fig. 33.8).

Distant disease: imaging characteristics

The second part of the staging procedure is determination of the distant extent of disease. Detection of distant metastases upstages the tumour to a Stage-4 or 4S. Neuroblastoma metastasizes to liver, cortical bone, and bone marrow. Skin metastases occur in 20–25% of tumours, almost always in association with Stage-4S disease. Hepatic metastases occur in 5–10% of children with neuroblastoma, usually in Stage-4S disease and rarely in Stage-4 disease. Skeletal metastases are found in over half of the children with neuroblastomas.[29] These can involve cortical bone or bone marrow. For practical purposes, differentiation is not possible on the basis of imaging studies. In fact, the two probably coexist. For the purpose of this presentation, cortical metastases and marrow metas-tases will be considered as one and referred to as skeletal metastases.

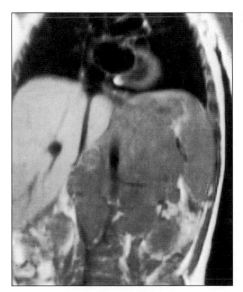

Figure 33.7. *Coronal T1-weighted MR image of abdominal NBL with encasement of major vessels.*

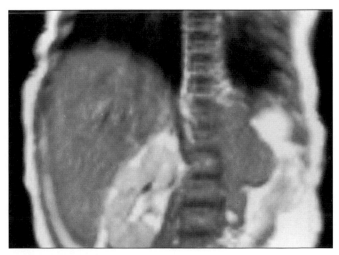

Figure 33.8. *Coronal T1-weighted MR image of left paraspinal tumour in a neonate.*

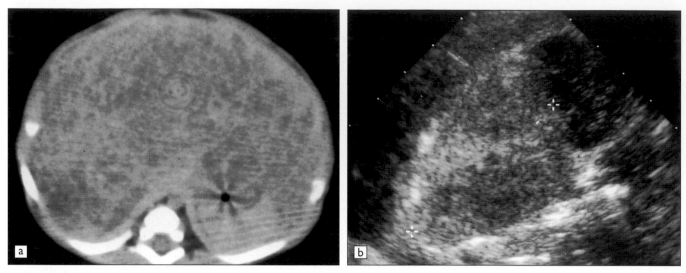

Figure 33.9. *Neuroblastoma 4S: (a) CT scan of diffuse liver infiltration and (b) ultrasound of small suprarenal primary.*

Hepatic metastases have a varying appearance depending on patient age. In older infants and children, the lesions tend to be well-defined and may be single or multiple. These lesions are equally well recognized on CT and MRI. Hepatic metastases in a patient under 1 year or age are more often diffuse, ill-defined and infiltrate the liver. When associated with a small renal primary this is Stage-4S (Fig. 33.9). Magnetic resonance appears superior to CT in detecting and determining extent of hepatic metastases in neonates.

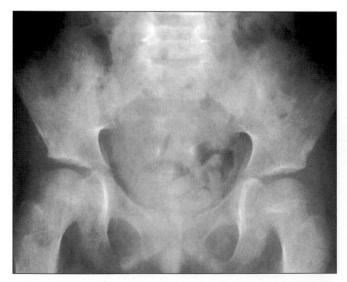

Figure 33.10. *Osteopenia with abnormal trabecular pattern due to diffuse marrow infiltration.*

Skeletal and bone marrow metastases

Neuroblastoma is the commonest paediatric tumour to metastasize to bone. Skeletal metastases occur in 50–60% of patients.[29] Whilst plain radiographs are not routinely used in the detection of bony metastases, the initial presentation to hospital in some patients may be with bone pain, and, therefore, it is important to recognize the appearances of neuroblastoma metastases on plain film. A generalized reduction in bone density and a mottled trabecular pattern due to marrow infiltration (Fig. 33.10) is seen sometimes with erosions, pathological fractures and periosteal reactions.

Characteristically, metastatic disease to the orbit with proptosis is demonstrated on CT and MR as soft tissue masses adjacent to involvement of the sphenoid wing with bony destruction and a spiculated periosteal reaction (Fig. 33.11a and b).

Rarely the presentation of a child with periorbital bruising and fractures with little obvious cause has led to an erroneous diagnosis of non-accidental injury due to failure to recognize metastatic neuroblastoma on skeletal radiographs. Skull radiographs demonstrate sutural diastasis and irregularity of the sutures secondary to infiltration of the meninges.

Isotope bone scanning with Tc-99m labelled dimercaptophosphonate (MDP) is the method of choice in the detection of bone metastases and many studies indicate that it is more sensitive than a conventional skeletal survey, detecting 50–70% more sites of disease.[30] The sensitivity of radionuclide imaging in detecting occult metastases is reported to be about 90% compared with a sensitivity of between 35 and 70% for radiographic skeletal survey.[30,31] Metastases will appear either as focal areas of increased radiopharmaceutical accumulation (Fig. 33.12); rarely, as photopenic or cold

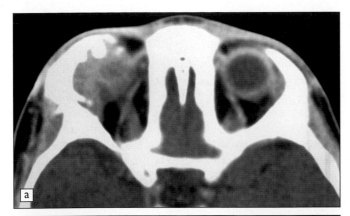

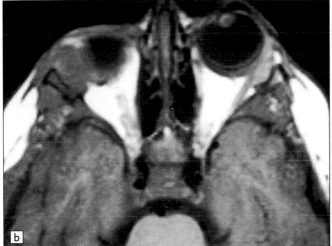

Figure 33.11. *Orbital neuroblastoma deposit. (a) CT scan of orbital metastasis with right sphenoid wing involvement; (b) MR image of same patient.*

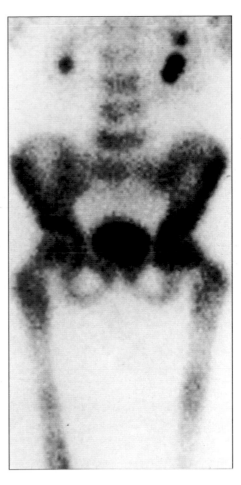

Figure 33.12. *Tc-99m MDP scan — extensive metastatic disease involving lumbar spine, iliac wing and femora.*

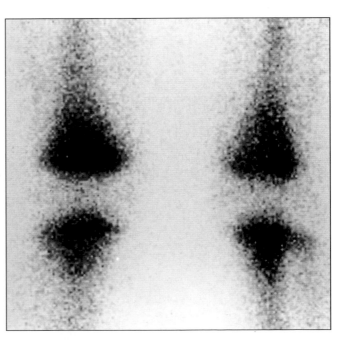

Figure 33.13. *Tc-99m MDP scan — bilateral, symmetrical knee involvement.*

lesions, and also as symmetrical metaphyseal uptake. This last characteristic pattern is produced by an appearance of blurring of the normally sharply demarcated epiphyseal growth plate and requires careful technique and positioning of the child, since it is often bilateral and symmetric, and may be mistakenly considered normal (Fig. 33.13). Lesions are also seen in the skull, facial bones, orbits, ribs and vertebral bodies. Abnormal activity is seen in the primary tumour and in bone, bone marrow and soft tissue metastases (Fig. 33.14). Cortical bony metastases often appear more focal than the diffuse appearance of marrow involvement (Fig. 33.15).

There are several other imaging techniques that are occasionally useful in an adjunctive setting for staging disease, particularly for assessing skeletal metastases. These include MRI,[32] MIBG imaging,[32–36] In-111 pentetreotide[37–39] and positron emission tomography (PET).[40]

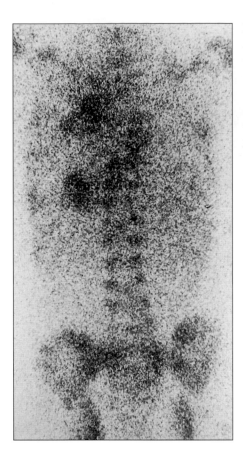

Figure 33.14.
Posterior image — MIBG scan, extensive marrow involvement and uptake in left suprarenal primary.

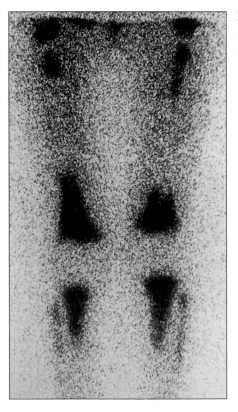

Figure 33.15.
MIBG scan — bilateral bony metastases.

MIBG was developed in the 1980s and has been shown to be extremely useful in imaging neuroblastoma. This agent is available in two forms: I-131 MIBG and I-123 MIBG. Both agents have a sensitivity for detection of the primary tumour of 90% or greater.[33] I-131 MIBG has a sensitivity of 70% or greater for detection of skeletal metastases.[36] Its major disadvantage is poor resolution. By comparison, I-123 MIBG has an 80–95% sensitivity for detection of skeletal metastases.[34] Its major drawbacks are cost and lack of availability. Abnormal activity is seen in the primary tumour and in bone, bone marrow and soft tissue metastases (Fig. 33.14). Cortical bony metastases often appear more focal than the diffuse appearance of marrow involvement (Fig. 33.15). MIBG often detects bone and bone marrow disease at diagnosis and at follow-up, not demonstrated by MDP bone scans, plain radiographs or marrow biopsy.[41]

Gordon et al.[34] found eight false-negative results with I-123 MIBG when compared with Tc-99m MDP in 44 children with neuroblastoma. Therefore, in some units both MIBG and Tc-99m MDP scans are used in the detection of skeletal metastases, whereas in others only MIBG scans are performed; in the latter a Tc-99m MDP scan will only be conducted if the MIBG scan is negative. The latter is the recommendation in the INSS for the detection of bony disease.

Magnetic resonance imaging is also playing an increasing role in the detection of marrow metastases.[32] Small series have shown that MRI has a sensitivity of approximately 85% in diagnosing skeletal metastases in neuroblastoma. The diagnosis of marrow metastases is based on either focal or diffuse change in marrow signal. On T1-weighted images, marrow disease produces a low signal intensity (Fig. 33.16). On T2-weighted and fat saturation images, the signal intensity increases. There are two limitations of MRI. First, it studies only a limited area. Secondly, the MRI findings are non-specific; normal or hyperplastic red marrow can have a similar appearance.

Corbett et al. reported that MIBG and MR showed abnormalities in 33% of cases not detected by bone marrow biopsy.[42] Occasionally, neuroblastoma will not take up MIBG and a negative scan is obtained. This is the case in some of the more mature tumours and also some very undifferentiated tumours.

The newest imaging studies for diagnosing metastases are In-111 pentetreotide (octreotide) and PET imaging with 2-[F-18] fluoro-2-deoxy-D-glucose (18-FDG). In-111 pentetreotide is a somatostatin receptor. It has a 80–100% sensitivity for detection of the primary tumour.[37,39] In addition to being useful for diagnosis, octreotide has the potential to provide information about prognosis. In small series, patients with receptor-positive tumours had 100% one-year survival, while those with receptor-negative tumours had <60% one-year survival.[37,39] Its limitation is that experience with skeletal metastases is unavailable. Larger, prospective studies are needed to assess the usefulness of octreotide for staging distant disease.

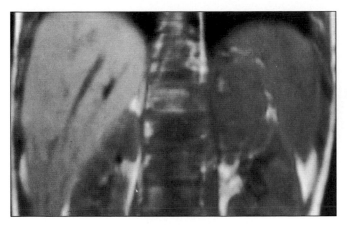

Figure 33.16. *Coronal T1-weighted MR image — left suprarenal NBL and vertebral body marrow metastases.*

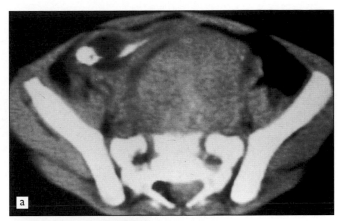

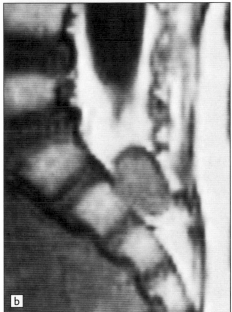

Figure 33.17. *(a) CT scan of pelvic NBL with extension into sacral foramina. (b) MR image of same patient.*

Key points: imaging of abdominal tumours

■ Ultrasound is used predominantly to confirm the presence of a mass lesion; CT and MRI are used to stage the disease

■ In the newborn, neuroblastomas are often cystic

■ The essential staging features that need to be assessed on CT/MRI are the presence of midline extension, vascular encasement, regional lymph node enlargement and intraspinal extension

■ There are no large series that compare CT with MRI for staging accuracy in neuroblastomas

■ Midline extension occurs in 50% of cases and is defined on CT/MRI as tumour extending to or across the contralateral pedicle

■ Tc-99m labelled MDP is the method of choice for detecting skeletal metastases

■ Several other imaging techniques play an adjunctive role in assessing skeletal metastases, including MIBG and MRI. In-111 pentetreotide and PET with 18-FDG are still being evaluated

EXTRA-ABDOMINAL TUMOURS

Pelvic neuroblastoma

Pelvic tumours are frequently presacral in location and are usually situated above or behind the bladder. Erosion of the sacrum and bony pelvis and extension into the lateral pelvic side walls, sacral foramina and sciatic notches is not uncommon and clearly seen on CT (Fig. 33.17a). The differential diagnosis includes pelvic rhabdomyosarcoma.

Thoracic neuroblastoma

A thoracic neuroblastoma is almost always paravertebral within the posterior mediastinum and may be associated with rib and vertebral body erosion and displacement. Approximately 25% demonstrate calcification (Fig. 33.18). A chest radiograph will demonstrate the tumour but CT and MR imaging will be required to show any extension into the spinal canal. Tumours may be asymptomatic and fairly small and well-defined, with mature histology and a good prognosis. As many thoracic neuroblastomas are Stage 1 or 2, and therefore amenable to treatment with surgical excision, it is important to look carefully at the extent of the tumour in relation to the vertebral bodies on the CT and MR images

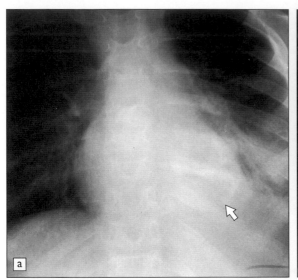

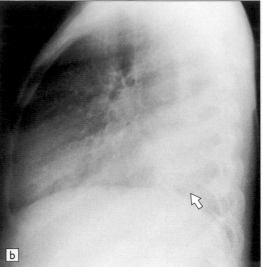

Figure 33.18.
Posteroanterior (a) and lateral (b) chest radiographs of calcified left paravertebral tumour (arrowed).

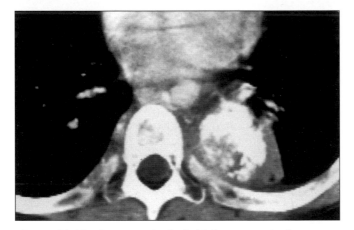

Figure 33.19. *CT scan of calcified left paravertebral tumour.*

(Fig. 33.19). The tumours may be small and encapsulated, or large and demonstrate vascular encasement and extension into the spinal canal.

Coronal MR imaging clearly demonstrates spinal involvement which may extend over several segments and, therefore, should be the imaging modality of choice. The differential diagnosis includes other causes of posterior mediastinal masses such as neurenteric and enteric duplication cysts and thoracic meningocoeles.

Cervical and apical neuroblastoma

Neuroblastoma presenting as a solid neck mass should be imaged with CT or MRI. If an ultrasound scan is performed, an irregular solid echogenic mass will be seen. Calcification is common. Displacement and compression of the pharynx and trachea with involvement of the carotid artery and jugular vein, and extension through the skull base into the infratemporal fossa is seen. It may be difficult to distinguish a cervical neuroblastoma from a rhabdomyosarcoma arising in the neck.

Cerebral neuroblastoma

Primary cerebral neuroblastoma is best imaged with MRI, or CT if MRI is unavailable. A cystic lesion with peripheral solid tumour or a mass with heterogeneous contrast enhancement is shown. Approximately 50% of tumours show calcification on CT. Extension outside the cranial vault and distant metastases are rare. Intracerebral neuroblastoma are usually considered in the spectrum of primitive neuro-ectodermal tumours and the conventional staging system is not applicable.

Key points: extra-abdominal tumours

■ Pelvic tumours are frequently presacral

■ Thoracic neuroblastomas are often Stage I or II and amenable to surgical excision

■ MRI is advisable to show extension into the spinal canal

■ Cerebral neuroblastoma rarely extend outside the cranial vault

RESPONSE TO TREATMENT

The International Neuroblastoma Response Criteria (INRC) were established in 1988 and subsequently modified

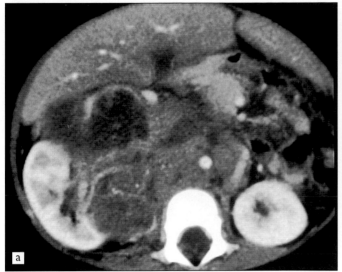

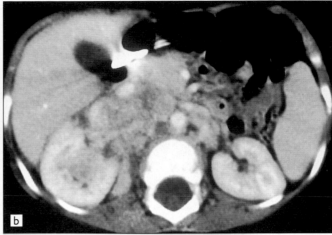

Figure 33.20. *CT scans pre- (a) and postchemotherapy (b) demonstrating greater than 50% shrinkage.*

in 1993. Response to treatment consists of response of the primary tumour and also the metastatic sites. The primary tumour is evaluated by CT and/or MRI and, because of the difficulties in making accurate measurements of a tumour with an irregular shape, it is recommended that the volume (rather than the product of the two largest diameters) should be used to assess response (Figs. 33.20a and 33.20b). Metastases are evaluated with MIBG scans, Tc-99m bone scans, CT and/or MR for the liver and lymph nodes, and bilateral posterior iliac crest marrow aspirates and trephine biopsies.

A complete response (CR) indicates complete disappearance of all primary and metastatic disease. A very good partial response (VGPR) indicates a 90–99% volume reduction in the primary tumour with clearing of all measurable metastatic disease. The only exception to this would be residual abnormalities on technetium bone scan attributable to incomplete healing of the bone at sites of previous metastases. The MIBG scan should be negative at all metastatic sites. A partial response (PR) indicates a greater than 50% reduction in both the primary tumour and all measurable metastatic sites. No response (NR) indicates a less than 50% reduction of some or all measurable lesions, but no increase of greater than 25% and no new lesions. Progressive disease (PD) indicates a greater than 25% increase in any pre-existing lesion or any new lesion.

Most tumours that are going to respond to treatment, do so by 3–4 months and therefore it is recommended that response is assessed at approximately 4 months from the initiation of chemotherapy, with an interim evaluation at approximately 2 months. Further evaluation at the end of

chemotherapy is recommended to determine the response to the particular drug regimen. The final response to treatment should be determined at the end of all treatment including delayed surgery.

Recurrent disease

There is little evidence that routine imaging of patients with disseminated disease following treatment is of benefit. Routine ultrasound, CT and isotope scans have not detected asymptomatic relapse and treatment for relapsed disseminated disease is poor. Therefore, routine regular follow-up is not recommended in these patients. Patients with localized disease should be followed up with appropriate chest radiography, CT and/or MRI.

Symptomatic relapse is best confirmed with plain radiographs, a Tc-99m MDP bone scan, an abdominal ultrasound, and demonstration of abnormal catecholamine levels in the urine.

Complications and late effects of neuroblastoma and its treatment

Some of the complications seen in neuroblastoma are not unique to this tumour. They include late effects of chemotherapy, radiotherapy and surgery. Chemotherapy with iphosphamide has been demonstrated to cause renal tubular damage and rickets resulting in bone pain which must be distinguished from recurrent disease (Fig. 33.21).[43] Extensive spinal surgery to remove tumour eventually leads to spinal scoliosis (Fig. 33.22).

Second malignant neoplasms such as phaeochromocytoma, brain tumours, acute leukaemia and renal cell carcinoma have been reported.

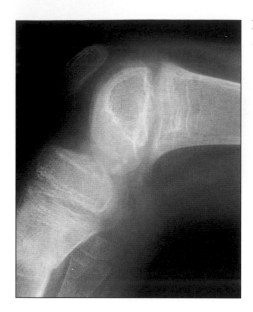

Figure 33.21. *Rickets.*

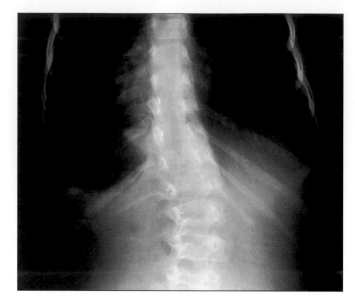

Figure 33.22. *Scoliosis associated with extensive laminectomy.*

Key points: follow-up

■ Measurement of response requires monitoring change in the primary tumour and in the metastases

■ The primary tumour, lymph nodes and liver metastases are monitored using CT and metastases using MIBG, Tc-99m bone scans and bone marrow biopsies

■ Response is assessed at approximately 4 months after initiation of chemotherapy, with an interim evaluation at approximately 2 months

■ Complications of the treatment of childhood tumours with radiotherapy, chemotherapy and surgery can all cause confusion on imaging

SPECIAL SITUATIONS

Myoclonic encephalopathy of infancy ('dancing-eyes' syndrome)

This clinical syndrome which includes opsoclonus, myoclonus, and cerebellar ataxia may be associated with neurogenic tumours of ganglion cell origin. The incidence of neurogenic tumours with myoclonic encephalopathy of infancy (MEI) is unknown, although it has been suggested that almost half of the children with MEI have associated neuroblastoma, ganglioneuroblastoma or ganglioneuroma. However, only 2% of patients with neuroblastoma have MEI. Patients with MEI must be evaluated for a neurogenic tumour even though the incidence is low. Neuroblastoma with MEI has a better prognosis than classic neuroblastoma.

Approximately 50% will have tumours in the posterior mediastinum and therefore a chest radiograph is essential. MIBG scanning is also suggested to locate a tumour prior to more specific imaging with ultrasound and CT. A negative MIBG scan with a normal CXR and normal abdominal ultrasound examination should indicate the absence of an occult neuroblastoma.

Antenatal neuroblastoma

Neuroblastoma *in situ* has been described in foetuses[44–47], with an incidence suggesting that many resolve spontaneously without progression to disease in childhood. The Japanese have advocated routine spot urine catecholamine screening of all neonates, but studies in Europe have not demonstrated any significant benefit from mass screening and early detection of tumours. Small suprarenal masses have been demonstrated in foetuses at routine antenatal ultrasound scans which have been thought to be neuroblastoma. Close clinical and radiological follow-up postnatally has demonstrated spontaneous resolution in all of these cases, confirming the benign nature of these antenatal tumours.

FUTURE CONSIDERATIONS

Neuroblastoma presents a complex and challenging problem with a poor response to treatment in many cases. Imaging has a well established role in diagnosis but new strategies must be developed in order to follow tumour response to treatment and to better determine prognosis.

With advances in PET technology, PET imaging may become more readily available for children. 2-[F-18]

fluoro-2-deoxy-D-glucose (18-FDG) imaging with PET provides an assessment of tumour metabolism and could play a clinical role in evaluating tumour response to treatment.[48]

Tumour spectroscopy with MRI has so far proved disappointing but may in the future prove to be helpful. Image registration and sophisticated computer software should enable radiologists to measures tumour volumes more accurately and to identify areas of active disease by combining anatomical and functional information.

Summary

- Neuroblastoma is the most common extracranial malignant tumour of childhood, accounting for 8–10% of all childhood cancers.

- Although in most cases the diagnosis is based on conventional staging with haematoxylin and eosin using light microscopy, it can also be made on the demonstration of bone marrow involvement combined with significantly raised urinary catecholamines or metabolites (VMA and HVA).

- 3 major staging systems have been in use, but the recently promulgated International Neuroblastoma Staging System is now the most widely used.

- The features that are essential for staging the tumour that need to be assessed on imaging are the presence of midline extension, vascular encasement, regional lymph node enlargement and intraspinal extension.

- Ultrasound is seldom used to demonstrate the full extent of a large tumour — this requires either CT or MRI.

- Although there are no large prospective series comparing CT with MRI for staging accuracy, MRI appears superior to CT in determining the full extent of local disease, and in showing vertebral abnormalities and intraspinal extension.

- Imaging is vital in the detection of distant metastases. For example, skeletal metastases occur in over half the children with neuroblastoma and Tc-99m-labelled MDP and MIBG remain the techniques of choice in their detection. MRI also plays a complementary role in the detection of bone lesions.

- The International Neuroblastoma Response Criteria (1993) require that the volume of the primary tumour, the liver and lymph nodes be evaluated by CT and/or MRI, and that metastases be evaluated with MIBG scans and Tc-99m MDP bone scans and the bone marrow by bilateral iliac crest marrow aspirates and trephine biopsies.

REFERENCES

1. Pritchard J, Kemshead J. Neuroblastoma. Recent developments in assessment and management. Recent Results in Cancer Res 1983; 88: 69–78

2. Pritchard J, Hickman J A. Why does stage 4S neuroblastoma regress spontaneously? Lancet 1994; 344: 869–870

3. Brodeur G M. Neuroblastoma and other neuroectodermal tumours. In: Fernbach D J, Vietti T J (eds) Clinical Pediatric Oncology. St Louis: C V Mosby Co, 1991; 437–464

4. Hayes F A, Smith E I. Neuroblastoma. In: Pizzo P A, Poplack D G (eds) Pediatric Oncology. Philadelphia: J B Lippincott Co, 1989; 607–622

5. Shimada H, Chatten J, Newton W A Jr et al. Histopathological prognostic factors in neuroblastic tumours: Definition of subtypes of ganglioneuroblastoma and an age-linked classification of neuroblastomas. J Natl Cancer Ins 1984; 73: 405–413

6. Look A T, Hayes A, Shuster J J et al. Clinical relevance of tumour cell ploidy and *N-myc* gene amplification in childhood neuroblastoma: A paediatric oncology group study. J Clin Oncol 1991; 9: 581–591

7. Friedland G W, Crowe J E. Neuroblastoma and other adrenal neoplasms. In: Parker B R, Castellino R A (eds) Pediatric Oncologic Radiology. St Louis: C V Mosby Co, 1977; 267–300

8. Hoffer F A, Chung T, Diller L et al. Percutaneous biopsy for prognostic testing of neuroblastoma. Radiology 1996; 200: 213–216

9. Evans A E, D'Angio G J, Randolph J. A proposed staging for children with neuroblastoma. Children's Cancer Study Group A. Cancer 1971; 27: 374–378

10. Hayes F A, Green A A, Hustu H O, Kumar M. Surgicopathologic staging of neuroblastoma: Prognostic significance of regional lymph node metastases. J Pediatr 1983; 102 59

11. UICC-TNM. Classification of malignant tumours (4th ed). Berlin: Springer Verlag, 1987

12. Brodeur G M, Seeger R C, Barrett A et al. International criteria for diagnosis, staging and response to treatment in patients with neuroblastoma. J Clin Oncol 1988; 6: 1874–1881

13. Brodeur G M, Pritchard J, Berthold F et al. Revision of the international criteria for neuroblastoma diagnosis, staging and response to treatment. J Clin Oncol 1993; 11: 1466–1477

14. Shimada H, Chatten J, Newton W A et al. Histopathologic prognostic factors in neuroblastic tumours: Definition of subtypes of ganglioneuroblastoma and age-linked classification of neuroblastomas. J Natl Cancer Inst 1984; 73: 405–416

15. Brodeur G M, Seeger R C, Schwab M, Varmus H E, Bishop J M. Amplification of *N-myc* in untreated human neuroblastomas correlates with advanced disease stage. Science 1984; 224: 1121–1124

16. Kiely E M. The surgical challenge of neuroblastoma. J Pediatr Surg 1994; 29: 128–133

17. Atkinson G O, Zaatari G S, Lorenzo R L, Gay B B, Garvin A J. Cystic neuroblastoma in infants: Radiographic and pathologic features. AJR 1986; 146: 113–117

18. Bousvaros A, Kirks D R, Grossman H. Imaging of neuroblastoma; An overview. Paediatric Radiol 1986; 16: 89–106

19. Stark D D, Moss A A, Brasch R C et al. Neuroblastoma: Diagnostic imaging and staging. Radiology 1983; 148: 101–105

20. Boechat M I. Adrenal glands, pancreas and retroperitoneal structures. In: Siegel M J (ed) Pediatric Body CT. New York: Churchill Livingstone, 1988; 177–217

21. Boechat M I, Ortega J, Hoffman A D et al. Computed tomography in stage III neuroblastoma. AJR 1985; 145: 1283–1287

22. Farrelly C, Daneman A, Chan H S L, Martin D J. Occult neuroblastoma presenting with opsomyo-clonus: Utility of computed tomography. AJR 1984; 142: 807–810

23. Cohen M D, Weetman R, Provisor A et al. Magnetic resonance imaging of neuroblastoma with a 0.15T magnet. AJR 1984; 143: 1241–1248

24. Dietrich R B, Kangerloo H, Lenarsky C et al. Neuroblastoma: The role of M R imaging. AJR 1987; 148: 937–942

25. Borrello J A, Mirowitz S A, Siegel M J. Neuroblastoma. In: Siegel B A, Proto A V (eds) Pediatric disease (fourth series) test and syllabus. Reston V A: American College of Radiology, 1993; 640–665

26. Dietrich R B, Kangarloo H, Lenarsky C, Feig S A. Neuroblastoma: The role of MR imaging. AJR 1987; 148: 937–942

27. Fletcher B D, Kopiwoda S Y, Strandjord S E, Nelson A D, Pickering S P. Abdominal neuroblastoma: Magnetic resonance imaging and tissue characterization. Radiology 1985; 155: 699–703

28. Siegel M J, Jamroz G A, Glazer H S, Abramson C L. MR imaging of intraspinal extension of neuroblastoma. J Comput Assist Tomogr 1986; 10: 593–595

29. Bostrom B, Nesbit M E, Brunning R D. The value of bone marrow trephine biopsy in the diagnosis of metastatic neuroblastoma. Am J Pediatr Hematol Oncol 1985; 303–305

30. Howman-Giles R B, Gilday D L, Ash J M. Radionuclide skeletal survey in neuroblastoma. Radiology 1979; 131: 497–502

31. Sty J R, Kun L E, Casper J T. Bone imaging as a diagnostic aid in evaluating neuroblastoma. Am J Pediatr Hematol Oncol 1980; 2: 115–118

32. Couanet D, Geoffray A, Hartmann O, Leclere J G, Lumbroso J D. Bone marrow metastases in children's neuroblastoma studied by magnetic resonance imaging. Prog Clin Biol Res 1988; 271: 547–555

33. Gelfand M J. Meta-iodobenzylguanidine in children. Semin Nucl Med 1993; 23: 231–242

34. Gordon I, Peters A M, Gutman A et al. Skeletal assessment in neuroblastoma. The pitfalls of iodine-123-MIBG scans. J Nucl Med 1990; 31: 129–134

35. Shulkin B L, Shapiro B, Hutchinson R J. Iodine-131-metaiodobenzylguanidine and bone scintigraphy for the detection of neuroblastoma. J Nucl Med 1992; 33: 1735–1740

36. Paltiel H J, Gelfand M J, Elgazzar A H et al. Neural crest tumors: I-123 MIBG imaging in children. Pediatr Radiol 1994; 117–121

37. Moertel C L, Reubi J C, Scheithauer B S, Schaid D J, Kvols L K. Expression of somatostatin receptors in childhood neuroblastoma. Am J Clin Pathol 1994; 102: 752–756

38. O'Dorisio M S, Hauger M, Cecalupo A J. Somatostatin receptors in neuroblastoma: Diagnostic and therapeutic implications. Semin Oncol 1994; 21: 33–37

39. Sautter-Bihl M L, Dorr U, Schilling F, Treuner J, Bihl H. Somatostatin receptor imaging: A new horizon in the diagnostic management of neuroblastoma. Semin Oncol 1994; 21: 38–41

40. Shulkin B L, Hutchinson R J, Castle V P et al. Neuroblastoma: Positron emission tomography with 2-[Fluorine-18]-Fluoro-2-deoxy-D-glucose compared with metaiodobenzylguanidine scintigraphy. Radiology 1996; 99: 743–750

41. Nadel H R. Nuclear Oncology in Children. Nuclear Medicine Annual. Philadelphia: Lippincott-Raven Publishers, 1996; 143–193

42. Corbett R, Olliff J, Fairly N et al. A prospective comparison between magnetic resonance imaging, meta-iodobenzyl guanidine scintigraphy and marrow histology/ cytology in neuroblastoma. Eur J Cancer 1991; 27: 1560–1564

43. Hall-Craggs M A, Shaw D, Pritchard J et al. Metastatic neuroblastoma: New abnormalities on bone scintigraphy may not indicate tumour recurrence. Skeletal Radiol 1990; 19: 33–36

44. Woods S G, Tuchman M, Robson L L et al. A population-based study of the usefulness of screening for neuroblastoma. Lancet 1996; 348: 1682–1687

45. Kanekoy Y, Kanda N, Maseka N et al. Current urinary screening for catecholamine metabolities at 6 months of age may be detecting only a small portion of higher risk neuroblastomas: A chromosome and *N-myc* amplification study. J Clin Oncol 1990; 8: 2005–2013

46. Yamatoo K, Hayashi Y, Hanada R et al. Mass screen-ing and age-specific incidence of neuroblastoma in Saitame Prefecture, Japan. J Clin Oncol 1995; 13: 2033–2038

47. Shulkin B L, Mitchell D S, Ungar D R et al. Neoplasms in a paediatric population: 2-[F-18]-fluoro-2-deoxy-D-glucose PET studies. Radiology 1995; 194: 495–500

Chapter 34

Uncommon paediatric neoplasms

Marilyn Siegel

INTRODUCTION

Leukaemias, lymphomas and cancers of the central nervous system comprise more than 60% of paediatric tumours, followed by tumours of the sympathetic nervous system, soft tissues, kidney, bone, liver, eye and germ cells.[1] As is true of adult malignancies, appropriate treatment of paediatric cancers is predicated primarily on tumour stage or extent at the time of diagnosis. This chapter reviews the staging of uncommon abdominal neoplasms in children. The following tumours are discussed:

- Hepatic neoplasms
- Rhabdomyosarcoma:
  bladder
  prostate
  vagina
- Testicular neoplasms
- Ovarian neoplasms
- Sacrococcygeal tumours

Guidelines for assessing metastatic disease and follow-up evaluation are presented.

HEPATIC NEOPLASMS

- Hepatoblastoma
- Hepatocellular carcinoma
- Embryonal sarcoma
- Fibrolamellar hepatocellular carcinoma

Incidence and clinical features

Primary hepatic tumours account for approximately 0.5–2% of paediatric tumours, with an annual incidence of 1.6 per million children.[1–3] They are the third most frequent neoplasm after Wilms' tumour and neuroblastoma. Malignant hepatic tumours are twice as frequent as benign tumours and most of these are hepatoblastomas and hepatocellular carcinomas.[1–3] Embryonal sarcoma and fibrolamellar hepatocellular carcinoma are rare malignant hepatic neoplasms in children.[4,5]

Hepatoblastoma almost always presents in infants and young children under 5 years of age, with the majority found in children under 2 years of age. In contrast, hepatocellular carcinoma is found most often in children between 5 and 15 years of age, with the peak incidence being after 10 years of age.[1–6] Common presenting signs of both tumours are abdominal mass, pain, anorexia, weight loss, and fever. Serum alpha-fetoprotein levels (AFP) are elevated in 65–90% of children with hepatoblastoma and in 50–60% of children with hepatocellular carcinoma.[1–4] Hepatoblastoma occurs in association with Beckwith–Wiedemann syndrome, foetal alcohol syndrome, polyposis coli, and hemihypertrophy. Hepatocellular carcinoma has been associated with chronic liver diseases, such as type-I glycogen storage disease, cystinosis, tyrosinemia, Wilson's disease, alpha-1-antitrypsin deficiency, extrahepatic biliary atresia, and giant cell hepatitis.[1,3] However, the majority of both tumours occur *de novo*.

Pathology

Pathological differentiation of hepatoblastoma and hepatocellular carcinoma is based on cellular maturity. Hepatoblastoma contains small, primitive epithelial cells, resembling foetal liver, and occasionally mesenchymal components, while hepatocellular carcinoma contains large, pleomorphic multinucleated cells with variable degrees of differentiation.[2,3] About 70% of patients with hepatocellular carcinoma and 40% of patients with hepatoblastoma have extrahepatic spread of tumour at presentation, usually to regional lymph nodes or lung.[2–4] Pulmonary metastases have been noted at the time of diagnosis in 15–20% of children.[4] Bone or bone marrow metastases are rare.

Fibrolamellar carcinoma is a rare variant of hepatocellular carcinoma, occurring in older children and young adults, with a mean patient age of 23 years. Pathologically, it is characterized by eosinophilic hepatocytes that are subdivided by fibrous bands arranged in a lamellar pattern, hence, the term 'fibrolamellar'. Serum AFP levels are usually normal. This tumour has a more favourable prognosis than the usual hepatocellular carcinoma.[7,8]

Clinical staging

There is no universally accepted staging system for hepatic malignancy in childhood, but the most widely utilized classification in the USA is that of the Children's Cancer Study Group and the Southwest Oncology Group (Table 34.1).[1]

This clinical staging classification, based on operative resection, has been shown to correlate well with survival in both hepatoblastoma and hepatocellular carcinoma.

Five-year survival after treatment is approximately:[2]

Group I (90%)
Group II (60%)
Group III (15%)
Group IV (10%)

Key points: hepatic neoplasms

■ Primary hepatic tumours are the third most common paediatric cancer

■ The majority of hepatic tumours are hepatoblastomas and hepatocellular carcinomas

■ Hepatoblastoma occurs in infants and young children whereas hepatocellular carcinoma is seen in older children

■ Alpha-foetoprotein is elevated in over 50% of patients with primary liver cancer

■ Pathological differentiation between hepatoblastoma and hepatocellular carcinoma is based on cellular maturity

■ Regional lymph node spread is common in both hepatoblastoma and hepatocellular carcinoma

■ Fibrolamellar carcinoma is rare and occurs in older children and young adults

Treatment options

Cure of malignant hepatic tumours is possible only with complete resection of the primary lesion. Tumours are considered resectable if the volume of liver left behind is adequate to support life and if the vascular supply and biliary and venous drainage of the remaining hepatic parenchyma is left intact. If tumour extends to the extraluminal margins of the inferior vena cava or the portal vein or if there is local spread to adjacent extrahepatic structures, resection may still be possible, although it is likely it will be technically difficult.[9] Tumours that involve all hepatic segments, encase or invade major vessels or the common hepatic duct, or spread to regional lymph nodes or distant sites are classified as unresectable. The four types of major resections most commonly performed are:

- Right lobectomy
- Trisegmentectomy
- Left lobectomy
- Left lateral segmentectomy

Complete resection is possible in 50–70% of hepatoblastomas and in one-third of hepatocellular carcinomas at time of diagnosis.[2–4] All patients with malignant neoplasms, both resectable and non-resectable, receive adjuvant chemotherapy, while radiation therapy is reserved for patients with Group-II or -III disease.[2,3] The use of preoperative chemotherapy for treatment of initially unresectable hepatoblastoma has improved survival rate.

Diagnostic imaging

The crucial criteria for assessing extent and resectability of hepatic neoplasms are:

- The extent of the primary tumour, most importantly the presence of tumour in surgically critical areas such as the porta hepatis, portal vein and inferior vena cava
- The presence of regional extrahepatic spread or distant metastases[9]

Hepatoblastoma and hepatocellular carcinoma have similar imaging features. Both usually appear as a solitary mass confined to a single lobe, with the right lobe involved twice as often as the left lobe. Less frequently, they are multifocal or diffusely replace hepatic parenchyma.

Diagnosis

Sonography with colour flow Doppler is the preferred examination to screen for the presence of an intrahepatic mass and to differentiate solid and cystic masses. It is also a useful study to identify the presence and extent of vascular involvement by tumour. Sonographic findings of malignant hepatic tumours include:

- A hyperechoic mass, occasionally with a hypoechoic rim
- Homogeneous or heterogeneous parenchyma
- Vessel invasion or amputation[10]
- Vascular thrombus which produces an echogenic intraluminal mass with peripheral hypervascularity

Localized staging: imaging findings

Both computed tomography (CT) and magnetic resonance imaging (MRI) have been used for diagnosis, staging and predicting resectability of hepatic neoplasms.[11–17] On CT, hepatocellular carcinoma and hepatoblastoma are either hypo- or isodense on non-contrast images and exhibit

Table 34.1. *Clinical grouping of malignant hepatic tumours*

I	Complete resection as initial treatment
IIA	Complete resection following initial irradiation or chemotherapy
IIB	Residual disease in one lobe
IIIA	Residual disease in both lobes
IIIB	Regional node involvement
IV	Distant metastases

transient, but intense, heterogeneous contrast enhancement. On T1-weighted images, malignant hepatic lesions appear hypointense relative to normal liver; on T2-weighted sequences the signal intensity increases and is similar to that of subcutaneous fat. Early enhancement with rapid wash-out is seen after administration of gadolinium-DTPA (Gd-DTPA). Tumour margins generally are well-defined and, in cases of hepatocellular carcinoma, there may be a low attenuation or low signal intensity rim, corresponding to a fibrous capsule. Tumour thrombus appears as a filling defect on CT and as a focus of increased signal within a normally echo-free vessel on spin-echo sequences or as a low intensity area on gradient-echo imaging.

Although large prospective studies comparing the ability of CT and MRI to stage hepatic malignancy in children are limited, a few small studies are available and have indicated the superiority of MRI.[11,12] In a study of 23 children comparing CT and intermediate field-strength MRI, retrospectively, Boechat et al. reported that MRI and CT were comparable for tumour detection, but MRI was superior to CT for detecting recurrence.[11] In a subsequent study of eight children, Finn et al. showed that high field-strength MRI was better than CT for defining parenchymal involvement and tumour margins, and hence, tumour resectability (Fig. 34.1).[12] Magnetic resonance imaging also more accurately evaluated vascular structures, such as the hepatic

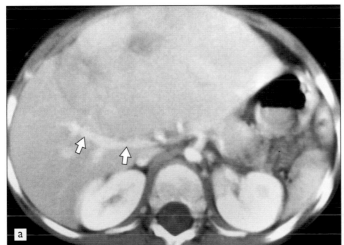

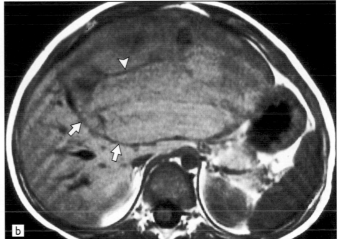

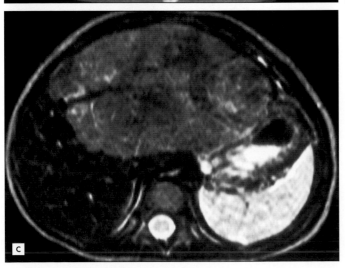

Figure 34.1. *Hepatoblastoma, Group I. (a) CT scan shows a mass replacing the left hepatic lobe and displacing the main portal vein (arrows) posteriorly. Except for small areas of haemorrhage or necrosis, the attenuation value of the tumour is similar to that of normal hepatic parenchyma; (b) T1-weighted axial MR image shows a slightly hypointense mass occupying the lateral and medial segments of the left lobe and surrounding the left portal vein (arrowhead), which courses through the centre of the mass. The main portal vein (arrows) is splayed and displaced posteriorly and to the right; (c) on T2-weighted MR image the signal intensity of the mass increases and approximates that of subcutaneous fat. Tumour margins and the relationship of tumour to hepatic vasculature are seen better on MRI than on CT. Because the tumour appeared to be confined to the left lobe, this patient was considered a surgical candidate. Subsequent left lobectomy was successful.*

and portal veins and inferior vena cava, even in very small children (Figs. 34.1 and 34.2). Computed tomography underestimated tumour in 25% of children. Moreover, MRI was superior in the evaluation of regional lymph nodes. Most neoplastic tissue on MRI, both nodal and primary tumour, has a higher signal intensity than normal parenchyma, resulting in improved contrast resolution compared with contrast-enhanced CT. Although MRI can accurately define portal adenopathy, it cannot distinguish between nodal involvement by tumour and hyperplastic adenopathy. Both can produce high signal intensity in enlarged nodes on T2-weighted images. Finn et al. also showed that MRI was able to detect postoperative recurrence that was not seen on CT.[12]

With the advent of CT and MRI, angiography is no longer performed for the initial staging evaluation of children with hepatic malignancy. On rare occasions, however, CT with arterial portography may be necessary for tumour mapping prior to trisegmentectomy.

Metastatic disease

Hepatic malignancy commonly metastasizes to portal lymph nodes and lung and on occasion to bone. Portal lymph nodes are easily evaluated by MRI at the same time that the primary tumour is imaged. Computed tomography is the best method to detect pulmonary metastases. Skeletal scintigraphy is recommended for assessing metastatic disease to bone. Brain metastases can occur, but are rare, and head CT or MRI is not recommended unless there are relevant clinical symptoms.

Key points: hepatoblastoma

■ Crucial criteria for determining resectability include the presence of spread into the portal vein, inferior vena cava, porta hepatis, regional lymph nodes and distal metastases

■ Hepatoblastoma and hepatocellular carcinoma have similar imaging features on sonography, CT and MRI

■ These tumours are usually solitary but occasionally are multifocal

■ MRI appears to be superior to CT for staging local tumour extent

■ MRI appears to be superior to CT for detecting vascular invasion

■ CT is the best technique for detecting pulmonary metastases

Follow-up

Computed tomography scans obtained after chemotherapy in children with initially unresectable tumour are not accurate for judging exact lobar involvement prior to definite tumour resection.[18] Areas of low attenuation are common and do not correlate well with tumour or necrosis. Follow-up evaluation of patients who have received preoperative chemotherapy, as well as those is have undergone resection, is best done by MRI because of its ability to demonstrate tumour margins better (Fig. 34.3).[12] Because most recurrences occur in the first two postoperative years, MRI of the liver and abdomen should be

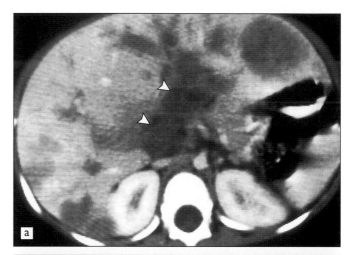

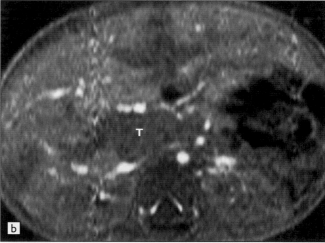

Figure 34.2. *Multifocal hepatoblastoma, Group IIIA. (a) Postcontrast CT scan shows multiple, low attenuation lesions in the right and left hepatic lobes. Low attenuation mass is also noted in the area of the porta hepatis (arrowheads), indicating either tumour thrombus or lymphadenopathy extrinsic to the porta; (b) axial gradient-echo MR image confirms that the porta hepatis disease is tumour thrombus (T). Collateral vessels are noted around the portal vein. Involvement of both lobes and the portal vein precludes resectability.*

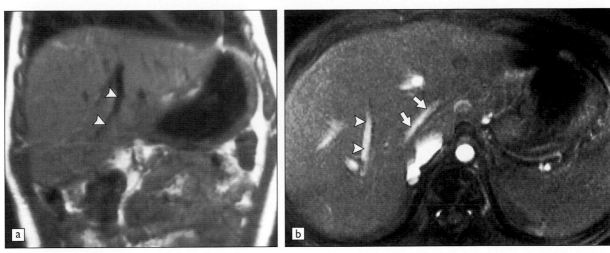

Figure 34.3. *MR images postresection of a right lobe hepatoblastoma. (a) Coronal T1-weighted and (b) axial gradient-echo images show regeneration of the left hepatic lobe and normal parenchyma without evidence of tumour recurrence. The remaining left lobe has regenerated to form a liver comparable to the preoperative liver in size. Note the distortion of the normal vascular anatomy; left-hepatic vein (arrowheads) and left portal vein (arrows).*

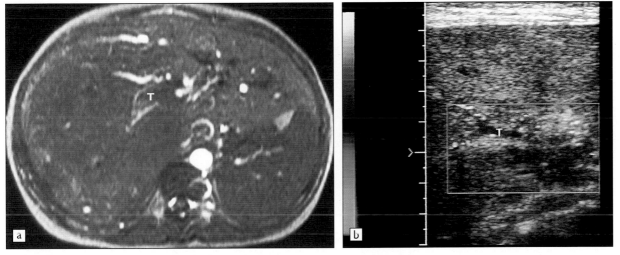

Figure 34.4. *Hepatocellular carcinoma invading the portal vein. (a) Axial gradient-echo MR image demonstrates increased signal intensity, consistent with tumour thrombus (T), in the right portal vein. The primary lesion occupies the entire right lobe and effaces vessels. The poor contrast between the primary tumour and adjacent normal tissues reflects the pulse sequence which was tailored for vascular imaging and not for demonstrating tumour margins; (b) colour Doppler image through the porta confirms tumour thrombus (T) in the right portal vein. Minimal flow is noted around the thrombosed vessel. Tumour was unresectable because of vascular invasion.*

obtained at regular intervals up to 2 years after surgery. The exact timing of the follow-up examinations is determined by the specific treatment protocol utilized.

Role of imaging

Magnetic resonance imaging with contrast enhancement should be the technique for staging hepatic tumours in chil-dren. It has replaced angiography in the preoperative staging evaluation. The detection of parenchymal extent of tumour, lymph node enlargement, vascular involvement, and invasion of adjacent abdominal organs is superbly displayed with multiplanar MRI. Ultrasonography, with colour flow Doppler imaging, is an excellent adjunctive technique to confirm vascular invasion (Fig. 34.4).

Differential diagnosis

Diagnosis and staging of hepatic cancer requires an understanding of the differential diagnostic considerations.

The major differential diagnoses are:

- Haemangio-endothelioma
- Mesenchymal hamartoma
- Embryonal sarcoma

Hepatic adenomas and nodular hyperplasia account for less than 5% of hepatic tumours in childhood.[4] Their imaging features are similar to those seen in adults and will not be discussed further.

Haemangio-endothelioma is the most common benign hepatic neoplasm in childhood. Most affected patients are diagnosed in the first 6 months of life and present with symptomatic hepatomegaly or congestive heart failure due to high-output overcirculation. Contrast-enhanced CT and MRI can definitely establish the diagnosis of haemangio-endothelioma and differentiate it from malignant hepatic tumours. Most haemangio-endotheliomas are solitary, but multicentricity can occur.[4] The lesion is usually well-circumscribed and has a low attenuation on CT, a low signal intensity (less than normal liver) on T1-weighted images and a high signal intensity (brighter than subcutaneous fat) on T2-weighted images (Fig. 34.5).[14,19] After intravenous administration of iodinated contrast medium or Gd-DTPA, there is peripheral enhancement during the early bolus phase and progressive centripetal filling-in on delayed images. If the typical findings of centripetal enhancement and filling-in are present, the diagnosis of haemangio-endothelioma can be made with certainty. Biopsy is not necessary. In contrast to adults, cavernous haemangiomas are rare in children.

Mesenchymal hamartoma is a benign lesion composed of cysts of varying size, separated by fibrous septations.[14,20] Median patient age at diagnosis is approximately 10 months. Diagnostic CT and MRI findings are a well-circumscribed multicystic lesion containing fluid-filled locules surrounded by thin septations. It has been observed, however, that the cysts are less apparent in very young children.[4]

Undifferentiated embryonal sarcoma is a hepatic malignancy that primarily affects older children and adolescents, usually between 6 and 10 years of age.[14,21] Clinical findings include fever, a painful mass, and normal levels of AFP.[14] Histologically, the tumour contains undifferentiated spindle cells that resemble embryonal cells with a myxoid matrix. Computed tomography findings are those of a predominantly solid mass with areas of cystic change and haemorrhage, in contrast to the benign mesenchymal hamartoma which is predominantly cystic.[21] On MRI, the tumour is heterogeneous and hypointense on T1-weighted images. The signal intensity on T2-weighted images reflects the cystic or solid internal contents of the lesion, but it is predominantly hyperintense.[14] Septations are particularly well seen on T2-weighted images. Patterns of spread are similar to other hepatic malignancies as is the staging evaluation.

GENITO-URINARY TUMOURS

- Rhabdomyosarcoma
- Bladder
- Prostate
- Vagina

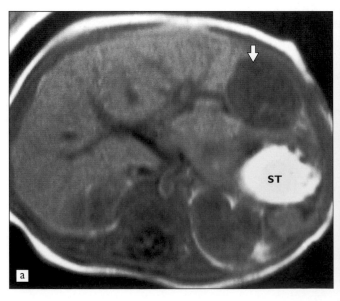

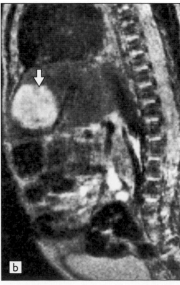

Figure 34.5. *Haemangio-endothelioma in a newborn girl with multiple cutaneous haemangiomas. (a) T1-weighted MR image shows a smoothly marginated, hypointense lesion (arrow) in the left lobe of the liver; (b) on the T2-weighted sagittal image, the lesion (arrow) is hyperintense to subcutaneous fat. The hyperintense signal intensity on T2-weighted images is typical of haemangio-endotheliomas. ST = stomach.*

Rhabdomyosarcoma is the most common tumour of the bladder, prostate and vagina, as well as the most common soft tissue tumour in childhood. It tends to affect children under 15 years of age and accounts for approximately 5% to 10% of all solid tumours in childhood.[22,23] The tumour has two age peaks of occurrence, with the first occurring between 2 and 6 years of age and the second between 14 and 18 years of age.[1] The embryonal and botryoid histological subtypes are the predominant subtypes in the genitourinary tract.

Clinical features

Symptoms of bladder neoplasms include a palpable pelvic mass, haematuria, increased frequency of urination, and urinary retention. Prostatic tumour frequently manifests as prostatism or urinary retention. Clinical symptoms of vaginal tumours include vaginal bleeding or mass or prolapse of polypoid tumour from the vaginal orifice onto the perineum. Rhabdomyosarcoma spreads by direct extension to contiguous structures or by hematogenous or lymphatic dissemination to lymph nodes, lungs, bone, bone marrow or liver.[1,22] Lymph node involvement or distant spread occurs at initial diagnosis in 10% to 20% of patients.[1]

Clinical staging

Several classifications have been used for staging rhabdomyosarcoma.[22,23] The two most frequently utilized systems are the Intergroup Rhabdomyosarcoma Study (IRS) which is based on surgical findings (Table 34.2) and the TNM (ie. tumour nodes, metastasis) system, based on pretreatment clinical assessment of tumour extent.

More recent trials are evaluating a system which combines the IRS system and a modified TNM system (below). Overall 3-year survival using the IRS classification system ranges from between 68 and 78%.[22]

Treatment options

Treatment of genito-urinary rhabdomyosarcoma is biopsy, followed by chemotherapy for 4 to 5 months, followed by excision of only residual disease. Radiation may be added if there is still residual tumour or if exenteration would be required. The desire is to do less radical surgery and preserve the major pelvic organs.[22]

Diagnostic imaging
Diagnosis

The purpose of diagnostic imaging is to delineate the extent of tumour for staging and treatment planning and to serve as a baseline for monitoring response to therapy. Since rhabdomyosarcoma often presents as a palpable mass, sonography is likely to be used in diagnosis. In the urinary tract, the tumour may be discovered incidentally on cystography or urography during the evaluation of non-specific symptoms, such as haematuria, increased frequency of urination, and

urinary retention. The cystographic and sonographic findings are bladder-wall thickening, a polypoid soft tissue mass at the bladder base, or a combination of both.[24] With deep invasion, the bladder wall is markedly deformed and rigid and bladder capacity is diminished.

Table 34.2. *Intergroup rhabdomyosarcoma study staging system*

I		Localized tumour, completely resected
II	A	Localized tumour, grossly resected with microscopic residual
	B	Tumour with regional disease or lymph node involvement, completely resected
	C	Tumour with regional disease or involved lymph nodes, grossly resected with microscopic residual
III	A	Gross residual tumour after biopsy only
	B	Gross residual tumour after incomplete resection
IV		Distant metastases present at diagnosis

Table 34.3. *Intergroup rhabdomyosarcoma study TNM system*

Summary of pretreatment clinical staging based on clinical, radiographic and laboratory examination (plus histological biopsy):

A Localized tumour with favourable histology and clinically negative nodes

B Locally extensive tumour with favourable histology and clinically negative nodes

C Any size tumour with clinically involved regional nodes and/or unfavourable histology

D Distant metastasis

Tumour

T1 Confined to anatomic site of origin
T1a <5 cm in size
T1b ≥5 cm in size
T2 Extension or fixation to surrounding tissues
T2a <5 cm in size
T2b ≥5 cm in size

Regional lymph nodes

N0 Regional nodes not clinically involved
N1 Regional nodes clinically involved by tumour
NX Clinical status of regional nodes unknown

Metastases

M0 No distant metastasis
M1 Metastases present

Local staging: imaging findings

Preoperative evaluation of tumour extent has included both CT and MRI.[25,26] On these studies, bladder rhabdomyosarcoma appears as a soft tissue mass deforming the bladder base, while prostatic rhabdomyosarcoma appears as an extravesical mass elevating the bladder base and elongating the prostatic urethra. Vaginal rhabdomyosarcoma arises in the upper third of the anterior vaginal wall and results in a soft tissue mass enlarging the vaginal lumen. Secondary findings include uterine enlargement and fluid collections in the endometrial cavity when there is obstruction of the cervix by tumour. Rhabdomyosarcoma has an attenuation value approximating that of muscle on CT, a low signal intensity on T1-weighted and a high signal intensity on T2-weighted MR images. Tumour necrosis and calcification are frequent. Signs of regional spread include lymph node enlargement and invasion of adjacent pelvic organs, pelvic side walls, and in girls the parametrium. T1-weighted images are useful for depicting the primary tumour, lymphadenopathy, and invasion of perivesical fat.

Although there are no large series in children comparing the ability of CT and MRI to stage pelvic rhabdomyosarcoma, the experience in adults with bladder, prostate and vaginal tumours suggests that MRI, especially with Gd-enhancement, is more sensitive than CT in assessing lymphadenopathy and invasion of perivisceral fat and adjacent organs (Fig. 34.6).[27–29]

Metastatic disease

Imaging of the abdomen is routinely performed to search for retroperitoneal adenopathy. The imaging tests that have been used for this assessment are lymphangiography, CT and MRI. Lymphangiography was the mainstay of evaluation of nodal disease prior to the advent of CT. Its major advantage is its ability to detect architectural changes in non-enlarged lymph nodes. However, it has a number of disadvantages: it is time consuming, it fails to demonstrate the superior extent of involvement and it cannot separate hyperplasia from tumour reliably. As a result it has been replaced by CT. Studies assessing the efficacy of CT in detecting nodal involvement by rhabdomyosarcoma are lacking, but experience in adults with bladder carcinoma has shown that CT has an accuracy ranging from between 70 and 90%.[27] The CT appearance of retroperitoneal lymph nodes ranges from small discrete nodules to large conglomerate masses (Fig. 34.7). Experience with MRI in the detection of retroperitoneal adenopathy is limited, although theoretically it has the ability to distinguish lymph nodes and blood vessels without the need for administration of contrast medium. At the present time, it does not have an important role in the evaluation of nodal metastases.

The lungs, bone and liver are common sites of metastatic spread. Computed tomography of the chest is recommended as the study of choice for detecting pulmonary metastases and mediastinal lymphadenopathy because it is more sensitive than chest radiography (Fig. 34.8). Metastases to bone are best detected by skeletal scintigraphy.

Studies comparing CT and MRI for detecting hepatic metastases in children, regardless of the site of primary tumour, have not been performed. Results of studies in adults in the late 1980s showed that CT and MRI were comparable for demonstrating liver metastases with sensitivities between 93 and 96%.[30,31] However, as technology has advanced MRI has become increasingly sensitive and now appears superior to CT (see Chapter 38). Currently, however, CT is still considered the method of choice in children for detecting hepatic metastases and for defining their extent because it is more readily available and has shorter scanning times.

Follow-up evaluation

Magnetic resonance imaging is the preferred study for evaluation of the response to chemotherapy or radiation therapy in children with initially unresectable tumours. After tumour resection or disappearance, CT can suffice for demonstrating local or distant recurrence. The timing of the follow-up imaging examination is determined by the specific protocol to which the patient is randomized.

Role of imaging

Magnetic resonance imaging is the study of choice in staging children with pelvic rhabdomyosarcoma and can provide the necessary morphological information regarding local tumour extent and respectability. Computed tomography of the chest and abdomen and skeletal scintigraphy are recommend to detect metastatic disease.

Key points: rhabdomyosarcoma

- Rhabdomyosarcomas of the genito-urinary tract arise in the bladder, prostate and vagina

- Rhabdomyosarcomas are the most common soft tissue tumour of childhood

- The predominant histological subtypes in the genito-urinary tract are embryonal and botryoid tumours

- Lymph node and distant metastases occur at presentation in 10–20% of patients

- Ultrasonography is useful for diagnosis but CT and MRI are the preferred methods for staging local spread and lymph node metastases

- CT is recommended to screen for pulmonary metastases

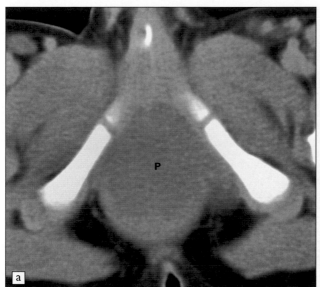

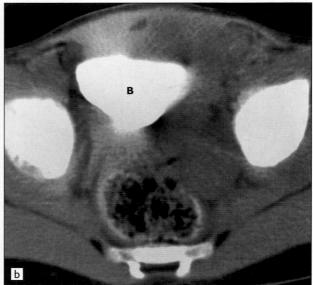

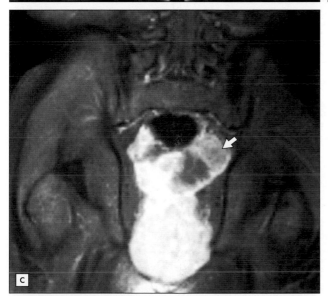

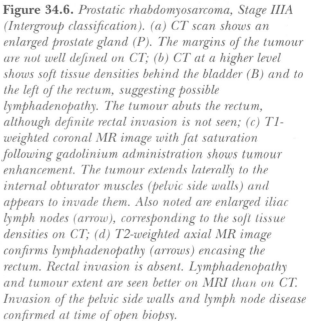

Figure 34.6. *Prostatic rhabdomyosarcoma, Stage IIIA (Intergroup classification). (a) CT scan shows an enlarged prostate gland (P). The margins of the tumour are not well defined on CT; (b) CT at a higher level shows soft tissue densities behind the bladder (B) and to the left of the rectum, suggesting possible lymphadenopathy. The tumour abuts the rectum, although definite rectal invasion is not seen; (c) T1-weighted coronal MR image with fat saturation following gadolinium administration shows tumour enhancement. The tumour extends laterally to the internal obturator muscles (pelvic side walls) and appears to invade them. Also noted are enlarged iliac lymph nodes (arrow), corresponding to the soft tissue densities on CT; (d) T2-weighted axial MR image confirms lymphadenopathy (arrows) encasing the rectum. Rectal invasion is absent. Lymphadenopathy and tumour extent are seen better on MRI than on CT. Invasion of the pelvic side walls and lymph node disease confirmed at time of open biopsy.*

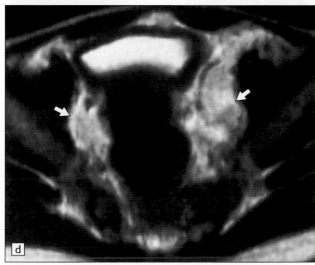

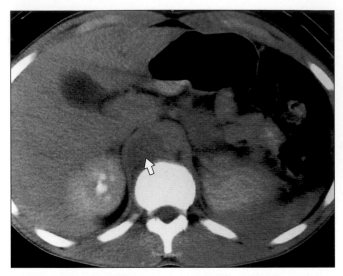

Figure 34.7. *Lymphadenopathy secondary to prostatic rhabdomyosarcoma. CT scan through the upper abdomen shows an enlarged lymph node (arrow) in the rectrocrural area.*

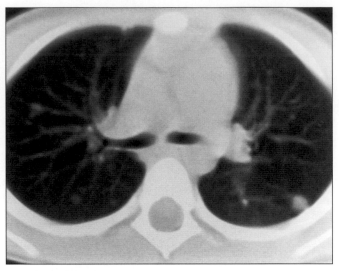

Figure 34.8. *Pulmonary metastases secondary to prostatic rhabdomyosarcoma. Several small nodules of varying size are seen in the pulmonary parenchyma bilaterally.*

TESTICULAR NEOPLASMS

- Yolk sac tumours
- Endodermal sinus tumours
- Embryonal carcinomas
- Teratocarcinoma
- Seminoma
- Choriocarcinoma

Testicular tumours account for approximately 1% of all childhood malignancies and for 2–3% of cancers in boys.[32,33]

Between 70% and 90% of testicular neoplasms originate from germ cells; 80% of these are malignant and 20% are benign and pure teratomas.[32,33] The most common malignant germ cell tumours of the testes in young boys are yolk sac and endodermal sinus tumours, comprising approximately 65% of the total, followed in frequency by embryonal carcinomas and teratocarcinomas. Most affected boys are under 4 years of age. Seminomas and choriocarcinomas are rare in young children, but increase in frequency in adolescents. Most patients with testicular tumours present with non-tender, scrotal or testicular enlargement.[33] More than 90% of boys with endodermal sinus or embryonal cell tumours have elevated serum AFP levels. The major sites of metastases from testicular tumours are the lymph nodes, lungs, and liver. Spread to regional or retroperitoneal lymph nodes is found in 10–20% of patients at presentation.[32,33]

Non-germinal or stromal tumours account for 10–30% of testicular neoplasms:[32,33]

- Leydig cell tumours
- Sertoli cell tumours
- Leukaemia
- Lymphoma

Sixty percent of these are Leydig cell tumours and 40% are Sertoli cell tumours. Sertoli cell tumours usually present as asymptomatic masses in the first year of life. Leydig cell tumours are found in patients between 3 and 6 years of age and present with precocious virilization or gynaecomastia. Both are benign in approximately 90% of cases. Leukemias and lymphomas account for fewer than 10% of testicular masses.[33] Disease is clinically symptomatic in 5–30% of boys, and is found at biopsy or autopsy.[34,35]

Testicular tumours in adults are discussed in detail in Chapter 16.

Clinical staging and treatment

Although a number of systems are available for staging testicular neoplasms, the most widely utilized is the germ cell tumour study from the Children's Cancer Study Group and Paediatric Oncology Group (Table 34.4).[32,33]

Approximately 80–90% of children have Stage I disease; the remainder usually have Stage-II or -III disease.[1,33] Patients with Stage-I disease are treated with radical orchidectomy alone. The overall survival rate ranges from 70 to 85% when the tumour is confined to the testis. In more advanced disease, treatment includes radical orchidectomy, retroperitoneal lymph node dissection, radiotherapy and chemotherapy.[1,32,33]

Diagnostic imaging
Diagnosis and local staging: imaging findings
Both ultrasonography and MRI have been used in the diagnosis of scrotal masses.[36–39] The sensitivity of both modalities in detecting testicular tumours and in distinguishing between intra- and extratesticular masses approaches 100%. This distinction is important because the vast majority of intratesticular lesions are malignant, whereas most extratesticular lesions are benign.

Sonographic findings of testicular neoplasms include:[36–39]

- A well-defined intratesticular mass
- Diffuse testicular enlargement, especially with leukaemic infiltration
- Variable echogenicity ranging from hypo- to hyperechoic
- Hypervascularity (85% of cases)

On T1-weighted images, malignant tumours are isointense to normal testis. On T2-weighted images, signal intensity is increased compared with the contralateral normal testis. Findings of extratesticular extension include irregularity of the tunica albuginea and reactive hydroceles. Scrotal skin thickening is rare. The combination of scrotal skin thickening and an intratesticular mass is more characteristic of an inflammatory process than a neoplasm.

Both MRI and sonography appear to be relatively insensitive in assessment of local tumour extension (63% vs 45%), although MRI may be more sensitive for demonstrating diffusely infiltrating tumours, such as leukaemia.[39] With both modalities, infiltration of the tunica albuginea and mediastinum testis is often difficult to recognize. In general, sonography is preferred for local staging because of its ease of performance and availability (Fig. 34.9).

Metastatic disease
Computed tomography is the study of choice to evaluate the pelvis and retroperitoneum for nodal spread. The sensitivity of CT in the detection of retroperitoneal lymph node involvement averages between 75 and 80% with a specificity between 75 and 85%, which is equivalent to lymphangiography (Fig. 34.10).[27,40] Although the results of published series are variable, CT is believed to be superior to sonography in detection of metastases. A major limitation of sonography is interference of penetration of the ultrasound beam by bowel gas. The use of MRI in the staging of extratesticular disease is limited, although in one study MRI was found to be comparable to CT in identifying retroperitoneal adenopathy, both examinations correctly detecting metastatic adenopathy in approximately 85% of cases.[41] Computed tomography, however, appeared superior to MRI in detecting other abdominal abnormalities.

Table 34.4. *Staging of testicular germ cell tumours (Children's Cancer Group; Paediatric Oncology Group)*

I	Limited to testis (testes), completely resected; tumour markers normal
II	Microscopic disease in scrotum or high in spermatic cord; retroperitoneal lymph node involvement (≤2 cm) and/or increased tumour markers
III	Retroperitoneal lymph node involvement (>2 cm), but no visceral or extra-abdominal involvement
IV	Distant metastases, including liver

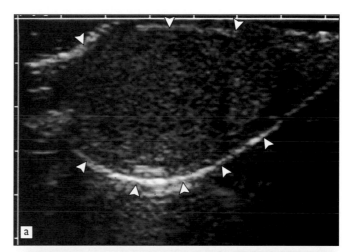

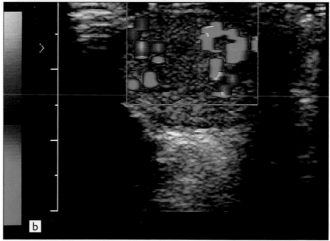

Figure 34.9. *Testicular yolk sac tumour, Stage I. (a) Longitudinal gray-scale sonogram shows an enlarged left testis. The echotexture is slightly increased, but there is no evidence of a discrete mass. The tunica albuginea (arrowheads) is intact; (b) colour Doppler flow image demonstrates abnormal tumour vascularity, although no discrete mass is seen. The number and size of vessels are increased for the patient's age. Tumour was localized to the central part of testis at surgery; no extratesticular spread was found.*

Because the lungs are a common site of metastatic spread, all patients with malignant testicular tumours undergo some form of chest imaging. Computed tomography of the chest is the most sensitive method for detecting pulmonary metastases as well as hepatic lesions.

Follow-up evaluation

After tumour resection or resolution following chemotherapy or radiation treatment, sonography usually suffices for defining local scrotal recurrence, as well as assessing the status of the contralateral testis. Although the frequency is unknown, patients with testicular cancers are at greater risk for developing a tumour in the contralateral testis. Chest and abdominal CT are performed for evaluation of lung and nodal metastases, respectively.

Key points: testicular tumours

■ Testicular tumours account for 1% of all childhood malignancy

■ The majority of testicular neoplasms in childhood are germ cell tumours, most being yolk sac and endodermal sinus neoplasms

■ Most children with a germ cell tumour have elevated serum alpha protein levels

■ Lymph node metastases are seen in 10–20% of patients at presentation

■ Ultrasound and MRI are highly accurate in detecting testicular tumours and in distinguishing between intra- and extratesticular masses

■ CT is the technique of choice for staging testicular cancer spread to lymph nodes and distant sites

Role of imaging

Sonography is the primary imaging study for detection and local staging of testicular disease. Computed tomography is firmly established as the imaging procedure of choice for detecting metastatic lymphadenopathy or distant spread to the lungs. At the present time, MRI does not have any advantage over CT in staging patients with testicular neoplasms.

Differential diagnosis

The differential diagnosis of testicular malignancy includes both benign intratesticular lesions and paratesticular lesions. Benign testicular lesions are not as frequent as malignant neoplasms. These include lipoma, haemangioma, neurofibroma, fibroma and cysts.

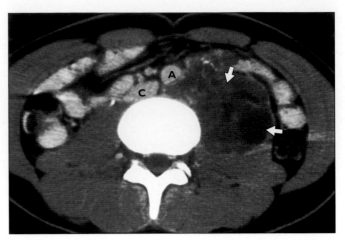

Figure 34.10. *Metastatic testicular tumour, Stage III. Postcontrast CT scan demonstrates enlarged para-aortic lymph nodes (arrows). Note that the attenuation value of these lymph nodes is lower than that of the abdominal wall and paraspinal muscles, which is typical of teratocarcinoma. A = aorta; C = inferior vena cava.*

Paratesticular tumours are more often benign than malignant. Benign lesions are usually:

• Adenomatoid tumours
• Spermatocoeles
• Cysts of the tunica albuginea

While the malignant ones are usually:

• Rhabdomyosarcoma
• Metastatic neuroblastoma
• Lymphoma
• Leiomyosarcoma
• Fibrosarcoma

The majority of intra- and paratesticular tumours appear as well-defined, complex or predominantly solid masses on sonography, CT and MRI. Final diagnosis requires tissue sampling. The staging evaluation of malignant lesions is similar to that of the intratesticular germ cell tumours.

OVARIAN TUMOURS

Ovarian tumours account for 1% of neoplasms in children under 17 years of age[1] Of these, 60–70% are benign, usually teratomas, and 30% are malignant.[1,32] Between 60 and 90% of malignant neoplasms are of germ cell origin. The most common subtypes of germ cell tumours are:

- Dysgerminoma
- Endodermal sinus tumour
- Malignant teratoma
- Embryonal carcinoma

Stromal tumours (Sertoli-Leydig cell, granulosa-theca cell, and undifferentiated neoplasms) have a 10–13% incidence.

Epithelial carcinomas account for 5–11% of malignant ovarian lesions.[32,33,42] Most malignant germ cell tumours are found in postmenarcheal girls. Abdominal mass and pain are the common presenting symptoms. Germ cell neoplasms spread by contiguous extension, regional and distant lymph node metastases, and distant dissemination to lungs or liver. Ovarian carcinomas spread directly by seeding the omental or peritoneal surfaces. Alpha-foetoprotein levels are elevated with endodermal sinus tumours, while beta human choriogonadotrophin (HCG) levels are elevated with embryonal carcinoma.

Clinical staging

The staging for ovarian tumours is not uniform. The two systems most often used are one from the Children's Cancer Study Group (Table 34.5) and one modified from the International Federation of Gynaecology and Obstetrics (FIGO) (Table 34.6).[1,32,33]

Seventy-five percent of cases are Stage I at diagnosis.[33] Survival rates are approximately 95% when the tumour is well encapsulated.[1] In more advanced disease (Stages II–IV), the survival rate is approximately 80%.[33] Treatment is complete resection when possible. Otherwise surgical debulking or biopsy is performed followed by chemotherapy and definitive resection.[32]

Diagnostic imaging

Diagnosis and local staging: imaging findings

The diagnosis of an ovarian mass is usually established by sonography. Sonographic findings suggesting malignancy include a solid mass with central necrosis and thickened irregular septae or papillary projections. By comparison, benign teratomas are predominantly cystic masses with hypo- or anechoic components, echogenic foci with acoustic shadowing, and a fat–fluid or fluid–fluid level.[43]

Computed tomography and MRI are superior to sonography in characterizing ovarian masses and more importantly, in determining their extent. A specific diagnosis of teratoma is easy on CT or MRI when fatty elements are

Table 34.5. *Staging of ovarian germ cell tumours (Children's Cancer Study Group; Paediatric Oncology Group)*

I	Limited to ovary (ovaries); tumour markers normal
II	Microscopic residual or positive lymph nodes (≤2 cm): negative peritoneal washings; tumour markers positive or negative
III	Lymph node involvement >2 cm; gross residual tumour; contiguous visceral involvement (omentum, intestine, bladder); peritoneal washings positive for malignant cells; tumour markers positive or negative
IV	Distant metastases including liver

Table 34.6. *Ovarian tumour staging system (after FIGO)*

Stage I	Tumour limited to the ovaries	
	IA	Tumour limited to one ovary; no ascites
		i. No tumour on the external surface; capsule intact
		ii. Tumour present on external surface
	IB	Growth limited to both ovaries; no ascites
		i. No tumour on the external surface; capsule intact
		ii. Tumour present on external surface and or capsule(s) ruptured
	IC	Stage IA or IB with obvious ascites present or positive peritoneal washings
Stage II	Tumour involving one or both ovaries with pelvic extension	
	IIA	Extension and/or metastases to the uterus and/or tubes
	IIB	Extension to other pelvic tissues including peritoneum and uterus
	IIC	Staging IIA or IIB with ascites or positive peritoneal washings
Stage III	Tumour involving one or both ovaries with metastases outside the pelvis and/or positive nodes.	
	Tumour limited to the true pelvis with extension to small bowel or omentum	
Stage IV	Tumour involving one or both ovaries with distant metastases	

identified within an ovarian mass.[44,45] Benign teratomas are predominantly cystic and fluid-filled, while malignant teratomas contain extensive soft tissue elements (>50% by volume), areas of haemorrhage or necrosis, thick septations, or papillary projections.[44,46] Findings indicating extra-ovarian spread of tumour are:

- Ascites
- Lymphadenopathy
- Omental cake
- Mesenteric nodules
- Peritoneal implants
- Hepatic metastases

Peritoneal tumour implants appear as soft tissue nodules on the lateral peritoneal surfaces of the abdomen. Omental implants appear as either discrete nodules or a sheet of soft tissue densities beneath the anterior abdominal wall. Computed tomography usually suffices for determining local tumour extent (Fig. 34.11). The role of MRI is still evolving, but it is excellent for demonstrating pelvic side wall extension or spread to pelvic organs if this information is important for staging or surgical planning.

Metastatic disease
Computed tomography is the study of choice to evaluate the common sites of intra-abdominal spread, such as the lymph nodes, subphrenic regions, omentum and cul-de-sac. It is more sensitive then MRI in identifying small lymph nodes and intraperitoneal implants, bowel encasement, and mesenteric infiltration (Fig. 34.12).[47] The superior spatial resolution of CT and its ability to obtain scans with oral contrast medium makes the detection of these abnormalities easier with CT than with MRI.

The most frequent sites of distant disease are lung and liver. If imaging findings suggest a benign teratoma at the time of diagnosis (i.e. fluid-filled mass with calcification or fat), evaluation of distant metastases is not warranted

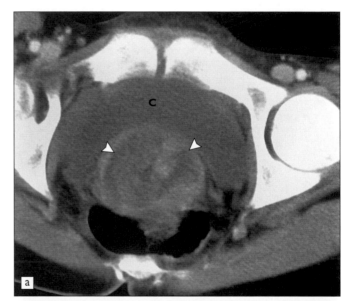

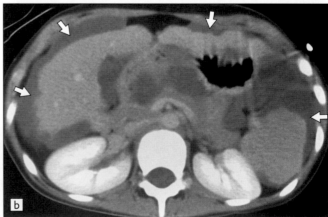

Figure 34.12. *Mucinous ovarian carcinoma with omental implants, Stage IV. Fourteen-year-old girl with abdominal distention and weight loss. (a) CT scan shows the primary tumour (arrowheads) is a complex mass with cystic and solid components. Peritoneal spread is indicated by an omental cake (C); (b) CT through the upper abdomen demonstrates diffuse implants along the lateral peritoneal surface (arrows).*

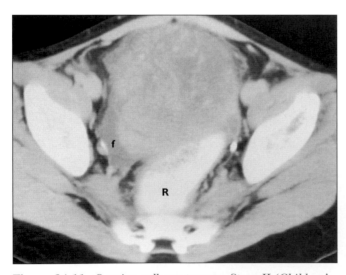

Figure 34.11. *Ovarian yolk sac tumour, Stage II (Children's Cancer Study Group). CT scan shows a large, complex mass anterior to the rectum (R). A small amount of fluid (f) is noted in the right hemipelvis. The fat planes around the tumour, except those adjacent to the rectum are well seen, and there are no local nodes. The primary tumour was grossly resected, but with microscopic residual.*

preoperatively. However, if malignancy is confirmed on histological examination, CT scanning of the chest and upper abdomen is needed to assess the presence or absence of metastatic disease.

Key points: ovarian tumours

■ Ovarian tumours account for 1% of neoplasms in children under the age of 17 years of which 30% are malignant

■ The majority of malignant neoplasms are germ cell tumours

■ Stromal cell tumours account for 10–13% and epithelial tumours for 5–11% of all ovarian masses

■ Alpha-foetoprotein levels are elevated in endodermal sinus tumours and HCG levels in embryonal carcinoma

■ CT and MRI are superior to sonography for characterizing ovarian masses and determining local spread

■ CT of the chest is required to detect pulmonary metastases

Follow-up evaluation

Computed tomography is the best study for follow-up evaluation after surgical or medical therapy to detect residual or recurrent local disease, abdominal nodal disease, and pulmonary and liver metastases.

Role of imaging

In children with malignant ovarian neoplasms, CT is the study of choice for providing information regarding tumour size extent, nodal disease and resectability in the chest and abdomen. Magnetic resonance imaging has a limited role in evaluating malignant ovarian tumours.

SACROCOCCYGEAL TUMOURS

Sacrococcygeal teratoma is the most common germ cell tumour in children, accounting for 40% of all teratomas. Other teratomas in order of decreasing frequency are:[1]

- Ovary (37%)
- Head and neck (6%)
- Retroperitoneum (5%)
- Mediastinum (4%)
- Testes (3%)
- Trunk (1%)

Of all sacrococcygeal tumours, 48% are benign, 19% are malignant, and 23% have immature but no malignant elements.[32] There are four types of sacrococcygeal teratomas based on location (Fig. 34.13):[32]

- Type I — predominantly external (47%)
- Type II — external and intrapelvic (34%)
- Type III — external, pelvic and abdominal (9%)
- Type IV — purely presacral (10%)

Teratomas with external components are usually detected on physical examination in the neonatal period. In fact, over 90% of sacrococcygeal teratomas are diagnosed before 2 months of age and of these, 90% are benign. Tumours that are entirely presacral are often overlooked until later childhood or adolescence when patients present with constipation. Over 50% of lesions are malignant in patients older than 2 months of age at time of diagnosis.[33,48] Approximately 20% of infants with malignant teratomas have pulmonary metastases at the time of diagnosis.[1]

Clinical staging

The staging for extragonadal teratomas is shown in Table 34.7.

Treatment for benign sacrococcygeal teratomas is complete resection. For malignant tumours with bowel or sacral involvement, chemotherapy is given prior to excisional surgery. The survival rate for benign sacrococcygeal tumours is over 95%.[33] In contrast, the long-term survival rates of children whose tumours have malignant elements is only 50%.[48]

Diagnostic imaging

Local staging: imaging features

The role of imaging is to determine surgical resectability. Radiological evaluation typically begins with the plain radiograph, which is useful for demonstrating calcification in the mass and sacral destruction or erosion. Both CT scanning and MRI are excellent methods for characterizing sacrococcygeal teratomas.[48] Computed tomography findings of sacrococcygeal teratoma are a complex mass containing fluid, fat, calcification, bone or teeth and soft tissue. The fluid component has a low signal intensity on T1-weighted images and a high signal intensity on T2-weighted MR images. Fat

Table 34.7. *Staging for extragonadal tumours*

I	Complete resection, negative tumour margins and nodes
II	Microscopic residual; lymph nodes negative; tumour markers positive or negative
III	Gross residual; retroperitoneal nodes negative or positive, tumour markers positive or negative
IV	Distant metastases including liver

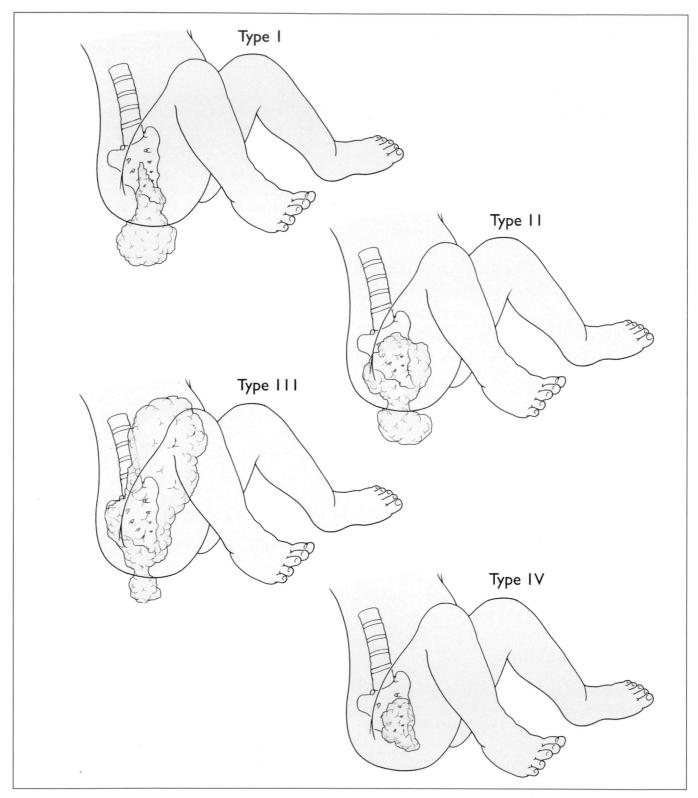

Figure 34.13. *Classification of sacrococcygeal teratomas. Type I: predominantly external with a small presacral component; Type II: external with a significant intrapelvic component; Type III: predominantly internal, both pelvic and intra-abdominal, with a smaller external component; Type IV: entirely presacral, without an external component or significant intra-abdominal extension (From ref. 49, with permission.)*

appears as a high signal intensity foci on T1-weighted images, and calcification, bone or hair as low signal foci on both T1 and T2-weighted images. In general, benign tumours are more likely to be cystic, while malignant tumours are more likely to be solid (Figs. 34.14 and 34.15).[44]

Magnetic resonance is the imaging study of choice to assess local extent of sacrococcygeal tumour because of its ability to evaluate the relationship of tumour to gluteal muscles and pelvic soft-tissue structures (Figs. 34.14 and 34.15) and to identify intraspinal involvement, without the need for intrathecal contrast medium. Therefore, it is recommended as the examination of choice to follow the plain radiograph if additional imaging is needed. It is controversial in neonates whether MRI is needed because most lesions are benign. Many surgeons advocate only plain radiographs and renal sonography prior to surgical resection. After 2 months of age, however, when the frequency of malignant change increases, cross-sectional imaging is recommended.

Metastatic disease

Metastases are to lung and occasionally to liver or retroperitoneal lymph nodes. Computed tomography scanning of the chest and upper abdomen is the best study to assess the presence or absence of metastatic disease (Fig. 34.16).

Follow-up evaluation

Magnetic resonance imaging is preferred for defining local recurrence of sacrococcygeal tumour after tumour resection, chemotherapy or radiation therapy. Computed tomography is the method of choice for evaluating pulmonary metastases.

Role of imaging

Most sacrococcygeal teratomas are quite large at presentation, but benign. Presacral teratomas are smaller, but often malignant. Magnetic resonance imaging in axial and sagittal planes is recommended as the study of choice for defining the primary tumour mass and for evaluating regional spread into adjacent structures.

Key points: sacrococcygeal tumours

- ■ Sacrococcygeal teratoma is the most common germ cell tumour of childhood

- ■ CT and MRI are excellent for characterizing sacrococcygeal teratomas

- ■ Most sacrococcygeal tumours are benign

- ■ MRI is the technique of choice for assessing local spread of malignant tumours

- ■ Long-term survival of malignant sacrococcygeal tumours is only 50%

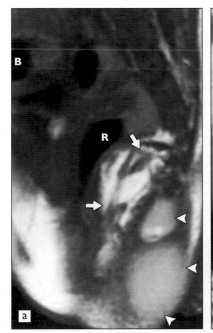 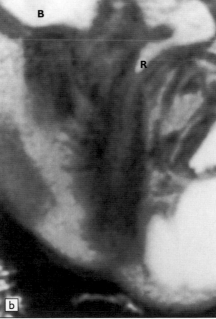

Figure 34.14. *Benign sacrococcygeal tumour. (a) T1-weighted MR image shows a large mass with external and intrapelvic component. The internal components (arrows) about the lower sacrum and have a high signal intensity similar to subcutaneous fat. The external portion of the mass (arrowheads) has an intermediate signal intensity; (b) on the T2-weighted image, the signal intensity of the intrapelvic portions of the mass is again similar to that of subcutaneous fat, whereas the extrapelvic portion is higher than that of fat, suggesting the presence of fluid. The high signal intensity of the external components on T1-weighted images reflected the presence of proteinaceous contents. The predominance of fluid and fat with an absence of significant soft tissue component is characteristic of benign teratomas. B = bladder, R = rectum. The tumour was easily resected. (Case courtesy of Andrew Landes, Hollywood, FL).*

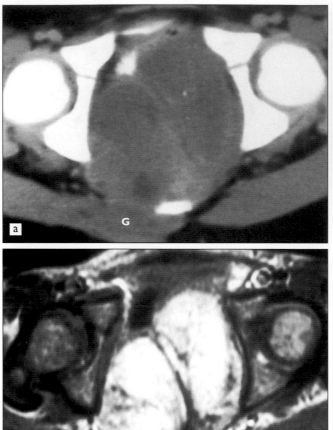

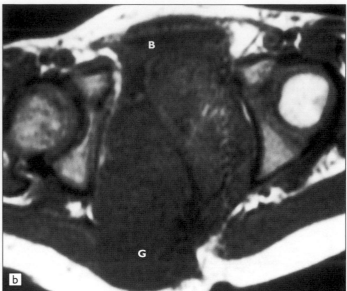

Figure 34.15. *Malignant sacrococcygeal tumour, Stage III. (a) CT scan shows a large soft tissue mass anterior to the sacrum. The mass is inseparable from the internal obturator muscles and appears to extend into the right gluteal muscle (G); (b) T1-weighted MR image shows a large mass lying behind the bladder (B) and displacing the right gluteal muscles (G) posteriorly. The predominant signal intensity of the mass is equal to that of muscle. The mass is well delineated from pelvic fat laterally; (c) on a proton-density weighted MR image the signal intensity of the mass increases. Internal heterogeneity is present. The tumour extends into the gluteal muscles bilaterally (arrowheads). Disease in the left gluteal muscle was not appreciated on CT scanning. The patient underwent biopsy for diagnosis followed by chemotherapy.*

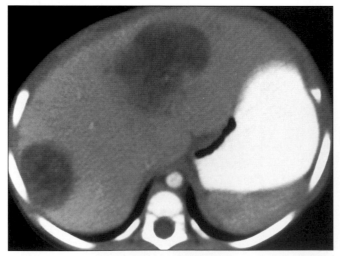

Figure 34.16. *Malignant sacrococcygeal tumour, Stage IV. Postcontrast-enhanced CT scan shows two large hypodense liver lesions with irregular borders, consistent with metastases.*

Differential diagnosis

Other presacral masses include:

- Neuroblastoma
- Anterior meningocoele
- Lymphoma

Anterior meningocoeles are herniations of spinal contents through a congenital defect in the vertebral body (anterior dysraphism) and are most common in the sacral region. The soft tissue contents of the herniated sac, especially the presence of a tethered cord, and the communication between the meningocoele and the thecal sac can be demonstrated best with MRI. Neuroblastoma and lymphoma appear as presacral soft tissue masses. When fat is present within a presacral mass, the diagnosis of teratoma can be suggested but otherwise, final diagnosis will require tissue sampling.

Summary

- Malignant hepatic tumours are more common than benign; most are hepatoblastomas or hepatocellular carcinomas.

- Hepatic malignancy metastasizes to portal lymph nodes, lungs and occasionally bone.

- MRI with contrast enhancement is the technique of choice for staging hepatic tumours in childhood.

- Rhabdomyosarcoma is the most common soft tissue tumour of childhood.

- Rhabdomyosarcoma metastasizes to the lungs, bone and liver.

- Testicular tumours account for 1% of all childhood malignancies.

- Metastases are predominantly to the abdominal lymph nodes and the lungs.

- Ovarian tumours account for 1% of all childhood malignancies below 17 years.

- 60–90% of malignant ovarian tumours are germ cell tumours.

- CT is the investigation of choice for staging ovarian tumours.

- Sacrococcygeal teratomas are the most common germ cell tumour of childhood.

- Treatment of malignant sacrococcygeal tumours is complete resection with or without neo-adjuvant chemotherapy depending on local extent.

- MRI is the best technique for assessing local extent of sacrococcygeal tumours.

REFERENCES

1. Pizzo P A, Poplack D G, Horowitz M E et al. Solid tumours of childhood. In: DeVita V T, Hellman S, Rosenberg S A (eds). Cancer: Principles and Practice of Oncology (4th ed). Philadelphia: J B Lippincott Co., 1993; 1738

2. Greenberg M, Filler R M. Hepatic tumours. In: Pizzo P A, Poplack D G (eds). Principles and Practice of Paediatric Oncology. Philadelphia: Lippincott-Raven, 1997; 717–732

3. Ortega J A, Malogolowkin M H. Epithelial and neuroectodermal tumours of the gastrointestinal, genitourinary, and gynecological tracts. In: Fernbach D J, Vietti T J (eds). Clinical Paediatric Oncology (4th ed). St. Louis: Mosby-Year Book, 1991; 611–626

4. Dehner L P. Liver, gallbladder, and extrahepatic biliary tract. In: Dehner L P (ed). Paediatric Surgical Pathology (2nd ed). Baltimore: Williams & Wilkins, 1987; 433–523

5. Weinberg A G, Finegold M J. Primary hepatic tumours of childhood. Hum Pathol 1983; 14: 512–537

6. Dachman A H, Pakter R L, Ros P R et al. Hepatoblastoma: radiologic–pathologic correlation in 50 cases. Radiology 1987; 164: 15–19

7. Stevens W R, Johnson C D, Stephens D H et al. Fibrolamellar hepatocellular carcinomas: stage at presentation and results of aggressive surgical management. Am J Roentgenol 1995; 164: 1153–1158

8. Titlebaum D S, Burke D R, Menanze S G et al. Fibrolamellar hepatocellular carcinoma: Pitfalls in non-operative diagnosis. Radiology 1988; 167: 25–30

9. Mukai J K, Stack C M, Tuner D A et al. Imaging of surgically relevant hepatic vascular and segmental anatomy, Part 2. Extent and resectability of hepatic neoplasms. Am J Roentgenol 1987; 149: 293–297

10. Brunelle F, Chaumont P. Hepatic tumours in children: ultrasonic differentiation of malignant from benign lesions. Radiology 1984; 150: 695–699

11. Boechat M I, Kangarloo H, Ortega J et al. Primary liver tumours in children: comparison of CT and MR imaging. Radiology 1988; 169: 727–732

12. Finn J P, Hall-Craggs M A, Dicks-Mireaux C et al. Primary malignant liver tumours in childhood: assessment of resectability with high-field MR and comparison with C T. Pediat Radiol 1990; 21: 34–38

13. Pobiel R S, Bisset G S III. Pictorial essay: imaging of liver tumours in the infant and child. Pediat Radiol 1995; 25: 495–506

14. Powers C, Ross P R, Stoupis C et al. Primary liver neoplasms: MR imaging with pathologic correlation. RadioGraphics 1994; 14: 459–482

15. Rummeny E, Weissleder R, Stark D D et al. Primary liver tumours: diagnosis by MR imaging. Am J Roentgenol 1989; 152: 63–72

16. Siegel M J. Paediatric liver and biliary tract. In: Freeney P C, Stevenson G W (eds). Alimentary Tract Radiology. St. Louis: Mosby-Year Book, 1989: 1958–1986

17. Weinreb J C, Cohen J M, Armstrong E, Smith T. Imaging the paediatric liver: MRI and CT. Am J Roentgenol 1986; 147: 785–790

18. King S J, Babyn P S, Greenberg M L, Phillips M J, Filler R M. Value of CT in determining the resectability of hepatoblastoma before and after chemotherapy. Am J Roentgenol 1993; 160: 793–798

19. Kesslar P J, Buck J L, Selby D M. Infantile hemangioendothelioma of the liver revisited. RadioGraphics 1993; 13: 657–670

20. Ros P R, Goodman A D, Ishak K G et al. Mesenchymal hamartoma of the liver: radiologic–pathologic correlation. Radiology 1986; 158: 619–624

21. Newman K D, Schisgall R, Rearman G, Guzzetta P C. Malignant mesenchymoma of the liver in children. J Pediat Surg 1989; 24: 781–783

22. Maurer H M, Ragab A. Rhabdomyosarcoma. In: Fernbach D J, Vietti T J (eds). Clinical Paediatric Oncology (4th ed). St Louis: Mosby-Year Book, 1991; 491–515

23. Wexler L H, Helman L J. Rhabdomyosarcoma and the undifferentiated sarcomas. In: Pizzo P A, Poplack D G (eds.) Principles and Practice of Paediatric Oncology. Philadelphia: Lippincott-Raven, 1997; 799–829

24. Bahnson R R, Zaontz M R, Maizels M et al. Ultrasonography and diagnosis of paediatric genitourinary rhabdomyosarcoma. Urology 1989; 33: 64–68

25. Bartolozzi C, Selli C, Olmastroni M et al. Rhabdomyosarcoma of the prostate: MR findings. Am J Roentgenol 1988; 150: 1333–1334

26. Tannous W N, Azouz E M, Homsy Y L et al. CT and ultrasound imaging of pelvic rhabdomyosarcoma in children. A review of 56 patients. Pediatr Radiol 1989; 19: 530–534

27. Heiken J P, Forman H P, Brown J J. Neoplasms of the bladder, prostate and testis. Radiol Clin North Am 1994; 32: 81–98

28. Friedman A C, Seidmon E J, Radecki P D et al. Relative merits of MRI, transrectal endosonography and CT in diagnosis and staging of carcinoma of prostate. Urology 1988; 35: 530–53

29. Tanimoto A, Yuasa Y, Imai Y U et al. Bladder tumour staging: comparison of conventional and gadolinium-enhanced dynamic MR imaging and CT. Radiology 1992; 188: 741–747

30. Chezmar J L, Rumancik W M, Megibow A L et al. Liver and abdominal screening in patients with cancer: CT versus MR imaging. Radiology 1988; 168: 43–47

31. Reinig J W, Dwyer A J, Miller D I. Liver metastases: Detection with M R imaging at 0.5 and 1.5 T. Radiology 1989; 170: 149–153

32. Castleberry R P, Cushing B, Perlman E, Hawkins E P. Germ cell tumours. In: Pizzo P A, Poplack D G (eds). Paediatric Oncology. Philadelphia: Lippincott-Raven, 1997; 921–945

33. Castleberry R P, Kelly D R, Joseph D B, Cain W S. Gonadal and extragonadal germ cell tumours. In: Fernbach D J, Vietti T J (eds). Clinical Paediatric Oncology (4th ed). St. Louis: Mosby-Year Book; 1991; 577–594

34. Askin F B, Land V J, Sullivan M et al. Occult testicular leukemia: testicular biopsy at three years continuous complete remission of childhood leukemia — a Southern Oncology Group study. Cancer 1961; 47: 470–475

35. Crist W M, Pullen J, Rivera G K. Acute lymphoid leukemia. In: Fernbach J D, Vietti T J (eds). Clinical Paediatric Oncology (4th ed). St. Louis: Mosby-Year Book, 1991; 305–335

36. Luker G D, Siegel M J. Paediatric testicular tumours: evaluation with gray-scale and color Doppler US. Radiology 1994; 191: 561–564

37. Mazzu D, Jeffrey R B, Ralls P W. Lymphoma and leukemia involving the testicles: findings on gray-scale and color Doppler sonography. Am J Roentgenol 1995; 164: 645–647

38. Siegel M J. Male genital tract. In: Siegel M J (ed). Paediatric Sonography (2nd ed). New York: Raven Press, 1995; 479–512

39. Thurnher S, Hricak H, Carroll P R et al. Imaging the testis: comparison between MR imaging and US. Radiology 1988; 167: 631–636

40. Tesoro-Tess J D, Pizzocaro G, Zanoni F et al. Lymphangiography and computerized tomography in testicular carcinoma: How accurate in early stage disease? J Urol 1985; 133: 967–970

41. Ellis J H, Bies J R, Kopecky K K et al. Comparison of NMR and CT imaging in the evaluation of metastatic retroperiotoneal lymphadenopathy from testicular carcinoma. J Comput Assist Tomogr 1984; 8: 709–719

42. Breen J L, Bonamo J F, Maxson W S. Genital tract tumours in children. Pediatr Clin North Am 1981; 28: 355–367

43. Surrattt J T, Siegel M J. Imaging of paediatric ovarian masses. RadioGraphics 1991; 11: 533–548

44. Quillin S P, Siegel M J. CT features of benign and malignant teratomas in children. J Comput Assist Tomogr 1992; 16: 722–726

45. Togashi K, Nishimura K, Itoh K et al. Ovarian cystic teratomas: MR imaging. Radiology 1987; 162: 669–673

46. Brammer H M, Buck J L, Hayes W S et al. Malignant germ cell tumours of the ovary: radiologic–pathologic correlation. RadioGraphics 1990; 10: 715–724

47. Ghossain M A, Buy N J, Ligneres C et al. Epithelial tumours of the ovary: Comparison of MR and CT findings. Radiology 1991; 181: 863–870

48. Kesslar P J, Buck J L, Suarez E S. Germ cell tumours of the sacrococcygeal region: radiologic–pathologic correlation. RadioGraphics 1994; 14: 607–620

49. Shackelford G S. Adrenal glands, pancreas, and other retroperitoneal structures. In: Siegel M J (ed). Paediatric Sonography, 2nd ed. New York: Raven Press, 1995; 301–355

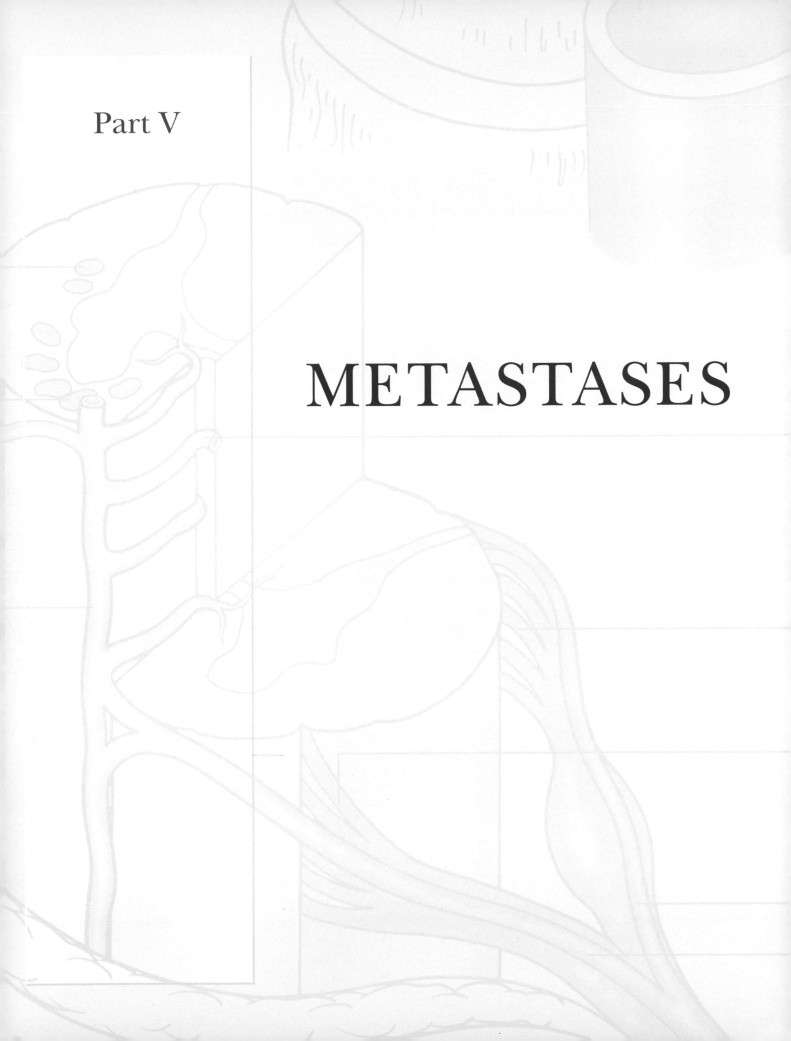

Part V

METASTASES

Chapter 35

Lymph nodes

Bernadette Carrington

INTRODUCTION

Lymphatic dissemination is one of the three principal pathways by which tumours escape from their organ of origin, the other two being direct local infiltration and haematogenous spread. Lymph node metastases are frequently identified in the commoner tumours, for example in bowel cancer locoregional lymph node involvement is seen in 40–50% of patients at the time of primary surgical resection.[1,2] For breast cancer the figure is 50%[3] and, of those patients considered to have surgically resectable non-small cell lung cancer, 40% are found to have positive nodes in the resected specimen.[4] The presence of lymph node metastases is an adverse prognostic indicator in all circumstances and may radically alter patient management. Therefore it is necessary to identify nodal metastases as part of any staging procedure before patients receive definitive treatment. In the treated patient, lymph node relapse is a common finding and involved nodes may be at the expected sites, or in more unusual locations due to treatment-induced modification of the disease process.

To identify abnormal nodes, radiologists should:

- Understand the physiological processes occurring in the lymphatic system
- Know the preferential lymphatic drainage of each primary tumour
- Have established criteria for normal lymph node size at specific anatomical sites
- Be able to distinguish lymph nodes from normal anatomical structures or normal variants
- Be aware of the more unusual sites of lymphadenopathy which can be identified on cross-sectional imaging

THE LYMPHATIC SYSTEM

The lymphatic system returns excess tissue fluid, deposited in the extracellular space due to high pressure capillary filtration, back to the vascular circulation. *En route* the lymph fluid passes through a series of lymphatic channels and lymph nodes before ultimately draining via the thoracic duct into the subclavian vein. Lymph nodes act as complex filters for antigenic material and are situated at the junction of several lymphatics where they lie parallel to adjacent blood vessels. The number of nodes may vary tremendously in superficial locations, for example the neck, but in visceral sites the number of nodes is more constant. Each node has multiple, afferent lymphatics passing through a collagenous capsule along the convex nodal surface with lymph draining directly into the subcapsular sinus (Fig. 35.1). This is located immediately deep to the capsule but also alongside the fibrous trabeculae of the node thereby extending through the cortex to the medulla. Lymph leaves the node via a small number of efferent ducts situated at the hilum of the node.

The composition of a lymph node varies with its anatomical site and degree of stimulation;[5] for example:

- Axillary nodes may be almost entirely replaced by fat with only a thin peripheral rim of lymphatic tissue (Fig. 35.2)
- Inguinal nodes may have a target appearance (Fig. 35.2)
- Inguinal nodes may demonstrate focal scarring and calcification in areas of hyaline fibrosis[5]
- Mesenteric nodes are extremely active manifesting as hypercellular nodes with large numbers of follicles[5]

In addition to site-specific structural variations, each node is also in a state of continual flux with inflow and outflow of lymph (up to 10 ml/hr/g nodal weight), blood (1 ml/min/g nodal weight) and lymphocytes (each node recirculates its own weight of lymphocytes every 4–12 days depending on antigenic stimulation).[5]

MECHANISM OF TUMOUR SPREAD TO LYMPH NODES

Although all neoplasms develop new blood vessels, most tumours cannot develop their own lymph vessels and tumour penetration of lymphatics is therefore by direct erosion of the tumour mass or by individual tumour cell invagination through

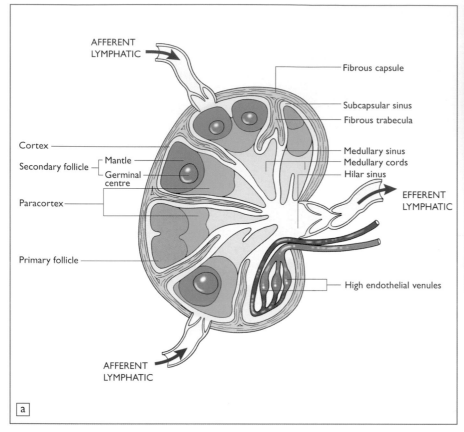

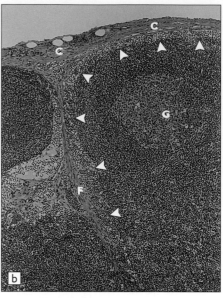

Figure 35.1. *The normal lymph node. (a) Cross-section through a normal lymph node. (b) Photomicrograph of a normal lymph node (Haematoxylin and Eosin). The capsule (C) is well seen as is the subcapsular sinus (arrowheads) which extends deep into the node alongside the fibrous trabecula (F). Germinal centre (G).*

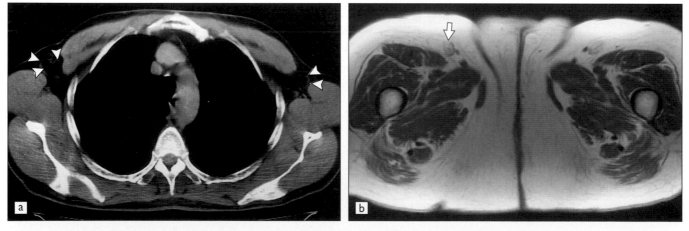

Figure 35.2. *Fatty lymph nodes. (a) Transaxial thoracic CT scan demonstrating crescents of lymphoid tissue (arrowheads) in otherwise fatty nodes; (b) transaxial T1-weighted MR image showing a target appearance to a right inguinal node (arrow).*

the lymphatic endothelium.[6] Either singly or in small groups, tumour cells then migrate to the nearest lymph node where they are usually arrested in the subcapsular sinus (Fig. 35.3).[5,6] Most tumour deposits die[6] but a small percentage initiate metastatic colonies which may ultimately replace the entire node and in some cases go on to penetrate the nodal capsule and extend into the adjacent tissue. Alternatively, the neoplastic cells may traverse the lymph node leaving via the efferent lymphatics or venules. Once a lymph node metastasis has been established there may be a reduction of the involved node's filtering capability allowing subsequent tumour emboli effectively to bypass that node and reach other sites more easily.[7]

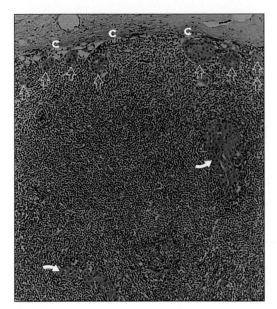

Figure 35.3. *Subcapsular sinus tumour deposits (Haematoxylin and Eosin). Multiple small tumour deposits (open arrows) are identified within the subcapsular sinus in a patient with metastatic breast cancer. Some of these deposits measure 5 μm or less. Larger deposits are seen (curved arrows) deeper within the substance of the gland.*

EVALUATION OF LYMPH NODE METASTASES WITH CROSS-SECTIONAL IMAGING

In clinical practice, the cross-sectional imaging modalities computed tomography (CT), ultrasound and magnetic resonance imaging (MRI) are widely used to assess lymph nodes and the diagnosis of abnormality rests on features such as nodal size together with limited assessment of tissue characteristics. Unfortunately, it is well recognized that, for most primary tumours, 10–20% of normal sized locoregional nodes will contain small tumour deposits[8–10] and conversely over 30% of enlarged nodes will show only inflammatory hyperplasia with no evidence of malignancy.[9,11] In certain tumour types the incidence of metastatic normal-sized nodes is even greater, for example in colorectal cancer two-thirds of nodal metastases occur in nodes less than 5 mm and 90% in nodes less than 1 cm.[1]

Ideally, therefore, imaging techniques should allow identification of small, even microscopic, tumour deposits. Historically lymphangiography has been used to detect tumour deposits in normal-sized nodes and newer functional imaging techniques may also be important in this regard, particularly positron emission tomography (PET), which detects metabolic changes in metastatic nodes. Nonetheless, most centres still primarily rely on cross-sectional imaging and the following discussion will concentrate on these techniques.

The choice of imaging will depend on local expertise but also on the primary tumour, for example high resolution ultrasound may be used for assessment of inguinal nodes in a patient with a peripheral melanoma, or for neck nodal status in a patient with a thyroid tumour. However, in patients with primary malignancies of the thorax, abdomen and pelvis, CT or MRI are the preferred investigations since, with satisfactory patient preparation and radiographic technique, these modalities provide the most reliable and least invasive means of lymph node evaluation.

Computed tomography (CT)

A meticulous radiographic technique is vital for proper interpretation and for CT there must be thorough bowel preparation, contiguous or near contiguous slices and standardized window levels and window widths for all hard copy images. Where there is potential confusion, for example from poorly opacified bowel loops, then the patient should be rescanned through the relevant area after an interval or scanned in the decubitus position to try and resolve any uncertainty. Because lymph nodes usually have a soft tissue density similar to vessels, intravenous contrast medium may be used as a problem-solving tool to help distinguish between lymph nodes and vessels. For a given tumour, the preferred lymphatic drainage needs to be covered in any radiological assessment. Thus, in patients with ovarian cancer, where spread may occur to diaphragmatic nodes,[12] it is important that patients are scanned from the xiphisternum to the pelvis, and for tumours of the anal canal, the inferior extent of any CT examination must include the inguinal nodes.

Magnetic resonance imaging (MRI)

On MRI, lymph nodes are seen on T1-weighted images as intermediate signal intensity structures, the node contrasting well with the high signal intensity of the surrounding fat.[13] Proton density images also show lymph nodes as intermediate intensity structures. On T2-weighted sequences lymph nodes have an intermediate to high signal intensity, they may therefore be difficult to visualize as there is little inherent contrast between the node and surrounding fat. Short tau inversion recovery (STIR) sequences are useful for demonstrating enlarged lymph nodes which appear as very high signal intensity structures against a background of low signal intensity. Occasionally, bowel loops may be confusing and delayed scans may be necessary. Magnetic resonance imaging specific bowel contrast medium is now available although it is not used routinely in most centres. As with CT, the entire pathway of locoregional spread must be covered and this may result in relatively long examination times, for example the abdomen and pelvis need to be imaged in pelvic malignancies and the entire neck for head and neck tumours.

Magnetic resonance imaging has the potential advantage that lymph nodes can be differentiated from blood vessels due to the intravascular signal void of flowing blood (Fig. 35.4). Sometimes slow blood flow in an ectatic vein may simulate an enlarged lymph node, but this diagnostic dilemma can be solved by use of flow-sensitive techniques such as gradient-recalled echo imaging.[14]

Key points: general features

■ Lymph node metastases are always an adverse prognostic indicator

■ Most tumours cannot develop their own lymphatic system

■ Tumours penetrate the lymphatic channels by direct erosion or tumour cell invagination through the lymphatic endothelium

■ Tumour cells migrate to the nearest lymph node when metastatic colonies develop in the subcapsular sinus

■ CT and MRI are the preferred imaging modalities for evaluation of lymph node metastases

IDENTIFICATION OF LYMPH NODES

Certain nodal sites are easily overlooked and several of these are illustrated in Figure 35.5; they are also summarized in Table 35.1. While abnormality at these sites does not usually represent the only nodal group involved in a particular pathological process, it is necessary to identify all disease sites so that the most appropriate treatment can be decided upon and to enable subsequent assessment of disease response.

Misdiagnosis of lymphadenopathy (Table 35.2)

In cross-sectional imaging, the most common diagnostic error results from mistaking vessels, particularly aberrant

Table 35.1. *Overlooked lymph node sites*[15–23]

Head and neck	Lateral retropharyngeal Facial
Thorax	Subpectoral/subscapular/interpectoral Internal mammary Posterior mediastinal Paracardiac Retrocrural
Abdomen	Diaphragmatic Hepatogastric ligament Peripancreatic Splenic hilar Porta hepatis Portacaval Paracaval Common iliac Psoas
Pelvis	Obturator Presacral Paracervical Perirectal Inguinal

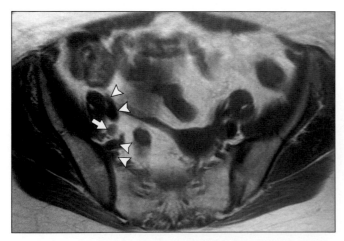

Figure 35.4. *Transaxial T1-weighted MR image demonstrating an enlarged right internal iliac lymph node (arrow) clearly seen separate from the external iliac and internal iliac vessels (arrowheads). The intermediate signal intensity of the node contrasts well with the surrounding high signal intensity fat.*

Table 35.2. *Structures which may be mistaken for lymph nodes*

Head and neck	Muscles — posterior belly of digastric; styloid; styloglossus; stylopharyngeus Thrombosed internal jugular vein Submandibular gland — deep portion
Thorax	Superior recess of pericardium Left atrial pericardial defect Aberrant vessels Coronary sinus
Abdomen	Bowel Vessels Other structures (ureters, lymphatic trunks)
Pelvis	Bowel Vessels Other structures (ovaries, lymphocoeles, iliopsoas bursae)

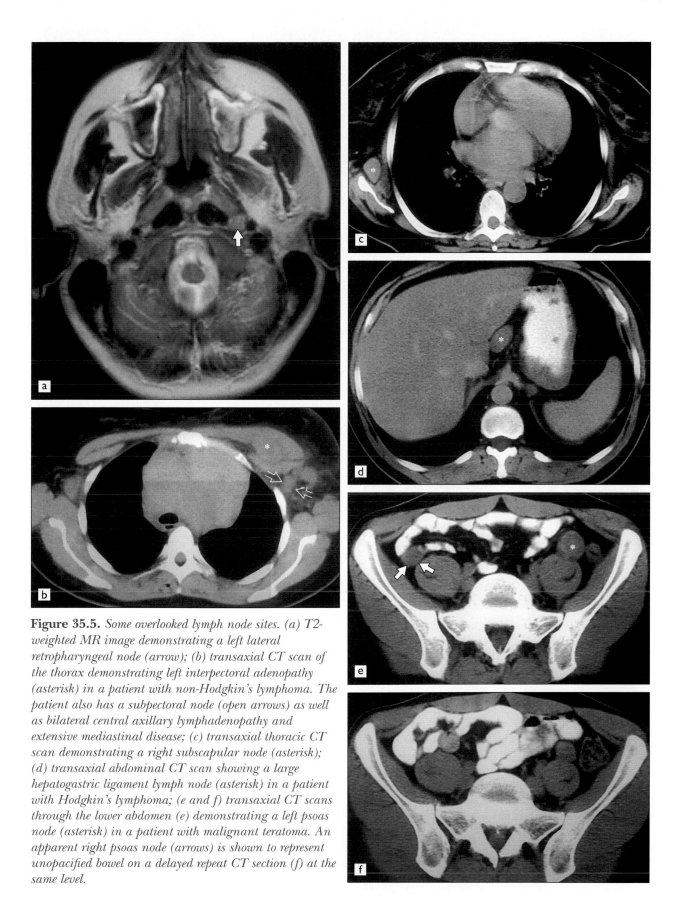

Figure 35.5. *Some overlooked lymph node sites. (a) T2-weighted MR image demonstrating a left lateral retropharyngeal node (arrow); (b) transaxial CT scan of the thorax demonstrating left interpectoral adenopathy (asterisk) in a patient with non-Hodgkin's lymphoma. The patient also has a subpectoral node (open arrows) as well as bilateral central axillary lymphadenopathy and extensive mediastinal disease; (c) transaxial thoracic CT scan demonstrating a right subscapular node (asterisk); (d) transaxial abdominal CT scan showing a large hepatogastric ligament lymph node (asterisk) in a patient with Hodgkin's lymphoma; (e and f) transaxial CT scans through the lower abdomen (e) demonstrating a left psoas node (asterisk) in a patient with malignant teratoma. An apparent right psoas node (arrows) is shown to represent unopacified bowel on a delayed repeat CT section (f) at the same level.*

vessels, for enlarged nodes (Fig. 35.6).[24,25] Other structures which may be confused with lymph nodes are the superior recess of the pericardium and posterior pericardial defects (Fig. 35.7), dilated lymphatic trunks in the thorax or abdomen,[26,27] lymphocoeles, retained or transposed ovaries (Fig. 35.8)[28,29] and, in the inguinal region, iliopsoas bursae (Fig. 35.9).[30] For this reason radiologists need good anatomical knowledge and access to relevant clinical information, for example previous surgical procedures.

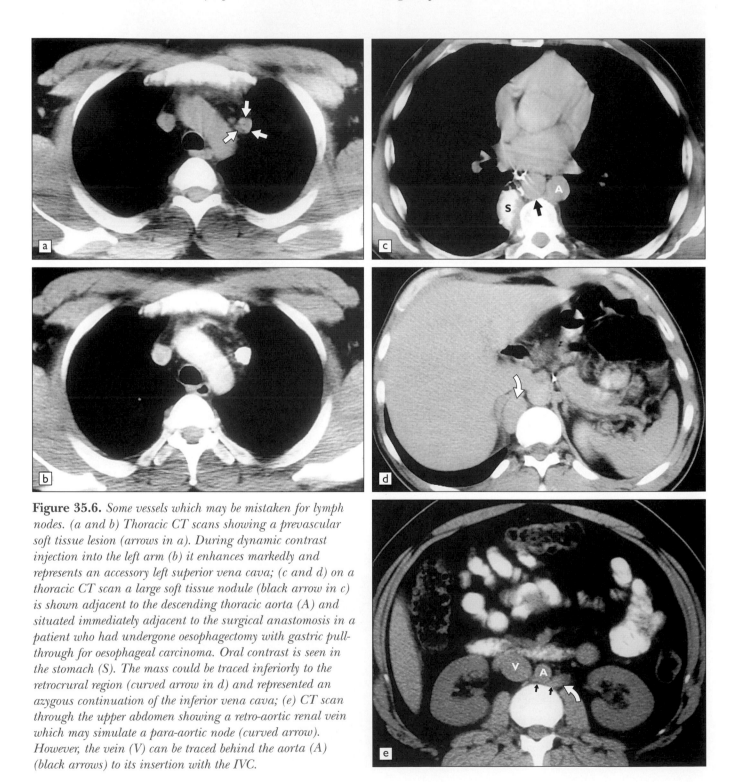

Figure 35.6. *Some vessels which may be mistaken for lymph nodes. (a and b) Thoracic CT scans showing a prevascular soft tissue lesion (arrows in a). During dynamic contrast injection into the left arm (b) it enhances markedly and represents an accessory left superior vena cava; (c and d) on a thoracic CT scan a large soft tissue nodule (black arrow in c) is shown adjacent to the descending thoracic aorta (A) and situated immediately adjacent to the surgical anastomosis in a patient who had undergone oesophagectomy with gastric pull-through for oesophageal carcinoma. Oral contrast is seen in the stomach (S). The mass could be traced inferiorly to the retrocrural region (curved arrow in d) and represented an azygous continuation of the inferior vena cava; (e) CT scan through the upper abdomen showing a retro-aortic renal vein which may simulate a para-aortic node (curved arrow). However, the vein (V) can be traced behind the aorta (A) (black arrows) to its insertion with the IVC.*

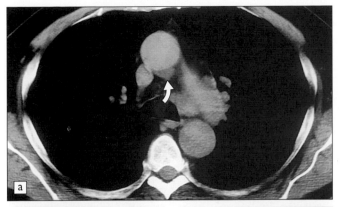

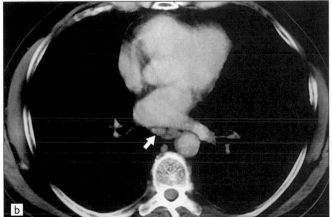

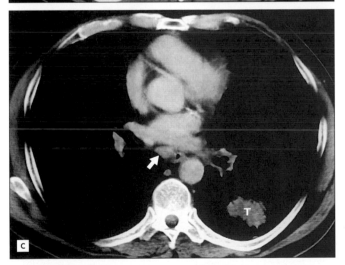

Figure 35.7. *Some structures which may be mistaken for lymphadenopathy. (a) The superior recess of the pericardium (curved arrow). On this non-contrast CT scan it is of low attenuation due to its fluid content and is always situated directly adjacent to the posterior aspect of the ascending aorta; (b and c) prolapse of the left atrium (white arrows) due to a localized pericardial defect shown on sequential CT scans. The lesion could easily be mistaken for a posterior mediastinal node, particularly in this patient with a bronchial tumour (T) seen in (c).*

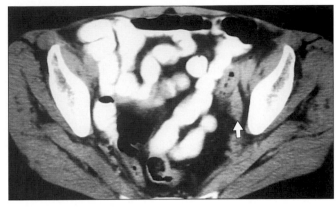

Figure 35.8. *CT scan through the pelvis demonstrating a retained ovary on the left pelvic side wall (arrow). This could easily be confused with a unilateral enlarged obturator node. The only clue that the mass may be an ovary is its pear shape, and full clinical information is required.*

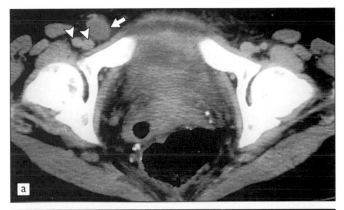

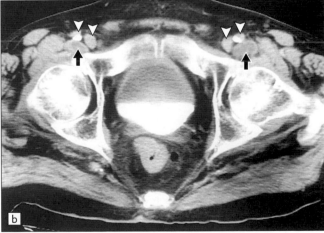

Figure 35.9. *(a) CT scan demonstrating a cystic right inguinal node in a patient with an anal tumour. Note the position of the node (white arrow) which is anterior and medial to the femoral vein and artery (arrowheads); (b) iliopsoas bursae (black arrows) are situated posterolateral to the inguinal vessels (arrowheads) on this transaxial enhanced CT scan.*

Key points: cross-sectional imaging

- Common sources of error are overlooked sites of lymph node involvement and misdiagnosis of lymph nodes as vessels

- Size, site, number and tissue characteristics of nodes are all important criteria for determining whether lymph nodes are normal or abnormal

Imaging features of abnormal lymph nodes

Once lymph nodes have been identified, the critical decision is whether the nodes are normal or abnormal. Currently there is one major radiological criterion and three minor criteria which are employed to differentiate between those nodes likely to be malignant and those considered to be benign:

Major criterion
- Size

Minor criteria
- Site
- Number
- Tissue characteristics
  — attenuation
  — signal intensity
  — echogenicity

Nodal size

Since there may be considerable interobserver variation in lymph node assessment[31], measurement of nodes should be performed in a standard fashion to maximize reproducibility within and between examinations. It is known that altering the window level and window width on CT can lead to marked variation in the apparent size of a nodule [32,33] so measurements should be made on images at a standard window level and window width. Hard-copy assessment is preferable since this allows improved edge appreciation. The maximum short-axis diameter (MSAD) should be measured (Fig. 35.10) since it has been demonstrated that the short-axis diameter of a lymph node remains relatively constant irrespective of its orientation in a vertical plane[34], and that an involved node is likely to become rounder before it enlarges longitudinally.[4] Use of the maximum short-axis diameter as a nodal measurement may increase sensitivity, specificity or both.[35–37]

The upper limits of normal lymph node size have been derived from many studies over the last 10–15 years. Some studies document postmortem values in normal populations[38–40] while others deal with pathological assessment of resected specimens.[1,2,9] The majority of papers correlate cross-sectional imaging findings with pathology, other imaging modalities, biochemistry or clinical outcome[8,10,11,35–37,41–68] and one paper measures nodal size on lymphangiography.[69] There have been inherent problems with some of the study populations which include:

- Small patient numbers
- Patient factors
- Nodal measurement technique
- Other causes of nodal enlargement

In the studies reported there is a preponderance of North American patient groups, little allowance for age and gender (which affect nodal size), and often, of necessity, the evaluation of oncological patient cohorts. Although the oncological patients studied may be in long-term remission or have tumours unlikely to affect the regions being studied, possible bias is still introduced. Other potential errors relate to technique, particularly which nodal axis has been measured and to which anatomical subgroup the measured nodes belong. There has been difficulty in identifying which histological nodes correspond with which imaged nodes, in maintaining the nodal axis between CT, surgical resection and pathological sectioning, and in quantifying the effect of histological fixation. Even in normal populations assessed at postmortem, or by CT,[46,50] possible factors influencing nodal size include air pollution, pneumoconiosis, granulomatous disease and HIV status. Despite all these problems,

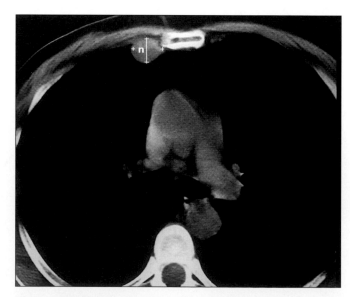

Figure 35.10. *Measurement of lymph nodes. The maximum short axis of a right internal mammary node (n) is the largest measurement perpendicular to the long axis (between the crosses).*

Table 35.3. *Size: recommendations on normal upper limit*

Site	Short axis diameter (mm)
Head and neck	10
Lateral retropharyngeal	<5
Facial	Not seen
Submental	11
Axilla	12
Mediastinum	10
Subcarinal	12
Retrocrural	6
Paracardiac	8
Abdomen	10
Gastrohepatic ligament	8
Porta hepatis	7
Upper para-aortic	9
Lower para-aortic	11
Pelvis	10
Common iliac	9
Internal iliac	7
Obturator	8
Presacral, paracervical, perirectal	Not seen
Inguinal	15

a reasonably clear consensus is emerging as to what constitutes upper limits of normal for lymph nodes in different areas of the body and this is detailed in Table 35.3.

Measurement ratios have been used to try and improved nodal assessment accuracy, for example maximum short axis:maximum long axis in the transaxial plane in patients with head and neck tumours[42,43,70] and, more recently, the maximal longitudinal to the maximal axial diameter using spiral (helical) CT reformations.[71] Results are variable with some authors reporting increased accuracy[42,43,70,71] and others maintaining that maximum short-axis diameter is the best measurement.[35,37]

Some lymph nodes are not usually visualized on cross-sectional imaging, for example, facial, splenic hilar, central pelvic (paracervical, perirectal) and posterior pelvic (presacral) nodes. When they are identified it is likely that they are abnormal (Fig. 35.11).

Nodal site

Knowledge of the normal pathways of lymphatic spread from a particular organ means that more emphasis can be placed on nodes of borderline size in a recognized drainage site for a particular primary tumour, for example, an asymmetrical, prominent obturator node is of great concern in bladder, prostate or cervical primary cancers. On the other hand, isolated contralateral lymphadenopathy in a patient being staged for a testicular tumour is extremely rare[72] and should be interpreted with caution.

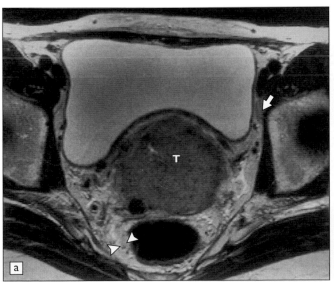
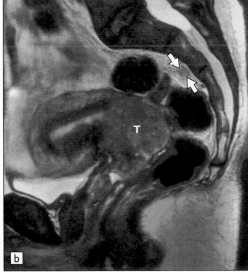

Figure 35.11. *(a) Axial T2-weighted MR image in a patient with a large cervical tumour (T). There is a right perirectal node (arrowheads) and a prominent left pelvic side wall node (arrow). (b) Sagittal T2-weighted MR image in a patient with a large cervical tumour (T), in whom there is a presacral node (arrows).*

Table 35.4. *Normal number of nodes*[45,54,67,68]

Site	Range	Mean
Axilla	1–21	5
Retroperitoneum	0–4	2
Pelvis	0–28	9
Inguinal	3–8	6

Nodal number

In daily practice radiologists are concerned by a cluster of normal sized nodes which are asymmetrical compared to the contralateral side of the body but there is a paucity of data about normal nodal number in most anatomical sites. The information that does exist is shown below in Table 35.4.[45,54,67,68]

It should be noted that, in every anatomical site, fewer nodes are identified on cross-sectional imaging than at surgery or in pathological specimens, perhaps not surprising when the smallest node may measure only 1 mm, but emphasizing our current inability to provide a complete radiological evaluation of lymph nodes. This fact is reinforced by recent work looking at pelvic CT in patients pre- and post-lymphangiography, where the number of identifiable nodes rose dramatically when lymphangiographic contrast was present.[67]

The advent of spiral CT has also resulted in increased detection of lymph nodes. For example on thoracic spiral CT scans it is now possible to identify normal hilar lymph nodes,[73] and 40% of nodes measuring 5–9 mm were seen in patients undergoing surgery for gastric cancer resection.[70] Nonetheless, even with spiral CT only 1% of nodes less than 5 mm were detected.[70]

Nodal tissue characteristics

Normal nodes may have a uniform appearance or may demonstrate characteristic features of central fat on ultrasound, CT and MRI (echogenic/low attenuation/high signal intensity, respectively) (Fig. 35.2). Fatty nodes are commonly seen in the axilla and occasionally in the groin, where there may be a target appearance to the node. They are less likely to be infiltrated with tumour but may become solid when involved by tumour (Fig. 35.12) and revert to the previous appearance after treatment. Sometimes the consistency of the node is a helpful pointer towards its involvement by tumour and may suggest a particular tumour type. For example, in testicular malignant teratoma, involved nodes are often of low attenuation on CT[74] (Fig. 35.13). Thus, in a patient known to have a malignant teratoma, a small node with a cystic central component may be a pointer to metastatic tumour involvement. Conversely, in a male patient being investigated for retroperitoneal adenopathy the presence of cystic nodes makes a non-seminomatous germ cell tumour (NSGCT) of the testis a likely diagnosis.

As a consequence of granulomatous disease, mediastinal or mesenteric nodes are often densely calcified. However, more speckled amorphous calcification may be seen in metastatic nodes due to gastro-intestinal neoplasms or ovarian tumours and this calcification may persist or resolve after treatment (Fig. 35.14). In certain tumours, for example testicular NSGCT, treated metastatic nodes may become densely calcified (Fig. 35.15).

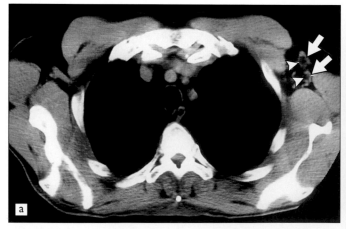 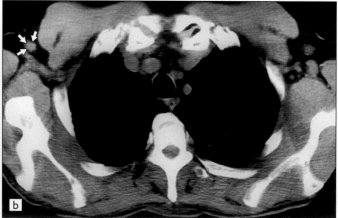

Figure 35.12. *(a) CT scan in a patient in remission with non-Hodgkin's lymphoma demonstrating normal left axillary nodes (large arrows) which are predominantly fatty with a thin soft tissue capsule medially (arrowheads). (b) On relapse the nodes become solid and a new node appears in the right axilla (small white arrows).*

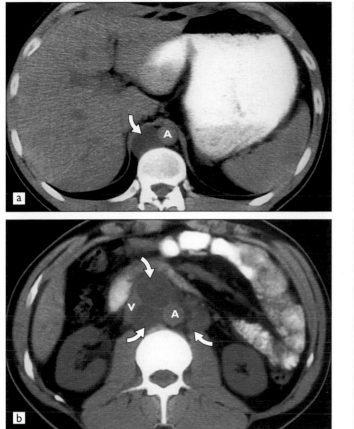

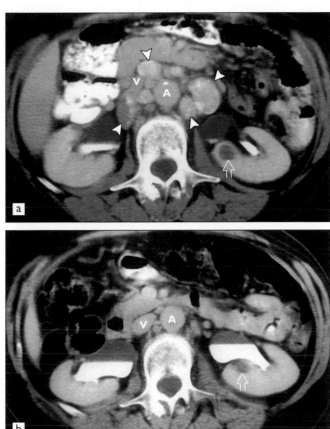

Figure 35.13. *CT scans of a patient with a testicular malignant teratoma demonstrating low attenuation cystic adenopathy in the retrocrural region (a) and retroperitoneum (b). The inferior vena cava (V) is displaced by the adenopathic masses (curved arrows). Abdominal aorta (A).*

Figure 35.14. *Abdominal CT scans at the same level in a patient with ovarian cancer before treatment (a) and after chemotherapy (b). Before treatment there is considerable upper retroperitoneal lymphadenopathy (arrowheads) which contains dystrophic calcification. After treatment not only do the nodes shrink but the dystrophic calcification resolves. Simple cyst in left kidney (open arrow). V = inferior vena cava; A = abdominal aorta.*

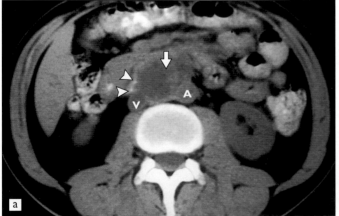

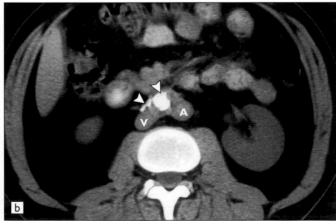

Figure 35.15. *(a) CT scan of a large cystic interaortocaval nodal mass (arrow) in a patient with metastatic testicular malignant teratoma. There is one small area of calcification*

(arrowheads) at the periphery of the nodal mass. (b) After treatment the residual mass is heavily calcified (arrowheads). A = abdominal aorta. V = inferior vena cava.

Central necrosis may occur in some metastatic nodes due to medullary invasion by tumour producing local ischaemia[17,75] and CT is superior to MRI in its identification,[75,76] although MRI detection rate is improved by the use of contrast agent (gadolinium-DTPA).[77] Central nodal necrosis is most frequently observed in squamous cell primary tumours of the head and neck (Fig. 35.16) where it is a recognized adverse prognostic sign,[17] and in the appropriate clinical setting necrotic normal-sized nodes are to be regarded as involved by tumour in patients with head and neck primaries.[17,35] In Hodgkin's lymphoma, however, nodal necrosis is not a poor prognostic feature.[78]

In vitro MRI work on axillary nodes from patients with breast cancer suggested that tissue relaxation times could be used to differentiate benign from malignant lymph glands.[79,80] Unfortunately, *in vivo* studies have shown that there are no absolute criteria for lymph node involvement on MRI since there is considerable overlap in the T1- and T2-relaxation times of cancerous, lymphomatous, hyperplastic and benign nodes.[81–83] Nonetheless, when the signal intensity of a node parallels the signal intensity of the primary lesion, then this sign increases diagnosticconfidence (Fig. 35.17).

High frequency ultrasound has been used to assess superficial lymph nodes, particularly in head and neck tumours, and certain factors may indicate a likely primary site. For example, posterior acoustic enhancement and lack of intranodal necrosis, together with a nodal distribution predominantly involving the submandibular and posterior triangle groups, are more in keeping with lymphoma than metastatic disease.[84] Metastatic papillary thyroid nodes are usually solid, hyperechoic masses, and 70% of these nodes have punctate calcification due to psammoma bodies.[85]

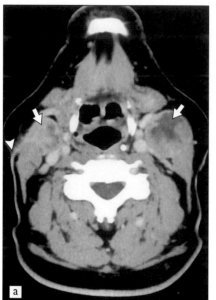

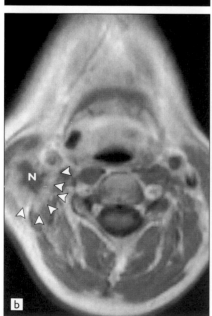

Figure 35.16. *Central nodal necrosis. (a) Contrast-enhanced CT scan demonstrating large partially necrotic deep cervical nodes in a patient with a head and neck tumour (white arrows). The patient has undergone a surgical biopsy on the right resulting in a scar (arrowhead); (b) T1-weighted postcontrast MR image through the neck at the level of the hyoid in a patient with a metastatic deep cervical node from a head and neck primary. Central nodal necrosis is apparent (N) and there is a spiculated margin to the node with enhancing strands of soft tissue extending into the adjacent musculature and fat (arrowheads) compatible with extracapsular extension.*

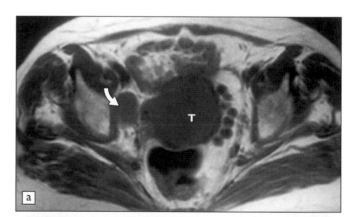

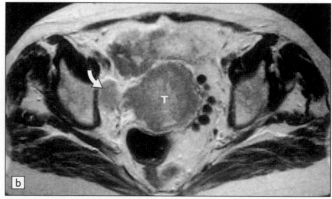

Figure 35.17. *(a) T1-weighted and (b) T2-weighted MR images in a patient with a large cervical tumour (T). The signal intensity of the enlarged right obturator node (arrows) parallels that of the primary tumour increasing diagnostic confidence that the node is metastatic.*

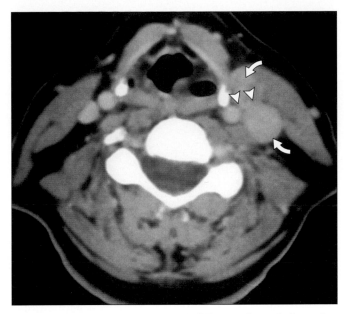

Figure 35.18. *Contrast-enhanced CT scan through the neck demonstrating enhancing left cervical lymph nodes (arrows) in a patient with a thyroid follicular carcinoma. The left internal jugular vein is compressed (arrowheads).*

Extracapsular tumour spread

When the margins of an enlarged lymph node are irregular, then it is likely that tumour has spread beyond the capsule of that node, providing that there is no evidence of acute inflammation in and around the nodal site (Fig. 35.16). This feature is of particular relevance in head and neck tumours since prognosis is considerably worse if it is present.[17] Unfortunately, by the time extracapsular tumour spread is identified, over 75% of nodes are already enlarged.[17,75] Computed tomography is more accurate than MRI in the identification of extracapsular nodal extension of tumour in neck nodes.[75,76]

The use of intravenous contrast medium in lymph node assessment

Just as lymph nodes were occasionally identifiable on angiography so some nodal masses are vascular and may enhance on CT[86] (Fig. 35.18). Adenopathy may also enhance with MRI contrast media (Fig. 35.19), but enhancement *per se* does not necessarily imply tumour involvement. However, the use of intravenous contrast medium may serve to highlight central nodal necrosis which may indicate malignant involvement of non-enlarged nodes (Fig. 35.19).

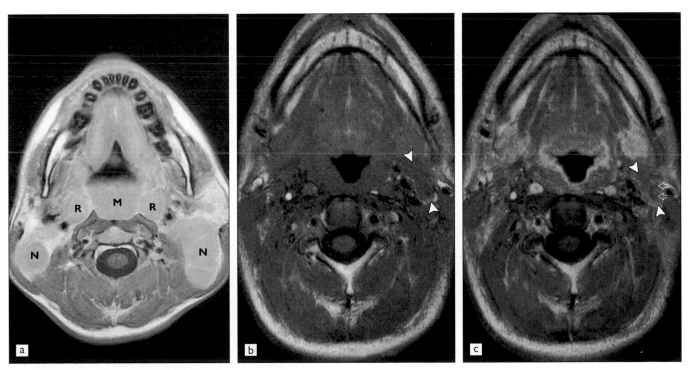

Figure 35.19. *(a) Axial T1-weighted contrast-enhanced MR image at the level of the inferior alveolar ridge. Bilateral solid enhancing deep cervical adenopathy is evident (N). In addition there is bilateral lateral retropharyngeal adenopathy (R) and a large pharyngeal tumour mass (M). This patient had non-Hodgkin's lymphoma. (b and c) T1-weighted precontrast image (b) and T1-weighted postcontrast image (c) in a patient with a squamous cell tumour of the nasopharynx. A deep cervical node is seen (arrowheads) but the central nodal necrosis is better appreciated after intravenous contrast (open arrows in c).*

More recently, dynamic contrast-enhanced MR imaging has been used to differentiate between enlarged benign and malignant mediastinal nodes in a small number of patients with promising results, and in bladder cancer it may help to detect tumour in normal sized nodes.[87,88] Obviously, this technique can only be employed over a limited area and could not be used to assess all nodal sites, since this would result in unacceptably long examination times.

Ultrafine superparamagnetic iron oxide particulate contrast has been used as an MRI lymph node-specific contrast medium which may be injected intravenously, or intra-arterially (after histamine). It is taken up within normal lymph nodes and produces a signal void, whereas the presence of tumour causes a failure of contrast uptake and persisting nodal signal intensity. This technique has the potential to allow differentiation between enlarged metastatic and hyperplastic benign nodes and may possibly permit the identification of metastases in normal-sized nodes. Most studies have been performed in animals[89–94] with only a few trials in humans[95,96] and short-term toxicity (proportional to the amount of injected iron) is low.[93] The technique awaits full translation into routine imaging practice.

Key points: nodal characteristics

■ Nodal size should be measured using the maximum short axis diameter (MSAD) or a ratio of orthogonal diameters, e.g. maximum longitudinal to the maximum axial diameter

■ Clusters of normal sized asymmetric nodes should be regarded with suspicion of harbouring metastases

■ Spiral (helical) CT identifies a greater number of normal nodes than conventional CT

■ Metastatic nodes may show central necrosis, cystic change or calcification on CT

■ On MRI there is considerable overlap between the T1- and T2-weighted relaxation times of cancerous and benign nodes

■ High frequency ultrasound may show nodal characteristics typical of a particular tumour type, e.g. lymphoma

■ Intravenous contrast medium may result in nodal enhancement on CT and MRI

■ Dynamic contrast-enhanced imaging has potential for differentiating enlarged benign from malignant lymph nodes

Accuracy of cross-sectional imaging

The available literature on cross-sectional imaging accuracy for lymph node metastases is confusing due to tremendous variation in:

- Patient populations
- Scanner sophistication
- Measurement methods
- Nodal identification
- Image correlation

For the most part, initial results have not been corroborated by large prospective multicentre studies. So, for colorectal disease, CT and MRI have accuracies of 62 and 64%, respectively[97] and for lung cancer sensitivities and specificities of 52 and 69% for CT and 48 and 64% for MRI have been reported.[98] The Diagnostic Oncology Group results for head and neck tumours indicate that CT is more sensitive than MRI with false-negative rates of 9 and 16%, respectively.[76] Results for pelvic lymph node evaluation are more encouraging and representative figures on CT and MRI accuracy are approximately 75%.[58,59]

In the final analysis all imaging assessment of nodes relies on probability rather than histological certainty and clinicians should appreciate that using the criteria outlined will inevitably result in a proportion of false-positive and false-negative reports.

Key point: accuracy

■ CT and MRI have comparable accuracies in the detection of lymph node metastases

RADIONUCLIDE LYMPH NODE IMAGING

Gallium-67 citrate

In the 1970s and early 1980s Ga-67 citrate was used extensively for the clinical evaluation of oncology patients. It accumulates within lymphomatous masses and some solid tumours, particularly bronchogenic carcinoma, with reported detection rates of 70 and 90% respectively.[99] For mediastinal and hilar node involvement Ga-67 scanning was reported to be 84% accurate for staging peripheral lung cancers and 60% accurate for staging paramediastinal primary lung tumours.[100] However, in other hands Ga-67 was disappointing when used as a prospective preoperative staging investigation with a sensitivity of only 55% for nodal metastases in lung cancer.[101] Other disadvantages are relative cost, the protracted nature of the test (taking up to one week to perform), the potential confusion with inflammatory conditions which are also Ga-67 avid and the relative lack of uptake in necrotic tumours. These factors have led to Ga-67 falling out of favour as a staging tool. In some centres it is still used as a predictor of disease-free status in treated lymphoma, when it is more accurate than CT[102] (Fig. 35.20).

Positron emission tomography (PET) imaging

Positron emission tomography is a functional imaging modality which detects metabolic alterations in diseased tissues. It utilizes positron-emitting substances, particularly radionuclides of carbon incorporated into organic compounds, the most commonly used being the glucose analogue 2-[F-18] fluoro-2-deoxy-D-glucose (18-FDG). Since PET units specifically count only the 2 annihilation photons emitted at 180° to each other during radionuclide decay, there is improved spatial resolution and mathematical accuracy compared with conventional radionuclide studies.[103] Most tumours take up 18-FDG avidly, resulting in a high signal-to-noise ratio and excellent tumour localization in a variety of tumours. Research confirms that PET is of value in the identification of metastatic nodal disease in breast and lung cancer, as well as in head and neck tumours and lymphoma.[103–107] Currently, PET can be used to image the whole body and, when PET images are superimposed on CT or MRI images to give so-called 'fusion' or 'anatometabolic' images, the reported accuracy of tumour localization is very high.[104] There is some uptake in inflammatory tissue but usually it can be distinguished from neoplastic lesions, and radiation-induced fibrosis can be differentiated from recurrent tumour in the treated patient.[108,109]

These initial clinical reports are encouraging although PET needs to be widely used before its true potential can be accurately assessed. Currently, the major disadvantage of PET is its limited availability due to high cost. Since PET is regarded as a complementary technique and will not replace imaging modalities such as MRI, it adds considerably to the expense of patient investigation.

Monoclonal antibody imaging

Radiolabelled-monoclonal antibodies have been raised against some tumour antigens, for example carcinoembryonic antigen (CEA), and used to detect tumour deposits *in vivo*.[110,113] In colorectal tumour patients the technique has been shown to be useful in differentiating between recurrent tumour and treatment-induced fibrosis. Its accuracy in detecting involved lymph nodes is less clear, although it is theoretically capable of identifying tumour in normal-sized nodes.[113] Recognized problems include non-uniform antigen expression by the tumour, the need for high quality radionuclide imaging and false-positive antibody scans due to normal radiopharmaceutical distribution and excretion.[110]

Key points: radionuclide studies

- 18-FDG-PET is valuable for the detection of metastatic lymph nodes

- Radiolabelled monoclonal antibodies are currently under investigation for the detection of tumour in normal sized nodes

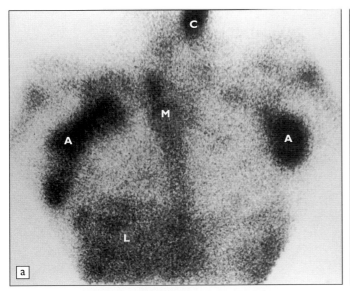
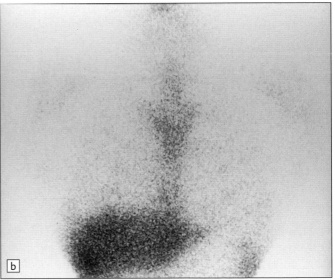

Figure 35.20. *Gallium-67 citrate radionuclide scan. (a) Pretreatment. Gallium-avid masses are seen in the axillae (A), mediastinum (M) and deep cervical chain (C) in a patient with Hodgkin's disease. Note the heterogeneous activity in the* liver (L) which was also infiltrated; (b) post-treatment. After chemotherapy there is no abnormal uptake and therefore this patient has a good prognosis.

Sentinel node imaging

An alternative approach to lymph node imaging is the identification of the gland at greatest risk of containing metastatic tumour — known as the sentinel node. This is the first lymph node to receive lymph drainage from a given primary tumour and, once identified, can be removed and histologically examined. Those patients who are sentinel node negative have no further surgery while those who are positive have more extensive lymph node dissection. Previously the sentinel node has been located using blue dye injected around tumours such as melanoma[111]; more recently lympho-scintigraphic methods have been used, for example injecting Tc^{99m} human serum albumin to image the nodal drainage sites and then performing sentinel node resection guided by a hand held γ-detector. In a large group of breast cancer patients, initial results have been excellent with sentinel node status correlating with total axillary nodal status in 97% of women[112].

LYMPHANGIOGRAPHY

Lymphangiography allows examination of the internal structure of lymph nodes (Fig. 35.21) and thereby offers the potential for identifying small tumour deposits in normal sized nodes and distinguishing between hyperplastic and malignant enlarged nodes.[52,114] Advocates of lymphangiography have claimed a significant advantage over CT in staging Hodgkin's disease,[115] but other studies show poor diagnostic information from lymphangiography in Hodgkin's patients,[116] and CT has been shown to be superior to lymphangiography in both staging and detection of disease-relapse in testicular tumours.[51,117] Moreover, lymphangiography is technically demanding and requires expertise in interpretation, which is fast vanishing due to the technique being superseded by cross-sectional imaging. A further drawback is that not all nodal sites opacify with contrast material.

THE ROLE OF IMAGE-GUIDED LYMPH NODE BIOPSY

After using all the accepted criteria for lymph node involvement by tumour, the final radiological interpretation may remain equivocal and in this situation there are three options:

- Adopt a cautious approach and treat the suspect site
- Rescan after an interval to look for new confirmatory evidence of nodal disease
- Perform a lymph node biopsy

The choice will be governed by the clinical circumstances but there is no doubt that if an aggressive biopsy policy is adopted, then there will be increased detection of metastatic nodes over and above the pick-up rate from imaging alone.[66,118,119] Percutaneous image-guided biopsy is relatively safe, well tolerated, easy to perform and should yield a diagnostic sample in 80% to 90% of patients[120] (Fig. 35.22).

ACKNOWLEDGEMENTS

I would like to acknowledge the help of the Cytology and Pathology Departments at the Christie Hospital. I would also like to thank Mrs Kami Ramnarain for assisting in the preparation of the manuscript and the Department of Medical Illustration for photographic assistance.

Summary

- ■ The accurate identification of lymph node metastases remains an ongoing problem in diagnostic radiology.

- ■ The radiologist should understand the physiology of the lymphatic system and lymphatic drainage of each primary tumour.

- ■ Using a combination of size, site, number of nodes and tissue characteristics the radiologist can indicate the likelihood of metastatic lymph node disease.

- ■ Percutaneous biopsy of suspicious nodal masses is required in some patients, yielding a diagnostic sample in 80–90% of patients.

- ■ In other instances it is the responsibility of the clinician to decide whether to modify the patient's treatment to encompass abnormal or suspect nodes.

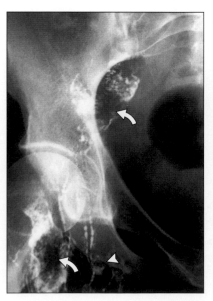

Figure 35.21. *Abnormal lymphangiogram. Right inguinal and iliac nodes are seen, some of which are enlarged (curved arrows) with large filling defects within them compatible with tumorous involvement. One smaller femoral node (arrowhead) demonstrates a similar internal filling defect compatible with involvement.*

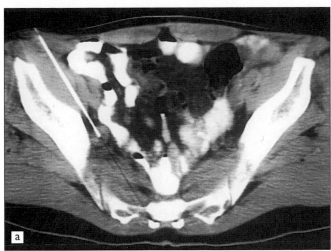

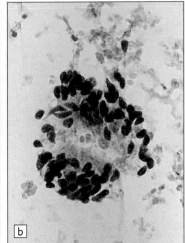

Figure 35.22. *(a) Percutaneous CT-guided biopsy of a right internal iliac node in a patient previously treated for rectal cancer. The needle tip is centrally positioned within the node. (b) Cytology sample of the same patient (Papanicolaou stain, magnification × 40) demonstrating pallisades of malignant glandular cells with a stromal core, compatible with a deposit of metastatic adenocarcinoma.*

REFERENCES

1. Herrera-Ornelas L, Justiniano J, Castillo N et al. Metastases in small lymph nodes from colon cancer. Arch Surg 1987; 122: 1253–1256

2. Jass J R, Morson B C. Reporting colorectal cancer. J Clin Pathol 1987; 40: 1016–1023

3. Sacks N P M, Baum M. Primary management of carcinoma of the breast. Lancet 1993; 342: 1402–1408

4. Minna J D, Pass H, Glatstein E, Ihde D. Cancer of the Lung. In: Devita V T, Hellman S, Rosenberg S A (eds). Cancer Principles and Practice of Oncology. Philadelphia: Lippincott, 1989; 591–705

5. Hall J G. The functional anatomy of lymph nodes. In: Stansfield A G, d'Ardenne A (eds). Lymph Node Biopsy Interpretation. London: Churchill Livingstone, 1992; 3–27

6. Liotta L A. Cancer cell invasion and metastasis. Sci Am February 1992; 34–41

7. Fajardo L F. Lymph nodes and cancer. In: Meyer J L (ed). The Lymphatic System and Cancer. Front Radiat Ther Oncol 1994; 28: 1–10

8. Gross B H, Glazer G M, Orringer M B et al. Bronchogenic carcinoma metastatic to normal-sized lymph nodes: frequency and significance. Radiology 1988; 166: 71–74

9. Kayser K, Bach S, Bulzebruck H et al. Site, size and tumour involvement of resected extrapulmonary lymph nodes in lung cancer. J Surg Oncol 1990; 43: 45–49

10. Staples C A, Muller N L, Miller R R et al. Mediastinal nodes in bronchogenic carcinoma: comparison between CT and mediastinoscopy. Radiology 1988; 167: 367–372

11. McLoud T C, Bourgouin P M, Greenberg R W et al. Bronchogenic carcinoma: analysis of staging in the mediastinum with CT by correlative lymph node mapping and sampling. Radiology 1992; 182: 319–323

12. Johnson R J. Radiology in the management of ovarian cancer. Clin Radiol 1993; 48: 75–82

13. Dooms G C, Hricak H, Crooks L E, Higgins C B. Magnetic resonance imaging of the lymph nodes: comparison with CT. Radiology 1984; 153: 719–728

14. Carrington B M, Hricak H. Anatomy of the pelvis. In: Hricak H, Carrington B M (eds). MRI of the Pelvis: A Text Atlas. London: Martin Dunitz, 1991; 43–91

15. Mancuso A A, Harnsberger H R, Muraki A S, Stevens M H. Computed tomography of cervical and retropharyngeal lymph nodes: normal anatomy, variants of normal, and applications in staging head and neck cancer. Radiology 1983; 148: 709–714

16. Tart R P, Mukherji S K, Avino A J et al. Facial lymph nodes: normal and abnormal CT appearance. Radiology 1993; 188: 695–700

17. Som P M. Lymph nodes of the neck. Radiology 1987; 165: 593–600

18. Callen P W, Korobkin M, Isherwood I. Computed tomographic evaluation of the retrocrural prevertebral space. Am J Radiol 1977; 129: 907–910

19. Balfe D M, Mauro M A, Koehler R E et al. Gastrohepatic ligament: normal and pathologic CT anatomy. Radiology 1984; 150: 485–490

20. Metreweli C, Ward S C. Ultrasound demonstration of lymph nodes in the hepatoduodenal ligament ('Daisy Chain Nodes') in normal subjects. Clin Radiol 1995; 50: 99–101

21. Okada Y, Yao Y K, Yunoki M, Sugita T. Lymph nodes in the hepatoduodenal ligament: US appearances with CT and MR correlation. Clin Radiol 1996; 51: 160–166

22. Zirinsky K, Auh Y H, Rubenstein W A et al. The portacaval space: CT with MR correlation. Radiology 1985; 156: 453–460

23. Williams M P, Cook J V, Duchesne G M. Psoas nodes — an overlooked site of metastasis from testicular tumours. Clin Radiol 1989; 40: 607–609

24. Royal S A, Callen P W. CT evaluation of the anomalies of the inferior vena cava and left renal vein. Am J Roentgenol 1979; 132: 763–769

25. Meanock I, Ward C S, Williams M P. The left ascending lumbar vein: a potential pitfall in CT diagnosis. Clin Radiol 1988; 39: 565–566

26. Gollub M J, Castellino R A. The cisterna chyli: a potential mimic of retrocrural lymphadenopathy on CT scans. Radiology 1996; 199: 477–480

27. Williams M P, Olliff J F C. Case Report: computed tomography and magnetic resonance imaging of dilated lumbar lymphatic trunks. Clin Radiol 1989; 40: 321–322

28. Reed D H, Dixon A K, Williams M V. Ovarian conservation at hysterectomy: A potential diagnostic pitfall. Clin Radiol 1989; 40: 274–276

29. Bashist B, Friedman W N, Killackey M A. Surgical transposition of the ovary: radiological appearance. Radiology 1989; 173: 857–860

30. Meaney J F, Cassar-Pullicino V N, Etherington R et al. Ilio-psoas bursa enlargement. Clin Radiol 1992; 45: 161–168

31. Guyatt G H, Lefcoe M, Walter S et al. Interobserver variation in the computed tomographic evaluation of mediastinal nodal size in patients with potentially resectable lung cancer. Chest 1995; 7: 116–119

32. Koehler P R, Anderson R E, Baxter B. The effect of computed tomography viewer controls on anatomical measurements. Radiology 1979; 130: 189–194

33. Harris K M, Adams H, Lloyd D C F, Harvey D J. The effect on apparent size of simulated pulmonary nodules using three standard CT window settings. Clin Radiol 1993; 47: 241–244

34. Glazer G, Gross B H, Quint L E et al. Normal mediastinal lymph nodes: number and size according to American Thoracic Society Mapping. Am J Radiol 1985; 144: 261–265

35. van den Brekel M W M, Stel H V, Castelijns J A et al. Cervical lymph node metastasis: assessment of radiologic criteria. Radiology 1990; 177: 379–384

36. Platt J F, Glazer G M, Orringer M B et al. Radiologic evaluation of the subcarinal lymph nodes: a comparative study. Am J Radiol 1988; 151: 279–282

37. Kim S H, Kim S C, Choi B I, Han M C. Uterine cervical carcinoma: evaluation of pelvic lymph node metastasis with M R imaging. Radiology 1994; 190: 807–811

38. Genereux G P, Howie J L. Normal mediastinal lymph node size and number: CT and anatomic study. Am J Radiol 1984; 142: 1095–1100

39. Quint L E, Glazer G M, Orringer M B et al. Mediastinal lymph node detection and sizing at CT and autopsy. Am J Radiol 1986; 147: 469–472

40. Kiyono K, Sone S, Sakai F et al. The number and size of normal mediastinal lymph nodes: a postmortem study. Am J Radiol 1988; 150: 771–776

41. Carvalho P, Baldwin D, Carter R, Parsons C. Accuracy of CT in detecting squamous carcinoma metastases in cervical lymph nodes. Clin Radiol 1991; 44: 79–81

42. Van Overhagen, Lameris J S, Berger M Y et al. Supraclavicular lymph node metastases in carcinoma of the oesophagus and gastro-oesophageal junction: assessment with CT, ultrasound and ultrasound-guided fine needle aspiration biopsy. Radiology 1991; 179: 155–158

43. Vassallo P, Wernecke K, Roos N, Peters P E. Differentiation of benign from malignant superficial lymphadenopathy: the role of high-resolution ultrasound. Radiology 1992; 183: 215–220

44. Ingram C E, Belli A M, Lewars M D et al. Normal lymph node size in the mediastinum: a retrospective study in two patient groups. Clin Radiol 1989; 40: 35–39

45. Parson V J, Carrington B M. Dougal M. Normal axillary lymph nodes as demonstrated by CT (Abstract). Radiology UK Congress 1996; 702: 237

46. Murray J G, O'Driscoll M, Curtin J J. Mediastinal lymph node size in an Asian population. Br J Radiol 1995; 68: 348–350

47. Libshitz H I, McKenna R J, Haynie T P et al. Mediastinal evaluation in lung cancer. Radiology 1984; 151: 295–299

48. Buy J N, Ghossain M A, Poirson F et al. Computed tomography of mediastinal lymph nodes in non-small cell lung cancer: a new approach based on the lymphatic pathway of tumour spread. J Comput Assist Tomogr 1988; 12: 545–552

49. Seeley J M, Mayo J R, Miller R R, Muller N L. T1 lung cancer: prevalence of mediastinal nodal metastases and diagnostic accuracy of CT. Radiology 1993; 186: 129–132

50. Dorfman R E, Alpern M B, Gross B H, Sandler M A. Upper abdominal lymph nodes: criteria for normal size determined with CT. Radiology 1991; 180: 319–322

51. Thomas J L, Bernadino M E, Bracken R B. Staging of testicular carcinoma: comparison of CT and lymphography. Am J Roentgenol 1981; 137: 991–996

52. Lien H H, Kolbenstvedt A, Talle K et al. Comparison of computed tomography, lymphography and phlebography in 200 consecutive patients with regard to retroperitoneal metastases from testicular tumour. Radiology 1983; 146: 129–132

53. Lien H H, Stenwig A E, Ous S, Fossa S D. Influence of different criteria for abnormal lymph node size on reliability of computed tomography in patients with non-seminomatous testicular tumor. Acta Radiol Diagn 1986; 27: 199–203

54. Taylor A, Carrington B M, Wong-You-Cheong J J. Prospective assessment of normal abdominal lymph node size and distribution (Abstract). Roentgen Centenary Congress 1995; 396

55. Hricak H, Lacey C G, Sandles L G et al. Invasive cervical carcinoma: comparison of MR imaging and surgical findings. Radiology 1988; 166: 623–631

56. Matsukuma K, Tsukamoto N, Matsuyama T et al. Preoperative CT study of lymph nodes in cervical cancer — its correlation with histological findings. Gynecol Oncol 1989; 33: 168–171

57. Greco A, Mason P, Leung A W L et al. Staging of carcinoma of the uterine cervix: MRI-surgical correlation. Clin Radiol 1989; 40: 401–405

58. Kim S H Choi B I Lee H P et al. Uterine cervical carcinoma: comparison of CT and MR findings. Radiology 1990; 175: 45–51

59. Hawnaur J M, Johnson R J, Buckley C H et al. Staging, volume estimation and assessment of nodal status in carcinoma of the cervix: comparison of magnetic resonance imaging with surgical findings. Clin Radiol 1994; 49: 443–452

60. Walsh J W, Amendola M A, Konerding K F et al. Computed tomographic detection of pelvic and inguinal lymph-node metastases from primary and recurrent pelvic malignant disease. Radiology 1980; 137: 157–166

61. Morgan C L, Calkins R F, Cavalcanti E J. Computed tomography in the evaluation, staging and therapy of carcinoma of the bladder and prostate. Radiology 1981; 140: 751–761

62. Weinerman P M, Arger P H, Coleman B G et al. Pelvic adenopathy from bladder and prostate carcinoma: detection by rapid-sequence computed tomography. Am J Roentgenol 1983; 140: 95–99

63. Amendola M A, Glazer G M, Grossman H B et al. Staging of bladder carcinoma: MRI–CT–surgical correlation. Am J Roentgenol 1986; 146: 1179–1183

64. Bryan P J, Butler H E, LiPuma J P et al. CT and MR imaging in staging bladder neoplasms. J Comput Assist Tomogr 1987; 11: 96–101

65. Buy J N, Moss A A, Guinet C et al. MR staging of bladder carcinoma: correlation with pathologic findings. Radiology 1988; 169: 695–700

66. Oyen R H, Van Poppel H P, Ameye F E et al. Lymph node staging of localized prostatic carcinoma with CT and CT-guided fine-needle aspiration biopsy: prospective study of 285 patients. Radiology 1994; 190: 315–322

67. Vinnicombe S J, Norman A R, Nicolson V, Husband J E. Normal pelvic lymph nodes: evaluation with CT after bipedal lymphangiography. Radiology 1995; 194: 349–355

68. Grey A, Carrington B M, Ryder D. The inguinal region: Normal anatomy and nodal distribution in an adult population. Submitted for publication

69. Magnusson A. Size of normal retroperitoneal lymph nodes. Acta Radiol Diagnos 1983; 24: 315–318

70. Steinkamp H J, Hosten N, Richter C et al. Enlarged cervical lymph nodes at helical CT. Radiology 1994; 191: 795–798

71. Fukuya T, Honda H, Hayashi T et al. Lymph-node metastases: efficacy of detection with helical CT in patients with gastric cancer. Radiology 1995; 197: 705–711

72. Dixon A K, Ellis M, Sikora K. Computed tomography of testicular tumours: distribution of abdominal lymphadenopathy. Clin Radiol 1986; 37: 519–523

73. Remy-Jardin M, Duyck P, Remy J et al. Hilar lymph nodes: identification with spiral CT and histologic correlation. Radiology 1995; 196: 387–394

74. Husband J E, Hawkes D J, Peckham M J. CT estimations of mean attenuation values and volume in testicular tumors: a comparison with surgical and histologic findings. Radiology 1982; 144: 553–558

75. Yousem D M, Som P M, Hackney D B et al. Central nodal necrosis and extracapsular neoplastic spread in cervical lymph nodes: MR imaging versus CT. Radiology 1992; 182: 753–759

76. Curtin H D, Ishwaran H, Mancuso A A et al. Comparative imaging of cancer metastasis to neck nodes: Report of radiologic diagnostic oncology Group III. Radiological Society of North America Scientific Program November 1995 Chicago (Abstract No 677), p. 238

77. Chong V F H, Fan Y F, Khoo J B K. MR features of cervical node necrosis in metastatic disease. Clin Radiol 1996; 51: 103–109

78. Hopper K D, Diehl L F, Cole B A et al. The significance of necrotic mediastinal lymph nodes on CT in patients with newly diagnosed Hodgkin Disease. Am J Roentgenol 1990; 155: 267–270

79. Fossel E T, Brodsky G, Delayre J L, Wilson R E. Nuclear magnetic resonance for the differentiation of benign and malignant breast tissues and axillary lymph nodes. Ann Surg 1983; 198: 541–545

80. Wiener J I, Chako A C, Merten C W et al. Breast and axillary tissue MR imaging: correlation of signal intensities and relaxation times with pathological findings. Radiology 1986; 160: 299–305

81. Glazer G M, Orringer M B, Chenevert T L et al. Mediastinal lymph nodes: relaxation times/pathologic correlation and implications in staging of lung cancer with MR imaging. Radiology 1988; 168: 429–431

82. Dooms G C, Hricak H, Moseley M E et al. Characterization of lymphadenopathy by magnetic resonance relaxation times: preliminary results. Radiology 1985; 155: 691–697

83. Lee J K T, Heiken J P, Ling D et al. Magnetic resonance imaging of abdominal and pelvic lymphadenopathy. Radiology 1984; 153: 181–188

84. Ahuja A, Ying M, Yang W T et al. The use of sonography in differentiating cervical lymphomatous lymph nodes from cervical metastatic lymph nodes. Clin Radiol 1996; 51: 186–190

85. Ahuja A T, Chow L, Chick W et al. Metastatic cervical nodes in papillary carcinoma of the thyroid: ultrasound and histological correlation. Clin Radiol 1995; 50: 229–231

86. Husband J E, Robinson L, Thomas G. Contrast enhancing lymph nodes in bladder cancer: a potential pitfall on CT. Clin Radiol 1992; 45: 395–398

87. Laissey J P, Gay-Depassier P, Soyer P et al. Enlarged mediastinal lymph nodes in bronchogenic carcinoma: assessment with dynamic contrast-enhanced MR imaging. Radiology 1994; 191: 263–267

88. Barentsz O, Jager G J, van Vierzen P B J et al. Staging urinary bladder cancer after transurethral biopsy: value of fast dynamic contrast-enhancing MR imaging. Radiology 1996; 201: 185–193

89. Weissleder R, Elizondo G, Josephson L et al. Experimental lymph node metastases: enhanced detection with MR lymphography. Radiology 1989; 171: 835–839

90. Weissleder R, Elizondo G, Wittenberg J et al. Ultrasmall superparamagnetic iron oxide: an intravenous contrast agent for assessing lymph nodes with MR imaging. Radiology 1990; 175: 494–498

91. Weissleder R, Elizondo G, Wittenberg, Rabito C A et al. Ultrasmall superparamagnetic iron oxide: characterization of a new class of contrast agents for MR imaging. Radiology 1990; 175: 489–493

92. Lee A S, Weissleder R, Brady T J, Wittenberg J. Lymph nodes microstructural anatomy at MR imaging. Radiology 1991; 178: 519–522

93. Vassallo P, Matei C, Heston W D W et al. AMI-227-enhanced MR lymphography: usefulness for differentiating reactive from tumor-bearing lymph nodes. Radiology 1994; 193: 501–506

94. Weissleder R, Heautot J F, Schaffer B K et al. MR lymphography: study of a high-efficiency lymphotrophic agent. Radiology 1994; 191: 225–230

95. Anzai Y, McLachlan S, Saxton R et al. Dextran-coated superparamagnetic iron oxide: the first human use of a new MR contrast agent for assessing lymph nodes of the head and neck. Am J Roentgenol 1994; 15: 87–94

96. Anzai Y, Blackwell K E, Hirschowitz S L et al. Initial clinical experience with dextran-coated superparamagnetic iron oxide for detection of lymph node metastases in patients with head and neck cancer. Radiology 1994; 192: 709–715

97. Zerhouni E A, Rutter C, Hamilton SR et al. CT and MR imaging in the staging of colorectal carcinoma: report of the Radiology Diagnostic Oncology Group II. Radiology 1996; 200: 443–451

98. Webb W R, Gatsonis C, Zerhouni E A et al. CT and MR imaging in staging non-small cell bronchogenic carcinoma. Report of the Radiologic Diagnostic Oncology Group. Radiology 1991; 178: 705–713

99. Bekerman C, Hoffer P B, Bitran J D. The role of Gallium-67 in the clinical evaluation of cancer. Semin Nucl Med 1984; XIV: 296–323

100. DeMeester T R, Golomb H M, Kirchner P. The role of Gallium-67 scanning in the clinical staging and preoperative evaluation of patients with carcinoma of the lung. Ann Thorac Surg 1979; 28: 5: 451

101. Neumann R, Merino M, Hoffer P B. Gallium-67 in hilar and mediastinal staging of primary lung carcinomas. J Nucl Med 1980; 21: 32

102. Front D, Ben-Haim S, Israel O et al. Lymphoma: predictive value of Ga-67 scintigraphy after treatment. Radiology 1992; 182: 359–363

103. Cook G J R, Maisey M N. Review — The current status of clinical PET imaging. Clin Radiol 1996; 51: 603–613

104. Wahl R L, Quint L E, Greenough R L et al. Staging of mediastinal non-small cell lung cancer with FDG PET, CT, and fusion images: preliminary prospective evaluation. Radiology 1994; 191: 371–377

105. Newman J S, Francis I R, Kaminski M S, Wahl R L. Imaging of lymphoma with PET with 2-[F-18]-fluoro-2-deoxy-D-glucose: Correlation with CT. Radiology 1994; 190: 111–116

106. Jabour B A, Choi Y, Hoh C K et al. Extracranial head and neck: PET imaging with 2-[18]fluoro-2-deoxy-D-glucose and MR imaging correlation. Radiology 1993; 186: 27–35

107. Wahl R L, Hawkins R A, Larson S M et al. Proceedings of a National Cancer Institute Workshop: PET in oncology — A Clinical research agenda. Radiology 1994; 193: 604–606

108. Anzai Y, Carroll W R, Quint D J et al. Recurrence of head and neck cancer after surgery or irradiation: prospective comparison of 2-deoxy-2-[F-18] fluoro-D-glucose PET and MR imaging diagnoses. Radiology 1996; 200: 135–141

109. Patz E F, Lowe V J, Hoffman J M et al. Persistent or recurrent bronchogenic carcinoma: detection with PET and 2-[F-18]-2-deoxy-D-glucose. Radiology 1994; 191: 379–382

110. Stomper P C, D'Souza D J, Bakshi S P et al. Detection of pelvic recurrence of colorectal carcinoma: prospective, blinded comparison of Tc-99m-IMMU-4 monoclonal antibody scanning and CT. Radiology 1995; 197: 688–692

111. Morton D, Wen D, Wong J et al. Technical details of intraoperative lymphatic mapping for early stage melanoma. Arch Surg 1992; 127: 392–399

112. Veronesi U, Paganelli G, Galimberti V et al. Sentinel-node biopsy to avoid axillary dissection in breast cancer with clinically negative lymph nodes. Lancet 1997; 349: 1864–1867

113. Rosen S. Innovations in monoclonal antibody tumor targeting. JAMA 1989; 261: 744–746

114. Fuchs W A, Böök-Hederström G. Lymphography in the diagnosis of metastases with special reference to the carcinoma of the uterine cervix. Acta Radiol Diagn 1964; 2: 161–171

115. Castellino R A, Hoppe R T, Blank N et al. Computed tomography, lymphography, and staging laparotomy: correlations in initial staging of Hodgkin Disease. Am J Roentgenol 1984; 143: 37–41

116. Libson E, Polliack A P, Bloom R A. Value of lymph-angiography in the staging of Hodgkin lymphoma. Radiology 1994; 193: 757–759

117. Williams M P, Husband J E. Computed tomography scanning and post-lymphangiogram radiography in the follow-up of patients with metastatic testicular cancer. Clin Radiol 1989; 40: 47–50

118. van den Brekel M W M, Casstelijns J A, Stel H V et al. Occult metastatic neck disease: detection with US and US-guided fine-needle aspiration cytology. Radiology 1991; 180: 457–461

119. Takes R P, Knegt P, Manni J J et al. Regional metastasis in head and neck squamous cell carcinoma: revised value of US with US-guided FNAB. Radiology 1996; 198: 819–823

120. Charboneau J W, Reading C C, Welch T J. CT and sonographically guided needle biopsy: current techniques and new innovations. Am J Roentgenol 1990; 154: 1–10

Chapter 36

Lung and pleura

Anwar Padhani

INTRODUCTION

Autopsy series show that pulmonary metastases are found in 20–54% of all patients who die of cancer.[1-3] The incidence of detected metastatic lung disease at initial presentation or during the clinical course for any given cancer will be less than that encountered in autopsy series.[4,5] Detection of pulmonary metastatic disease is critical for the planning of effective therapy of cancer patients. Routine thoracic imaging by any imaging modality should take into account the propensity of the tumour to metastasize to the lungs. Gilbert and Kagan[6] have studied the incidence of lung metastases for various primary neoplasms documented on chest X-ray at presentation and at autopsy (Table 36.1). Tumours such as choriocarcinoma, osteosarcoma, Ewing's sarcoma, testicular teratomas, melanomas and thyroid cancer have a higher incidence of pulmonary metastatic disease at presentation. However, these are not the most common cancers; the most common sources of metastases to the lungs are therefore common tumours, e.g. breast, colon, prostate, head and neck, and renal cancer.[7]

METASTASES TO THE LUNG

METASTATIC PATHWAYS

The most common pathway for pulmonary metastatic spread is by way of blood-borne tumour emboli arising from invasion of thin-walled and defective tumour capillaries.[8] The lungs serve as the primary filter site for those tumours whose venous drainage is into the systemic venous circulation.[9] Therefore, cancers of the head and neck, kidney and testes, choriocarcinoma, bone and soft tissue sarcomas and endocrine tumours (e.g. thyroid and adrenal glands) primarily metastasize to the lungs. For this reason, major paediatric tumours, with the exception of neuroblastoma, also first metastasize to the lung.[10,11] For other tumours draining via the portal venous system (e.g. stomach, pancreas and colon cancer), the liver is the initial filter site; the lungs being secondarily affected. Either the lungs or the liver may be involved first by oesophageal or rectal cancers as these tumours drain either into the portal venous or systemic venous circulations. Familiarity with these general principles

Table 36.1. *Incidence of pulmonary metastases from extrathoracic primary tumours (at presentation and autopsy)*[*]

Primary lesion	Frequency (%)	
	Presentation	Autopsy
Rhabdomyosarcoma	21	25
Wilms' tumour	20	60
Ewing's sarcoma	18	77
Osteosarcoma	15	75
Neuroblastoma	<5	25
Kidney	5–30	50–75
Bladder	5–10	25–30
Prostate	5	13–53
Testis (germ cell)	12	70–80
Choriocarcinoma (female)	60	70–100
Hepatoma	–	20
Ovary	5	10
Uterus	<1	30–40
Cervix	<5	20–30
Breast	4	60
Bronchus (unresected)	34	20–40
Thyroid	5–10	65
Melanoma	5	66–80
Head and neck	5	13–40
Oesophagus	–	20–35
Stomach	–	20–35
Pancreas	–	25–40
Colon/rectum	<5	25–40
Hodgkin's lymphoma	5	50–70
Non-Hodgkin's lymphoma	1–10	30–40

*Modified from ref. 6.

is helpful when evaluating patients for pulmonary metastatic disease. For example, if there are no detectable liver metastases in patients with gastro-intestinal cancer or bony metastases in patients with prostatic cancer, the likelihood of detecting pulmonary metastases is relatively low.[7,12]

Metastases via direct lymphatic spread, transbronchial aspiration and bronchial arterial spread[4,13,14] are less common. Lymphangitic spread almost always results from haematogenous metastases to small capillaries in the lung with secondary invasion of peripheral pulmonary lymph channels. In a few instances, however, retrograde extension from central mediastinal or hilar nodes or direct invasion through diaphragmatic lymphatics[3,15] may also occur. The most common tumours resulting in lymphangitis are breast, lung, stomach, pancreas, prostate, cervix and thyroid cancer.[4,16] Endobronchial metastases are rare and associated with cancers of the breast, colon or kidney; sarcomas or melanomas.[4,16] Tumour embolization into the pulmonary arteries through the right side of the heart is associated with renal cancer, hepatoma, choriocarcinoma and hepatic metastases. This entity is distinct from haematogenous dissemination in that embolic tumours proliferate within the vascular compartment.

PATHOLOGY OF PULMONARY METASTATIC DISEASE

Haematogenous dissemination of metastatic disease results in the formation of pulmonary nodules. Such nodules are usually multiple and circular but of variable size.[2,7,17] Postmortem series indicate that metastases are frequently small. Crow[2] observes that 59% were less than 5 mm in size. They are generally bilateral and peripheral; predominantly in the outer one-third of the lung, often in a subpleural distribution. In pathological series 82–92% of metastases are in the periphery of the lung and 59–67% subpleural.[2,18] The mid and lower zones are affected in preference to the lung apex. This distribution is as a result of normal blood flow patterns. Lymphangitis carcinomatosis refers to tumour growth in lymphangitic channels, and in the peribronchovascular and interlobular connective tissue that surrounds them.

PATIENT'S SYMPTOMATOLOGY

Eighty to ninety-five percent of patients with metastatic disease are asymptomatic. Breathlessness may develop due to airways obstruction, pleural effusion or parenchymal replacement. Sudden shortness of breath may be related to haemorrhage into a lesion or the rapid development of a pleural effusion or pneumothorax. Patients with lymphangitis, endobronchial metastases or tumour emboli are usu-

ally symptomatic. Lymphangitis carcinomatosis is associated with increasing breathlessness, dry cough or chest pain. Endobronchial metastases result in wheezing or haemoptysis. Tumour embolism can cause the acute or subacute symptoms of pulmonary thrombo-embolism.

RADIOLOGICAL APPEARANCES OF METASTASES

Lung metastases usually appear as well-defined nodules (Fig. 36.1). Occasionally, edges are ill-defined as in metastatic adenocarcinoma, haemorrhage (e.g. choriocarcinoma) or following treatment (Fig. 36.2).[19,20] Cavitation can occur in metastases from any malignancy,[21–23] but particularly those originating from tumours of squamous cell type. Sarcomas cavitate frequently, particularly after treatment. Common sites of cavitating metastases include cervix, colon, head and neck.[21,22] The wall of cavities vary from thick and irregular to thin. Cavitation of a subpleural metastasis may result in a pneumothorax; indeed spontaneous pneumothorax in a patient with a sarcoma should raise the possibility of a metastasis even if the plain chest X-ray fails to show metastatic disease.[23–25] Cavitation is not related to the size of metastases and may be related to liquefaction of keratin in squamous cell carcinoma and mucoid degeneration in adenocarcinoma (Fig. 36.3).

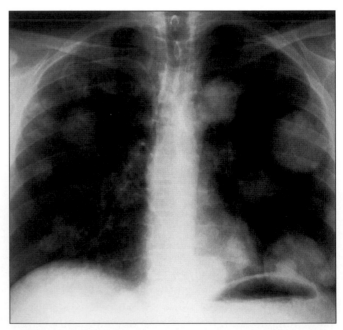

Figure 36.1. *Typical lung metastases. 50-year-old male with Stage-IV testicular teratoma. The chest radiograph shows bilateral lung masses of variable size in the periphery of the lungs. Lesions are well-defined, some have lobulated margins.*

Calcification may be seen in metastases *de novo* or as a result of treatment. Calcification in osteosarcomas or chondrosarcoma metastases occur as part of the tumour matrix (Fig. 36.4). Metastatic synovial sarcoma, giant cell tumours, carcinomas of colon, breast, ovary and thyroid also calcify. Both chemotherapy and radiotherapy can cause degeneration of metastases, resulting in calcification.[26–31]

Thin-walled air cysts (pulmonary lacunae) at the site of treated metastases is most frequently seen with germ cell tumour metastases (Fig. 36.5).[32] These represent healed tumours with no viable tumour and are characterized by a thin cyst wall and no mural nodule. Treated metastases from non-seminomatous germ cell tumours may also become smaller, stabilize, or enlarge despite successful

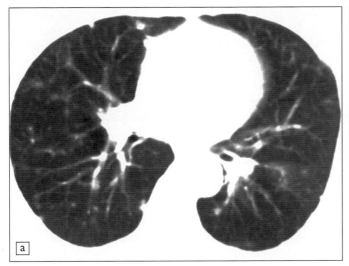

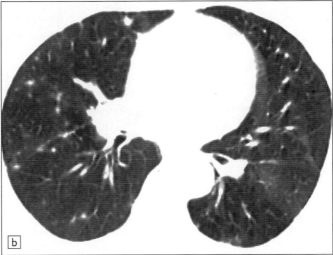

Figure 36.2. *Metastases from breast cancer with ill-defined margins. (a) CT scan (8 mm collimation) showing bilateral small lung nodules with ill-defined margins. Many nodules are associated with pulmonary vessels; (b) 2 mm collimation CT of* the same patient at the same table position as (a), showing fewer lung nodules. The ill-defined edges of the nodules are better seen. However, the association of the lung nodules with vessels is less clear.

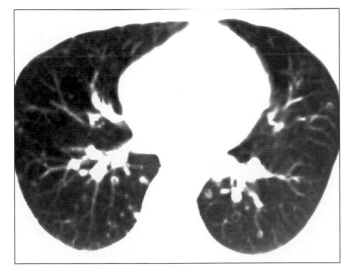

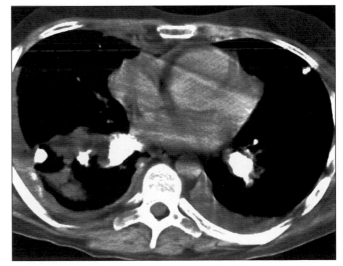

Figure 36.3. *Cavitating lung metastases. Cavitating lung metastases from adenocarcinoma of the rectum. Small lesions are seen bilaterally, many showing cavitation with thin walls. Cavitation is not related to the size of metastases.*

Figure 36.4. *Ossification in pulmonary metastases. Ossified pleural and pulmonary metastatic deposits from osteosarcoma is seen. Bilateral pleural effusions with minimal air from aspiration is present on the right side. Artefacts are due to the inability to raise the diseased left arm.*

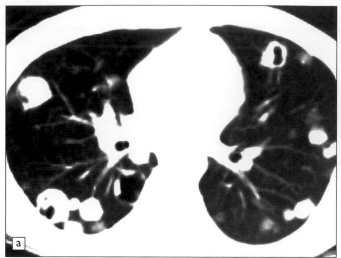 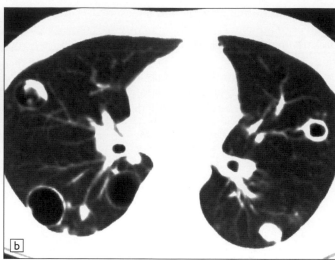

Figure 36.5. *Cavitation in testicular teratoma. (a) 25-year-old male with Stage-IV testicular teratoma. Bilateral cavitating lung metastases are seen; (b) same patient 2 months later. With chemotherapy some lesions have resolved, others are smaller and some metastases have become thin walled cavities. Mural nodularity is present in some lesions.*

chemotherapy. The latter have transformed into mature teratoma and serum tumour markers can be helpful in determining the activity of residual disease.

Lymphangitis carcinomatosis may occur from a variety of tumours, most commonly in lung, gastric, breast, pancreatic and prostate cancer. Findings at high resolution CT include:

- Interlobular septal thickening and nodularity
- A prominent reticular pattern
- Nodular thickening of bronchovascular bundles
- Polygonal structures (Fig. 36.6)

Interlobular septal thickening, a highly specific sign, is attributed to irregular tumour growth with septae with or without fibrosis. Lobar or lung collapse is associated with endobronchial metastases from kidney, breast, colon, rectal, thyroid and female genital cancers. Metastatic involvement of the bronchi is seen in approximately 2–28% of cancer patients (Fig. 36.7).[33–35]

ACCURACY OF COMPUTED TOMOGRAPHY (CT) EVALUATION IN PULMONARY METASTATIC DISEASE

The standard chest X-ray is the initial test for the detection of pulmonary metastases. High-kilovoltage techniques (>125 kV) show more lesions than low-kilovoltage films. Although an abnormal X-ray demands comparison with previous chest X-ray films and delineation of the morphological features, CT has become standard for the detection, operative planning and follow-up of patients with metastatic lung disease.

CT, particularly spiral (helical) is currently the most sensitive technique for the detection of pulmonary lesions compared to chest radiography or conventional linear tomography. The greater sensitivity of CT is attributable to the lack of superimposition of intrathoracic structures and the high contrast resolution of soft tissue attenuation nodules and air-containing lung.[4,7] Lesions in the lung apices, the extreme lung bases, against the heart and mediastinum, and those adjacent to their pleura are visualized at CT but may be obscured by conventional radiographic techniques.

Computed tomography in patients with known extrathoracic malignancies detects more lesions than conventional linear tomography or radiography.[36–38] It is true to say that nodules exceeding 3 mm in size are visible on CT, whereas the lower limit for uncalcified lesions on plain radiographs is between 7 and 9 mm.[37] It is now generally accepted that the increased sensitivity of CT is accompanied by a decrease in specificity.[7,36,37,39–42] Schaner[37] showed that 60% of additional nodules seen at CT were granulomata or pleural-based lymph nodes at resection. The precise sensitivity and specificity of CT on the basis of existing clinical studies is difficult to assess. Sensitivity cannot be assessed since surgical correlation has only been obtained in a limited number of studies. Palpation of the lungs for nodules at surgery is not a reliable standard.[37] Schaner found six nodules greater than

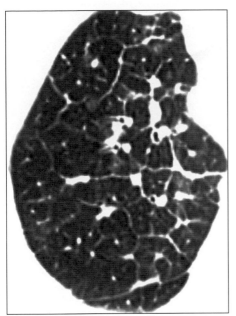

Figure 36.6. *Lymphangitis carcinomatosis. High-resolution CT (2 mm slice thickness) targeted to the right lung. Metastatic lymphangitic carcinoma from prostate cancer is seen. Thickening and nodularity of the interlobular septae with prominent polygonal structures is seen.*

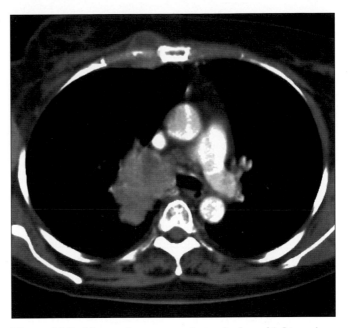

Figure 36.7. *Metastatic cancer to the tracheobronchial tree. A large metastatic lesion from breast cancer is seen occluding the right main bronchus. The patient had marked air trapping in the right lung (not shown). Metastatic deposits in regional lymph nodes are also seen in the right lower axilla and in the right internal mammary region extending through the chest wall.*

6 mm in size seen at CT, and at linear tomography, that were not palpable at surgery. Small lesions are a real dilemma as they cannot be biopsied percutaneously and are not palpable at surgery. Wire localization and thorascopic excision is an option in these cases.[42]

The specificity of CT is not only influenced by the type and stage of the underlying extrathoracic malignancy but also by the frequency of benign entities in a population. False-positive results may occur with conditions such as:

- Hamartoma
- Sarcoidosis
- Silicosis
- Histoplasmosis
- Tuberculosis
- Intrapulmonary lymph nodules
- Small areas of fibrosis
- Small pulmonary infarcts

All of these may be indistinguishable from metastatic disease.[36,39,43–46] Similarly, surgical resections of pulmonary metastases may result in nodular scarring and suture granulomata. Infections or pulmonary toxicity from chemotherapy may also result in nodular lung opacities. Clinical considerations of epidemiology, patient age and previous treatment will help to reduce incidence of false-positive results. Granulomas, frequently due to histoplasmosis, feature prominently in studies from the USA.[36,37,39] In contrast, fungal granulomatous disease is less prevalent in European countries.[47,48]

Unfortunately, the differentiation between metastases and benign lesions remains difficult on CT. Morphological features, distribution, size, number and densitometry have been used to improve specificity. Most metastatic lesions are smaller than 2 cm in size, having a smooth rounded contour. Gross et al.[49] found that most metastatic lesions were likely to be spherical or ovoid in shape. Linear, triangular or irregular shaped or multiple ill-defined lesions, particularly when centrally located, were less likely to represent metastases. The number of lesions is generally unhelpful. Gross et al.[49] found that if non-calcified lesions were greater than 2.5 cm, or if more than 10 lesions were present, the likelihood of metastatic disease was very high. Other morphological clues include a frequently observed sign in which CT demonstrates a connection between a metastatic nodule and an adjacent branch of the pulmonary artery (Fig. 36.8). Pathological correlation in inflated lung specimens have shown the frequent presence of a pulmonary vessel leading to a metastatic lesion.[50,51] Vascular connection cannot always be demonstrated and partial volume effects may make a lesion appear connected to an adjacent but unrelated vessel. Another sign that is infrequently seen is a zone of decreased density distal to the metastatic nodule, presumably related to underperfusion due to occlusion of the pulmonary vessel (Fig. 36.9). The presence of reticular changes around a metastatic lesion may also be a helpful sign. The pathological basis of this is neoplastic growth in capillaries and lymphatic vessels with secondary perivascular and interstitial oedema and fibrosis.[52] Gross beading of the septal interstitium on high resolution CT is highly suggestive of metastatic disease. The growth rate of a nodule is also a reliable indicator of its nature. Nathan et al.[53] measured the doubling times of 177 malignant and 41 benign nodules. The longest doubling time for a malignant nodule was 6–7 months. The lesions that had doubling times of 18 months or more were invariably benign. Weiss[54] found that the doubling times of malignancies ranged from between 1.8 and 10 months. Doubling times of less than a month are unlikely in malignancy and are usually seen with active inflammatory lesions. However, aggressive primary carcinomas, such as choriocarcinomas and sarcomas, may sometimes grow rapidly. When questionable metastases are present, monitoring the growth rate over 4–6 weeks is reasonable to establish a diagnosis. Minimal or moderate growth, or a decrease in size, under specific chemotherapy is considered to be reliable evidence of the metastatic nature of pulmonary lesions.

Key points: factors favouring metastases

- ■ Close relationship to adjacent vessel
- ■ Decreased density distal to lesion
- ■ Reticular changes around lesion
- ■ Gross 'beading' of septal interstitium
- ■ Spherical/ovoid versus linear or irregular shapes
- ■ Non-calcified lesions >2.5 cm are likely to be metastatic

SOLITARY NODULE IN A PATIENT WITH KNOWN MALIGNANCY

In a study of 800 patients who presented with an apparently solid nodule a year or more after detection and treatment of an extrathoracic malignancy, 63% proved to be a new primary tumour and less than 25% solitary metastases.[55] The likelihood of metastatic disease in such solitary lesions depends on the histology of the primary carcinoma. In a patient over 35 years, if the primary extrathoracic tumour is a squamous carcinoma, the likelihood of a new primary lung cancer is about 65%. If the extrathoracic malignancy is an adenocarcinoma, then the likelihood of a new tumour is about 50%. For extrathoracic sarcoma, a new solitary nodule is most likely to represent metastatic

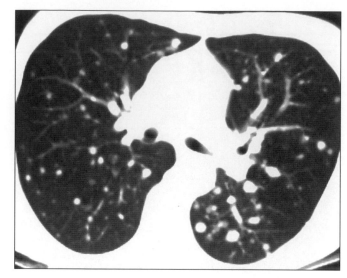

Figure 36.8. *The nodule vessel sign. Bilateral small lung metastases from colonic cancer are visible, the majority demonstrating proximity to pulmonary vessels.*

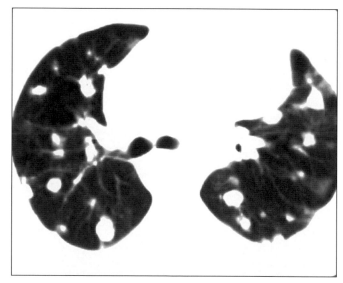

Figure 36.9. *Distal hypoperfusion sign. Several metastatic nodules appear connected to vessels in this patient with Stage-IV testicular teratoma. Zones of hypointensity distal to the deposits are seen. This sign is presumed to be due to hypoperfusion of the parenchyma due to occlusion of the feeding artery by the metastasis.*

disease. Computed tomography performed in a patient with a new pulmonary nodule seen on radiography is primarily indicated to determine whether other nodules are present which would make the diagnosis of metastatic disease more likely.

COMPUTED TOMOGRAPHY TECHNIQUE

Spiral CT is the method of choice for the detection of nodules because of its ability to scan the entire lungs without slice-to-slice misregistration. This is particularly valuable at the lung bases where the potential for respiratory misregistration is greatest. Respiratory motion artefacts that occasionally degrade image quality in conventional CT examinations are also significantly reduced. Costello et al.[56] compared standard and spiral CT in 20 patients with suspected lung nodules less than 1 cm in size. Spiral CT with overlapping sections (8 mm thick with 50% overlap) detected 4 of 22 nodules in 55 patients that were missed by standard CT due to respiratory misregistration. Similarly, Heywang-Koebrunner et al.[57] also showed that the nodules missed were usually small (<5 mm in size). Even without overlapping sections, contiguous sections will also detect more lesions.[58] An important disadvantage of spiral CT is that despite an increased sensitivity there is decreased specificity partly due to decreased sensitivity to the presence of calcium within the lesions. Thus, potentially many calcified granulomata can be misinterpreted.

Despite these advantages, it is unclear whether all routine metastatic surveys require spiral CT. Spiral CT with overlapping sections may be more time-consuming on some spiral CT scanners and the cost of additional films and data storage are important considerations. We reserve the use of spiral CT for those patients in whom there is a high index of suspicion that nodules are present, and for those in whom the detection of solitary or additional nodules is clinically significant.

In general, thinner sections (<5 mm) are not routinely used as the distinction of nodules and vessels can be problematic, particularly in the subpleural areas (Fig. 36.2). However, thin sections may be useful for densitometry.

High-resolution CT (HRCT) should be used for the evaluation of lymphangitis carcinomatosa. Our technique involves 1–2 mm thick sections every 10 mm through the chest. Two factors greatly enhance the spatial resolution of HRCT images: narrow columnation (1–2 mm thick scans) and a high spatial resolution reconstruction algorithm (bone). The high spatial resolution algorithm provides optimal edge enhancement of small structures, such as the interlobular septae and the walls of bronchi and cystic spaces. We rarely perform targeted reconstruction, a time-consuming technique whereby an entire lung is reconstructed to make the best use of the image matrix and so improve spatial resolution. In some cases, however, targeting may provide useful information (Fig. 36.10).

GENERAL INDICATIONS FOR CT

A chest X-ray is always performed in patients with known intrathoracic malignancy. The indication for CT will depend on the findings on the chest radiograph and on several other factors including:

- The likely influence on management
- The nature of the underlying neoplasm and its propensity to spread to the lungs

Clearly CT is only necessary in selected cases because it is rarely necessary to demonstrate further metastases once the presence of definite metastatic disease has been established. General indications include:[59]

- In patients with a normal chest X-ray, with a tumour which has a propensity to metastasize to the lungs, with an absence of metastatic disease elsewhere and in whom the discovery is likely to alter the patient's management. Testicular germ cell tumours and osteosarcomas are such examples, with a high incidence of lung metastases in the absence of metastatic disease elsewhere. Conversely, patients with malignancy of the gastro-intestinal tract or prostate are unlikely to have pulmonary metastases in the absence of spread to other organs such as liver or bones. In these patients CT is not routinely performed
- When a chest X-ray shows a solitary lung lesion and the dilemma is between a solitary lung metastasis, a bronchial carcinoma or other lesion, the documentation of multiple lesions will favour metastases
- In patients in whom surgery is being contemplated, CT is clearly indicated so that the true number and extent of lesions can be assessed

In screening for the development of early metastases, surveillance should be most intense during the time these metastatic lesions are most likely to occur. Computed tomography scans every 3–6 months for at least 2 years has been recommended for high risk tumours, e.g. bone and soft tissue sarcomas, paediatric tumours, choriocarcinomas and non-seminomatous germ cell tumours.

BIOPSY

A tissue diagnosis with definite histology of a lung mass is important in planning optimal clinical management. In view of the limited tissue specificity of CT, parenchymal lung nodules may be biopsied percutaneously. This may be done under fluoroscopic or CT guidance. CT is helpful in planning the optimal approach by localizing the largest and most accessible lesions. The yield of fibre-optic bronchoscopy is generally poor. If CT suggests endobronchial or lymphatic metastatic disease, bronchoscopy is more successful. Endobronchial lesions can be directly visualized and sampled. For lymphangitis carcinomatosis, transbronchial biopsy has a higher yield than percutaneous needle biopsy.

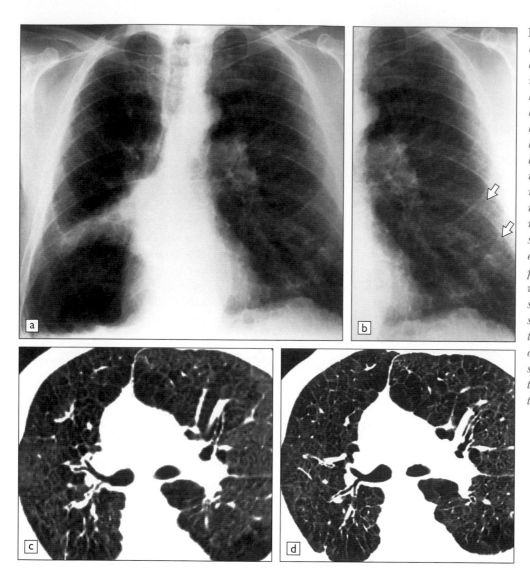

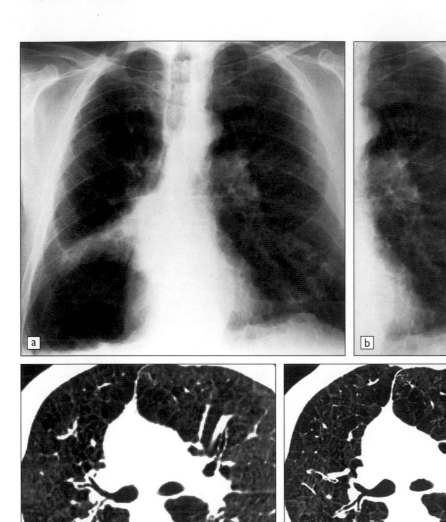

Figure 36.10. *Lymphangitis carcinomatosis with lung emphysema. (a) Frontal chest radiograph showing a right hilar mass (adenocarcinoma of lung) with atelectasis of the lateral segment of the middle lobe; (b) coned view of the left lung showing prominent interstitial lines with some nodularity (arrows). The lung is hyperinflated; (c) high-resolution CT scan of the lungs showing bilateral lung emphysema. Prominent polygonal structures are visible with thickened interlobular septae. There is apparent hazy shadowing in both lungs; (d) targeted CT reconstruction is able to resolve the hazy shadowing. This is due to thickening and nodularity of the interlobular septae.*

SURGICAL RESECTION OF METASTASIS

The operative mortality of pulmonary metastectomy is low (0–4%).[60–64] Resection of pulmonary metastases appears to be most beneficial in tumours of the urinary tract, testicular and uterine neoplasms, colon and rectal carcinoma, tumours of the head and neck and various sarcomas, particularly osteogenic sarcoma. Although surgical resection was initially performed for solitary lesions, it is now evident that favourable survival rates may be obtained in patients with multiple lesions and even after repeat resections. In general, patients should be able to tolerate the operation; there must be absence of tumour at the primary site; no extrapulmonary metastases should be present; the pulmonary metastatic disease must be resectable. Alternative therapy would not be as effective. Surgical resection of pulmonary metastases should be per-

formed primarily to cure patients and not for debulking. Surgery may also be required for staging, in order to plan future therapy and to determine prognosis. However, with the use of fine-needle aspiration, resection for diagnosis alone is now rarely done.

METASTASES TO THE PLEURA

The presence of a malignant pleural effusion implies advanced disease with a poor prognosis; prompt diagnosis and effective treatment is therefore required. Chest radiography remains the first examination in the initial assessment of these patients, but depending on the clinical context, further studies with ultrasound or CT may be required. Magnetic resonance imaging (MRI) currently plays a minor role in the assessment of metastatic pleural disease.

PATHOLOGY OF MALIGNANT PLEURAL EFFUSIONS

Fifty percent of patients with advanced cancer eventually develop a pleural effusion and of these 10% have an effusion at diagnosis.[65–69] Twenty-four to fifty percent of exudative effusions are due to malignant disease.[66] Metastatic pleural disease most frequently originates from cancers of the lung, breast, pancreas and stomach and has a tendency to be associated with adenocarcinoma histology.[67,70] In a review of 1783 patients with malignant pleural effusions, lung cancer accounted for 36%, breast cancer for 25%, lymphoma for 10% and ovarian and gastric carcinoma for 5% or less.[71] In approximately 10% of patients with malignant pleural effusions, the primary site is unknown. Women are more likely to be affected due to the preponderance of effusions in breast and gynaecological cancers. Raju et al. reported that pleural effusions are the most common manifestations of pleural metastases in patients with breast carcinoma.[72] Canto reported that in patients with breast cancer the pleural space was involved on the same side as the breast primary in 77% and on the contralateral side in 24%.[73]

The mechanism of pleural effusions in patients with cancer is multifactorial:

- Direct invasion of the pleura causing an inflammatory response with increased capillary permeability
- Tumour invasion of pulmonary and pleural lymphatics with central mediastinal, hilar and bronchopulmonary lymph node invasion
- Central bronchial obstruction with increased negative intrapleural pressure and increased transudation
- Hypoproteinaemia
- Infective obstructive pneumonitis and parapneumonic effusion
- An immune complex phenomenon with increased capillary permeability[74,75]

Clinically, it is important to determine whether an effusion is a transudate or an exudate.[76] Exudates most commonly result from increased permeability of the microvascular circulation due to inflammatory or neoplastic processes involving the pleura. An exudate is present when the pleural fluid meets at least one of the following criteria proposed by Light:[77]

- A pleural fluid total protein/serum total protein ratio of more than 0.5
- A pleural fluid lactic dehydrogenase (LDH)/serum LDH ratio of more than 0.6
- Pleural fluid LDH greater than two-thirds of the upper limit of normal for serum LDH

Features suggesting a malignant pleural effusion are lymphocytic predominance although polymorphonuclear leucocytes may be prominent. A minority are grossly bloody. The majority have normal glucose levels and pH above 7.30.[78] Malignant effusions with low glucose and a pH less than 7.30 are more likely to have a positive cytology and carry a poorer prognosis.[79]

The prognosis of patients who have malignant pleural effusions varies with the histological type of the primary tumour. When all patients are considered, 65% die within 3 months and 80% within 6 months. In patients with breast cancer the mean survival is 7–15 months after effusion and a 3-year survival of 20% has been reported.[78] The prognosis in lung cancer is much worse with a mean survival of 2 months from the diagnosis of a malignant pleural effusion and two-thirds of patients die within 3 months.[78] Diagnosis should therefore be rapid and relatively non-invasive and treatment should palliate symptoms in a reliable and durable manner.

Key points: malignant pleural effusions

- A malignant pleural effusion implies a poor prognosis
- 80% of all patients with malignant pleural effusions die within 6 months of diagnosis
- Metastatic pleural effusion most commonly originates from lung and breast cancer
- In 10% of patients the primary tumour site is unknown

DIAGNOSTIC TECHNIQUES

Radiography

A pleural effusion is the most common manifestation of metastatic disease to the pleura. A small amount of fluid can readily be identified within the pleural space. An opacified hemithorax without mediastinal shift should alert the radiologist to the possibility of:

- Main stem bronchial obstruction
- Mediastinal fixation with malignant lymph nodes or malignant mesothelioma. In most cases, it is very difficult to distinguish between malignant and nonmalignant pleural effusions unless irregular thickened plaques or pleural nodules are visible (Figs. 36.11 and 36.12)

When widespread metastatic encasement of the hemithorax is seen this may mimic mesothelioma[67] but this pattern has also been described with lymphoma.[80] Metastatic thymoma can also result in pleural nodules or plaques.[81–86]

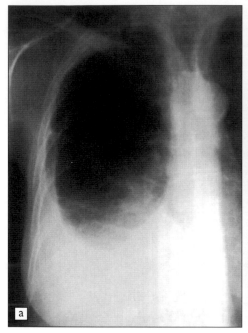

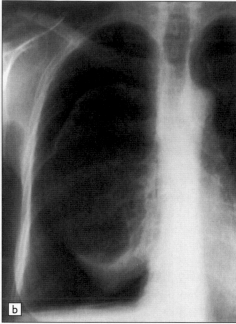

Figure 36.11. *Malignant pleural effusion from metastatic adenocarcinoma. (a) A large right pleural effusion with fluid tracking in the minor fissure is seen. Some volume-loss of the right lower lobe is seen without depression of the minor fissure; (b) following drainage of the pleural fluid the atelectatic lung has failed to re-expand with a large right hydropneumothorax. The pleural surface is only minimally thickened. The chest tube is in situ.*

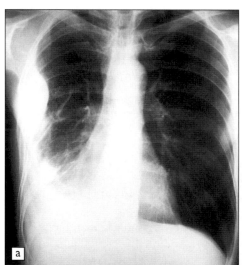

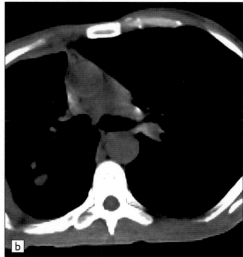

Figure 36.12. *(a) Malignant right pleural effusion from metastatic anaplastic carcinoma from an unknown primary source. Lobulated tumour mass can be seen with a right pleural effusion. There is volume-loss of the right hemithorax with a right lower lung mass adjacent to the pleural effusion. (b) Unenhanced CT scan confirms the presence of pleural tumour (of soft tissue attenuation) with involvement of the mediastinal pleura.*

Pleural cytology and biopsy

The presence of malignant cells within a pleural aspirate is indicative of a malignant pleural effusion. The results of cytological evaluation vary with the size of the effusion, the type and site of the primary neoplasm and the methods of processing of specimens. Cytological specimens from patients known to have neoplasms give positive results in 42–96% of patients with low false-positive results.[82–86]

Closed pleural biopsy should be performed before fluid aspiration to avoid lung injury. Cytological examination of pleural fluid alone has a higher sensitivity than pleural biopsy[87,88] with the yield of pleural cancer by needle biopsy ranging from 40–70%.[89–91] Pleural biopsy and cytology are complementary procedures with a high combined diagnostic yield of between 80 and 90%.[92,93]

Thoracoscopy

When a pleural effusion in a cancer patient is persistently cytologically negative, thoracoscopy may occasionally be useful in establishing the diagnosis. Visual inspection of the pleural surface with biopsy can then be performed with the synchronous sclerosis of malignant pleural effusions at the time of thoracoscopy.

Ultrasound

Ultrasound is a major imaging modality in determining the presence and nature of a pleural effusion. Ultrasound features suggesting an exudate include:

- Complex septations
- Complex non-septated collections
- Echogenic fluid
- Thickened pleura
- Associated parenchymal lesions

While these findings can be helpful, isoechoic effusions may be either transudates or exudates.[94,95] Ultrasound, like CT, has a low yield in confirming the presence of pleural metastases because most are too small (<1 mm) to be detected. Pleural metastases that can be detected appear as small hypoechoic masses forming obtuse angles with the chest wall or as large masses with a complex echogenic pattern.[96] Pleural metastases can simulate the appearance of malignant mesothelioma. The combined use of radiography and ultrasound is more accurate than either of these modalities alone in differentiating pleural fluid from solid pleural lesions.[97] Ultrasound is also important for directing interventional procedures of the pleural space[98] due to its speed, low cost and availability.[99] Under ultrasound guidance the best and safest site for the procedure and the depth of the pleural lesion to be biopsied can be determined. Because aerated lung is not penetrated using this method, pneumothorax uncommonly results. Since the differentiation of malignant from benign pleural disease can be difficult, histological samples should be obtained using large calibre cutting needles.

Computed tomography (CT)

Both benign and malignant pleural diseases result in pleural thickening, calcification and effusions with similar radiographic manifestations. Recently, Leung et al. have shown that CT can play a major role in distinguishing malignant from benign pleural disease.[100] Features that are helpful in distinguishing malignant from benign disease include:

- Circumferential involvement
- Nodularity
- Parietal pleural thickening of more than 1 cm (Fig. 36.13)

These features may also be seen in mesothelioma but are unusual in benign pleural disease. The presence of pleural calcification in general suggests a benign process.[100] Even in mesothelioma, calcified plaques are uncommon. Malignant pleural disease extends over the entire pleural surface whereas reactive pleurisy in general does not affect the mediastinal pleura with the main exception being tuberculous empyema.[101] Additional morphological features that can help discriminate malignant from benign disease include:

- An irregular external pleural border
- Extrapleural extension (chest wall, mediastinum and pericardium)
- Associated lymphadenopathy

Computed tomography can be helpful in determining the gross distribution of the disease and in determining whether thoracotomy or needle biopsy is most likely to yield a positive diagnosis (Fig. 36.14).

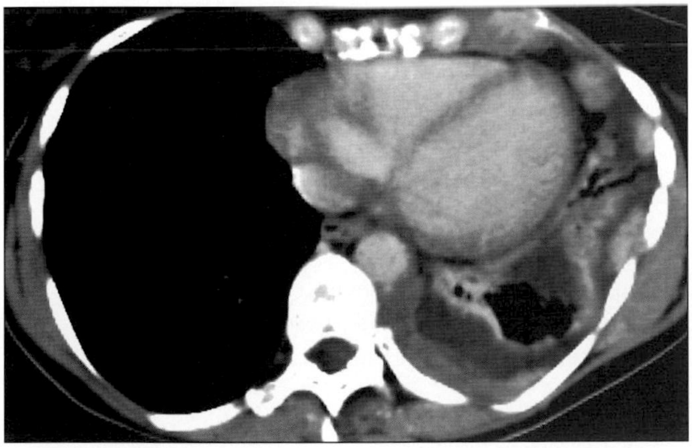

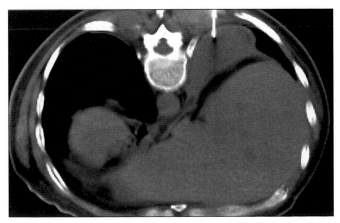

Figure 36.13. *CT scan of pleural metastases shown as enhancing tumour nodules and diffuse irregular pleural thickening in a patient with metastatic adenoid cystic carcinoma. A pleural effusion with atelectasis of the left lower lobe and volume-loss of the left hemithorax is noted.*

Figure 36.14. *CT-guided biopsy of a pleural mass performed with the patient prone. Direct spread to the pleural space of a chest wall carcinosarcoma occurred following resection of the primary tumour.*

Key point: CT

■ Circumferential involvement, nodularity and parietal pleural thickening greater than 1 cm are signs of malignancy on CT

Magnetic resonance imaging (MRI)

In most patients, the clinical issues necessary for management are adequately evaluated by chest radiography, ultrasound and CT. Magnetic resonance imaging appears to be superior to CT in the characterization of pleural fluid, showing different signal intensities in three types of effusions:

• Transudates
• Simple exudates
• Complex exudates with malignant cells or infection[102]

Signal hypointensity on T2-weighted images is a reliable predictor of benign pleural disease.[103] The multiplanar capability of MRI has been shown to be useful in differentiating parenchymal or pleural neoplasms from pleural fluid collections.[104] Coronal and sagittal images may be useful in demonstrating:

• The extent of pleural disease
• Mediastinal invasion
• Chest wall invasion
• Abdominal extension by malignant pleural disease

Contrast enhancement may also be helpful in distinguishing an exudative from a transudative pleural effusion.[105] Exudative effusions show significantly greater enhancement than transudative effusions after the administration of gadolinium-DTPA. The transport of Gd-DTPA into pleural effusions is possibly facilitated through the increased permeability of the pleural surfaces involved by metastatic disease.

Key point: MRI

■ MRI is superior to CT for characterization of pleural fluid

CONCLUSIONS

The management of patients with malignant pleural effusions from diagnosis to treatment is a difficult task with the prime consideration being palliation. The role of radiography is in the diagnosis of pleural effusions. Ultrasound guidance can be particularly useful in directing the site of aspiration and for pleural interventions. Computed tomography can more fully diagnose and document the extent of disease and has a role in pleural biopsy. Magnetic resonance imaging may provide additional useful information in selected patients.

Summary

■ Tumours with the highest incidence of lung metastases include choriocarcinoma, osteosarcoma, Ewing's sarcoma, testicular teratomas and thyroid cancer.

■ Spread of tumour to the lungs is usually haematogenous, less commonly lymphatic.

■ Over 80% of lung metastases are in the periphery of the lung (>60% subpleural), more commonly in the mid and lower zones.

■ Lymphangitis carcinomatosa arises most commonly from tumour of the lung, breast and prostate. Characteristic findings are demonstrated on HRCT.

■ Spiral CT is currently the most sensitive technique for the detection of lung metastases but is less specific than conventional CT.

■ Indications for CT must take into consideration the findings on chest X-ray, the likely influence of the results on management, and the propensity of the tumour to metastasize to the lungs.

■ Malignant pleural effusions occur in 50% of patients with malignancy during the course of disease.

■ Most pleural effusions are seen in patients with lung cancer, breast cancer and gastro-intestinal malignancy.

■ Malignant pleural effusions carry a poor prognosis.

■ Plain radiographs and ultrasound are the imaging investigations of first choice to demonstrate pleural effusions. Ultrasound is the best technique for directing biopsy and drainage.

■ CT and MRI may provide additional information, particularly in the distinction of benign from malignant pleural effusions and in determining the extent of disease.

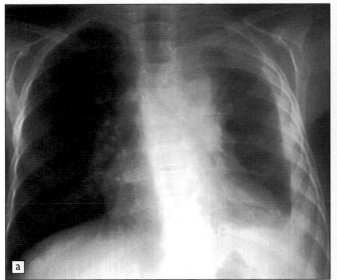

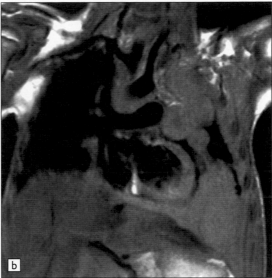

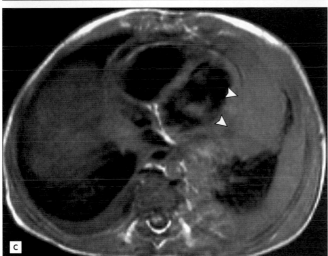

Figure 36.15. *Metastatic rhabdomyosarcoma. (a) Chest radiograph shows volume loss of the left hemithorax with larger left pleural effusion and gross thickening of the mediastinal pleura; (b) coronal spin-echo T1-weighted MR image shows the pleural deposits to advantage. Central mediastinal and left hilar lymphadenopathy is present. Note the sharp delineation of the left hemidiaphragm compared to the right side. (c) Axial T1-weighted MR image demonstrates bilateral pleural effusions with loss of the dark line of the pericardium posteriorly (arrowheads) indicating pericardial invasion. The pleural tumour is of intermediate signal intensity compared to the lower signal of the effusion on the right side.*

REFERENCES

1. Abrams H L, Spiro R, Goldstein N. Metastases in carcinoma: analysis of 1000 autopsied cases. Cancer 1950; 2: 74–85

2. Crow J, Slavin G, Kreel L. Pulmonary metastasis: a pathologic and radiologic study. Cancer 1981; 47: 2595–2602

3. Spencer H. Secondary tumours in the lung. In: Spencer H (ed.) Pathology of the Lung (4th ed). Oxford: Pergamon Press 1985; 1085–1096

4. Libshitz H I, North L B. Pulmonary metastases. Radiol Clin North Am 1982; 20: 437–451

5. Davis S D. CT evaluation for pulmonary metastases in patients with extrathoracic malignancy. Radiology 1991; 180: 1–12

6. Gilbert H A, Kagan A R. Metastases: incidence, detection and evaluation without histologic confirmation. In: Weiss L (ed). Fundamental Aspects of Metastases. Amsterdam: Holland, 1976; 385–405

7. Coppage L, Shaw C, Curtis A M. Metastatic disease to the chest in patients with extrathoracic malignancy. J Thorac Imag 1987; 2: 24–37

8. Liotta L A, Kleinerman J, Saidel M G. The significance of hematogenous tumour cell clumps in the metastatic process. Cancer Res 1976; 36: 889–894

9. Morgan-Parkes J H. Metastases: mechanisms, pathways and cascades. Am J Roentgenol 1995; 164: 1075–1082

10. Romansky S G, Landing B H. Metastatic patterns in childhood tumours. In Weiss L, Gilbert H A (eds). Pulmonary Metastasis. Boston: Hall, 1978: 114–125

11. Jaffe N, Schwartz L, Vawter G F. Childhood malignancy: patterns of metastases to the lungs and other target organs. In: Weiss L, Gilbert H A (eds). Pulmonary Metastasis. Boston: Hall, 1978: 126–141

12. Dodds P R, Caride V J, Lytton B. The role of the vertebral veins in the dissemination of prostatic carcinoma. J Urol 1981; 126: 753–755

13. Berg H K, Petrelli N J, Herrera L et al. Endobronchial metastases from colorectal carcinoma. Dis Colon Rectum 1984; 27: 745–748

14. Slapshay S M, Strong M S. Tracheobronchial obstruction from metastatic distant malignancies. Ann Otol Rhinol Laryngol 1982; 91: 648–651

15. Janower M L, Blennerhassett J B. Lymphangitic spread of metastatic cancer to the lung. A radiologic–pathologic classification. Radiology 1971; 101: 267–273

16. Filderman A E, Coppage L, Shaw C, Matthay R A. Pulmonary and pleural manifestations of extrathoracic malignancies. Clin Chest Med 1989; 10: 747–807

17. Muller K M, Respondek M. Pulmonary metastases: pathologic anatomy. Lung 1990; 168 (Supp.): 1137–1144

18. Scholten E T, Kreel L. Distribution of lung metastases in the axial plane. Radiol Clin North Am 1977; 46: 248–265

19. Benditt J O, Faber H W, Wright J, Karnad A B. Pulmonary haemorrhage with diffuse alveolar infiltrates in men with high volume choriocarcinoma. Ann Intern Med 1988; 109(8): 674–675

20. Hirakata K, Nakata H, Haratake J. Appearance of pulmonary metastases on high resolution CT scans: comparison with histopathologic findings from autopsy specimens. Am J Rocntgenol 1993; 161: 37–43

21. Chauduri M R. Cavitating pulmonary metastases. Thorax 1970; 25: 375–381

22. Dodd G D, Boyle J J. Excavating pulmonary metastases. Am J Roentgenol 1961; 85: 277–293

23. Wright F W. Spontaneous pneumothorax and pulmonary malignant disease: a syndrome sometimes asociated with cavitating tumours. Clin Radiol 1976; 27: 211–222

24. D'Angio G J, Iannaccone G. Spontaneous pneumothorax as a complication of pulmonary metastases in malignant tumour of childhood. Am J Roentgenol 1961; 86: 1092–1102

25. Dines D E, Cortese D A, Brennan M D et al. Malignant pulmonary neoplasm predisposing to spontaneous pneumothorax. Mayo Clin Proc 1973; 48: 541–544

26. Morse D, Reed J O, Bernstein J. Sclerosing osteogenic sarcoma. Am J Roentgenol 1963; 88: 491

27. Fraser R G, Pare J A P. Neoplastic disease of the lung. In: Fraser R G, Pare J A P (eds). Diagnosis of Diseases of the Chest. Philadelphia: W B Saunders, 1989; 1630

28. Zollikofer C, Castaneda-Zuniga W, Stenlund R et al. Lung metastases from synovial sarcoma simulating granulomas. Am J Roentgenol 1980; 135: 161–163

29. Rosenfield A T Sanders R C Custer L E. Widespread calcified metastases from adenocarcinoma of the jejunum. Am J Dig Dis 1975; 20: 990–993

30. Fraley E E, Lange P H, Kennedy B J. Germ cell testicular cancer in adults. New Engl J Med 1979; 301: 1370–1377

31. Panella J, Mintzer R A. Multiple calcified pulmonary nodules in an elderly man. JAMA 1980; 244: 2559

32. Charig M J, Williams M P. Pulmonary lacunae: sequelae of metastases following chemotherapy. Clin Radiol 1979; 43: 913–916

33. King D S, Castleman B. Bronchial involvement in metastatic pulmonary malignancy. J Thorac Surg 1943; 12: 305

34. Braman S S, Whitcomb M E. Endobronchial metastases. Arch Intern Med 1975; 135: 543–547

35. Shepherd M P. Endobronchial metastatic disease. Thorax 1982; 37: 362–365

36. Muhm J R, Brown L R, Crowe J R et al. Comparison of whole lung tomography for detecting pulmonary nodules. Am J Roentgenol 1978; 131: 981–984

37. Schaner E G, Chang A E, Doppman J L et al. Comparison of computed and conventional whole lung tomography in detecting pulmonary nodules: a prospective radiologic–pathologic study. Am J Roentgenol 1978; 131: 51–54

38. Chang A E, Schaner E G, Conkle D M et al. Evaluation of computed tomography in the detection of pulmonary metastases: a prospective study. Cancer 1979; 43: 913–916

39. Peuchot M, Libshitz H I. Pulmonary metastatic disease: radiologic/surgical correlation. Radiology 1987; 164: 719–722

40. Wellner L J, Putman C E. Imaging of occult pulmonary metastases: state of the art. Cancer 1986; 36: 48–58

41. Dinkel E, Mundinger A, Schopp D et al. Diagnostic imaging in metastatic lung disease. Lung 1990; 168 (Suppl): 1129–1136

42. Shah R M, Sprin P W, Salazar M A et al. Localization of peripheral pulmonary nodules for thoracoscopic excision: value of CT guided wire placement. Am J Roentgenol 1993; 161: 279–283

43. Lund G, Heilo A. Computed tomography of pulmonary metastases. Acta Radiol Diagn 1982; 23: 617–620

44. Kalifa L G Schimnel R H, Gamsu G. Multiple chronic benign pulmonary nodules. Radiology 1976; 121: 275–279

45. Webb W R, Cooper C, Gamsu G. Interlobar pleural plaque mimicking a lung nodule in a patient with asbestos exposure. J Comput Assist Tomogr 1983; 7: 135–136

46. Kagan A R, Steckel R J. Radiologic contribution to cancer management: lung metastases. Am J Roentgenol 1986; 147: 473–476

47. Husband J E, Macdonald J S, Peckham M J. Computed tomography in testicular disease: a review. J R S Med 1981; 74: 441–447

48. Vanel D, Henry-Amar M, Lumbroso J et al. Pulmonary evaluation of patients with osteosarcoma: roles of standard radiography, tomography, CT, scintigraphy and tomoscintigraphy. Am J Roentgenol 1984; 143: 519–523

49. Gross B II, Glazer G M, Backstein F L. Multiple pulmonary nodules detected by computed tomography: diagnostic implications. J Comput Assist Tomogr 1985; 9: 880–885

50. Meziane M A, Hruban R H, Zerhouni E A et al. High resolution CT of the lung parenchyma with pathologic correlation. Radiographics 1988; 8: 27–54

51. Milne E N, Zerhouni E A. Blood supply of pulmonary metastases. J Thorac Imag 1987; 2: 15–23

52. Ren H, Hruban R H, Kuhlman J E et al. Computed tomography of inflation-fixed lungs: the beaded septum sign of pulmonary metastasis. J Comput Assist Tomogr 1989; 13: 411–416

53. Nathan M H, Collins V P, Adams R A. Differentiation of benign and malignant pulmonary nodules by growth rate. Radiology 1962; 79: 221–227

54. Weiss W, Boucot K E, Cooper D A. Survival of men with peripheral lung cancer in relation to histologic characteristics and growth rate. Am Rev Resp Dis 1968; 98: 75–86

55. Cahan W G, Shah J P, Castro E B. Benign solitary lung lesions in patients with cancer. Ann Surg 1978; 187: 241–244

56. Costello P, Anderson W, Blume D. Pulmonary nodule: evaluation with volumetric CT. Radiology 1991; 179: 875–876

57. Heywang-Koebrunner S H, Lommatzsch B, Kloeppel R et al. Comparison of spiral and conventional CT in the detection of pulmonary nodules (Abstract). Radiology 1993; 189(P): 263

58. Remy-Jardin M, Remy J, Giraud F et al. Pulmonary nodules: detection with thick section spiral CT versus conventional CT. Radiology 1993; 187: 513–520

59. Armstrong P. Neoplasms of the lungs, airways, and pleura. In: Armstrong P, Wilson A G, Dee P, Hansell D M (eds). Imaging of Diseases of the Chest (2nd ed). Mosby-Year Book, Inc. 1995; 272–368

60. McCormack P M, Martini N. The changing role of surgery for pulmonary metastases. Ann Thorac Surg 1979; 28: 139–145

61. Mountain C F, McMurtrey M J, Hermes K E. Surgery for pulmonary metastasis: a 20-year experience. Ann Thorac Surg 1984; 38: 323–330

62. Putnam J B, Roth J A, Wesley M N et al. Analysis of prognostic factors in patients undergoing resection of pulmonary metastases from soft tissue sarcomas. J Thorac Cardiovasc Surg 1984; 87: 260–268

63. Fallon R H, Roper C L. Operative treatment of metastatic pulmonary cancer. Ann Surg 1967; 166: 263–265

64. Vogt Moykopf I, Meyer G. Surgical technique in operations on pulmonary metastases. Thorac Cardiovasc Surg 1986; 34: 125–132

65. Rusch V W, Harper G R. Pleural effusions in patients with malignancy. In: Roth J A, Ruckdeschel J C, Weisenburger TH (eds). Thoracic Oncology. Philadelphia: W B Saunders, 1989; 594

66. Light R W, Erozan Y S, Ball W C. Cells in pleural fluid: their value in differential diagnosis. Arch Intern Med 1973; 132: 854–860

67. Matthay R A, Coppage L, Shaw C, Filderman A E. Malignancies metastatic to the pleura. Invest Radiol 1990; 25: 601–619

68. Monte S A, Ehya H, Lang W A. Positive effusion cytology as the initial presentation of malignancy. Acta Cytol 1987; 31: 448–452

69. van de Molegraft F J, Vooijs G P. The interval between the diagnosis of malignancy and the development of effusion with reference to the role of cytological diagnosis. Acta Cytol 1988; 32: 183–187

70. Meyer P C. Metastatic carcinoma of the pleura. Thorax 1966; 21: 437–443

71. Sahn S A. Malignant pleural effusion. In: Fishman A P (ed). Textbook of Respiratory Medicine. Philadelphia: W B Saunders, 1988; 1770–1780

72. Raju R N, Kardinal C G. Pleural effusion in breast carcinoma. Analysis of 122 cases. Cancer 1981; 48: 2524–2527

73. Canto-Armengod A. Macroscopic characteristics of pleural metastases arising from the breast and observed by diagnostic thoracoscopy. Am Rev Resp Dis 1990; 142: 616–618

74. The Pleura. In: Fraser R S, Parre J A P, Fraser R G, Parre P D (eds). Synopsis of Diseases of the Chest (2nd ed). Philadelphia: W B Saunders Co., 1994; 868–894

75. Andrews B S, Arora N S, Shadforth M F et al. The role of immune complexes in the pathogenesis of pleural effusions. Am Rev Resp Dis 1981; 124: 115–120

76. Light R W. Diseases of the pleura, mediastinum, chest wall and diaphragm. In: George R B, Light R W, Matthay M A, Matthay R A (eds). Chest Medicine. Baltimore: Williams & Wilkins, 1990: 381–412

77. Light R W, MacGregor M I, Luchsinger P C, Ball W C. Pleural effusions: the diagnostic separation of transudates and exudates. Ann Intern Med 1972; 77: 507–513

78. Chernow B, Sahn S A. Carcinomatous involvement of the pleura: an analysis of 96 patients. Am J Med 1977; 63: 695–702

79. Sahn S A, Good J T Jr. Pleural fluid pH in malignant effusions. Diagnostic, prognostic and therapeutic implications. Ann Intern Med 1988; 108: 345–349

80. Libshitz H I. Metastases to the thorax. In: Greene R, Muhm J R (eds). Syllabus: A Categorical Course in Diagnostic Radiology. Chest Radiology. Oak Brook, IL: RSNA Publications, 1992; 235–244

81. Ellis K, Wolff M. Mesotheliomas and secondary tumours of the pleura. Semin Roentgenol 1977; 12: 303–311

82. Lopes-Cardozo P L. A critical evaluation of 3000 cytological analyses of pleural fluid, ascitic fluid and peritoneal fluid. Acta Cytol 1966; 10: 455

83. Jervi O H, Kunnas R J, Laitio M T, Tyrkko J E. The accuracy and significance of cytologic cancer diagnosis of pleural effusions (a follow-up of 338 patients). Acta Cytol 1972; 16: 152–158

84. Johnson W D. The cytologic diagnosis of cancer in serous effusions. Acta Cytol 1966; 10: 161–172

85. Melamed M R. The cytologic preparation of malignant lymphomas and related disease in effusions. Cancer 1963; 16: 413

86. Ceelan G H. The cytologic diagnosis of ascitic fluid. Acta Cytol 1964; 8: 175

87. Prakash U B. Malignant pleural effusions. Postgrad Med 1986; 80: 201–209

88. Prakash U B S, Reiman H M. Comparison of needle biopsy with cytologic analysis for the evaluation of pleural effusion: analysis of 414 cases. Mayo Clin Proc 1985; 60: 158–164

89. Hanson G, Philip S T. Pleural biopsy in diagnosis of thoracic disease. Br Med J 1962; 2: 300

90. Sisson B S, Weiss W. Needle biopsy of the parietal pleura in patients with pleural effusion. Br Med J 1962; 2: 298–299

91. Scerbo J, Keltz H, Stone D J. A prospective study of closed pleural biopsies. JAMA 1971; 218: 377–380

92. Salyer W R, Eggleston J C, Erozan Y S. Efficacy of pleural needle biopsy and pleural fluid cytopathology in the diagnosis of malignant neoplasm involving the pleura. Chest 1975; 67: 536–539

93. Winkelmann M, Pfitzer P. Blind pleural biopsy in combination with cytology of pleural effusions. Acta Cytol 1981; 25: 373–376

94. Hirsch J H, Rogers J V, Mack L A. Real time sonography of pleural opacities. Am J Roentgenol 1981; 136: 297–301

95. Yang P C, Luh K T, Chang D B et al. Value of sonography in determining the nature of pleural effusion: Analysis of 320 cases. Am J Roentgenol 1992; 159: 29–33

96. Wernecke K. Sonographic features of pleural disease. Am J Roentgenol 1997; 168: 1061–1066

97. Lipscomb D J, Flower C D R, Hadfield J W. Ultrasound of the pleura: an assessment of its clinical value. Clin Radiol 1981; 32: 289–290

98. Boland G W, Lee M J, Silverman S, Mueller PR. Interventional radiology of the pleural space. Clin Radiol 1995; 50: 205–214

99. O'Moore P V, Mueller P R, Simeone J F et al. Sonographic guidance in diagnostic and therapeutic interventions in the pleural space. Am J Roentgenol 1987; 149: 1–5

100. Leung A N, Muller N L, Miller R R. CT in the differential diagnosis of diffuse pleural disease. Am J Roentgenol 1990; 154: 487– 492

101. Muller N L. Imaging of the pleura. Radiology 1993; 186: 297–309

102. Davis SD, Henschke CI, Yankeleritz D F et al. MR imaging of pleural effusions. J Comput Assist Tomogr 1990; 14: 192–198

103. Falaschi F, Battolla L, Mascalchi M et al. Usefulness of MR signal intensity in distinguishing benign from malignant pleural disease. Am J Roentgenol 1996; 166: 963–968

104. Lorigan J G, Libshitz H I. MR imaging of malignant pleural mesothelioma. J Comput Assist Tomogr 1989; 13: 617–620

105. Cantoni S, Ropolo F, Serrano J et al. MR enhancement of pleural effusions after IV administration of Gd-DTPA in patients with bronchogenic carcinoma. Eur Radiol 1995; 5(Suppl.): 286

Chapter 37

Bone

Anwar Padhani and Janet Husband

INTRODUCTION

Bone is a complex composite tissue that has an important role in human physiology as it is the site of immunological, haematological and metabolic processes.[1,2] Evaluation of the bone marrow in patients with cancer is important for determining treatment and prognosis. Traditionally, bone marrow biopsy has been used to evaluate metastatic involvement, but this is prone to sampling errors and unguided biopsy may yield results that are not representative of changes in the rest of the bone marrow.[3]

The purpose of imaging is to identify bone metastases, to determine the extent of disease, to evaluate complications such as spinal cord compression or fractures, and to monitor therapeutic response. Imaging may be undertaken for routine screening in those tumours which have a high incidence of bone metastases such as breast and prostate cancer. It is also frequently employed in symptomatic patients presenting with pain or neurological deficit. Imaging studies complement clinical examination, serum tumour marker estimations which may point to disseminated disease, such as prostatic specific antigen levels in prostate cancer, and trephine bone marrow biopsy. Imaging studies are able to detect bone metastases non-invasively. These include:

- Radionuclide scintigraphy
- Plain radiography
- Computed tomography
- Magnetic resonance imaging

Radionuclide scintigraphy can provide a survey of bone marrow directly (using radiolabelled colloid or iron)[4] or the supporting bone (diphosphonate bone scan). The latter is the most commonly used radionuclide study for the assessment of bone but lacks anatomical detail and has low specificity. Detection of lesions by plain radiography and computed tomography (CT) requires the presence of bone destruction.[1,5]

Magnetic resonance imaging is an important technique for evaluating the bone marrow because it has excellent spatial and contrast resolution, multiplanar imaging capability, and the unique ability to separate haemopoietic (red) marrow from non-haemopoietic (yellow) marrow.[5] It also provides the opportunity to survey large volumes of bone marrow at a single examination.

NORMAL BONE MARROW

The vast majority of bone metastases are intramedullary lesions which develop within the cellular marrow of cancellous bone. An appreciation of the morphology of normal bone marrow is therefore important for understanding the development and distribution of metastatic disease and may be helpful for interpreting imaging studies, particularly magnetic resonance imaging (MRI).

The normal bone marrow is composed of three major components (fat, water and proteins) (Table 37.1). The osseous component of marrow is cancellous bone which acts as a supporting structure for the cellular marrow constituents. The cellular elements include all stages of erythrocytic and leucocytic development as well as fat and reticulum cells.[6] The red bone marrow is considered haemopoietically active, producing red blood cells, white blood cells and platelets.

The vascular supply of red marrow differs from yellow marrow. The red marrow has a rich sinusoidal system,[7] whereas the vascular network of yellow marrow is more sparse with thin walled capillaries, venules and veins.

During development from birth to adulthood, conversion of red to yellow marrow occurs in a predictable and orderly manner. At birth, virtually all marrow is of the haemopoietic (red) type. Conversion begins in the postnatal

Table 37.1. *Major components of normal bone marrow*

Component	Red marrow (%)	Yellow marrow (%)
Water	40	15
Fat	40	80
Protein	20	5

period, first in the extremities, progressing from the peripheral towards the axial skeleton and from diaphysis to the metaphysis of individual long bones. The epiphyses and apophyses lack bone marrow until they begin to ossify. Rapid conversion occurs and as a result, ossification centres are characterized as yellow marrow areas.[1] By the age of 25 years, marrow conversion is usually complete and an adult pattern has been established.[1,8] At this time, the red marrow is predominantly seen in the axial skeleton and in the proximal part of the appendicular skeleton (Table 37.2; Fig. 37.1).[1,9] It is not unusual, however, to see red marrow persisting in the lower two-thirds of the femora.[1,3] Indeed, islands of residual red marrow within yellow marrow may simulate pathology.[10] With ageing the volume of red marrow continues to decrease, reducing from a mean of 58% in the first decade of life to 29% in the 8th decade.[11] The increase of proportion of yellow marrow is attributed not only to a decrease in red marrow but also to age-related osteoporosis. A change in the balance of red and yellow marrow may occur during life due to an increased demand for haemopoiesis which may result from chronic anaemia, in smokers or in patients with diffuse infiltrative disorders involving haemopoietically active marrow. Rarely this is seen in extensive metastatic disease.[12] Reconversion takes place from the axial to the peripheral skeleton.[8,13,14]

BONE METASTASES

Clinical features

Most bone metastases are asymptomatic and are detected on routine screening which is mainly undertaken in patients with breast and prostate cancer, these being the tumours with the highest incidence of bone metastases. Symptoms occur when lesions reach a certain size, when destruction of trabecular bone leads to bone weakening and collapse, or when a fracture from a metastasis occurs in a long bone.

Table 37.2. *Red marrow distribution in adults and distribution of bone metastases by anatomical site*

Anatomical site	% of total red marrow*	% of total bone metastases**
Head	13.1	7.3
Cranium	12.0	6.8
Mandible	1.1	0.5
Upper limbs	8.3	10.1
Humeri	2.0	4.7
Scapulae	4.8	2.8
Clavicles	1.5	2.6
Sternum	2.3	2.6
Ribs	7.9	12.2
Vertebrae (exc. sacrum)	28.4	33.5
Pelvis and sacrum	35.9	19.9
Femurs	4	12.3
Other sites	N/A	2.1

*Extracted from: Ellis R E. The distribution of active bone marrow in adults. Phys Med Biol 1961; 5: 255.
**Extracted from: Clain A. Secondary malignant disease of bone. Br J Cancer 1965; 19: 15–29. Based on 2001 autopsied cases.

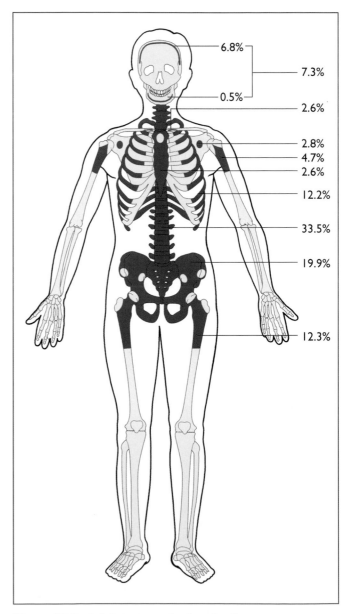

Figure 37.1. *Adult pattern of red and yellow marrow distribution with incidence of metastatic disease, from Table 37.2. (Adapted from refs. 1 and 23.)*

Pain may also occur when a metastasis has broken through the cortex of a vertebra to produce a paravertebral soft tissue mass and may be associated with neurological deficit if there is compression of nerve roots or the spinal cord. Vertebral collapse causing spinal cord compression is seen in 5–10% of patients with vertebral body metastases. Vertebral instability occurs when the dorsal elements of vertebrae are also involved.

Treatment of bony metastatic disease depends on:

- The nature of the primary tumour
- The presence of soft tissue disease
- Complications
- The presence of other bony metastases

For example, treatment of a solitary bone metastasis in an asymptomatic patient with advanced local disease and other soft tissue metastases may not be indicated whereas a patient with a solitary bone metastasis and no other evidence of disseminated malignancy may be given radiotherapy or chemotherapy depending upon the sensitivity of the primary tumour to different therapy regimes. Thus if a solitary metastasis is found within a vertebral body it is important to determine whether other lesions are present, as this will significantly alter management. Localized spinal cord compression may be treated with radiotherapy if there is a significant soft tissue component, alternatively surgical intervention with a laminectomy may prevent irreversible neurological damage.

Incidence

The most common focal bone marrow pathology in cancer patients is metastatic disease. Metastatic cancer to the skeletal bone occurs in 30–70% of all cancer patients.[15,16] Recently, with improved patient survival, the overall incidence of metastatic bone disease has increased. In 1950 Abrams[16] reported an incidence of 27% from 1000 consecutive autopsy patients who died from epithelial cancers. The sites of the primary tumours most commonly associated with bony metastases were:

- Breast (73%)
- Lung (32%)
- Kidney (24%)

Other sites included:

- Rectum
- Pancreas
- Stomach
- Colon
- Ovary

Today breast and prostate cancer are the most common causes of bone metastases. Overall breast cancer is responsible for approximately 70% of all bone metastases in women and prostate cancer represents the primary site in 60% of bone metastases in men.[17]

Distribution

Bone involvement by cancer occurs most commonly by haematogenous spread although direct extension of tumour in adjacent soft tissues into bone is not uncommon.[18,19] Over 90% of metastatic lesions are found in the distribution of the red marrow in adults (Table 37.2) (Fig. 37.1).[20–22] In a series of 2001 cases, Clain[23] reported the percentage of patients with metastases to different sites as follows:

- Vertebrae (69%)
- Pelvis (41%)
- Femur, especially the proximal femora, (25%)
- Skull (14%)

The upper extremity is much less commonly involved (10–15%).[16] For most cancers, the pattern of involvement is similar although some tumours show a predilection for specific sites (e.g. pelvic bones in prostate and bladder cancer). Peripheral long bone metastases are most commonly seen in lung and breast cancer and occasionally in renal and thyroid cancer. Metastases usually involve multiple sites although approximately 10% are solitary most frequently from renal or thyroid primary tumours.[24] It may be difficult on occasion to differentiate these metastases from a primary bone tumour. In general, metastatic deposits are small (1–3 cm); however, deposits in the pelvis are often very extensive by the time of diagnosis. Extra-osseous tumour extension into the adjacent soft tissues is rare in metastatic disease and is a useful distinguishing feature between primary and metastatic malignant lesions.

Metastases in long bones initially involve the metaphysis which is the site of residual red marrow. Less commonly, the mid-diaphysis is first affected. Primary cortical metastases are rare but have been reported in lung cancer[25] as well as in metastatic melanoma and sarcomas.[26]

Pathophysiological features

The venous system is the main pathway for transport of cancer cells to the skeleton as bone does not contain lymphatic channels.[27] It is well established that the network of vertebral epidural and perivertebral veins plays a significant role in the transport of cancer cells to the vertebral bone marrow.[28–31] The system parallels, joins and bypasses the normal venous system and its presence, in part, explains the frequency of distribution of metastases within the vertebral column, pelvis and shoulder girdles.

In addition, the increased susceptibility of the red marrow compared with yellow marrow is related to haemodynamic factors which contribute to tumour extravasation and hence the development of metastases.[18]

Tumour cells may destroy bone directly or by the production of mediators that stimulate reabsorption by osteoclasts. Prostaglandins and other tumour-derived growth factors also appear to be important.[32,33] As metastatic lesions enlarge within the marrow, the surrounding bone undergoes osteoclastic (resorptive) and osteoblastic (depositional) activity. The level of these activities differs between tumour types and sometimes for the same tumour at different skeletal locations. The balance of these two processes determines the final radiographic appearance of lytic, sclerotic or mixed lesions.

IMAGING TECHNIQUES FOR DETECTION OF METASTASES

Accurate assessment of bony metastases requires the combination of clinical evaluation, biochemical parameters and appropriate imaging studies. A flow diagram for evaluating bone metastatic disease is shown in Fig. 37.2. Radionuclide bone scans and plain radiographs remain key investigations but CT and MRI have important supplementary roles. Both of these techniques have strengths and weaknesses which should be recognized so that they are used appropriately in a cost-effective manner.

Key points: general features

- Most bone metastases are asymptomatic

- Over 90% of metastases occur within the distribution of the red marrow

- Approximately 10% of metastases are solitary

- Extra-bony spread into the soft tissues is rare

- In long bones metastases usually occur in the metaphysis

- The network of vertebral, epidural and perivertebral veins plays a significant role in transport of cancer cells to the vertebral column

Radionuclide scintigraphy

Scintigraphic methods provide a physiological survey of either the bone marrow elements or the surrounding osseous structures. The haemopoietic elements within the marrow are imaged using radiolabelled iron. The reticuloendothelial system may be imaged using a radioactive colloid, (e.g., technetium-99m sulphur colloid). Bone marrow scintigraphy (BMS) has been replaced by MRI due to the greater sensitivity and spatial resolution of the latter. Bone marrow scintigraphy depicts pathological areas of bone marrow replacement as cold spots. These photopenic areas have to be large (>2–4 cm) before becoming detectable.

Figure 37.2. *Evaluating the skeleton for metastatic disease.*

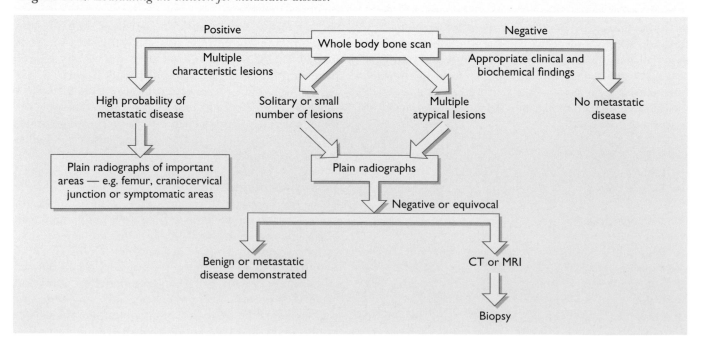

Since large amounts of tracer accumulate in the liver and spleen, some vertebral bone marrow is obscured.

Bone may be imaged using Tc-99m diphosphonate scanning (MDP). The bone scan image reflects skeletal metabolic activity and the major factors affecting diphosphonate uptake by the skeleton are osteoblastic activity and to a lesser extent, skeletal vascularity.[34] The Tc-99m-diphosphonate bone scan is an extremely useful imaging modality for the diagnosis and management of patients with skeletal metastases.[22,35–39] It is used for detection and staging of cancer but is less useful for following the response of bony lesions to treatment (Fig. 37.2). The major advantages of bone scans are excellent sensitivity for lesion detection and visualization of the whole skeleton. In general, bone scans will detect metastatic lesions before they are evident on plain radiographs.[40–42] As little as a 5–10% change in lesion-to-normal bone ratio is required before an abnormal focus is seen on scintigraphy.[43–45] Wilner[45] estimated that bone scans detected lesions 3 months earlier than plain radiographs. Galasko[19] reported a range of 2 to 18 months.

Despite its high sensitivity, bone scans have low specificity and cannot distinguish benign from malignant causes of increased tracer uptake. Bone scans are reliable for the detection of metastases from the breast, prostate, lung and kidney. However, bone scans are less reliable for the diagnosis of round cell tumours, myeloma, lymphoma and the leukaemias.[19,46,47] Photopenic areas are observed with myeloma and aggressive metastatic lesions that have rapid lytic bony destruction, e.g. renal cancer. Overall, false-negative results are uncommon.[40] False-positive results may occur from traumatic, infectious or metabolic causes as well as from benign bone tumours.

The relative distribution of bony metastatic disease detected by bone scans is similar to pathological specimens. Thus, most metastatic deposits are seen in the axial skeleton. Osteoblastic metastases are more easily detected than osteolytic disease. When large volume metastatic disease is present in the axial skeleton reconversion of peripheral marrow occurs which may be visible on bone scans as diffuse juxta-articular uptake of activity. Metastatic superscans may be seen in breast and prostate cancer (Fig. 37.3). The uptake of MDP is intense and irregular with minimal uptake in the soft tissues, distal extremities and the kidneys.

A common problem encountered with bone scans is that of the solitary lesion in a patient with known malignancy. This occurs in 5–8% of all patients.[22] McNeil[22] reviewed 273 such patients and reported that 55% were due to metastatic disease. Trauma (25%), infection (10%) and miscellaneous factors (10%) accounted for non-malignant causes. The anatomical site is important; 80% of vertebral lesions compared with 18% of rib lesions proved to be metastatic. If scintigraphy reveals a solitary lesion plain radiographs, CT or MRI may aid in the differential diagnosis (Fig. 37.4).

Radionuclide bone scans are relatively insensitive for evaluating treatment response but in general healing is indicated by a decrease in activity. However, in 10–15% of patients a 'flare phenomenon' is seen in which increased bony uptake is due to stimulation of osteoblastic activity in response to treatment.[36,48] In rare cases, previously undetected lesions may become visible due to the same phenomenon, thus simulating progressive disease.

Key points: radionuclide scintigraphy

- ■ Tc-99m-diphosphonate (MDP) bone scanning has excellent sensitivity in the detection of bone metastases and visualizes the whole skeleton

- ■ MDP bone scans are unreliable in myeloma, lymphoma and leukaemia

- ■ Osteoblastic metastases are more easily detected than osteolytic lesions

- ■ False-positive results occur with trauma, infection and degenerative change

- ■ MDP bone scans are relatively insensitive for evaluating treatment response

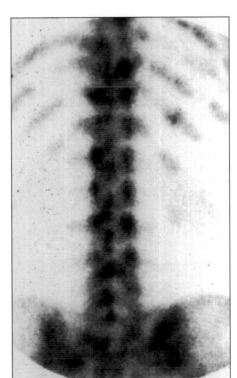

Figure 37.3. *Metastatic superscan. Posterior view of Tc-99m-MDP bone scan in a patient with metastatic breast cancer. Multiple irregular focal areas of increased tracer uptake are seen and are characteristic of metastatic disease. There is minimal uptake of the tracer in the soft tissues and kidneys.*

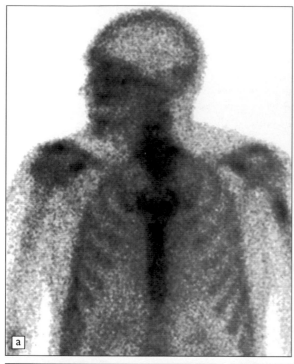

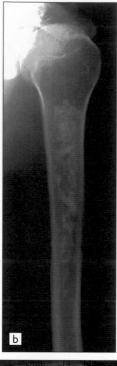

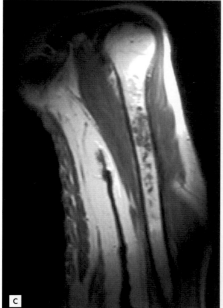

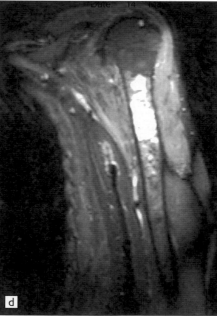

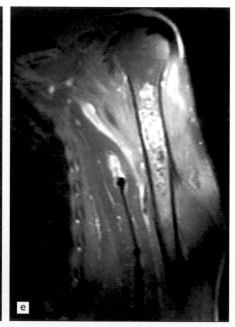

Figure 37.4. *Solitary bone lesion (enchondroma). (a) Tc-99m-MDP bone scan. Anterior view of the upper torso of a 75-year-old male with prostate cancer (MR image Stage T4, PSA 28) with an asymptomatic left humeral lesion. Poor uptake of MDP into the skeleton is seen but there is a high activity lesion in the upper left humerus. No other lesions are seen; (b) plain radiograph of the left humerus shows a lesion at the corresponding site to the abnormal bone scan with irregular areas of calcification; (c–e) paracoronal T1, STIR and post-gadolinium-DTPA T1 MR images with fat suppression show an intermediate signal intensity lesion on T1-weighted images that extends into the diaphysis. The upper part of the lesion is of very high signal intensity on STIR images. Contrast enhancement is seen on the fat-suppressed T1-weighted images. Histological examination revealed islands of cartilage, calcification and sclerotic bone consistent with an enchondroma.*

Plain radiography

Conventional plain radiographs provide important information about cortical and trabecular bone, but little information regarding the presence of lesions confined to the bone marrow. Radiographic sensitivity is dependent on the presence of bone destruction and the type and degree of host response. Considerable bone destruction must be present before a bone metastasis is evident radiographically and indeed it has been estimated that a 30–50% reduction in bone density is required to visualize a lesion in cancellous bone.[42–44] Plain radiographs are therefore an insensitive method of detecting metastatic bone disease but have the major advantage of high specificity. Plain radiographs are an excellent method of differentiating metastatic cancer from benign lesions of bone although on occasion there may be considerable overlap of appearances, particularly if a lesion is solitary.

On plain radiographs bone metastases are seen as osteolytic, osteoblastic or less commonly mixed lesions (Table 37.3). Combinations of all three types may also be observed. In general, osteoblastic metastases are more easily detected than osteolytic metastases which may reach considerable size before detection, particularly in large bones, e.g. sacrum or pelvis, or when bone superimposition is present, e.g. skull base, cervicothoracic junction.

Osteolytic metastases (Fig. 37.5) show three different appearances on plain radiographs which include:

- Moth-eaten appearance — multiple small–medium sized lesions coalescing to form larger defects:
    - Ill-defined zone of transition
    - No sclerotic margins
    - No periosteal reaction
    - Soft tissue mass absent or small
    - *typically seen in breast cancer*
- Diffuse infiltration — lesions infiltrating the whole bone:
    - Ill-defined zone of transition
    - No sclerotic margins
    - No peristeal reaction
    - No soft tissue mass
    - *typically seen in neuroblastoma*
- Large bubbly expansile lesions — may be solitary
    - well-defined
    - sharp zone of transition
    - may have sclerotic margin
    - periosteal reaction sometimes seen
    - soft tissue mass may be present
    - *typically seen in thyroid and renal cancer*

Osteoblastic lesions are less common and are most frequently seen in patients with breast and prostate cancer. Osteoblastic metastases may be:

- Round discrete lesions of uniform high density
- Irregular lesions showing a mottled appearance due to varying degrees of sclerosis (Fig. 37.6)
- Diffuse large lesions of high density with poorly defined borders

The osteoblastic component of the metastasis represents a reaction of normal bone to the metastatic process and thus the degree and pattern of sclerosis varies between different tumours and in the same tumour at different sites. The degree of sclerosis is considered to indicate the rate of tumour growth and hence dense reactive sclerosis usually reflects slow tumour growth. In fast growing tumours with a tendency to induce sclerosis, a mixed lytic and sclerotic pattern may be seen. Increasing sclerosis is also a sign of repair following treatment (Fig. 37.7).

Table 37.3. *Radiographic appearance of skeletal metastases*

Primary tumour	Radiographic appearance
Common primary cancer	
Breast	Lytic; also mixed; frequently blastic
Lung	Lytic; also mixed; occasionally blastic
Kidney	Invariably lytic
Thyroid	Invariably lytic
Prostate	Usually blastic; occasionally lytic
Head and neck	Usually lytic
Gastro-intestinal tract	
Oesophagus	Lytic or mixed
Stomach	Lytic or mixed; occasionally blastic
Colon	Lytic or mixed; infrequently blastic
Rectum	Lytic or mixed; infrequently blastic
Pancreas	Lytic or mixed; occasionally blastic
Liver	Lytic or mixed
Gallbladder	Lytic or mixed
Genito-urinary tract	
Urinary bladder	Lytic; infrequently blastic
Adrenal	Lytic
Reproductive system	
Uterine cervix	Lytic or mixed; occasionally blastic
Uterine corpus	Lytic
Skin	
Squamous and basal cell carcinoma	Lytic
Malignant melanoma	Lytic
Carcinoid tumours	Bronchial and abdominal blastic; frequently mixed

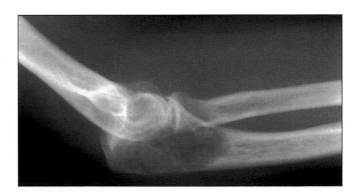

Figure 37.5. *Osteolytic metastasis. Well-defined lytic metastasis from breast cancer in the olecranon and proximal ulnar bone. There is predominant involvement of the medulla with thinning of the cortex. A pathological fracture is present. There is a small associated soft tissue mass.*

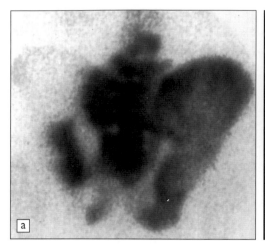

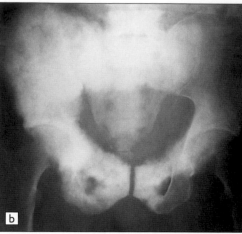

Figure 37.6. *Diffuse lytic metastases. (a) Posterior view of pelvis of Tc-99m-MDP bone scan in a patient with metastatic prostate cancer. Marked tracer uptake is seen in the lower lumbar and sacral spine and both iliac bones; (b) pelvic radiograph shows corresponding mottled sclerotic deposits with expansion of the bones and irregularity and poor definition of the cortical outlines.*

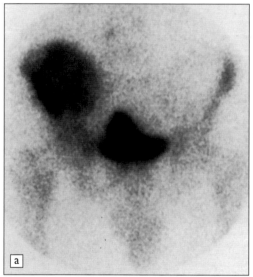

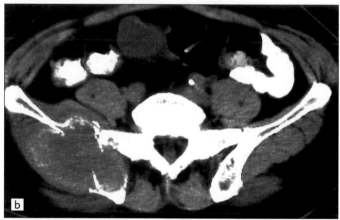

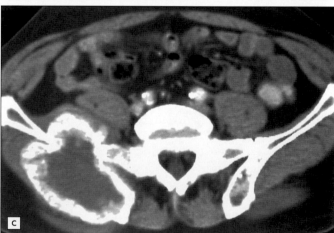

Figure 37.7. *Calcifying metastatic bladder cancer. (a) Tc-99m MDP bone scan of pelvis showing marked focal increased tracer uptake in the right iliac bone; (b) CT scan demonstrates a lytic lesion with a large soft tissue component with some matrix calcification in the soft tissue component; (c) CT scan 4 months after commencement of chemotherapy demonstrates marked calcification/ossification of the metastatic deposit, indicating response to therapy.*

Plain radiographs are primarily used to:

- Establish the diagnosis
- Determine the target volume for radiotherapy
- Assess treatment response
- Evaluate bones for structural integrity

Fractures may occur when >50% of the thickness of the cortex in a long bone is involved radiographically.[49] Prophylactic therapy at appropriate sites should be considered for lesions that are >2.5 cm in size, when >50% of the cortical bone is compromised and for pain.

Key points: plain radiographs

■ A 30–50% reduction in bone density is required before a lesion in cancellous bone will be visible on plain films

■ Osteolytic lesions are more difficult to identify than osteoblastic lesions

■ Fractures may occur when greater than 50% of the thickness of the cortex of the long bone is involved radiographically

Computed tomography

Computed tomography (CT) is not used in the routine evaluation of metastatic bone cancer although its role in the diagnosis and management of benign and malignant primary bony neoplasms is well established. The advantages of CT are excellent anatomical resolution, good soft tissue contrast and tomographic display. The excellent definition of trabecular and cortical bone is useful for the assessment of the structural integrity of bone. Computed tomography allows some separation of yellow from red marrow but is limited in assessing bone marrow infiltration. When bony metastases are suspected but not confirmed radiographically, CT can help establish the diagnosis, particularly in areas of complex anatomy or in those bones that are difficult to assess radiographically, for example the sternum, sacrum (Fig. 37.8) and craniovertebral junction. Computed tomography may demonstrate bone metastases as incidental findings in patients undergoing staging of the chest, abdomen and pelvis primarily for the evaluation of the soft tissues such as the liver and lymph nodes. Both lytic and sclerotic metastases can be demonstrated on CT down to

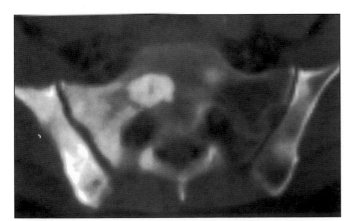

Figure 37.8. *Sclerotic sacral metastases. Coned view of a CT scan of the sacrum in a patient with metastatic prostate cancer. Multiple focal areas of sclerosis are seen. There is no associated soft tissue mass.*

the size of approximately 1 cm. In the vertebral bodies difficulties in differentiating metastases from benign pathology occur, particularly near to the vertebral end-plates where sclerotic areas may be misinterpreted as deposits. Dense bone islands may also be misinterpreted as metastases, particularly in patients with prostate cancer.

Before MRI was introduced, CT proved to be a useful method of evaluating solitary focal areas of increased tracer uptake in patients with positive bone scans and negative radiographs.[27,50,51] Muindi[51] studied 20 patients with breast cancer who had abnormal bone scans and normal radiographs. Of 28 sites examined with CT, metastases were diagnosed in 13 and benign lesions detected in 7. Computed tomography remains a valuable diagnostic technique, particularly in centres where MRI facilities are not available. Computed tomography is also useful for preoperative planning in patients with metastatic lesions to the spine where decompression surgery is required to alleviate spinal cord or neural compression and in defining the extent of metastatic involvement to the femur when prophylactic intramedullary pinning is being considered.

Computed tomography continues to play an important role in the evaluation of vertebral metastases when dural compression is suspected and for distinguishing benign from malignant causes of vertebral collapse by demonstrating the presence or absence of an associated soft tissue mass or involvement of posterior vertebral body elements[52] (vide infra). An important use of CT is to provide guidance for percutaneous bone biopsy. Computed tomography not only demonstrates the most appropriate route for biopsy but also demonstrates the presence of an associated soft tissue mass which may be easier to biopsy than the bone itself. If no soft tissue mass is seen then CT may demonstrate areas of destruction of the cortex, again depicting the most suitable biopsy site. In summary, the role of CT in evaluating bone metastases is:

• Detection of bone metastases if MRI is not available, e.g. a solitary hot spot on a bone scan
• Preoperative planning for decompression for spinal metastases
• Distinction of benign from malignant vertebral collapse
• Guidance of percutaneous biopsy

Magnetic resonance imaging

Magnetic resonance imaging is ideally suited for the evaluation of bone marrow because the technique:

• Visualizes bone marrow and bone marrow disorders directly
• Has excellent soft tissue contrast
• Provides good anatomical detail
• Has multiplanar imaging capabilities[5,47, 53–60]

Magnetic resonance imaging is highly sensitive for the detection of bone marrow metastases demonstrating lesions in the presence of normal radiographs and negative radionuclide bone scans.[61–64] Not uncommonly, MRI demonstrates incidental bone marrow metastases in patients undergoing MRI for primary tumour staging, e.g. prostate cancer. The appearance of the bone marrow on MRI is dependent on a number of factors including mineral, fat and water composition.

Both trabecular and cortical bone produce little or no signal due to a lack of mobile protons. In addition, the mineral matrix creates local field inhomogeneity (magnetic susceptibility) which interferes with signal from fat and water. Where trabecular bone is present, marrow signal intensity is altered accordingly. As yellow marrow predominates in the appendicular skeleton, the T1 and T2 relaxation patterns are those of fat. Similarly, haemopoietic (red) marrow has increased cellularity and therefore, the T1 and T2 characteristics of red marrow differ from that of yellow marrow. However, as 25–50% of red marrow is composed of fat (depending on patient age and anatomical site), the short T1 and moderately long T2 relaxation times of fat are averaged with longer T1 and T2 relaxation times of cellular marrow. The resulting signal from red marrow is therefore intermediate with a T1 relaxation longer than that of fat and the T2 relaxation time depending on the proportion of water, fat and cells. Most benign and malignant bone marrow disorders have long T1 and T2 relaxation times with the exception of fibrotic and blastic lesions, haemangiomas, bone islands and haematomas.

The appearances of bone marrow metastases are dramatically influenced by the pulse sequences used (Fig. 37.9). In general, T1-weighted spin-echo images are obtained complemented by short tau inversion recovery (STIR) or T2-weighted images (either spin echo or fast spin-echo [FSE]). Fat saturation is useful when obtaining fast spin-echo T2-weighted images. Gradient-echo sequences have important disadvantages when evaluating the bone marrow since susceptibility artefacts from trabecular bone may mask the presence of metastatic disease. In general, we prefer to obtain T1-weighted images followed by STIR images in the evaluation of metastatic disease and FSE T2-weighted images for the evaluation of spinal cord compression because the latter sequence provides better spatial resolution.

T1-weighted sequences (short TR and TE) have particular advantages in bone marrow imaging. The signal from fatty marrow is optimized and contrasts with red marrow and pathological processes. Excellent anatomical and contrast information is obtained with relatively short image acquisition times. With longer TR/TE spin-echo sequences, greater T2-weighting in image contrast is obtained. The differentiation of pathological processes from fat on T2-weighted images can be difficult as the T2 relaxation time for pathological processes may not differ from that of fat. As a result, imaging bone marrow pathology with T2-weighted spin-echo images is less reliable with variable contrast.[1,65] Large lytic lesions with high water content, e.g. metastases from bladder, kidney, thyroid cancers and myeloma, may be detectable on T2-weighted spin-echo sequences. However, diffuse or mixed lytic/blastic lesions may be isointense with normal bone marrow on T2-weighted spin-echo sequences. [5,66,67] Fast spin-echo T2-weighted sequences are equivalent to conventional T2-weighted spin-echo imaging [68] for detecting bone metastases in the axial skeleton and may be combined with fat suppression. With STIR sequences the T1 and T2 contrast of lesions (other than fat which is nulled) are additive and thus greater sensitivity to pathological processes is obtained.

Chemical shift sequences demonstrate changes in fat/water ratio allowing increased sensitivity for the detection of bone marrow infiltrative processes on opposed-phase sequences (Fig. 37.10). Although initial results have been encouraging, they are not yet in routine use.[69]

Contrast enhancement can be a useful parameter when evaluating focal bone marrow pathology. Low signal intensity lesions on T1 images that enhance following injection of intravenous contrast medium (gadolinium-DTPA) are potentially active (due to tumour neovascularity). Exceptions include sclerotic lesions (e.g. sclerotic metastases) and treated lesions. The intensity of contrast uptake by lesions can be compared with the surrounding marrow. Active lesions enhance to a greater level than surrounding normal marrow which allows the differentiation of marrow oedema (e.g. due to osteoporotic collapse or bone fractures) from tumour involvement. T1-weighted images obtained by subtracting images before and after gadolinium enhancement allow an appreciation of the pattern of contrast enhancement (Fig. 37.11).

Key points: MRI

■ MRI visualizes large portions of the bone marrow directly and has excellent soft tissue contrast resolution and multiplanar capabilities

■ MRI is highly sensitive in the detection of bone marrow metastases

■ Both trabecular and cortical bone produce little or no signal due to the lack of mobile protons

■ Bone marrow metastases are seen because they have longer T1 and T2 relaxation times than normal marrow

■ Bone marrow metastases are well-demonstrated on T1- and T2-weighted images. Short tau inversion recovery sequences often show metastases as very high signal intensity lesions

■ Gradient-echo sequences are prone to susceptibility artefacts from trabecular bone

■ Bone marrow metastases usually enhance following injection of intravenous contrast medium

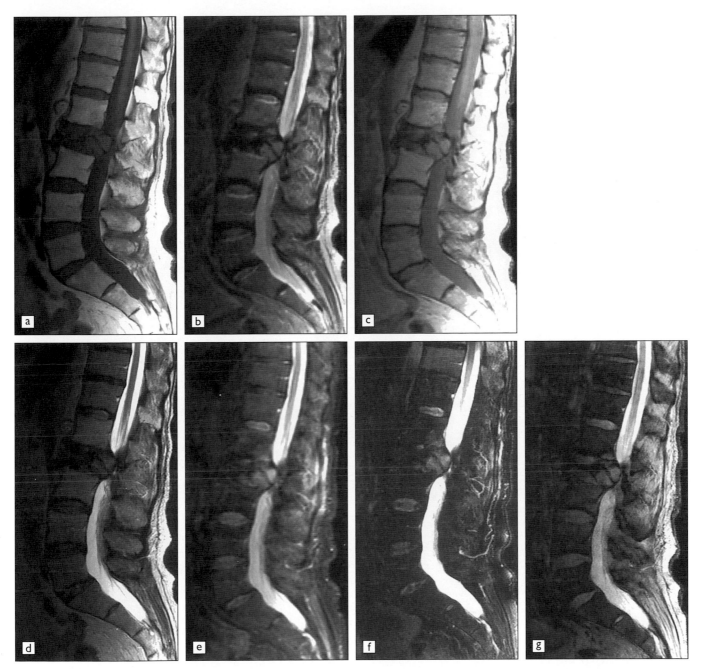

Figure 37.9. *Appearances of normal and metastatic marrow (prostatic cancer) on different imaging sequences. (a) Conventional T1-weighted (780/12); (b) T2-weighted (2000/80) and (c) proton density-weighted (2000/20) spin-echo images demonstrate a metastatic deposit causing vertebral collapse of the L2 vertebral body. The bone marrow signal intensity (intermediate to high) on T1-weighted and (low) on T2-weighted images in the other vertebral bodies is normal. A significant proportion of the normal marrow is of yellow type; (d) fast/turbo T2-weighted spin-echo image provides conventional spin-echo contrast with higher signal-to-noise ratio. Note that fat is of higher signal intensity compared to conventional T2-* weighted images; (e) STIR sequence is very sensitive to marrow pathology due to additive T1 and T2 contrast. The normal fat is nulled by this technique and the spatial resolution is poor compared with turbo/fast spin-echo images; (f) fast/turbo T2-weighted spin-echo image with spectral fat suppression shows excellent sensitivity for marrow disease while maintaining high spatial resolution (note poor fat suppression of T10/T11 vertebrae at the edge of the receiver coil); (g) gradient-echo FLASH image provides alternative T2*-weighting. Magnetic field inhomogeneity caused by intact trabecular bone results in low signal intensity from normal bone marrow increasing the conspicuity of the metastatic lesion at L2.*

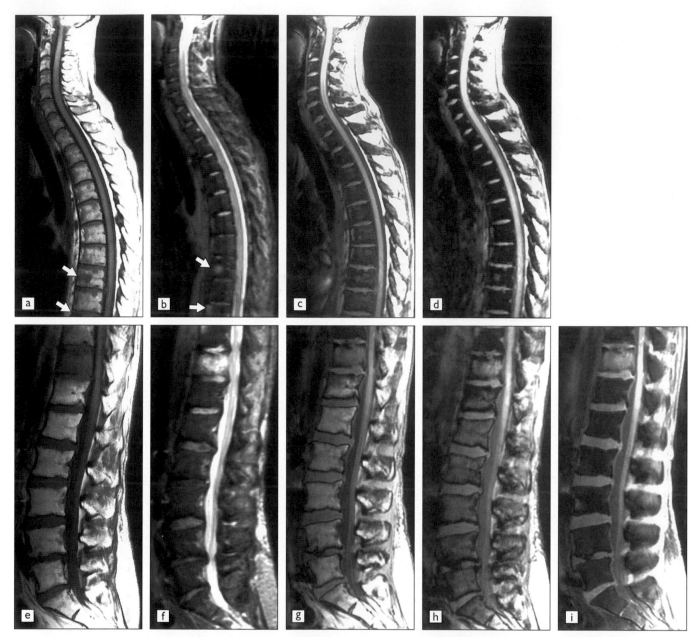

Figure 37.10. *MR images of various sequences showing metastatic disease. (a) T1-weighted (TR 500/TE 12) spin-echo and (b) turbo-STIR (TR 2385/TI 150/TE 30) sagittal images of the cervicodorsal spine in a 48-year-old female with metastatic caecal cancer. Low signal intensity areas on T1-weighted and high signal intensity areas on STIR in T8 and T10 (arrows) are typical of metastatic disease. (c) Opposed-phase T1-weighted gradient-recalled MR image (TR 100/TE 6.7/90° flip angle) shows decrease in signal intensity in normal marrow areas with higher signal from metastatic deposits which are not very conspicuous. (d) Opposed-phase T2*-weighted gradient-recalled MR image (500/15.7/90° flip angle) now shows further darkening of normal marrow areas and increased conspicuity of metastatic lesions due to the higher sensitivity of this weighting due to T2* effects. (e) T1-weighted (605/12) spin-echo and (f) turbo-STIR (TR 2385/TI 150/TE 30) images in the same patient's lumbar spine. (g) Paradoxically both the opposed-phase T1-weighted (120/6.7/90° flip angle) and (h) T2*-weighted (500/15.7/90° flip angle) gradient-recalled echo MR images do not show darkening of the bone marrow (compared with thoracic spine). This is due to complete fatty replacement of the marrow secondary to para-aortic radiation treatment 3 years previously. This is confirmed on the opposed-phase T1-weighted (120/6.7/90° flip angle) gradient-recalled image, with spectral fat suppression (i). A shift in the fat/water ratio (more fat due to radiation treatment in this patient) may result in an increased sensitivity for bone marrow infiltrating processes.*

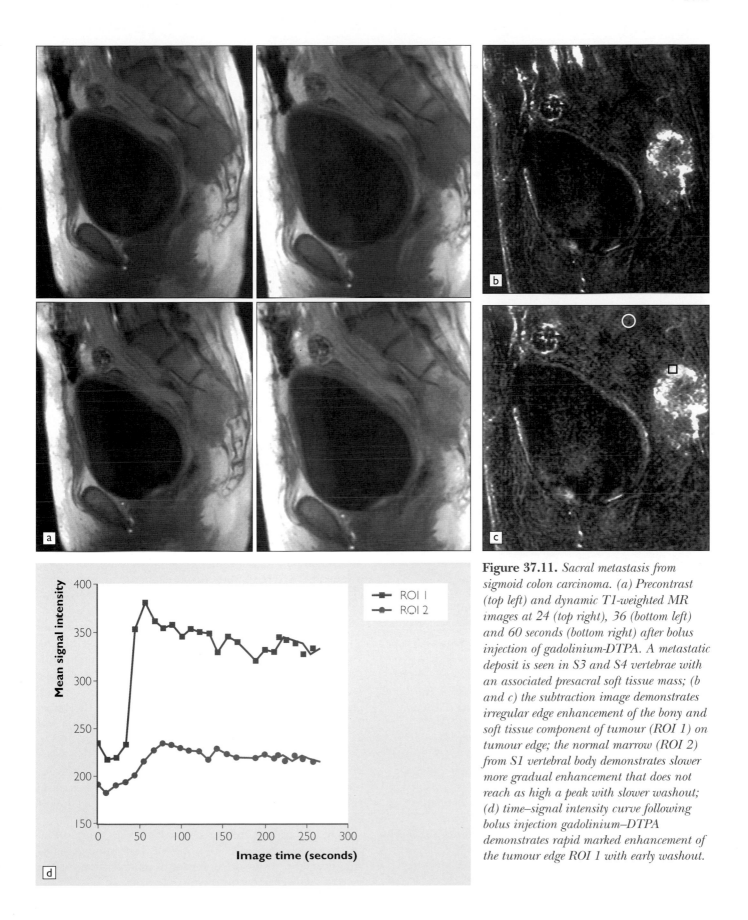

Figure 37.11. *Sacral metastasis from sigmoid colon carcinoma. (a) Precontrast (top left) and dynamic T1-weighted MR images at 24 (top right), 36 (bottom left) and 60 seconds (bottom right) after bolus injection of gadolinium-DTPA. A metastatic deposit is seen in S3 and S4 vertebrae with an associated presacral soft tissue mass; (b and c) the subtraction image demonstrates irregular edge enhancement of the bony and soft tissue component of tumour (ROI 1) on tumour edge; the normal marrow (ROI 2) from S1 vertebral body demonstrates slower more gradual enhancement that does not reach as high a peak with slower washout; (d) time–signal intensity curve following bolus injection gadolinium–DTPA demonstrates rapid marked enhancement of the tumour edge ROI 1 with early washout.*

Technique

The area of the body examined will depend on the reason for referral. This is usually pain, neurological deficit or inconclusive radionuclide, radiographic or CT studies. If the questionable area is in the spine it is important to examine the whole vertebral column as multiple lesions may be identified which might then alter patient management. Sagittal images throughout the spine should be obtained using T1-weighted as well as STIR or T2-weighted images. Axial images should be taken through areas where further information is required, for example for radiotherapy planning. Suspected lesions in the pelvis or proximal femora are best evaluated using a combination of axial and coronal scans.

Normal bone marrow

The MR imaging features of normal and abnormal marrow are dependent upon the sequence used. On T1-weighted images, yellow marrow exhibits a signal intensity similar to that of subcutaneous fat. Normal red marrow is hypointense compared with the yellow marrow (Fig. 37.12), although its signal intensity is still greater than that of muscle.

The MR appearances of marrow in any particular bone reflect the relative composition of red and yellow marrow and the presence of trabecular bone. In the spine, for example, the red marrow fraction remains high throughout life and marrow signal will remain lower than in locations where little red marrow remains. On T1-weighted images older patients have higher signal intensity of bone marrow when compared with younger patients due to the process of fatty conversion. This variation can affect the visibility of lesions on T1-weighted sequences, focal lesions being better seen in older patients than in children.[70]

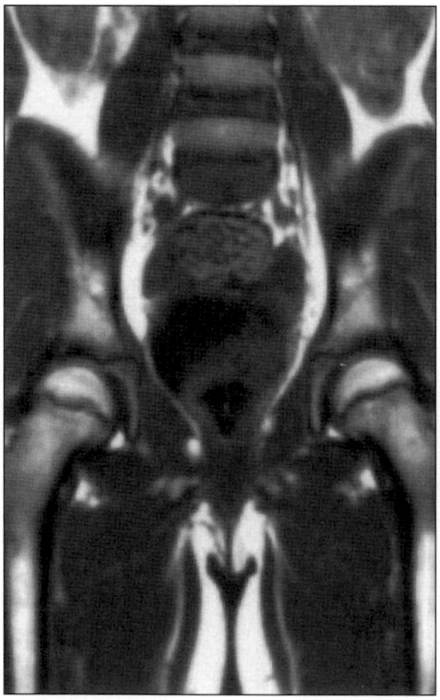

The vertebral marrow is of higher signal intensity than the adjacent disc on T1-weighted images in subjects over 10 years of age. Marrow signal lower than the adjacent disc suggests diffuse bone marrow infiltration.[16] Other conditions which lower bone marrow signal compared with the intervertebral disc include obesity, smoking, chronic cardiac failure, marked anaemia, anorexia nervosa (due to depletion of fat cells from marrow[71]) and AIDS.[72]

The appearance in any given bone can also be influenced by local factors. For example, the conversion of red to yellow marrow in the vertebral bodies may be focal. Several patterns of fatty replacement of the vertebral marrow have been described including:

- Linear areas of fatty high signal intensity paralleling the basivertebral vein
- A diffuse pattern
- Focal spotty areas of conversion are seen as bright spots on T1-weighted images[73] usually peripherally near the end-plates and in the posterior elements

Alteration in red marrow pattern can also occur adjacent to degenerative intervertebral discs.[74] The marrow changes have a band-like configuration that parallels the end-plate, presumably, as a result of ischemic changes. Adjoining dark areas adjacent to the end-plates as a result of sclerosis or fibrosis may also be seen.

The yellow marrow of the appendicular skeleton usually exhibits diffuse homogeneous high signal intensity on T1-weighted images. Nodules of intermediate or low signal corresponding to remnants of normal red marrow are occasionally seen, particularly in the proximal metaphysis of the femora and humeri and around the knee. These are frequently seen in premenopausal women and in marathon runners.[75]

The presence of trabecular bone affects the appearance of the appendicular marrow. Low signal intensity bands are seen on all sequences, particularly in the proximal femora (Fig. 37.13). Similarly, epiphyseal scars also give a band of low signal intensity.

On gadolinium-enhanced MR sequences, the normal red marrow exhibits a mild, diffuse and homogeneous enhancement, while no significant enhancement can be seen in yellow marrow on these sequences.

Figure 37.12.
Normal bone marrow distribution in a child. T1-weighted spin-echo coronal pelvic image (650/15) in a 9-year-old male with normal low signal intensity (red) bone marrow in the metaphysis of the proximal femora, pelvis and spine. Normal red marrow signal intensity is greater than muscle. Yellow marrow signal intensity is similar to subcutaneous fat. This appearance in an adult can simulate a bone marrow disorder by replacement or hyperproliferation. In a child this is a normal finding. Note the yellow marrow signal of the femoral heads.

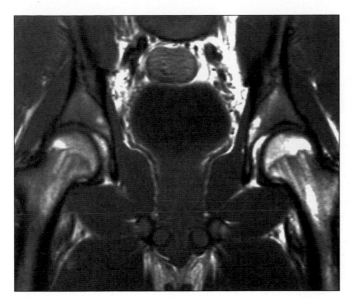

Figure 37.13. *Normal trabecular bone causing low signal intensity. T1-weighted spin-echo (TR758/TE12) coronal MR image in a 20-year-old male with normal distribution of red bone marrow in the proximal femora and in the pelvis. The presence of trabecular bone can be seen as low signal intensity bands in both proximal femora. The epiphyseal line is also seen as a low signal intensity band.*

Metastatic disease

Several patterns of bony marrow involvement have been described using T1-and T2-weighted sequences (Figs. 37.14 and 37.15). Metastatic lesions are typically focal with low signal on T1-weighted images and high signal intensity (greater than marrow fat) on T2-weighted sequences (Fig. 37.15). On fat-suppressed STIR images lesions are often of very high signal, particularly lytic metastases such as those from the kidney, thyroid or bladder cancer. Sclerotic lesions are of low signal intensity on T1-and T2-weighted weighted images (Fig. 37.14) typically seen in metastases from prostate and breast cancer. Similar changes may also be seen in sclerotic myeloma. A third pattern is a diffuse inhomogeneous low signal involving the whole bone. Very rarely, a diffuse homogeneous low signal is seen on T1-weighted images and homogeneous increased signal is seen on T2-weighted images.[76–79] This pattern can also be identified in lymphoma, leukaemia and other bone marrow infiltrating disorders. Metastases enhance following injection of intravenous contrast material. The T1 shortening with the administration of Gd-DTPA produces a high signal intensity on T1-weighted images and hence tumour enhancement. This reduces the contrast between tumour and normal marrow fat, making lesions less conspicuous and producing nearly normal-appearing marrow even in the presence of extensive disease.[66] If intravenous contrast medium is used, T1-weighted images should be combined with fat suppression. Studies using dynamic MR imaging after the administration of Gd-DTPA demonstrate a sharper more rapid peak in enhancement for malignant lesions compared with benign masses (Fig. 37.11).[79]

The differentiation of metastatic or malignant marrow processes from benign and traumatic conditions remains a problem.[80,81] Non-malignant conditions which may be confused with neoplastic involvement include:

- Normal haemopoietic marrow
- Degenerative disc disease
- Fatty deposits
- Schmorl's nodes
- Osteomyelitis
- Primary bone tumours
- Compression fractures
- Bone islands
- Infarcts

Features more likely to be seen in malignant vertebral disease are discussed below.

Key points: MRI findings

- The MRI appearances in any bone reflect the relative composition of red and yellow marrow

- The vertebral body has a higher signal intensity than the intervertebral disc on T1-weighted images and this is a useful guide for detecting early infiltrative processes

- Osteolytic metastases have a low signal intensity on T1 weighting and a high signal intensity on T2 weighting

- Sclerotic metastases have a low signal intensity on both T1 and T2 weighting

- Normal marrow shows mild diffuse homogeneous enhancement after administration of intravenous contrast medium

- Metastases enhance following injection of intravenous contrast medium to a greater degree than normal marrow

- Metastases may have a similar appearance to a variety of benign lesions

- Abnormal signal intensity in the posterior aspect of the vertebral body extending into the posterior elements should suggest metastatic disease

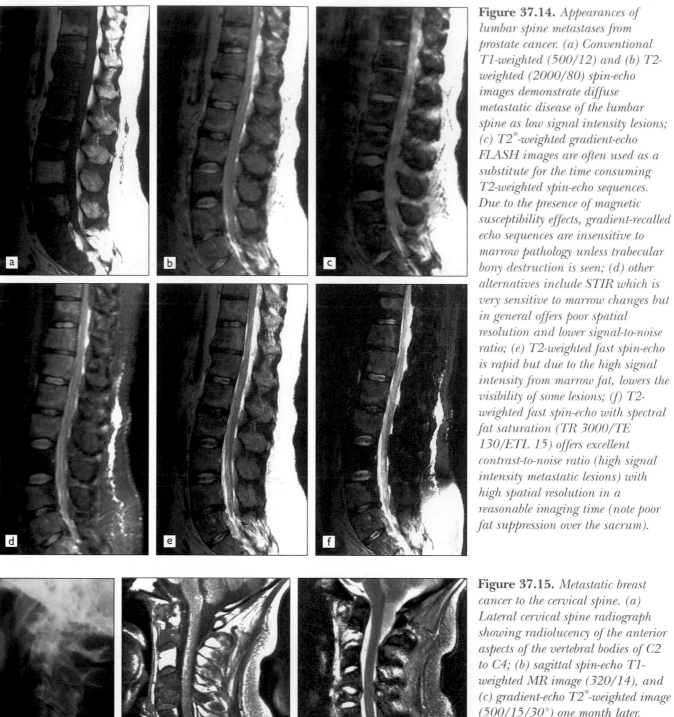

Figure 37.14. *Appearances of lumbar spine metastases from prostate cancer. (a) Conventional T1-weighted (500/12) and (b) T2-weighted (2000/80) spin-echo images demonstrate diffuse metastatic disease of the lumbar spine as low signal intensity lesions; (c) T2*-weighted gradient-echo FLASH images are often used as a substitute for the time consuming T2-weighted spin-echo sequences. Due to the presence of magnetic susceptibility effects, gradient-recalled echo sequences are insensitive to marrow pathology unless trabecular bony destruction is seen; (d) other alternatives include STIR which is very sensitive to marrow changes but in general offers poor spatial resolution and lower signal-to-noise ratio; (e) T2-weighted fast spin-echo is rapid but due to the high signal intensity from marrow fat, lowers the visibility of some lesions; (f) T2-weighted fast spin-echo with spectral fat saturation (TR 3000/TE 130/ETL 15) offers excellent contrast-to-noise ratio (high signal intensity metastatic lesions) with high spatial resolution in a reasonable imaging time (note poor fat suppression over the sacrum).*

Figure 37.15. *Metastatic breast cancer to the cervical spine. (a) Lateral cervical spine radiograph showing radiolucency of the anterior aspects of the vertebral bodies of C2 to C4; (b) sagittal spin-echo T1-weighted MR image (320/14), and (c) gradient-echo T2*-weighted image (500/15/30°) one month later. Multiple metastatic lesions are seen as low signal intensity areas on T1-weighted and as high signal intensity on T2-weighted images. A lytic metastasis of the anterior arch of C1 with involvement of C2 vertebral body is seen resulting in craniospinal instability.*

COMPARISON OF IMAGING TECHNIQUES

Several studies have now demonstrated that MRI is more sensitive than radionuclide bone scanning for detecting bone marrow metastases. In a study of 84 patients from the Royal Marsden Hospital, Jones et al.[82] reported a 7% yield of MRI over Tc-99m diphosphonate bone scans and plain radiographs in patients with primary breast cancer. Although MRI may demonstrate metastases in the presence of negative bone scans, the converse is also occasionally true.[83] Radionuclide scanning and MRI are highly sensitive techniques but radionuclide scanning clearly lacks specificity. Magnetic resonance imaging also has limitations due to non-specificity of signal patterns but morphological features outlined above may point to a malignant process. Plain radiographs are insensitive to the detection of metastases but are highly specific; a major role of plain radiography being to determine the nature of increased tracer uptake demonstrated on radionuclide bone scans. Plain radiographs may also yield metastatic bone disease in tumours in which radionuclide scanning has a low yield such as myeloma, renal carcinoma, lymphoma and some sarcomas. Computed tomography is a highly sensitive method of evaluating cortical and trabecular bone showing areas of early destruction not visible on plain radiographs. The technique has been shown to be more sensitive than plain radiography in evaluating patients with abnormal bone scans and provides complementary information to plain radiographs, particularly in areas where plain films are difficult to interpret, such as the sacrum and skull base.

EVALUATION OF VERTEBRAL COLLAPSE

The loss of vertebral height in a patient with a known malignancy poses a diagnostic problem since the distinction between malignant and osteoporotic vertebral collapse cannot always be made on standard radiographs. The clinical history, age and radiographic changes are important. A history of trauma and multiple areas of involvement in an elderly person suggest non-metastatic disease (Fig. 37.16). The location of the lesion is also important as a vertebral collapse in the upper thoracic spine is more likely to be malignant than post-traumatic.[84,85] On plain radiographs uniform compression of the end-plates is more likely to be due to osteopenia or trauma whereas irregularity is more commonly seen with metastases. Multiple levels of vertebral involvement, a soft tissue mass and destruction of pedicles are more likely to indicate metastases. However, a paravertebral soft tissue mass can also be seen with trauma.[86]

Both CT and MRI can be used for distinguishing benign from malignant causes of acute vertebral collapse.[52]

Computed tomography features suggesting benign vertebral collapse include:

- Cortical fractures
- Retropulsion of bone fragments into the spinal canal
- Fractures within cancellous bone
- Absence of bony destruction
- Thin diffuse paraspinal soft tissue mass

Malignant acute vertebral collapse is characterized by:

- Anterolateral or posterior cortical bone destruction
- Destruction of cancellous bone
- Destruction of pedicles
- Focal paraspinal soft tissue mass (Fig. 37.17)

Magnetic resonance imaging also provides important information on the nature of collapse. In benign vertebral collapse the features depend on the age of the injury. In the acute setting, the vertebral marrow is oedematous with uniform loss of signal on T1-weighted images, and an increased signal on T2-weighted and STIR sequences.[85,87–89] The absence of other focal lesions and of a soft tissue mass makes the diagnosis of a benign fracture more likely. When the collapse is longstanding, the marrow signal is similar to that of normal vertebral bodies (Fig. 37.18). Bone marrow oedema following a benign fracture usually returns to normal or nearly normal signal after 1–3 months. Involvement of the posterior elements of a vertebra is also more likely in malignant involvement (Fig. 37.18).

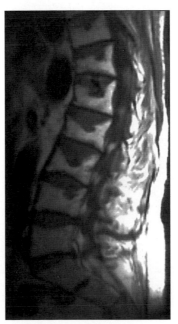

Figure 37.16. *Osteoporotic vertebral collapse of T11–L4 in a 65-year-old female patient. The marrow signal intensity on this T1-weighted spin-echo MR image is normal for a patient of this age with colon cancer. Note anterior wedging together with superior end-plate depression by disc bulges.*

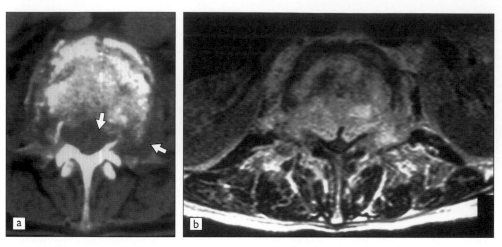

Figure 37.17. *Colon cancer metastatic to the 12th thoracic vertebra showing destruction of the cancellous and cortical bone of the vertebral body, pedicles and a soft tissue mass (arrows) on CT (a). On T1-weighted axial MR image (b) the vertebral involvement is obvious and the perivertebral soft tissue mass and compression of the thecal sac can be seen. Bony destruction is less well appreciated than on CT.*

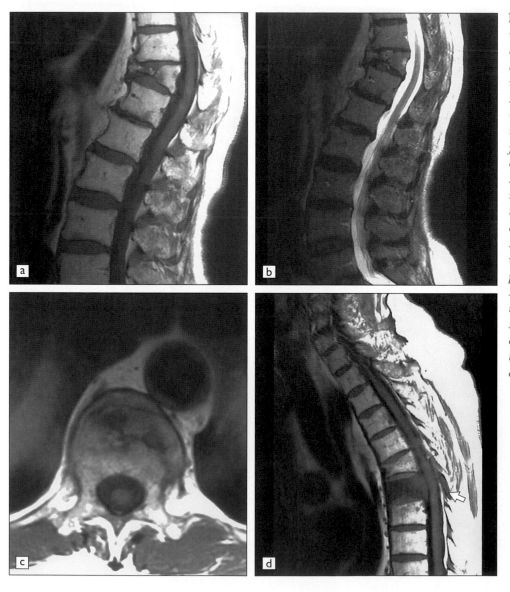

Figure 37.18. *Osteoporotic vertebral collapse and metastatic disease in a patient with prostate cancer. (a) Sagittal spin-echo T1-weighted (587/12) and (b) turbo spin-echo T2-weighted (TR 4000/TE 130/ETL 15) MR images through the lumbodorsal junction. Loss of vertebral height of T11 with anterior wedging is seen. (c) The axial T1-weighted image shows cortical fractures, the absence of bony destruction and preserved normal marrow signal characteristic of benign vertebral collapse. (d) Same patient at a higher level. The sagittal T1-weighted spin-echo image shows a uniform decreased signal intensity with expansion of the T7 vertebral body causing thecal compression. The posterior elements are involved (arrow).*

Magnetic resonance imaging features suggestive of malignant vertebral collapse include:

- Involvement of the posterior vertebral body and posterior elements
- Associated soft tissue mass
- Diffuse involvment of the whole vertebra
- Contrast enhancement of the abnormal area
- Multiple lesions

MONITORING TUMOUR RESPONSE TO TREATMENT

Tumours in bone marrow respond to treatment with a reduction in size of tumour and a change in signal intensity. Changes in lesion size are best demonstrated on T1-weighted images but signal intensity changes are often better appreciated on T2-weighted or STIR images. Following treatment of primary bone tumours an increase in signal intensity of lesions is seen on T2-weighted images.[90] An increase in bone marrow oedema may also be noted.[91] Areas of intermediate and low signal intensity within the marrow represent areas of fibrosis, haemorrhage, or residual disease on T1- and T2-weighted images. Focal areas of increased signal on T2-weighted images may remain for some time corresponding to areas of cyst formation or necrosis. It is not possible to identify residual active disease following treatment within the bone marrow on signal intensity changes alone. However, the use of dynamic intravenous contrast enhancement in assessing tumour response is currently undergoing evaluation.[86,92,93,94]

THE ROLE OF IMAGING

The accurate assessment of bone metastases in cancer patients requires a combined multidisciplinary approach of clinical and biochemical assessment in combination with imaging studies. In patients with breast and prostate cancer in which the incidence of bone metastases is high, routine screening is justified and radionuclide scanning is the most cost-effective initial test. Unfortunately, between 20 and 30% of positive bone scans represent benign disease, including degenerative change. Thus in patients with inconclusive radio-isotope scans other methods of imaging with higher specificity are required such as plain radiographs. Plain radiographs will usually be undertaken first, followed by MRI or CT depending upon the availability of equipment. In patients with lung cancer, renal cancer or bladder cancer, the incidence of skeletal metastases is only about 10% in the absence of symptoms; routine screening with bone scintigraphy is not recommended. However, in patients with symptoms of pain, the yield of bone scintigraphy rises to between 75 and 85% and is therefore the initial investigation of choice.

In patients with a solitary bone lesion considered to represent a metastasis, biopsy is indicated in the absence of metastases elsewhere. This is best performed under fluoroscopic or CT guidance (see Chapter 20).

The use of CT is declining as it is only of value in certain well-defined circumstances. Conversely the use of MRI is increasing as it is able to evaluate a wide variety of neoplastic and non-neoplastic bone marrow diseases. Magnetic resonance imaging is the most sensitive method for evaluation of the bone marrow as it is able to visualize the individual marrow components directly.

Summary

- Imaging plays a complementary role to clinical and biochemical evaluation in the detection of metastases.

- Radionuclide bone scans are the initial investigation of choice in the majority of patients.

- Screening with radionuclide studies for bone marrow metastases has a high yield in breast and prostate cancer.

- Plain radiographs should be used to elucidate inconclusive radionuclide abnormalities.

- CT has a role in detecting lesions at sites difficult to evaluate on plain radiographs.

- CT is useful for guidance of percutaneous biopsy.

- MRI is the most sensitive technique currently available for the detection of bone metastases and is moderately specific.

- CT and MRI are both useful in the evaluation of the cause of vertebral collapse.

- Response to treatment of bone marrow metastases is usually identified as a reduction in size of the lesion and a change in signal intensity.

REFERENCES

1. Vogler J B, Murphy W A. Bone marrow imaging. Radiology 1988; 168: 679–693
2. Ehman R L. MR imaging of medullary bone. Radiology 1988; 167: 867–868
3. Jones R J. The role of bone marrow imaging. Radiology 1992; 183: 321–322
4. Datz F L, Taylor A. The clinical use of radionuclide bone marrow imaging. Semin Nucl Med 1985; 15: 239–259
5. Porter B A, Sheilds A F, Olson D O. Magnetic resonance. Imaging of bone marrow disorders. Radiol Clin North Am 1986; 24: 269–289
6. Snyder W S, Cook M J, Nasset E S et al. Report of the task group on reference man. Oxford: Pergamon, 1974: 79–98
7. Steinbach H L, Jergesen F, Gilfillan R S et al. Osseous phlebography. Surg Gynaecol Obstet 1957; 104: 215–226
8. Piney A. The anatomy of the bone marrow. Br Med J 1922; 2: 792–795
9. Moore S G, Dawson K L. Red and yellow marrow in the femur: age related changes in appearance at MR imaging. Radiology 1990; 175: 219–223
10. Daffner R H, Lupetin A, Dash N et al. MRI in the detection of malignant infiltration of bone marrow. Am J Roentgenol 1986; 146: 353–358
11. Dunnill M S, Anderson J A, Whitehead R. Quantitative histological studies on age changes in bone. J Pathol Bacteriol 1967; 94: 275–291
12. Poulton T B, Murphy W D, Duerk J L et al. Bone marrow reconversion in adults who are smokers: MR imaging findings. Am J Roentgenol 1993; 161: 1217–1221
13. Custer R P, Ahlfeldt F E. Studies on the structure and function of bone marrow – II. Variations in cellularity in various bones with advancing years of life and relative response to stimuli. J Lab Clin Med 1932; 17: 960–962
14. Custer R P. Studies on the structure and function of bone marrow – I. Variability of the haemopoietic pattern and consideration of method for examination. J Lab Clin Med 1932; 17: 951–959
15. Silverberg E, Lubera J. Cancer statistics, 1987. CA Cancer J Clin 1987; 37: 2–19
16. Abrams H L, Spiro R, Goldstein N. Metastases in carcinoma. Analysis of 1000 autopsied cases. Cancer 1950; 2: 74–85
17. Napoli L D, Hansen H H, Muggia F M. The incidence of osseous involvement in lung cancer with special reference to the development of osteoblastic changes. Radiology 1973; 108: 17–21
18. Berrettoni B A, Carter J R. Mechanisms of cancer metastasis to bone. J Bone Joint Surg (Am) 1986; 68: 308–312
19. Galasko C S. Skeletal metastases. Clin Orthop 1986; 210: 18–30
20. Krishnamurthy G T, Tubis M, Hiss J et al. Distribution pattern of metastatic bone disease. A need for total body skeletal image. JAMA 1977; 237: 2504–2506
21. Tofe A J, Francis M D, Harvey W J. Correlation of neoplasms with incidence and localization of skeletal metastases: an analysis of 1355 diphosphonate bone scans. J Nucl Med 1975; 16: 986–989
22. McNeil B J. Value of bone scanning in neoplastic disease. Semin Nucl Med 1984; 14: 277–286
23. Clain A. Secondary malignant disease of bone. Br J Cancer 1965; 19: 15–29
24. Willis R A. The spread of tumours in the human body. London: Butterworth, 1973; 229–250
25. Deutsch A, Resnick D. Eccentric cortical metastases to the skeleton from bronchogenic carcinoma. Radiology 1980; 137: 49–52
26. Pagani J J, Libshitz H I. Imaging bone metastases. Radiol Clin North Am 1982; 20: 545–560
27. Malawer M M, Delaney T F. Treatment of metastatic cancer to bone. In: DeVita V T, Hellman S, Rosenberg S A (eds). Cancer Principles and Practice of Oncology. Philadelphia: Lippincott Co., 1993; 2225–2245
28. Batson O V. The function of the vertebral veins and their role in the spread of metastases. Ann Surg 1940; 112: 138–149
29. Batson O V. Role of vertebral veins in metastatic processes. Ann Intern Med 1942; 16: 38–45
30. Dodds P R, Caride V J, Lytton B. The role of the vertebral veins in the dissemination of prostatic carcinoma. J Urol 1981; 126: 753–755
31. del-Regato J A. Pathways of metastatic spread of malignant tumors. Semin Oncol 1977; 4: 33–38
32. Galasko C S B. Mechanisms of lytic and blastic metastatic disease of bone. Clin Orthopaed 1982; 169: 20–27
33. Manishen W J, Sivananthan K, Orr F W. Resorbing bone stimulates tumour cell growth. A role for the host microenvironment in bone metastasis. Am J Pathol 1986; 123: 39–45
34. Francis M D, Fogelman I. ^{99m}Tc-diphosphonate uptake mechanisms in bone. In: Fogelman I. (ed). Bone Scanning in Clinical Practice. London: Springer-Verlag, 1987; 1–6
35. Little A G, DeMeester T R, Velchik M G et al. Guided biopsies of abnormalities on nuclear bone scans: technique and indications. J Thorac Cardiovasc Surg 1983; 85: 396–403
36. Goris M L, Bretille J. Skeletal scintigraphy for the diagnosis of malignant metastatic disease of bone. Radiother Oncol 1985; 3: 319–329
37. Pollen J J, Witztum K F, Ashburn W L. The flare phenomenon of radionuclide bone scan in metastatic prostate cancer. Am J Roentgenol 1984; 142: 773–776
38. Hortobagyi G N, Libshitz H I, Seabold J E. Osseous metastases of breast cancer. Clinical, biochemical, radiographic and scintigraphic evaluation of response to therapy. Cancer 1984; 53: 577–582

39. Hayward R B, Frazier T G. A re-evaluation of bone scans in breast cancer. J Surg Oncol 1985; 28: 111–113

40. Tofe A J. Francis M A, Harvey W J. Correlation of neoplasms with incidence and localisation of skeletal metastases. An analysis of 1,355 diphosphonate bone scans. J Nucl Med 1975; 16: 986–989

41. Pistenma D A, McDougall I R, Kriss J P. Screening for bone metastases. Are only scans necessary? JAMA 1975; 231: 46–50

42. Citrin D L, Bessent R G, Greig W R. A comparison of the sensitivity and accuracy of the ^{99m}Tc-phosphonate bone scan and skeletal radiograph in the diagnosis of bone metastases. Clin Radiol 1977; 28: 107–117

43. Copeland M M. Metastases to bone from primary tumours in other sites. Proc NAH Cancer Conf 1970; 6: 743–756

44. Edelstyn G A, Gillespie P J, Grebbell F S. The radio-logical demonstration of osseous metastases: experimental observations. Clin Radiol 1967; 18: 158–162

45. Wilner D. Cancer metastasis to bone. In: Wilner D (ed). Radiology of Bone Tumors and Allied Disorders. Philadelphia: W B Saunders, 1982; 3641–3908

46. Weaver G R, Sandler M P. Increased sensitivity of magnetic resonance imaging compared to radionuclide bone scintigraphy in the detection of lymphoma of the spine. Clin Nucl Med 1987; 12: 333–334

47. Ludwig H. Fruhwald F, Tscholakoff D et al. Magnetic resonance imaging of the spine in multiple myeloma. Lancet 1987; 2: 364–366

48. Janicek M J, Hayes D F, Kaplan W D. Healing flare in skeletal metastases from breast cancer. Radiology 1994; 192: 201–204

49. Fidler M. Incidence of fracture through metastases in long bones. Acta Orthop Scand 1981; 52: 623–627

50. Durning P, Best J J, Sellwood R A. Recognition of metastatic bone disease in cancer of the breast by computed tomography. Clin Oncol 1983; 9: 343–346

51. Muindi J, Coombes R C, Golding S et al. The role of computed tomography in the detection of bone metastases in breast cancer patients. Br J Radiol 1983; 56: 233–236

52. Laredo J D, Lakhdari K, Bellaiche L et al. Acute vertebral collapse: CT findings in benign and malignant non-traumatic cases. Radiology 1995; 194: 41–48

53. Hudson T M, Hamlin D J, Enneking W F et al. Magnetic resonance imaging of bone and soft tissue tumours: early experience in 31 patients compared with computed tomography. Skel Radiol 1985; 13: 134–146

54. Porter B A. MR may become routine for imaging bone marrow. Diagnos Imag 1987; 9: 104–108

55. Shields A F, Porter B A, Churchley S et al. The detection of bone marrow involvement by lymphoma using magnetic resonance imaging. J Clin Oncol 1987; 5: 225–230

56. Olson D O, Shields A F, Scheurich C J et al. Magnetic resonance imaging of the bone marrow in patients with leukaemia, aplastic anaemia and lymphoma. Invest Radiol 1986; 21: 540–546

57. Colman L K, Porter B A, Redmond J et al. Early diagnosis of spinal metastases by CT and MR studies. J Comput Assist Tomogr 1988; 12: 423–426

58. Moon K L, Genant J H, Helms C A et al. Musculoskeletal applications of nuclear magnetic resonance. Radiology 1983; 147: 161–171

59. Ehman R L, Berquist T H, McLeod R A. MR imaging of the musculoskeletal system: a 5-year appraisal. Radiology 1988; 166: 313–320

60. Sartoris D J, Resnick D. MR imaging of the mus-culoskeletal system: current and future status. Am J Roentgenol 1987; 149: 457–467

61. Metha R C, Wilson M A, Perlmann S B. False negative bone scan in extensive metastatic disease: CT and MR findings. J Comput Assist Tomogr 1989; 13: 717–719

62. Arrahami E, Tadmor R, Dally O et al. Early MR demonstration of spinal metastases in patients with normal radiographs and CT and radionuclide bone scan. J Comput Assist Tomogr 1989; 13: 598–602

63. Kattapuram S V, Khurana J S, Scott J A et al. Negative scintigraphy with positive magnetic resonance imaging in bone metastases. Skel Radiol 1990; 19: 113–116

64. Algra P R, Bloem J L, Tissing H et al. Detection of vertebral metastases: Comparison between MR imaging and bone scintigraphy. RadioGraphics 1991; 11: 219–232

65. Zimmer W D, Berquist T H, McLeod R A et al. Bone tumours: magnetic resonance imaging versus computed tomography. Radiology 1985; 155: 709–718

66. Stimac G K, Porter B A, Olson D O et al. Gadolinium-DTPA-enhanced MR imaging of spinal neoplasms: Preliminary investigation and comparison with un-enhanced spin-echo and STIR sequences. Am J Roentgenol 1988; 151: 1185–1192

67. Porter B A, Redmond J, Dunning D M et al. Low field STIR imaging of spinal malignancies. Radiology 1988; 169(P): 65

68. Hanbold-Reuter B, Duewell S, Schilcher B et al. Fast spin-echo MRI and bone scintigraphy in the detection of skeletal metastases. Eur Radiol 1993; 3: 316–320

69. Rosen B R, Fleming D M, Kushner D C et al. Haematologic bone marrow disorders: quantitative chemical shift MR imaging. Radiology 1988; 169: 799–804

70. Moore S G, Gooding G A, Brasch R C et al. Bone marrow in children with acute lymphocytic leukaemia: MR relaxation times. Radiology 1986; 160: 237–240

71. Vande Berg B, Malghem J, Devuyst O et al. Anorexia nervosa: correlation between MR appearances of bone marrow and severity of disease. Radiology 1994; 193: 859–864

72. Eustace S J, McGrath D, Buff B R et al. Spectrum of skeletal marrow changes in the presence of HIV infection (Abstract). Radiology 1994; 193(P): 411

73. Hajek P C, Baker L L, Goobar J E et al. Focal fat deposition in axial bone marrow: MR characteristics. Radiology 1987; 162: 245–249

74. de Roos A, Kressel H, Spritzer C et al. MR imaging of marrow changes adjacent to end plates in degenerative lumbar disc disease. Am J Roentgenol 1987; 149: 531–534

75. Shellock F G, Morris E, Deutsch A L et al. Haematopoietic bone marrow hyperplasia: high prevalence on MR images of the knee in asymptomatic marathon runners. Am J Roentgenol 1992; 158: 335–338

76. Algra P, Bloem J L, Verboom L J et al. Sensitivity for MRI of vertebral metastases: A comparison of MRI and bone scintigraphy. Presented at the Society of Magnetic Resonance in Medicine, Amsterdam, The Netherlands, 1989

77. Berquist T H. Magnetic resonance imaging of musculo-skeletal neoplasms. Clin Orthopaed 1989; 244: 101–118

78. Thomsen C, Sorensen P G, Karle H et al. Prolonged bone marrow T1 relaxation in acute leukaemia. In vivo characterisation by magnetic resonance imaging. Mag Res Imag 1987; 5: 251–257

79. Erlemann R, Reiser M F, Peters P E et al. Musculoskeletal neoplasms. Static and dynamic Gd-DTPA enhanced MR imaging. Radiology 1989; 171: 767–773

80. Dooms G C, Fisher M R, Hricak H et al. Bone marrow imaging: Magnetic resonance studies related to age and sex. Radiology 1985; 155: 429–432

81. Doom G, Mathwin P, Cornelis G et al. MR differential diagnosis between benign and malignant vertebral collapse. Presented at Society of Magnetic Resonance in Medicine, Amsterdam, The Netherlands, 1989

82. Jones A L, Williams M P, Powles T J et al. Magnetic resonance imaging in the detection of skeletal metastases in patients with breast cancer. Br J Cancer 1990; 62: 296–298

83. Gosfield E, Alavi A, Kneeland B et al. Comparison of radionuclide bone scans and magnetic resonance imaging in detecting spinal metastases. J Nucl Med 1993; 34: 2191–2198

84. Hayes C W, Jensen M E, Conway W F. Non-neoplastic lesions in vertebral bodies. Findings in magnetic resonance imaging. RadioGraphics 1989; 9: 883–901

85. Yuh W T, Zachar C K, Barloon T J et al. Vertebral compression fractures: distinction between benign and malignant causes with MR imaging. Radiology 1989; 172: 215–218

86. de Baere T, Vanel D, Shapeero L G et al. Osteosarcoma after chemotherapy: evaluation with contrast material enhanced subtraction MRI. Radiology 1992; 185: 578–592

87. Berquist T H, Deutsch A L. Musculoskeletal neoplasms. In: Mink, J (ed). MRI of the Musculoskeletal System: A Teaching File. New York: Raven Press, 1990

88. Baker L L, Goodman S B, Perkash I et al. Benign versus pathological compression fractures of vertebral bodies: assessment with conventional spin-echo, chemical shift and STIR MR imaging. Radiology 1990; 174: 495–502

89. Berquist T H, Ehman R L, King B F et al. Value of MR imaging in differentiating benign from malignant soft tissue masses: study of 95 lesions. Am J Roentgenol 1990; 155: 251–255

90. Holscher H C, Bloem J L, Nooy M A et al. The value of MR imaging in monitoring the effects of chemotherapy on bone sarcomas. Am J Roentgenol 1990; 154: 763–769

91. Stoller D W, Genant H K, Lang P. The spine. In: Stoller D W (ed). Magnetic Resonance Imaging in Orthopaedics and Rheumatology. Philadelphia: Lippincott Co., 1989

92. Fletcher B D, Hanna S L, Fairclough D L et al. Paediatric musculo-skeletal tumours: use of dynamic, contrast enhanced MR imaging to monitor response to chemotherapy. Radiology 1992; 184: 243–248

93. Erlemann R, Sciuk J, Bosse A et al. Response of osteosarcoma and Ewing's sarcoma to pre-operative chemotherapy: assessment with dynamic and static MR imaging and skeletal scintigraphy. Radiology 1990; 175: 791–796

94. Erlemann R. Dynamic Gadolinium-enhanced MR imaging to monitor tumour response to chemotherapy (Letter). Radiology 1993; 186: 904

Chapter 38

Liver

Philip Robinson

INCIDENCE AND SOURCES OF LIVER METASTASES

Almost one half of all patients dying with malignant disease have metastatic tumours in the liver. The incidence of liver metastasis from various primary tumours, derived from autopsy series[1-3] is shown below.

These data reflect endstage disease whereas clinical interest for imaging will focus on the detection of liver metastases at the time of initial presentation of the primary tumour, and also on the likelihood of development of liver metastases during follow-up. About 25–40% of patients with gastro-intestinal primary neoplasms and small cell lung cancers have liver metastases at the time of first clinical presentation, but with other common primary tumours, liver metastases are rarely found at initial staging. Different primary malignancies can be classified into high-risk, intermediate, and low risk groups with reference to the likelihood of metachronous liver metastases developing after the initial presentation and treatment of the primary lesion.

In considering the clinical management of patients who have or who are at risk of developing liver metastases, it is important to take into account the progression of disease elsewhere. The presence of liver lesions becomes less significant if patients already have widespread metastatic disease in bones, lungs or central nervous system. Also, when multiple liver lesions are discovered in a patient under surveillance following treatment of a primary malignancy, it should not be assumed automatically that the liver lesions arise from the same pathology as the initial tumour, particularly if the combination is biologically unlikely. For example, liver metastases discovered during surveillance of a patient who has been successfully treated for prostatic cancer are more likely to arise from a second malignancy in the gastro-intestinal tract than from recurrence of prostate cancer.

BIOLOGY OF METASTATIC LIVER TUMOURS

The liver is a fertile ground for seeding of metastatic tumours. The reasons for this are not fully established but probably include the following:[4]

- The vast majority of liver metastases arrive via the blood stream, and the liver receives about 25% of the cardiac output
- The dimensions of liver sinusoids are suitable for entrapping small clumps of cells and gaps exist in the subendothelial basement membrane which in other organs provides a barrier to spread
- Continuous regeneration of liver cells is a normal phenomenon probably controlled by local humoral mechanisms which may also stimulate the growth of neoplastic cells once *in situ*
- Some tumours which commonly metastasize to the liver carry specific receptors for host endothelial cells

Table 38.1. *Incidence of liver metastases from various primary tumours at autopsy*

Primary site	Patients with liver metastases (%)
Oesophagus	30–100
Stomach	38–100
Colorectal	40–100
Pancreas	50–73
Bile ducts and gall bladder	45–80
Small cell lung cancer	38–67
Breast	49–73
Melanoma	69
Ovary	48–68
Uterus	24–75
Renal cell cancer	40
Urothelial cancer	37–38
Thyroid	20
Prostate	9–74

Table 38.2. *Likelihood of developing liver metastases during follow-up according to site of primary tumour*

High risk	Intermediate	Low risk
Oesophagus	Breast	Prostate
Stomach	Melanoma	Renal cell
Large bowel	Ovary	Cervix
Carcinoids	Soft tissue sarcoma	Head/neck (squamous cell)
Pancreas		Testis
Primary liver		Thyroid
Gall bladder/biliary		Bone sarcoma
Lung (small cell)		

Routes of spread

Primary tumours arising in the lower oesophagus, stomach, small bowel, colon, rectum and pancreas metastasize via lymphatics to local nodes and via portal venous spread to the liver. Ovarian malignant tumours and some gastro-intestinal and retroperitoneal neoplasms produce surface metastases on the liver by transperitoneal spread (Fig. 38.1). Hepatocellular carcinomas and cholangiocarcinomas tend to spread by seeding along portal veins and bile ducts. Liver metastases from tumours elsewhere arrive via the hepatic arterial route.

At the time of presentation or discovery, liver metastases from melanoma, testicular non-seminomatous germ cell tumours, and carcinomas of lung, breast, and kidney appear, typically, as numerous small deposits scattered throughout the liver. There is rarely, if ever, any indication for local treatment of the liver lesions. Similarly, patients with surface metastasis from transperitoneal spread of abdominal and pelvic tumours are treated with chemotherapy, either systemic or intraperitoneal. However, patients with liver metastasis from gastro-intestinal primary tumours often have a small number of overt lesions at the time of diagnosis and more detailed imaging is required to assess the possibility of local or regional treatment.

Growth rates

Since all metastases start out as individual cells or as clumps of cells, it follows that there is a latent period of occult disease between the seeding and the time when the lesions become manifest on imaging or by clinical presentation. The duration of this latent period varies with:

- Site of the primary tumour
- Histological cell type
- Grade of malignancy
- Local extent of the primary tumour
- Presence of subpopulations of different cell types within the primary

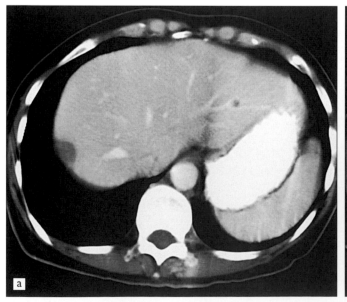
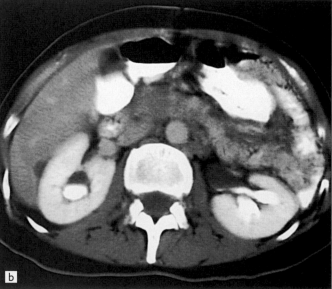

Figure 38.1. *(a, b) Portal-phase CT scans in a patient with ovarian carcinoma showing small metastases on the liver surface.*

In addition, tumour growth rates are affected by local factors, incompletely described and understood. Because surgical attempts to cure liver metastases have focused largely on patients with colorectal cancer, much more is known about the natural history of colorectal lesions than about other types of liver metastases. Surveillance studies after removal of colorectal primary tumours have shown that about one-third of patients whose livers appear normal to visual inspection and palpation at the time of laparotomy for removal of the primary tumour, are harbouring occult metastases which become overt over the next 2 years.[5,6] Techniques for detecting occult disease at this stage have been piloted but have not yet reached widespread acceptance (see below).

Blood supply of liver metastases

Histopathological studies suggest that metastases develop from clumps of tumour cells which lodge in the presinusoidal arterioles, terminal portal venules, in the sinusoids themselves, or in the adjacent spaces of Disse. For micrometastases up to about 100 μm diameter, surface diffusion probably provides sufficient nutrients for continuing growth. Further growth depends upon the development of a blood supply within the lesion and this is thought to be promoted by angiogenesis factors stimulated by the tumour itself. This neovascularity arises from the hepatic arterial circulation and rarely involves the portal venules. The blood supply of larger metastases is derived almost totally from the hepatic arterial route[7–9] although with some lesions there is a portal venous supply to the tumour periphery[10,11] which may develop further after hepatic artery ligation.[12] Shunting of blood between the arterial and portal elements is a well recognized feature of the normal hepatic microvasculature, and is usually increased in cirrhosis. Recent experimental work suggests that even in those tumours which have anatomically demonstrable portal venous branches, arterial inflow effectively replaces portal inflow via high pressure arterio-portal shunts around the tumour periphery.[13] This may account for the demonstrable change in arterial/portal flow ratio which occurs soon after the implantation of micrometastases in the liver.[14]

The vascular supply to liver metastases is of particular interest in relation to local treatment by chemo-embolization, arterial ligation or local infusion of chemotherapeutic or radioactive agents. In most types of liver disease there is a relative increase in hepatic arterial inflow and a decrease in portal venous inflow to the liver. This phenomenon has been used to detect liver metastases at a stage when they are too small for detection by anatomic imaging methods. The arterial blood supply of tumours is also a major consideration in imaging techniques using intravenous contrast agents with computed tomography (CT), magnetic resonance imaging (MRI), and also recently with sonography.

Key points: biology of liver metastases

- The majority of tumours metastasize to the liver via the bloodstream

- There is a latent period between the seeding of a metastasis and the time it becomes manifest on imaging or clinical evaluation

- Metastases develop from clumps of cells which lodge in presinusoidal arterioles, terminal portal venules, sinusoids or spaces of Disse

- The growth of a metastasis depends on the development of neovascularity

- The blood supply of larger metastases is derived almost totally from the hepatic arterial route

- Arterio-portal shunts develop around the tumour periphery

- There is an increase in the hepatic arterial blood flow/portal venous blood flow ratio which develops soon after the implantation of micrometastases

PATHOPHYSIOLOGY OF LIVER METASTASES RELEVANT FOR IMAGING

Physical characteristics

Imaging focal mass lesions within the liver depends on the demonstration of anatomical or physiological characteristics which are distinctly different from those of the surrounding liver tissue. With sonography, detection of lesions relies on microscopic structural differences which produce an increased or decreased number of reflective surfaces or an alteration in their architecture; these changes result in hyper- or hypoechogenicity, or heterogeneity respectively. Most tumours have a greater water content than the surrounding liver which accounts for their reduced attenuation on unenhanced CT, and the typical MRI findings of reduced signal on T1-weighted and increased signal on T2-weighted images. Other influential factors include fat or melanin within the tumour, matrix calcification and haemorrhage. Tumour necrosis, which occurs at a surprisingly early stage in some rapidly growing lesions, tends to produce a central area with fluid characteristics on imaging.

Contrast enhancement

Using CT, MRI and sonography, rapid imaging techniques with intravascular contrast media show unique enhancement patterns owing to the dual vascular supply of the liver. When a bolus of contrast medium is injected intravenously, the hepatic arterial component arrives at the liver 6–15 seconds before the portal venous component, allowing the recognition of four distinct phases of enhancement, classified as:

- Arterial-dominant
- Sinusoidal or portal venous-dominant
- Equilibrium
- Delayed

Lesions with increased arterial flow relative to normal liver (most hepatocellular cellular tumours and a minority of metastases) are best seen on the arterial-dominant phase of enhancement. Lesions with normal or sluggish flow but a large blood pool (e.g. vascular areas within haemangiomas, aneurysms and arteriovenous malformations) show rapid arterial-phase enhancement which declines in parallel with that of the major vessels. The inflow of contrast medium from the portal venous supply to tumours is negligible so those lesions which do not have increased arterial inflow become most conspicuous during the sinusoidal enhancement phase when the uptake of contrast by normal liver is at its peak. The majority of hypervascular tumours show a rapid washout of contrast and some become indistinguishable from adjacent liver in the later phases of enhancement. Where fibrous tissue forms a major component of a liver tumour (e.g. cholangiocarcinoma, central scars in focal nodular hyperplasia and in larger haemangiomas) enhancement is typically slow and prolonged, owing to diffusion of the contrast agent into the extracellular space of the tissue. These areas appear hypovascular on early images, but continue to enhance on delayed images when contrast is already washing out of other tissues.

Rim enhancement of a liver tumour in the arterial phase indicates a well vascularized lesion with a necrotic centre. With some lesions, slow diffusion of contrast into the centre may be seen. Rim enhancement which first appears on late phase or delayed images suggests the presence of a fibrous capsule, typically seen with hepatocellular carcinoma. A broad and ill-defined ring of transient or sustained enhancement may also be seen in liver tissue surrounding some metastases, probably a result of local oedema or inflammatory reaction. Although metastases rarely spread along the main portal veins, local occlusion of portal branches is a common pathological finding. This accounts for the fairly common feature of wedge-shaped areas of arterial hyperperfusion which are shown on CT and MRI as transient areas of hyperattenuation or increased signal during the arterial-dominant phase of enhancement, often in association with liver tumours.[15]

Key points: contrast medium enhancement and metastases

- Following a bolus injection of intravenous contrast medium, the hepatic arterial component arrives at the liver 6–15 seconds before the portal venous component

- The four main phases of enhancement are arterial, portal, equilibrium and delayed

- Lesions with an increased arterial flow, relative to normal liver, are best seen in the arterial phase of enhancement, e.g. hepatocellular carcinoma and a minority of metastases

- Lesions which do not have an increased arterial flow are most conspicuous during the portal phase of enhancement when the uptake of contrast medium by normal liver is at its peak

- In those tumours where fibrous tissue forms a major component, enhancement is slow and prolonged

- Rim enhancement of a liver tumour in the arterial phase indicates a well-vascularized lesion with a necrotic centre

- A broad or ill-defined ring of enhancement may result from oedema/inflammation around the lesion

- Local occlusion of portal branches is a common pathological finding and may produce wedge-shaped areas of arterial hyperperfusion on CT

OBJECTIVES OF IMAGING

Two attributes of metastatic disease determine the applications of imaging — firstly, the presence or absence of liver metastasis has a major influence on the prognosis and treatment of patients with primary tumours, and secondly, improved surgical and other locoregional forms of treatment for liver tumours require precise preoperative imaging. In the context of metastatic disease, the primary objectives of imaging the liver are:

- Detecting the presence of liver lesions
- Characterizing known or suspected liver abnormalities
- Establishing the likely resectability of liver tumours
- Assessing disease progression or response to treatment

DETECTING AND CHARACTERIZING LIVER METASTASES

Computed tomography

Dual-phase acquisition is recommended for patients in whom hepatocellular tumours or hypervascular metastases are suspected. With primary tumours at sites which usually give rise to hypovascular liver lesions, and for screening purposes, a single-phase volume acquisition is adequate.

Single-phase volumetric CT[16]

For optimum images, helical volume acquisition through the whole of the liver should be obtained in a single breath-hold, and should be timed so as to capture the period of peak enhancement of liver parenchyma after a bolus injection of IV contrast. The ratio of table speed to beam collimation (pitch) can be extended to 1.6–1.8 without significant loss of resolution. Routinely, sections are reconstructed at intervals equal to the beam collimation but for more detailed analysis of small areas of anatomy, or for 3D or multiplanar reformatting, thinner slices or overlapping slices can be reconstructed. The parameters chosen will vary according to the craniocaudal extent of the liver, the patient's breath-holding capability, and any restrictions imposed by the CT device itself. Typical settings would be: beam collimation 8 mm, table speed 10 mm per second, reconstruction interval 8 mm (5 mm for reformats). This allows a liver of 20 cm craniocaudal extent to be covered with a breath-hold of 20 seconds. Technique prescription also includes the volume and rate of injection of contrast medium, and the delay time between start of injection and start of CT acquisition. Typical factors for an average adult with no evidence of heart failure would be 100–150 ml at 2–3 ml per second, delay time 40–50 seconds.

Dual-phase computed tomography technique[17]

Two consecutive volume acquisitions using parameters similar to those above are timed so as to encompass arterial enhancement — about 20–40 seconds after injection — and portal venous or sinusoidal-phase enhancement — about 50–70 seconds after injection (Fig. 38.2). With dual-phase imaging, timing of acquisition is critical. Since the circulation time of individual patients varies considerably, it may be helpful to carry out a preparatory estimate of delay time using a small volume (5 ml) of IV contrast agent and obtaining serial low-dose scans through the descending aorta to detect the time of arrival of the injected contrast. With some CT devices, this procedure can be automated by initiating a series of low-dose scans through the lower thoracic aorta shortly after the main contrast injection, and preprogramming a threshold of increased attenuation within the aorta to trigger the arterial phase acquisition sequence so as to coincide with the arrival in the hepatic arteries of the main bolus of contrast medium.

Other computed tomography techniques

Delayed images, acquired 5–20 minutes after contrast injection, are rarely useful for lesion detection but may help to characterize haemangiomas and hypervascular metastases. Where helical CT is not available, a dynamic incremental contrast-enhanced technique can be used. Sequential contiguous slices are obtained to encompass the liver during the peak period of hepatic enhancement. It is important to complete the examination within 2–3 minutes because some lesions become indistinguishable from normal liver in the equilibrium phase. Non-contrast images are not routinely necessary for lesion detection and characterization, except for focal fatty liver, but if spiral (helical) CT is unavailable they may help to localize questionable liver lesions before injection of contrast material.

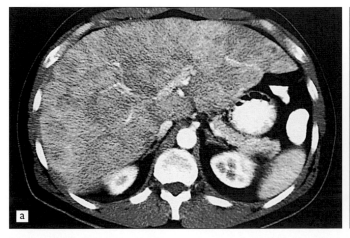 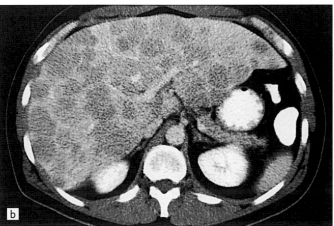

Figure 38.2. *Dual-phase CT scans in a patient with carcinoid metastases — in the arterial phase (a) the lesions show greater attenuation than the adjacent liver, whilst in the portal phase (b) the normal liver has enhanced more than the lesions.*

Computed tomography arteriography (CTA) requires rapid sequential or volume acquisition after a bolus of contrast medium is delivered through a catheter placed in the hepatic artery. The technique is invasive but sensitive for tumours with arterial hypervascularity. Its main application has been in detecting hepatocellular carcinoma in patients with cirrhosis, and so far there seems little place for this technique in dealing with metastatic liver disease. Ethiodised oil emulsion (EOE) was investigated as a liver specific contrast medium for CT with some promising results[18] but owing to a fairly high incidence of adverse reactions, has not come into widespread use. The technique of high-dose contrast infusion with CT images obtained immediately, and also after a delay of several hours, takes advantage of the observation that 1–2% of injected intravenous contrast medium is excreted by hepatocyte secretion into the biliary tract. Delayed images showed some advantages over immediate dynamic sequential CT[19] but this technique has been overtaken by multiphase CT with volume acquistion.

Computed tomography with arterial portography (CTAP)
Intense and specific enhancement of the liver parenchyma can be achieved by injecting the contrast medium directly into the superior mesenteric or splenic arteries.[20,21] Since liver tumours receive their blood supply via the hepatic arterial route, portal inflow of contrast material enhances only the normal liver parenchyma and therefore tumour to liver differentiation is maximized (Fig. 38.3a). Although this technique is highly sensitive for lesion detection, it requires the placement of an arterial catheter and it is also subject to false-

positive results caused by focal perfusion anomalies. Accessory or replaced right hepatic arteries arise from the superior mesenteric artery (SMA) in 15–20% of patients, and these reduce the sensitivity of CTAP in the affected parts of the liver. Placement of the catheter in the splenic artery is technically more difficult than SMA placement, owing to the relatively frequent occurrence of asymptomatic coeliac axis compression in older patients, but is thought by some users to give a more even distribution of contrast medium into the liver. Acquisition factors are similar to those used for intravenous bolus helical CT, using 75–100 ml contrast injected at 2–3 ml/second with a time delay of about 40 seconds before starting the volume acquisition. A second volume acquisition 2–3 minutes later is useful to aid discrimination between tumours and focal perfusion disturbances shown on the initial series.

Key points: CT detection

- Dual-phase CT is recommended for the detection of hepatocellular carcinoma and hypervascular liver metastases

- Single-phase volumetric CT is adequate for detection of hypovascular liver lesions and for screening purposes

- Computed tomography arteriography (CTA) is invasive; its main indication is for the detection of hepatocellular carcinoma in patients with cirrhosis

- Computed tomography with arterial portography (CTAP) is a highly sensitive method of detecting liver lesions

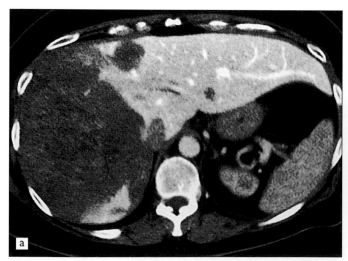
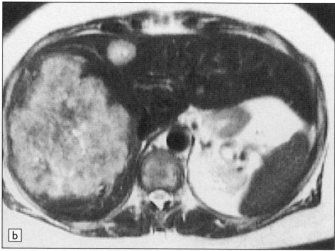

Figure 38.3. *(a) CT scan with arterial portography in a patient with three colorectal metastases. Note the disturbance of perfusion in liver tissue adjacent to the large tumour, which may lead to overestimation of tumour size by this technique. (b) T2-weighted MR image with SPIO enhancement showing the same three lesions.*

Appearances of liver metastases on computed tomography

A substantial proportion of small lesions are indistinguishable from normal liver on unenhanced CT but most larger lesions and a minority of small tumours show reduced attenuation. Calcification is not uncommon in larger lesions, particularly metastases from mucin-secreting tumours of the gastrointestinal tract (Fig. 38.4). After chemotherapy, calcification is more common, particularly in slow-growing lesions e.g., carcinoids, islet cell metastases. Small lesions are usually round and homogeneous, larger tumours often become irregular in shape and heterogeneous. The unsharp margin, which is typical of most metastases, is explained by a combination of volume averaging with irregularity of the interface between tumour surface and adjacent liver. In the sinusoidal phase of contrast enhancement, the majority of lesions are more conspicuous since they are hypovascular compared with adjacent liver (Fig. 38.5a). The transcoelomic spread of ovarian tumours typically produces deposits on the peritoneal surfaces of the liver, usually associated with ascites. Hypervascular tumours show a contrast blush during the arterial-dominant phase of enhancement which may persist into the sinusoidal phase. However, most hypervascular tumours show a fairly rapid washout of contrast and become hypoattenuating on delayed images. Hypervascular tumours with central necrosis produce a 'bull's eye' appearance with a peripheral ring of early enhancement.

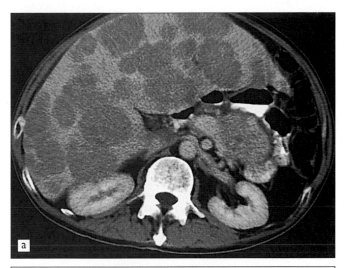

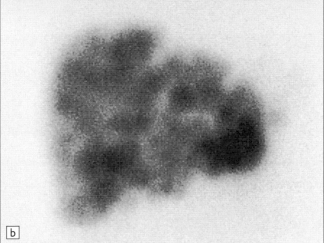

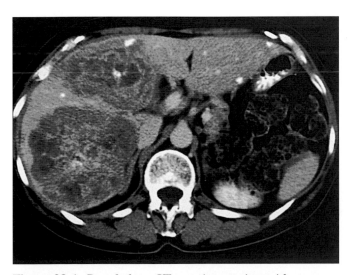

Figure 38.4. *Portal-phase CT scan in a patient with metastases from mucin-secreting colorectal cancer. The large tumours contain some central calcification and several small surface lesions are densely calcified following chemotherapy. All the lesions shown here were successfully resected.*

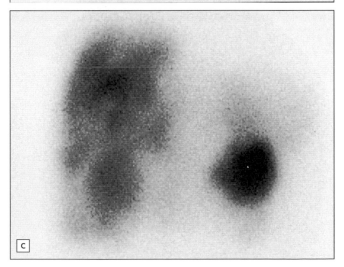

Figure 38.5. *(a) Portal-phase CT scan showing multiple low-attenuation metastases in the liver and a large tumour in the tail of the pancreas. (b and c) Labelled octreotide study in the same patient showing multiple functioning liver metastases and a large primary glucagonoma in the pancreatic tail.*

Primary tumours which commonly produce hypervascular liver metastases include:

- Islet cell tumours of the pancreas
- Carcinoids
- Phaeochromocytoma
- Melanoma
- Renal cell cancer

However, all of these tumours may also give rise to hypovascular liver metastases (Figs 38.6a,b). A small minority of liver secondaries from carcinomas of bronchus, breast, colorectal and other gastro-intestinal primaries appear hypervascular. Attempts to correlate the pathology of individual tumours with the imaging characteristics of liver metastases have been unsuccessful.[22]

Key points: appearance on CT

- The majority of metastases have an ill-defined margin due to irregularity of interface between tumour and adjacent liver

- The majority of metastases are more conspicuous in the sinusoidal (parenchymal) phase of contrast enhancement

- Hypervascular metastases show a contrast blush during the arterial phase and most have a relatively rapid washout

Magnetic resonance imaging

Optimum technique requires the usual trade-off between spatial resolution, contrast resolution and temporal resolution.

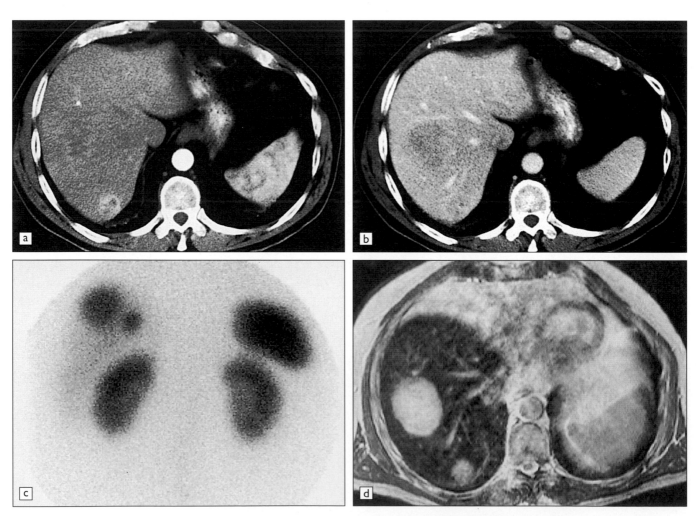

Figure 38.6. *Dual-phase CT scan in a patient with carcinoid metastases. (a) The smaller lesion is hypervascular and is best seen in the arterial phase, the larger lesion is hypovascular and is only seen in the portal phase (b). Labelled octreotide study (c) in the same patient shows normal uptake in kidneys and spleen, with two functioning metastases in the liver. (d) T2-weighted MR image shows the same two lesions.*

Chapter 39

Metastatic effects on the nervous system

David MacVicar

INTRODUCTION

Neurological complications in the cancer patient are an increasingly common problem. A simplistic explanation for this is that patients survive longer with their tumour and therefore develop more metastases at all sites, but it is also possible that the central nervous system (CNS) is a genuine sanctuary site for malignant cells from common solid tumours treated with systemic chemotherapy, just as it is in leukaemia. A recent study of nearly 12,000 patients identified neurological complaints including altered mental state, headache, back pain and leg weakness in 15% of patients with a variety of tumours.[1] In small cell lung cancer, the incidence of neurological disorder caused by the disease is 29%,[2] and a report from the Johns Hopkins Cancer Centre identified neurological problems as the cause of 50% of unplanned hospital admissions, with changes in mental status, brain metastases and epidural spinal cord compression being the major problems.[3] The effects of metastatic disease on the nervous system can be severely disabling, with a catastrophic effect on the quality of life of a patient whose tumour may be eminently treatable. This is partly because the brain and spinal cord are enclosed in bone, and thus relatively small-volume disease can cause disproportionately severe symptoms. In addition, the CNS lacks lymphatics, making removal of oedema and biological detritus difficult, and the capacity for regeneration of nervous tissue after damage is very limited.

A further difficulty is the sometimes bewildering clinical presentation of neurological problems in the cancer patient. An apparently simple symptom such as leg weakness has a wide differential diagnosis in a patient with systemic cancer, including:

- Cerebral deposits
- Compression of the spinal cord or cauda equina
- Leptomeningeal metastatic disease
- The effects of therapy such as cytotoxic drugs or steroids
- General debility

The effects of cancer on the nervous system may be classified into:

- Metastatic or direct effects of cancer
- Mass lesions compressing or infiltrating nervous tissues
- Indirect effects — non-metastatic or paraneoplastic syndromes

Paraneoplastic phenomena include vascular disorders, infections, metabolic effects, sequelae of treatment and the unusual but fascinating paraneoplastic syndromes. For the radiologist, a more useful approach is to classify by site in an attempt to narrow the area to be examined.

Once the area of greatest clinical suspicion has been identified, the majority of important differential diagnoses can be addressed using the most appropriate technique. The principal causes of neurological presentation in cancer patients according to site are listed in Table 39.1.

BRAIN

Clinical presentation

Brain metastases may arise from any primary systemic cancer, but the majority of brain metastases originate from:

- Cancer of the lung (especially small cell and adenocarcinoma)
- Carcinoma of breast
- Melanoma

Less common primary sites include renal and gastro-intestinal tumours and a significant number of brain metastases develop from a primary source which remains unknown even at autopsy.[4] The following tumours rarely metastasize to the brain:

- Prostate
- Ovary
- Osteosarcoma
- Hodgkin's lymphoma

Table 39.1. *Major neurological problems (classified by site)*

Site	Differential diagnosis
Brain	Parenchymal metastasis
	Leptomeningeal metastasis
	Infection (meningitis, brain abscess)
	Radiation encephalopathy
	Cerebral haemorrhage or infarction
	Metabolic and toxic encephalopathy
	Primary brain tumours
Cranial neuropathy	Parenchymal deposits (false localizing signs)
	Leptomeningeal metastases
	Bony lesions of skull base
Spinal cord and cauda equina	Epidural compression
	Leptomeningeal metastasis
	Intramedullary metastasis
	Epidural abscess or haematoma
	Radiation myelopathy
	Myelopathy following intrathecal chemotherapy
	Paraneoplastic myelopathy
Peripheral nerves and plexuses	Extrinsic compression by tumour mass
	Direct infiltration by tumour
	Drug toxicity
	Varicella zoster infection
	Radiation plexopathy
	Paraneoplastic neuropathy
Neuromuscular junction and muscle	Drugs
	Paraneoplastic disorders (Eaton–Lambert myasthenic syndrome, myasthenia gravis)
	Corticosteroid-induced myopathy
	Cachectic myopathy
	Paraneoplastic polymyositis or dermatomyositis

Most brain metastases, particularly those which arise from primary neoplasms other than the lung, occur at a late stage in dissemination of malignancy, and the presence of brain deposits is commonly associated with more widespread disease. Autopsy series have shown that asymptomatic brain metastases are present in patients dying of disseminated cancer in as many as 30% of cases.

The commonest presenting symptoms are:

• Headache
• Focal weakness
• Mental disturbance
• Seizures

Unsteadiness of gait is a prominent presenting complaint when the tumour lies in the cerebellum or brain-stem but may occasionally occur as a result of a large frontal lobe metastasis or hydrocephalus caused by obstruction of cerebrospinal fluid (CSF) pathways. Less common presenting symptoms are:

• Difficulty with speech
• Visual disturbance
• Sensory disturbance

Signs of visual field loss and sensory abnormalities may be elicited by neurological examination. Some physical signs are present in most, but not all, patients with brain metastases. The onset of symptoms is frequently insidious.

Pathophysiology of brain metastases

Metastasis is a complicated pathophysiological process which is not completely understood. For malignant cells to metastasize from, for example, breast to brain, they must first enter the blood stream, then cross the pulmonary capillary bed to enter the arterial blood supply of the brain. The tumour embolus, if large enough, is likely to lodge in the watershed areas of the brain at the terminations of the major end-arteries, and also in the grey/white junction where penetrating arterioles separate into capillary beds. This simple haemodynamic model should result in a predictable distribution of metastases within the brain, but there is clearly some variation in the distribution of metastases from certain tumours. The fertile soil hypothesis proposes that the host organ may synthesize and secrete factors which attract certain clones of circulating tumour cells and promote their growth.[5] Delattre et al. have drawn attention to the preferential distribution of metastatic lesions to watershed areas, but also noted that in patients with gastro-intestinal and pelvic tumours, there was predominant involvement of the posterior fossa, whereas with other tumours, the cerebral hemispheres were more likely to be involved.[6] It appears that infiltrating ductal carcinoma of the breast has a predilection to cause parenchymal brain metastases, whereas infiltrating lobular carcinoma is said to preferentially affect meningeal surfaces.[7] Melanoma frequently metastasizes to the grey matter, and experimental mouse melanoma lines have been developed which have specific predilection for brain parenchyma or the leptomeninges.[8] Although these preferential distributions are fascinating, in practice virtually any tumour can metastasize to any part of the brain or meninges, and variance with the expected pattern of distribution should not discourage the diagnosis of metastatic disease.

Imaging techniques

In 1972, the introduction of computed tomography (CT) by Hounsfield and Ambrose revolutionized the diagnosis of brain tumours. Twenty five years later it remains a viable method of establishing the presence of brain deposits. Ideally, CT scans should be performed before and after intravenous contrast administration, but if a patient has a known primary tumour and a clinical presentation strongly supporting a diagnosis of metastasis, little is lost by performing postcontrast scans only. Contiguous slices should be obtained through the posterior fossa at 4–5 mm intervals, continuing in the supratentorial brain using 8–10 mm slice intervals.

Although CT is sufficient for diagnosis in many cases, there is little doubt that magnetic resonance imaging (MRI) is a more sensitive technique than contrast-enhanced CT scanning for the detection of metastases to the brain parenchyma. T2-weighted unenhanced scans are slightly more sensitive than contrast-enhanced CT, but further sensitivity in detection is available with the use of T1-weighted sequences before and after intravenous gadolinium administration.[9,10] A suitable protocol would include axial T2-weighted spin-echo and T1-weighted spin-echo images using contiguous 6–7 mm slices from foramen magnum to skull vault, supplemented by gadolinium-enhanced T1-weighted spin-echo sequences. The use of the coronal plane for the T1-weighted sequences is preferred by some, particularly if surgery is being considered, but the key factor is to ensure that the entire brain is covered. There is controversy over the dosage of gadolinium, particularly in the US. Some authorities consider a dosage of 0.1 ml/kg body weight to be adequate, while others recommend a high-dose technique using three times this dose. Advocates of the high-dose technique point out the increased sensitivity as its chief advantage; in practical terms this is only important if local therapy is being considered for an ostensibly solitary metastasis, and the cost implications of trebling the dose prevent routine use of this technique. Most European centres routinely administer an intermediate dose of gadolinium of 0.2 mg/kg body weight.[11–13]

Newer imaging methods involving inversion recovery, e.g. fluid attenuation inversion recovery (FLAIR), or magnetization transfer, have been advocated as sensitive methods of detecting focal brain abnormalities. These methods are currently being evaluated, and are not available on every MR unit, but may result in a reduced utilization of contrast material in the future.[14]

Other modalities are not useful; cerebral angiography is rarely helpful and plain radiographs and electroencephalography are obsolete. Isotope studies, including positron emission tomography (PET) and single photon emission computed tomography (SPECT), lack the sensitivity and spatial resolution to challenge MRI as the investigation of choice.[15]

Screening for asymptomatic brain metastases

Cranial CT and MRI are only occasionally used as a staging technique at initial presentation of disease in a patient with no neurological symptoms. One clinical situation in which the brain is staged is where thoracotomy is being considered with curative intent for non-small cell lung cancer. Despite its rather disappointing sensitivity and specificity in diagnosis of lymph node involvement in the mediastinum, CT of the chest has become a recommended technique for preoperative staging of lung cancer;[16,17] many specialist centres now perform a CT of the brain as part of the same investigation. This reflects the propensity of lung cancer to metastasize to the brain relatively early in the disease compared with other common malignancies. Many series, mostly using CT as the staging technique, have investigated the incidence of asymptomatic brain metastases. The reported incidence varies between 5 and 30%.

One series has drawn attention to the variation of incidence of asymptomatic metastases at presentation, depending on histology and local tumour stage. In patients with Stage-I and Stage-II squamous cell carcinoma, no brain metastases were found, but in potentially resectable Stage-III disease the incidence was 8%. For Stage-III localized adenocarcinoma the incidence was 23%, for Stage-III large cell carcinoma 57%. For Stage-III non-small cell tumours of all histological types the overall incidence of asymptomatic brain deposits was 17.5%, which is clearly relevant when considering such patients for surgery. In patients with small cell carcinoma and apparently limited disease, the incidence of asymptomatic brain deposits was 14%.[18] Although very few patients with small cell lung cancer are suitable for surgery, cranial irradiation can palliate, and some centres include brain scanning as a staging investigation for this disease.[19]

Computed tomography or MRI of the brain is included as a staging investigation in selected patients with non-seminomatous germ cell tumours of the testis (NSGCT). Asymptomatic brain metastases may be seen at presentation in patients with aggressive disseminated disease and are more common in patients with trophoblastic teratoma than with any other histological type.[20] Those patients considered at high risk will have grossly elevated serum tumour markers (human chorionic gonadotrophin [HCG] >20 000 IU) or multiple pulmonary metastases (more than 50). Asymptomatic brain deposits may also be seen at the time of large-volume pulmonary relapse following chemotherapy, and any patient being put forward for high-dose salvage chemotherapy for multiple relapses of non-seminomatous germ cell tumour should have a brain scan. If cerebral deposits are present, any residual mass following treatment is likely to contain differentiated tumour, and will be resected if accessible.

Notwithstanding these exceptions, and acknowledging that brain lesions may be the presenting symptom of unknown primaries, the majority of brain metastases present late in the natural history of the disease, and are usually associated with some symptomatology, however vague. Early diagnosis of asymptomatic brain lesions rarely influences the outcome of disease, and brain imaging is not recommended as a staging investigation in most clinical circumstances.[19]

General imaging features

The majority of metastases in the brain grow as spherical masses, displacing rather than destroying brain tissue. Some metastases are more irregular, and all create oedema in the surrounding white matter. The amount of oedema is extremely variable, and its extent is not a reliable sign in differential diagnosis of metastasis from other pathological entities. Brain metastases are usually solid, but if they grow rapidly, they may undergo central necrosis. 'Cystic' lesions occasionally occur, particularly from primary breast carcinoma and squamous cell carcinoma from any site. At a pathological level, metastatic brain tumours usually show extensive neovascularization, and are accompanied by breakdown of the blood–brain barrier. Some tumours, for example melanoma and NSGCT, have a tendency to be haemorrhagic. The typical appearance of a metastasis from carcinoma on CT is a mass of similar attenuation to normal brain, associated with surrounding oedema and brisk enhancement following intravenous contrast injection. On MRI, most metastatic lesions are masses with a signal intensity higher than that of normal brain on T2-weighted sequences and surrounded by very high signal intensity oedema. On T1-weighted sequences they are isointense with brain and show enhancement with gadolinium-DTPA (Fig. 39.1). Metastases are usually discrete masses but are not necessarily multiple. The maxim that not all metastases are multiple, and not all multiple lesions are metastases remains valid in clinical practice.

Differential diagnosis of brain metastases

In general, the diagnosis of brain metastasis in a patient known to have cancer presents few difficulties. The most difficult differential diagnosis is with primary tumours such as:

- Meningioma
- Pituitary adenoma
- Acoustic neuroma
- Glioma

Gliomas tend to be more diffuse in their growth pattern, but metastases in an appropriate anatomical situation may mimic meningioma and other primary tumours almost exactly. In one study, 6 of 54 patients with known cancer and solitary brain lesions did not have metastases on biopsy, and 3 of these had non-neoplastic lesions.[21] However, if the clinical history and appropriate imaging features, especially with multiple lesions, are present, the diagnosis of brain metastases can be established with reasonable certainty. Other clinical differential diagnoses include:

- Cerebral haemorrhage
- Cerebral embolus
- Abscess
- Viral infections
- Cytotoxic leucoencephalopathy
- Radiation injury

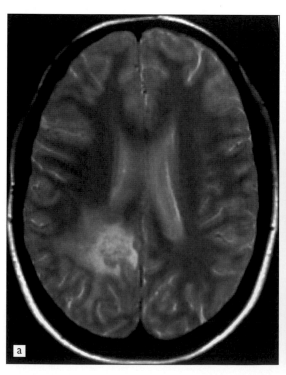 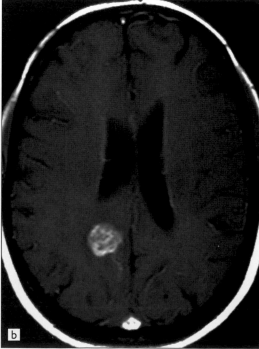

Figure 39.1. *(a) T2-weighted MR image, axial plane. Typical appearance of cerebral metastatic disease. The tumour mass is of higher signal intensity than surrounding brain. Extensive oedema returns a very high signal intensity; (b) T1-weighted MR image following gadolinium-DTPA.*

Cerebral haemorrhage or embolus will have characteristic imaging features. Infections, particularly abscess formation, can cause problems of differential diagnosis, especially in patients with lymphoma. Viral infections have a tendency to diffuse involvement of the brain without mass formation and often have a characteristic clinical syndrome. Examples are herpes simplex encephalitis (Fig. 39.2) and progressive multifocal leucoencephalopathy (Fig. 39.3), which is thought to be a result of reactivation of papova virus infection during prolonged suppression of cellular immunity. Cytotoxic leucoencephalopathy may be seen with drug regimens involving 5-fluorouracil and levamisole, or intrathecal methotrexate.[22,23] Focal changes, detectable as high signal lesions in the deep cerebral white matter on MRI, have also been demonstrated with a variety of high-dose intravenous chemotherapy regimens, particularly those involving bone marrow transplantation. These lesions do not enhance with gadolinium-DTPA, and clinically present with non-specific problems such as headache and seizures. The changes are reversible, and should not be confused with metastases.[24]

Radiation necrosis may be difficult to differentiate from recurrent brain metastases as it tends to enhance and may form ring lesions. However, it is rarely a problem at initial diagnosis of brain metastases. Occasionally, intercurrent common diseases, such as multiple sclerosis, are seen in patients known to have cancer. In the absence of typical imaging features of metastatic disease, a review of the clinical features is of paramount importance, and will frequently influence image interpretation.

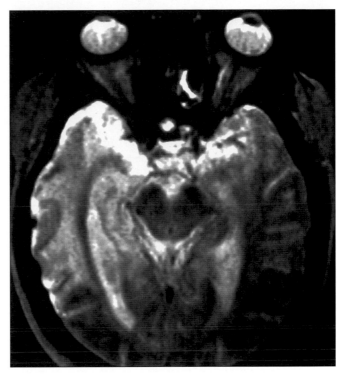

Figure 39.2. *T2-weighted MR image, axial plane. Herpes simplex encephalitis. There is diffuse high signal intensity in both temporal lobes. There is no discrete mass lesion, the abnormality affects grey and white matter and is asymmetrical. The features are typical of herpes simplex encephalitis and are unlikely to be confused with metastatic disease.*

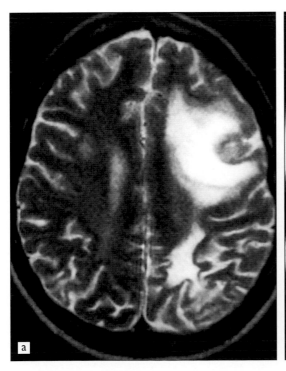

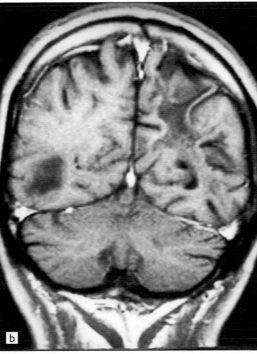

Figure 39.3. *(a) T2-weighted MR image, axial plane. Areas of diffuse grey and white matter abnormality are seen bilaterally. (b) T1-weighted MR image, coronal plane. Rather than mass effect, there is loss of substance within the grey and white matter. These appearances are typical of progressive multifocal leucoencephalopathy, which may be seen following prolonged suppression of cellular immunity in patients on treatment for malignancy, particularly lymphoma.*

Key points: brain metastases

- Most brain metastases occur late in the natural history of malignant disease

- Gadolinium-enhanced MRI is more sensitive than CT for detecting brain metastases

- Screening for brain metastases in non-small cell lung cancer prior to thoracotomy is recommended since 5–30% of patients harbour asymptomatic brain metastases

- Screening for brain metastases is also recommended in patients with (trophoblastic) non-seminomatous germ cell tumours of the testis

- The differential diagnosis of brain metastases includes primary brain tumours, cerebral haemorrhage, infection, cytotoxic-leucocephalopathy and radiation injury

Imaging features of some common brain metastases

Metastases from all primary tumours may look identical, but some of the common causes have 'trademark' features, which if present, may increase confidence in diagnosis. Virtually all cancers are capable of metastasizing to the brain. Lung and breast are the commonest organs of origin, followed by melanoma.

Bronchial tumours are the single commonest cause of metastastic deposits in the brain. Adenocarcinoma of the lung and squamous cell carcinoma typically metastasize to the grey/white junction, and both may produce ring-like enhancement on both CT and MRI (Fig. 39.4). A small cell lung cancer may produce large masses, but frequently produces innumerable small metastases throughout the brain (Fig. 39.5). These small lesions are best seen on enhanced T1-weighted MRI, emphasizing the increased sensitivity available with this technique.

Carcinoma of the breast has a tendency to metastasize to the periphery of the brain. An association between breast cancer and meningioma has created considerable interest in the literature. Some authors report a higher incidence of meningioma in women with breast cancer, although this has been disputed.[25–27] Meningiomas have a relative lack of peritumoral oedema, and show homogeneous contrast enhancement and attachment to the dura. However, the practical problem is that metastases from breast carcinoma may mimic in every way the features of meningioma, and vice versa. Oncologists are naturally keen to establish the definitive diagnosis and consider surgery. An early follow-up scan is frequently helpful as it will establish the tempo of disease; a rapidly enlarging lesion, with

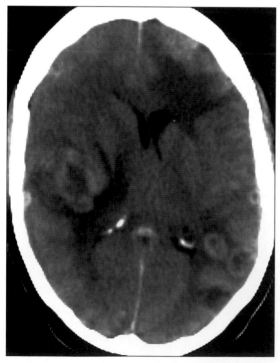

Figure 39.4. *Contrast-enhanced CT scan. Squamous cell carcinoma. Ring-like enhancement is common with squamous cell carcinoma deposits, but may also be seen with adenocarcinoma and melanoma.*

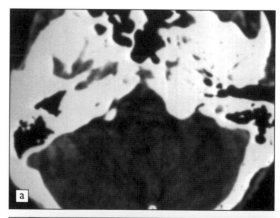
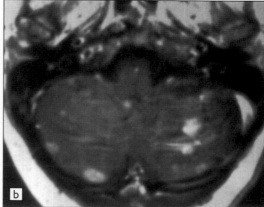

Figure 39.5. *(a) Small cell lung cancer. Contrast-enhanced CT scan through posterior fossa is equivocal. Individual metastases cannot be reliably identified. (b) T1-weighted MR image following gadolinium performed 2 days later. Multiple small lesions were scattered throughout the posterior fossa.*

or without new lesions, will confirm a diagnosis of metastatic disease and will avoid inappropriate craniotomy (Fig. 39.6). Breast carcinoma also has a tendency to metastasize to the pituitary where it can mimic an adenoma.

Metastases from *malignant melanoma* can exhibit some characteristic features. Like metastases from malignant testicular tumours and renal carcinoma, these tumours can be large and may have a prominent haemorrhagic component.

The breakdown products of blood may have paramagnetic or superparamagnetic effects. In addition, melanin pigments have intrinsic paramagnetic properties as a result of their molecular structure.[28] This can result in melanoma deposits having a high signal intensity on unenhanced T1-weighted images and a low signal intensity on T2-weighted images owing to the paramagnetic effect of pigments on proton relaxation (Fig. 39.7).

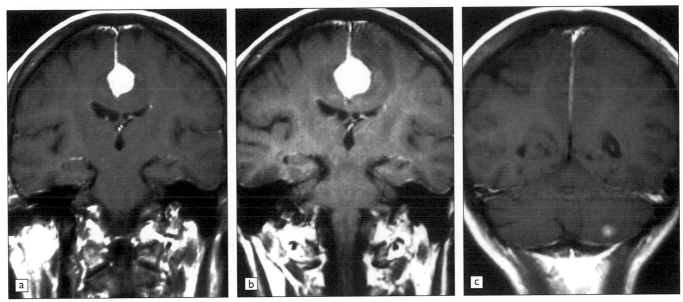

Figure 39.6. *Patient with carcinoma of breast, presenting with headaches. (a) T1 weighted spin-echo MR image following gadolinium administration, coronal plane. There is an enhancing mass apparently centred on the falx. The differential diagnosis lies between a deposit from carcinoma of the breast and a falx meningioma; (b, c) rather than immediate craniotomy, a follow-up scan was obtained after a 4-week interval. This shows a clearly discernible enlargement of the falx lesion over a 4-week period and further small lesions became detectable within the cerebellum during the interval. A diagnosis of cerebral metastatic disease was made.*

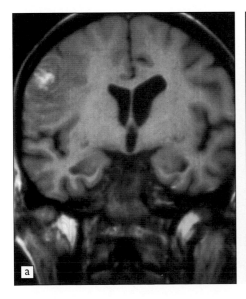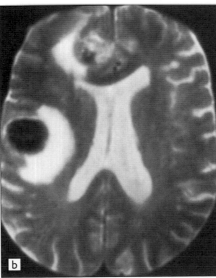

Figure 39.7. *(a) T1-weighted spin-echo MR image, coronal plane. A mass in the posterior frontal lobe returns signal hyperintense to surrounding brain. (b) T2-weighted spin-echo MR image, axial plane. The mass lesion is hypointense to normal brain. Surrounding oedema is present. The appearance is due to the paramagnetic effect of melanin within a deposit of metastatic melanotic melanoma.*

Colon cancer deposits may also exhibit paramagnetic effects, with a high signal intensity on T1-weighted images and a low signal intensity on T2 weighting. This is presumed to be caused by mucinous macromolecules (Fig. 39.8). Very

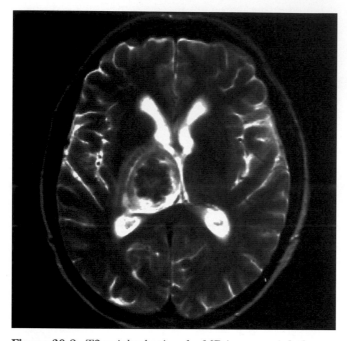

Figure 39.8. *T2-weighted spin-echo MR image, axial plane. Carcinoma of colon. Marked signal hypointensity is present in the central part of the deposit, which was not calcified on CT scanning. This appearance may be seen with mucinous adenocarcinoma deposits.*

occasionally, a similar appearance is seen with mucinous adenocarcinomas of ovary and breast.

Involvement of the brain by lymphoma is becoming very common, particularly in patients with human immuno-deficiency virus (HIV) infection and other forms of immuno-suppression. Lymphoma deposits are typically of higher attenuation than normal brain on unenhanced CT images and show only slight contrast enhancement (Fig. 39.9). There is relatively little oedema, and the lesions are situated characteristically around the midline. On T2-weighted MRI, lesions are often hypointense compared with normal brain.

INTRACRANIAL MENINGEAL DISEASE

Cancer may reach the meninges by direct contact with tumour in brain or bone, or by haematogenous dissemination. Once contact is made with the cerebrospinal fluid (CSF), tumour cells are likely to be shed and will float along CSF pathways to seed elsewhere in either a diffuse pattern or as multiple individual foci. Meningeal metastases are increasingly recognized, and are common in the leukaemias. They are sometimes seen in:

- Non-Hodgkin's lymphoma
- Breast carcinoma
- Lung carcinoma
- Malignant melanoma

Meningeal deposits have also been described in a wide variety of other tumours. The clinical presentation can be obscure with non-specific symptoms, such as headache,

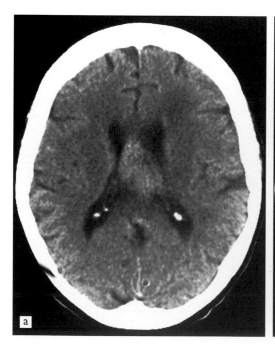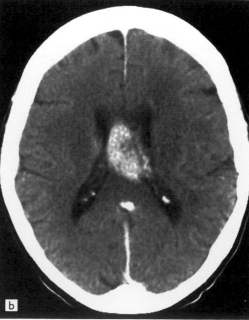

Figure 39.9. *(a, b) Pre- and post-contrast CT scans. There is a mass involving the corpus callosum associated with little oedema and of attenuation slightly higher than normal brain. Modest enhancement is present after IV contrast. The distribution and appearance are characteristic of lymphoma. The patient had suffered several relapses of non-Hodgkin's lymphoma before presenting with headache.*

mental change, nausea and vertigo predominating. It can be difficult to diagnose with imaging studies, particularly if diffuse. Meningeal metastases enhance with contrast medium, but can be demonstrated on CT only if gross. MRI is more reliable but false-negative examinations are common. There are several causes of false-positive results:

- Some meningeal enhancement can frequently be demonstrated in normal patients without meningeal disease
- Lumbar puncture with or without intrathecal chemotherapy can cause the meninges to enhance abnormally
- Previous surgery and radiation also result in diffuse abnormality for months or years

However, despite these difficulties, MRI is the most useful imaging technique, since its multiplanar imaging capability allows the demonstration of meningeal masses around the calvarium and skull base more readily than CT. A meningeal mass lesion in the appropriate clinical setting is adequate confirmation of diagnosis of meningeal disease (Fig. 39.10). If imaging is negative, lumbar puncture may then be utilized to confirm positive malignant cytology in the CSF.[29]

A further advantage of the use of MRI is its ability to demonstrate metastasis to the bones of the skull base. Cranial nerve abnormalities are not usually the presenting feature of meningeal disease, although subtle signs are frequently detectable. The main differential diagnosis is between involvement of the cranial nerves at the meningeal level or tumour deposits within bone. When seen, meningeal metastases are usually small, although occasionally they are large enough to mimic extrinsic tumours such as acoustic neuromas and meningiomas (Fig. 39.11). If skull base deposits are suspected as the cause of cranial neuropathy, sequences such as short tau inversion recovery (STIR) are frequently useful in highlighting bony pathology.

Key points: cerebral meningeal metastases

- ◼ Meningeal deposits are seen in the leukaemias, non-Hodgkin's lymphoma, breast cancer, lung cancer and malignant melanoma

- ◼ The clinical features are often non-specific

- ◼ Meningeal metastases enhance with contrast medium and are best demonstrated on MRI

- ◼ Meningeal enhancement may be seen in normal patients

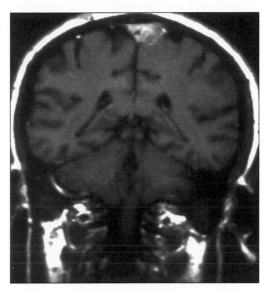

Figure 39.10. *T1-weighted spin-echo MR image following gadolinium, coronal plane. The patient presented with headache following treatment for acute myeloid leukaemia. There is a plaque of tissue involving the meninges close to the falx. Cytology revealed blasts, confirming meningeal recurrence. The CNS is an established 'sanctuary site' for recurrence of leukaemia and lymphoma.*

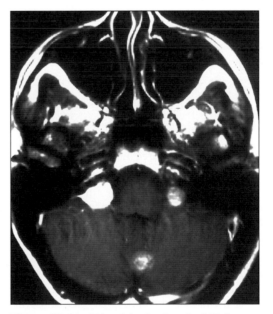

Figure 39.11. *T1-weighted spin-echo MR image following gadolinium, axial plane. Bilateral enhancing masses are present in the cerebello-pontine angles mimicking acoustic neuromas. There is a further lesion between the cerebellar hemispheres. Postmortem examination confirmed meningeal metastases from melanoma.*

SPINAL CORD AND CAUDA EQUINA

Epidural spinal cord compression

While most symptomatic intracranial metastases involve the brain parenchyma, in the spinal canal, most symptomatic tumours compress the spinal cord or cauda equina from the epidural space, while intramedullary and meningeal disease is more unusual.

Most epidural compression is caused by a tumour that has metastasized to the vertebral body; the most frequent cancers are:

- Carcinoma of breast
- Carcinoma of lung
- Carcinoma of prostate
- Multiple myeloma

In patients with systemic cancer, incidences of symptomatic spinal cord compression reported in the literature vary from 1–5%, and at autopsy approximately 5% of patients dying from cancer exhibit spinal cord or cauda equina compression.[30–33]

Clinical presentation

Pain is the earliest and most frequent presenting symptom of spinal cord compression. It is usually mild at first but becomes progressively more severe. However, absence of pain does not mean absence of cord compression. The pain may be of several types:

- Local
- Radicular
- Funicular

In most patients the initial pain is local and perceived as a steady ache at the site of the involved vertebral body. Compression of nerve roots within the spinal canal or within the exit foraminae generates radicular pain, which may precede local pain, and is typically band-like if the lesion is in the thoracic region and radiates to arms and legs in cervical and lumbar regions respectively. Funicular pain is caused by compression of ascending (sensory) spinal cord tracts, causing symptoms which are apparently remote from the lesion and in a non-dermatomal distribution. For example, upper thoracic or cervical cord compression can cause funicular pain in the lower extremities, or band-like pain around the thorax and abdomen.

Following the prodrome of pain which may be prolonged, other symptoms and signs develop rapidly, including:

- Weakness
- Sensory loss
- Autonomic dysfunction

Weakness is the second most common finding. It usually results from damage to the corticospinal tracts. The weakness begins in the legs, regardless of the level of compression and is more marked proximally early in the course of development of symptoms. The patient usually complains of difficulty walking and climbing stairs, and this symptom should precipitate a sense of urgency in the investigative chain, as treatment at this stage may enable full recovery of power. In the early stages, typical signs of upper motor neurone weakness may be absent, with spasticity and hyper-reflexia developing later. If the onset of spinal cord compression is sudden and leads to complete paraplegia, most patients are flaccid with areflexia, as a result of distal spinal reflex inhibition.

Lower motor neurone weakness results from compression of the cauda equina, and is characterized by hypotonia, atrophy and areflexia. Dysfunction of anterior horn cells in the spinal cord may also be seen, possibly as a result of vascular abnormality rather than true mechanical compression. The presence of lower motor neurone weakness will mask upper motor neurone signs at a higher level, so it should be remembered that in the presence of cauda equina compression, which explains lower motor neurone signs in the legs, an additional level of true cord compression may also be present.

Sensory loss follows shortly after the development of weakness, and the level will rise to arrive at the true level of compression given time. However, at the time of imaging the sensory level may be several segments below the compressive lesion. Sensory loss is rarely as profound or disabling as weakness. Autonomic dysfunction causes bladder and bowel dysfunction, and impotence in men in more than 50% of patients by the time of diagnosis of spinal cord or cauda equina compression. Bladder dysfunction predominates, with urinary retention being associated with sudden onset of compression while urgency with incontinence is a relatively frequent complaint if major symptoms are evolving slowly.

Key points: spinal cord compression

- Most tumours that compress the spinal cord are situated in the epidural space
- Pain is the earliest presenting feature and may be local, radicular or funicular
- In the early stages of spinal cord compression, upper motor neurone weakness may be absent
- Lower motor neurone weakness will mask upper motor neurone signs at a high level
- The sensory level may be several segments below the compressive lesion
- Bladder dysfunction is the predominant autonomic disturbance

Pathophysiology

The neurological presentation of spinal cord compression can be variable and occasionally confusing, and this is partly explained by consideration of the site of the epidural compressive lesion, and its relationship with the blood supply of the cord and the site of motor and sensory tracts within the cord.

The advent of MRI has clearly demonstrated that the vertebral body is involved more often than the posterior elements in patients with spinal cord compression, but all parts of the vertebra are susceptible. Some tumours, notably lymphoma, can invade the epidural space without involving the vertebrae. The dura is up to a millimetre thick and relatively resistant to penetration. Epidural tumours rarely breach the dura to invade the cord, but may interfere with the delicate blood supply. The cord receives its blood supply predominantly from the anterior spinal artery which forms an anastomotic chain running the length of the cord and breaking into cauda equina arteries in the lumbar region (Fig. 39.12). The anterior spinal artery is supplied by radicular arteries which are branches of the vertebral artery in the cervical region. In the thoracic region the anterior spinal artery is supplied via the anterior radicular arteries which come off the dorsal branch of the posterior intercostal arteries which in turn emanate directly from the aorta. The anatomy is variable and some major anterior radicular arteries, such as the artery of Adamkiewicz are well known to angiographers. The blood supply of the cord is vulnerable where the anterior radicular artery penetrates the neural foramen, and where the anterior spinal artery runs immediately behind the vertebral body. The anterior spinal artery may be occluded by a deposit in the vertebral body growing posteriorly on to the anterior aspect of the cord. At each segment the anterior spinal artery gives off branches supplying the anterior part of the cord which carries the anterior horn cells and major corticospinal pathways, and the damage resulting from ischaemia and infarction is responsible for clinically catastrophic power loss. A small volume of epidural disease at these critical sites can cause vascular compromise.

Some deposits grow from the posterior elements, compressing the cord from a lateral or posterior direction. Since the sensory tracts occupy a peripheral position in the lateral and posterior cord, sensory symptoms may predominate in this instance. A limited part of the cord's blood supply comes from the posterior radicular artery which branches from the anterior radicular artery in the neural foramen to form a posterior anastomotic chain. If the direction of compression is from the lateral or posterior aspect, the major part of the blood supply to the cord, from the anterior spinal artery, is likely to be preserved.

Technique of examination with imaging

Given the potential complexity of the neurological presentation, an imaging technique must take account of the fact that the clinically relevant lesion may be some distance away from the site suggested by the neurological signs. Abnormalities may be present within the vertebral bone marrow, epidural soft tissue, or both. As a result of its versatility in imaging the whole spine and surrounding soft tissues, MRI has replaced myelography (with or without CT myelography) as the investigation of choice in suspected spinal cord compression. Only when MRI is contraindicated should myelography be performed.

Plain radiographs remain a worthwhile investigation. If clinical signs point to a fairly definite level, many radiotherapists are prepared to commence steroids and plan an initial radiation field on a discrete bony abnormality if present. The sensitivity of plain radiographs in detecting lesions at other levels is low, and soft tissue extension can rarely be evaluated accurately. However, little is lost by obtaining plain radiographs while MRI is scheduled at the earliest opportunity. Isotope studies are sensitive in detecting bony deposits, but less so than MRI.[34] They are unlikely to be helpful in the acute management of spinal cord compression unless MRI is unavailable.

When MRI cannot be performed myelography with water soluble contrast agents should include the entire spine, with cervical as well as lumbar puncture if necessary. Subsequent CT scans (CT myelography) can identify paravertebral lesions growing into the spinal canal, and also bony lesions and herniated discs. For maximum information, CT myelography should be performed within a few hours, by the same radiologist or a radiologist with full access to the myelographic findings so that all appropriate levels can be imaged.

While MRI is relatively expensive it should now be considered as the first investigation since it avoids a series of increasingly sophisticated imaging techniques which may result in significant delay. Once the patient is in the MRI scanner the exact technique will depend on which sequences are available on the machine, but it is important to obtain a set of images of the entire spine. Levels of compression should be readily identifiable; most up-to-date scanners should be able to cover the spine from sacrum to foramen magnum in two sequences with a sufficient degree of overlap to identify levels confidently. If this is not possible some form of skin marker will be necessary so that adequate overlap can be ensured and exact levels of compression accurately identified. A T1-weighted spin-echo sequence in the sagittal plane should be obtained initially. Contrast between normal marrow and metastatic deposits will normally allow detection of malignant infiltration of the vertebral bodies and posterior elements. If doubt exists, a high contrast sequence, for example short tau inversion recovery (STIR), a gradient-echo sequence with T2*-weighted or a T2-weighted spin-echo

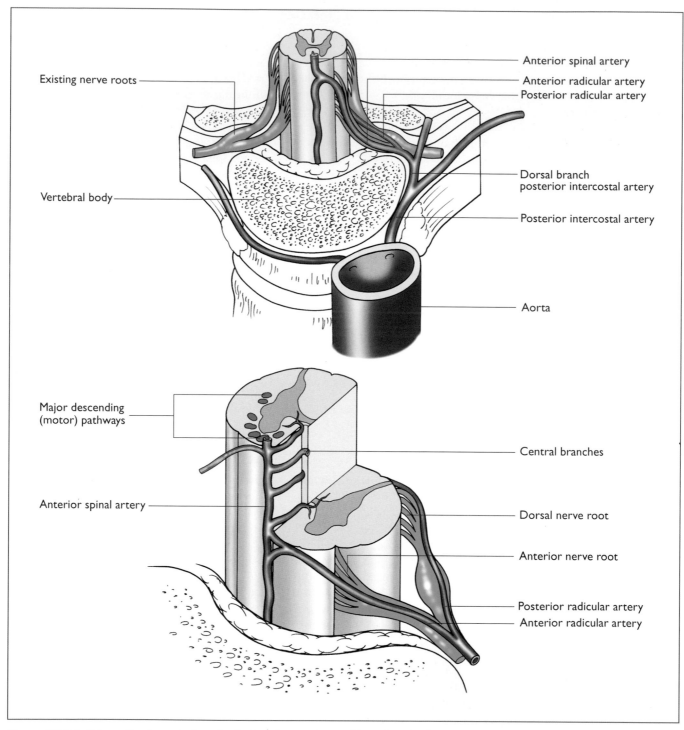

Figure 39.12. *Schematic representation of spinal cord anatomy demonstrating the blood supply. The major component of the cord's blood supply comes via the anterior radicular artery which emanates from the dorsal branch of the posterior intercostal artery. The anterior radicular artery runs through the neural foramen where a smaller posterior radicular artery comes off. The anterior radicular artery feeds the anterior spinal artery which forms a single anastomotic chain running the length of the cord.*

From the anterior spinal artery penetrating central branches supply the functionally crucial descending motor pathways. Some posterior and peripheral parts of the cord have some blood supply from a plexus of small pial vessels coming directly from the anterior and posterior radicular arteries. Interruption of the blood supply by compression of anterior radicular or anterior spinal arteries can cause infarction of the cord even in the absence of major mechanical compression.

sequence may indicate the site of metastatic bony lesions. T2*-weighted gradient-echo sequences produce an excellent myelographic effect with high signal intensity CSF and a low signal intensity cord. Sagittal scans should be 4–5 mm thick, but the neural foraminae must be covered, if necessary by widening slice thickness, inserting interslice gaps or obtaining two blocks. After review of sagittal images the radiologist should maintain a low threshold for obtaining sequences in orthogonal planes, as important lesions in the paravertebral region and intervertebral foraminae are easier to detect and interpret using the axial, or occasionally the coronal, plane. Gadolinium enhancement is not used routinely, but if the clinical presentation is suggestive of intramedullary or leptomeningeal disease, contrast-enhanced T1-weighted spin-echo sequences, initially in the sagittal plane, are mandatory.

Typical imaging features and differential diagnosis

The differential diagnosis of myelopathy includes:

- Epidural cord compression
- Meningeal metastases
- Intramedullary deposits
- Glioma of the spinal cord
- Meningioma
- Neurofibroma
- Radiation myelopathy
- Postinfection transverse myelitis
- Bone abscess, e.g. TB
- Osteoporotic vertebral collapse

Most causes of myelopathy which may be confused clinically with epidural cord compression can be accurately diagnosed by MRI. In the patient with systemic cancer, meningeal metastases and intramedullary tumours are the principal differentials. Glioma of the cord, meningioma and neurofibroma are rare. Radiation myelopathy is unusual, and requires an appropriate history. Like postinfectious transverse myelitis, it will be seen as an enhancing area without mass effect. Epidural haematoma usually has a precipitant such as recent lumbar puncture, epidural abscess should be associated with clinical signs of sepsis, and both should have recognizable morphological features and signal intensity characteristics to enable differential diagnosis. However, a bacterial abscess involving bone, for example a tuberculous abscess, may be extremely difficult to differentiate from tumour. An osteoporotic acute vertebral collapse should be suspected if it is the solitary spinal lesion, particularly if the posterior elements of the vertebra are entirely normal and there is no evidence of a soft tissue mass. A herniated degenerative disc and malignant involvement of the spine may coexist, but the two are rarely confused.

Tumour tissue in the epidural space typically returns low signal on T1-weighted sequences, intermediate to high signal on T2-weighted-spin-echo sequences, and high signal on T2* and STIR images. When bony lesions are discrete and focal, they are easy to discern. When very extensive diffuse bony metastatic disease is present, epidural spread of disease can be more difficult to identify. Where there is gross disease, several levels of compression may be present, underlining the necessity to cover the whole spine (Fig. 39.13). In the presence of diffuse disease, any subtle abnormality of cord morphology identified on the sagittal images

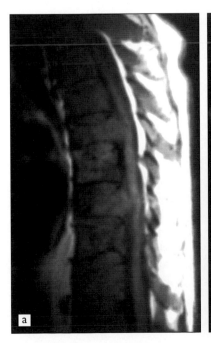
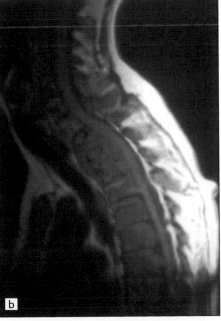

Figure 39.13. *(a, b) T1-weighted spin-echo MR images, sagittal plane. Extensive bony disease is present, metastatic from carcinoma of breast. Multiple levels of cord compression are identified in the lower thoracic region and cervicothoracic junction. It is unlikely that all of these levels would have been demonstrated by myelography. Magnetic resonance imaging should include the whole spine, as discovery of a level in the lower thoracic region does not exclude higher levels of compression, particularly in the presence of extensive bony metastatic disease.*

should raise the index of suspicion, and orthogonal plane imaging should be performed, which may reveal lateral compression of the cord from expanded pedicles (Fig. 39.14). This type of compression is not infrequently seen in metastatic prostate and breast cancer.

Bony changes may be subtle or even absent. Soft tissue extension of tumour (in a 'dumbell' fashion) may occur with a variety of tumours:

- Lymphoma
- Neurofibroma
- Neuroblastoma
- Malignant thymoma
- Mesothelioma
- Lung cancer

Apart from the classical but uncommon neurofibroma and neuroblastoma, bronchial carcinoma can penetrate the intervertebral foramen while causing little bony destruction, particularly in superior sulcus tumours. Malignant thymoma and mesothelioma may also compress the cord by soft tissue extension.

One of the most important dumbell tumours is lymphoma in the posterior mediastinum, retrocrural region and retroperitoneum. The tendency of lymphoma to involve the epidural spaces has been recognized for many years.[35] The incidence of spinal cord compression by lymphoma reported in the literature varies between 1 and 7%. Epidural masses may be small and subtle (Fig. 39.15) but any symptomatology should be vigorously investigated, since early treatment should result in a favourable response to treatment in keep-

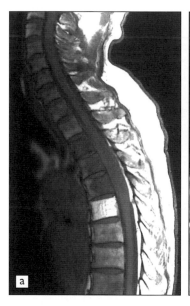
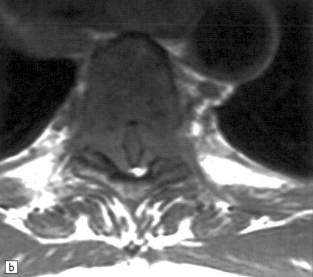

Figure 39.14. *(a) T1-weighted spin-echo MR image, sagittal plane. Extensive bony disease is present, metastatic from carcinoma of lung. This midline sagittal image shows apparent widening of the cord in the anteroposterior direction. (b) Axial imaging shows expansion of the pedicles, squeezing the cord predominantly from a lateral direction. This appearance is especially associated with deposits from carcinoma of breast and prostate and may result in atypical clinical features early in the presentation of spinal cord compression.*

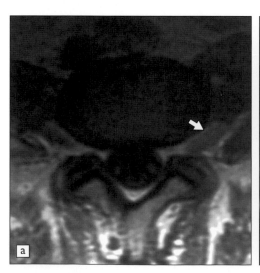
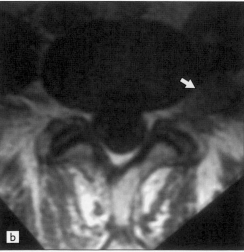

Figure 39.15. *A patient previously treated for non-Hodgkin's lymphoma, presenting with left-sided radicular pain interpreted clinically as disc disease. (a) In the left L5 neural foramen there is a small plaque of soft tissue tumour, suspected of being lymphoma recurrence (arrow); (b) interval scanning 6 weeks later confirms growth of the lesion (arrow). A diagnosis of epidural lymphoma was made, and following appropriate chemotherapy, the symptoms and the MRI abnormality resolved.*

ing with the overall prognosis of the disease. If paraplegia is allowed to develop, it is unlikely to recover.[36] In current practice it is most likely that a patient known to have lymphoma presenting with back pain and neurological symptoms will be referred for MRI. The same principles apply as for any tumour; the entire spine should be imaged, using orthogonal planes as necessary to elucidate soft tissue disease. In addition, when CT scans are performed as staging investigations for lymphoma, the epidural spaces should be an area subjected to special scrutiny as subtle signs, such as the obliteration of fat planes in the intervertebral foraminae, may give early warning of epidural space invasion and incipient neurological dysfunction (Fig. 39.16).

Key points: imaging features of spinal cord compression

■ MRI is the investigation of choice in suspected spinal cord compression

■ The entire spine should be evaluated as many tumours produce multiple levels of compression

■ T2-weighted sequences provide an excellent 'myelographic' effect

■ Most causes of myelopathy that mimic spinal cord compression can be accurately diagnosed with MRI

■ Lymphoma is the most common malignant tumour to invade the spinal canal through the intervertebral foraminae without any bony destruction

Spinal meningeal disease

As is the case with leptomeningeal disease in the cranial cavity, disease may spread to the meninges by:

- The haematogenous route
- Cerebrospinal fluid pathways
- Direct extension along peripheral nerves

The clinical presentation may be somewhat obscure. Symptoms can be divided into two broad categories, namely those caused by invasion of spinal nerve roots (i.e. neural dysfunction) and those caused by invasion of the leptomeninges alone (i.e. meningeal irritation).

Neural dysfunction is likely to result in a constellation of symptoms and signs which are anatomically remote owing to the selective involvement of individual nerve roots. If an isolated lumbar nerve root is involved, radicular pain will result, mimicking a herniated lumbar disc. However, there are usually some vague symptoms attributable to meningeal

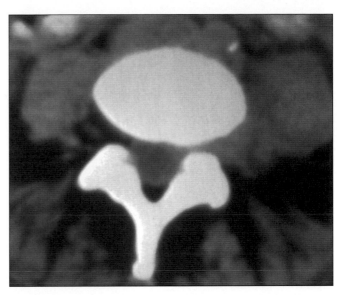

Figure 39.16. *Staging CT scan for non-Hodgkin's lymphoma. There is obliteration of the fat plane in the neural foramen on the left. This is due to lymphomas behaving as a 'dumb-bell tumour'. The patient had minor backache, but if such lesions are neglected, they will progress to cause cord compression.*

irritation such as back pain, neck pain or headache. When the referring clinician describes a neurological presentation verging on the bizarre, it is important to consider the diagnosis of leptomeningeal disease, since the MRI technique must involve T1-weighted sagittal sequences of the entire spine before and after intravenous gadolinium-DTPA administration. In distinction to the situation within the cranial cavity, any enhancement of the meninges in the spinal canal should be considered abnormal. Some tumours, notably carcinomas of lung and breast, produce enhancing masses within the meninges (Fig. 39.17). Leukaemia and lymphoma tend to result in plaques or sheets of enhancing tissue (Fig. 39.18). Melanoma, which frequently metastasizes to the meninges may do either (Fig. 39.19). When present, the appearance of enhancing plaques or masses of tumour is sufficiently characteristic to allow confident diagnosis. However, MRI is a distinctly insensitive technique, particularly in leukaemia and lymphoma. If MRI is negative, lumbar puncture can be used subsequently and may yield positive cytology.[29]

Primary brain tumours which have a tendency to seed spinal meninges via CSF-spread include:

- Medulloblastoma
- Pinealoblastoma
- Intracranial germ cell tumours
- Intracranial primitive neuro-ectodermal tumours (PNET)

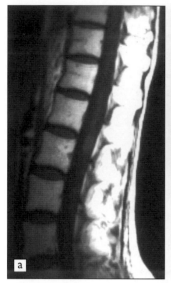
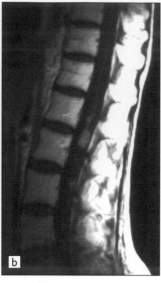

Figure 39.17. *T1-weighted spin-echo MR images before (a) and after (b) intravenous gadolinium-DTPA. Meningeal deposits from carcinoma of the breast. Some thickening of the meninges is just discernible before contrast. After administration of gadolinium, enhancing masses on the meninges are clearly identifiable. This is the characteristic appearance of carcinoma metastatic to the meninges.*

Magnetic resonance imaging is frequently used as a staging technique, notwithstanding its relative lack of sensitivity. Changes may be subtle, and it is important to ensure coverage of the meninges in the neural foraminae. An enhancing mass is diagnostic of drop metastases, but myelography is still used owing to its increased sensitivity in cases where clinical suspicion is particularly high (Fig. 39.20).

Key points: spinal meningeal and cord involvement

- Spinal meningeal disease is caused by invasion of spinal nerve roots or by haematogenous spread to the leptomeninges

- Patients frequently present with neurological features which do not point to a single specific site

- T1-weighted sagittal sequences of the entire spine before and after intravenous contrast medium are mandatory

- MRI is an insensitive technique and if negative, lumbar puncture is indicated

- Primary brain tumours produce spinal seedlings

- Intramedullary metastases most frequently occur in breast and lung cancer and malignant melanoma

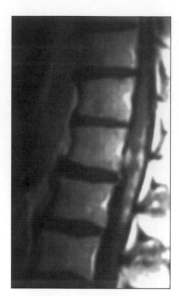

Figure 39.18. *T1-weighted spin-echo MR image following gadolinium. Meningeal spread of lymphoma. The tumour appears as an enhancing sheet of tissue in the lumbar meninges. The patient had presented with backache and leg weakness as the initial manifestation of non-Hodgkin's lymphoma. Biopsy at lumbar laminectomy confirmed the diagnosis. Staging CT scan revealed lymphadenopathy in mediastinum and retroperitoneum.*

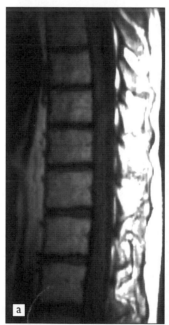
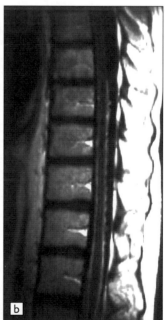

Figure 39.19. *T1-weighted spin-echo MR images before (a) and after (b) gadolinium-DTPA, sagittal plane. Diffuse nodular enhancement extends throughout the thoracic meninges. The appearance is due to diffuse meningeal involvement by melanoma (b) seen better following contrast injection.*

Intramedullary deposits

Tumour deposits are occasionally identified within the spinal cord. In these circumstances, clinical presentation is similar to meaningeal disease, giving neurological symptoms and signs which cannot be unified to a single anatomical site. Carcinoma of breast and lung and malignant melanoma are once again the most frequent culprits. Metastases to the

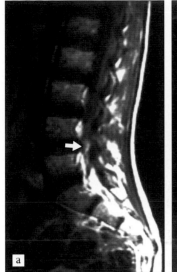
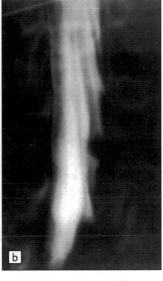

Figure 39.20. *(a) T1-weighted spin-echo MR image following gadolinium-DTPA, sagittal plane. Staging investigation in a patient diagnosed as medullablastoma of the roof of the fourth ventricle. There is a small mass in the neural foramen at L5 which showed enhancement following gadolinium (arrow). A drop metastasis was suspected, which was confirmed by myelography (b).*

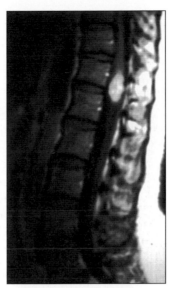

Figure 39.21. *T1-weighted spin-echo MR image following gadolinium-DTPA. An enhancing intramedullary mass is expanding the conus. This is a metastasis from carcinoma of the breast.*

spinal cord are seen as enhancing masses on MRI following gadolinium-DTPA injection, and appear to have a predilection for the conus (Fig. 39.21). Small cell lung cancer may give multiple small enhancing lesions throughout the cord, of similar appearance to small cell deposits metastatic to the brain parenchyma (Fig. 39.22).

METASTATIC INVOLVEMENT OF PERIPHERAL NERVES AND MUSCLE

Major nerve plexuses

The two major areas of nerve plexus formation are the brachial plexus and the lumbosacral plexus. The brachial plexus is most commonly involved, by superior sulcus tumours invading directly, or by lymph nodes metastatic from breast carcinoma. Both of these pathologies usually invade the plexus from below, affecting those fibres that begin as C8 and T1 roots and end as the ulnar nerve. The primary symptom is pain, which may localize to the posterior aspect of the shoulder or around the elbow; this pain may sometimes lead the physician to instigate fruitless investigations of the bony and soft tissue structures of the shoulder and elbow. Paraesthesia and numbness are often present, particularly affecting the medial part of the hand. The differential diagnosis from radiation fibrosis of the

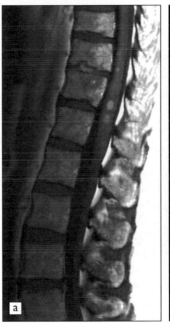
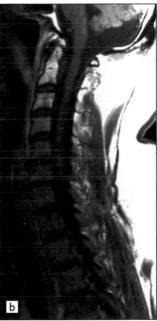

Figure 39.22. *(a and b) T1-weighted MR images following gadolinium-DTPA, sagittal plane. Very small enhancing lesions are identified within the cord. Those intramedullary lesions were scattered through the spinal cord and brain, and were due to metastases from small cell carcinoma.*

brachial plexus can be difficult, and CT and MRI can both be used to detect soft tissue masses in this region. MRI, as a result of its multiplanar imaging capability, has greater versatility, but it may be impossible to discriminate between radiation fibrosis and infiltrative forms of tumour which do not present as a morphological mass.[37–39] Brachial plexopathy is further discussed in Chapter 22.

Tumours that frequently affect the lumbosacral plexus include carcinomas of rectum, cervix, bladder and prostate. The clinical presentation is dominated by pain, usually in a radicular distribution. Radiation damage to the lumbosacral plexus is less common than in the brachial plexus. Often, the crucial question is to establish whether the plexus is involved by a soft tissue mass or by bony involvement of the lumbosacral spine. Computed tomography is frequently adequate for detecting a soft tissue mass extending from the pelvic organs into the sacral plexus. However, in the absence of a soft tissue mass, MRI is more sensitive at detecting malignant involvement of the sacrum (Figs. 39.23 and 39.24).

Key points: peripheral nerves

■ The brachial plexus is most commonly involved in breast and lung cancer by direct soft tissue invasion

■ The lumbosacral plexus is usually involved by direct extension of bone metastases, e.g. carcinoma of the prostate

Peripheral nerves

Peripheral neuropathy in a patient with systemic cancer is usually due to chemotherapy. Diffuse or focal involvement of nerves by tumour, resulting in a sensorimotor neuropathy, is rare and usually associated with lymphoma, leukaemia and other haematological malignancies.[40,41] Isolated mononeuropathies may result from invasion by adjacent tumour, particularly if a nerve is located at a point where it passes directly over a bone, or through a bony canal. The radial and ulnar nerves may be affected by bony metastatic disease around the elbow or within the axilla. The sciatic nerve is also vulnerable to involvement by bony or soft tissue tumour at several sites in the pelvis, and the obturator nerve may be compressed or invaded as it passes through the obturator canal. Imaging studies are only likely to be useful if there is a strong clinical indication that an individual nerve has been affected by metastatic disease; in these circumstances cross-sectional techniques including MRI, CT and ultrasound can give useful confirmation that there is a pathological mass in the vicinity of the affected nerve.

Muscle

Soft tissue metastases involving muscles are unusual, but may occasionally be seen in lymphoma and leukaemia (chloroma). Some solid tumours may also metastasize to the muscle:

• Melanoma
• Lung cancer
• Rhabdomyosarcoma

Such lesions are usually obvious clinically, and cross-sectional imaging techniques can be used to determine the extent of the abnormality, but these lesions rarely have specific diagnostic features.

THE ROLE OF IMAGING

As is the case in non-malignant neurological disease, MRI is assuming an increasingly central role in the investigation of the effects of metastatic disease on the CNS, although CT remains a valid and useful technique in many clinical circumstances. Interpretation of images of metastatic disease is often straightforward, but the radiologist must remain mindful of the protean manifestations of metastatic disease, and endeavour to ensure that the most appropriate imaging technique is used sooner rather than later.

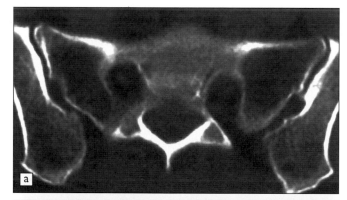

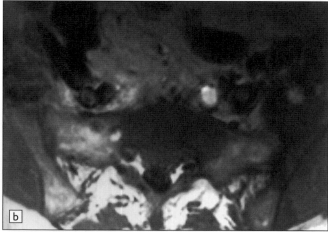

Figure 39.23. *This patient with a history of melanoma, presented with lower back pain radiating to the left leg. (a) CT scan with bony windows failed to reveal any explanation for the symptoms; (b) T1-weighted spin-echo MR image, axial plane. Involvement of the sacral marrow cavity and impingement on the nerve root is clearly demonstrated, owing to the high sensitivity of MRI in detecting bony lesions.*

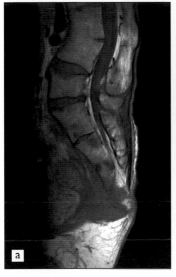
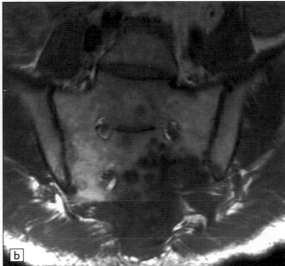

Figure 39.24. *The patient had a history of transitional cell carcinoma of the bladder treated by cystectomy. He presented with radicular pain. (a) T1-weighted spin-echo MR image, sagittal plane. There is a presacral soft tissue abnormality due to pelvic soft tissue recurrence; (b) T1-weighted spin-echo MR image, paracoronal plane. Bony invasion affecting the sacrum and involving the nerve roots is clearly demonstrated.*

Summary

- Neurological disorders are an increasingly common problem in the cancer patient.

- The radiologist should focus on the clinical findings so that the most appropriate investigation is performed.

- Most brain metastases arise from cancers of the lung, breast and melanoma.

- Other sources of primary tumour include the kidneys and gastro-intestinal tract.

- In a significant number of patients the primary source is unknown.

- MRI is the most sensitive imaging technique available for detecting brain metastases but screening is only undertaken in selected tumours (e.g. lung cancer pre-operatively).

- Symptomatic spinal cord compression is seen in 1–5% of patients with disseminated malignancy.

- Imaging of spinal cord compression should include the whole spine. MRI is the preferred investigation.

- Spinal meningeal disease results in a wide range of neurological symptoms which cannot be unified to a single anatomical site.

- The brachial plexus is most commonly involved in breast cancer and apical lung cancer by direct soft tissue invasion.

- The lumbosacral plexus is usually involved by direct extension of bone metastases.

- Peripheral neuropathy is usually due to chemotherapy but occasionally a bone metastasis may involve an adjacent nerve.

- Muscle deposits are unusual. They may be seen in lymphoma, leukaemia, melanoma, lung cancer and rhabdomyosarcoma.

REFERENCES

1. Clouston P D, de Angelis L M, Posner J B. The spectrum of neurologic disease in patients with systemic cancer. Ann Neurol 1992; 31: 268–273

2. Sculier J P, Feld R, Evans W K et al. Neurological disorders in patients with small cell lung cancer. Cancer 1987; 60: 2275–2283

3. Gilbert M R, Grossman S A. Incidence and nature of neurological problems in patients with solid tumours. Am J Med 1986; 81: 951–954

4. Eapen L, Vachet M, Catton G et al. Brain metastases with an unknown primary: A clinical perspective. J Neurooncol 1988; 6: 31–35

5. Nicholson G L. Organ specificity of tumour metastasis: Role of preferential adhesion, invasion and growth of malignant cells at specific secondary sites. Cancer Metastasis Rev 1988; 7: 143–188

6. Delattre J-Y, Kroll G, Thaler H T et al. Distribution of brain metastases. Arch Neurol 1988; 45: 741–744

7. Smith D B, Howell A, Harris M et al. Carcinomatous meningitis associated with infiltrating lobular carcinoma of the breast. Eur J Surg Oncol 1985; 11: 33–36

8. Nicholson G L, Kawaguchi T, Kawaguchi M et al. Brain surface invasion and metastasis of murine malignant melanoma variants. J Neurooncol 1987; 4: 209–218

9. Sze G, Milano E, Johnson C et al. Detection of brain metastases: Comparison of contrast-enhanced with unenhanced MR and enhanced CT. Am J Neuroradiol 1990; 11: 785–791

10. Cherryman G R, Olliff J F C, Golfieri R et al. A prospective comparison of Gadolinium-DTPA enhanced MRI and contrast-enhanced CT scanning in the detection of brain metastases arising from small cell lung cancer. Medicom. Contrast media in MRI. 1990

11. Hussman K C, Sze G. MR imaging of cerebral metastatic disease. Ad MRI cont 1996; 4: 2–12

12. Yuh W T C, Tall T E, Nguyen H D et al. The effect of contrast dose, imaging time and lesion size in the MR detection of intracerebral metastases. Am J Neuroradiol 1995; 16: 73–80

13. Black W C. High dose MR in evaluation of brain metastases: Will increased detection decrease costs? Am J Neuroradiol 1994; 15: 1062–1064

14. Boorstein J M, Wong K T, Grossman R I et al. Metastatic lesions of the brain imaging with magnetisation transfer. Radiology 1994; 191: 799–803

15. Griffeth L K, Rich K M, Dehashiti F et al. Brain metastases from non-central nervous system tumours: Evaluation with PET. Radiology 1993; 186: 37–44

16. Armstrong P, Vincent J N. Staging non-small cell lung cancer. Clin Radiol 1993; 48: 1–10

17. Whitehouse J M A (ed). Management of lung cancer. Current clinical practices (1994). Standing Medical Advisory Committee of Department of Health: Working Group Report

18. Salbeck R, Grau H C, Artmann H. Cerebral tumour staging in patients with bronchial carcinoma by computed tomography. Cancer 1990; 66: 2007–2011

19. Royal College of Radiologists. The use of computed tomography in the initial investigation of common malignancies (1994)

20. MacVicar D. Staging of testicular germ cell tumours. Clin Radiol 1993; 47: 149–158

21. Patchell R A, Tibbs P A, Walsh J W et al. A randomised trial of surgery in the treatment of single metastases to the brain. N Eng J Med 1993; 22: 495–500

22. Asato R, Akiyama Y, Ito M et al. Nuclear magnetic resonance abnormalities of the cerebral white matter in children with acute lymphoblastic leukaemia and malignant lymphoma during and after central nervous system prophylactic treatment with intrathecal methotrexate. Cancer 1992; 70: 1997–2004

23. Hook C C, Kimmel D W, Kvols L K et al. Multifocal inflammatory leuko-encephalopathy with 5-flurouracil and levamisole. Ann Neurol 1992; 31: 262–267

24. Stemmer S M, Stears J C, Burton B S et al. White matter changes in patients with breast cancer treated with high dose chemotherapy and autologous bone marrow support. Am J Neuroradiol 1994; 15: 1267–1273

25. Rubinstein A B, Schein M, Reichenthal E. The association of carcinoma of the breast with meningioma. Surg Gynaecol Obstet 1989; 169: 334–336

26. Smith F P, Slavik M, Macdonald J S. Association of breast cancer with meningioma: Report of two cases and review of the literature. Cancer 1978; 42: 1992–1994

27. Jacobs D H, Holmes F F, McFarlane N J. Meningiomas are not significantly associated with breast cancer. Arch Neurol 1992; 49: 753–756

28. Enochs W S, Hyslop W B, Bennett H F et al. Sources of the increased congenital longitudinal relaxation rates oberved in melanotic melanoma. An in vitro study of synthetic melanins. Invest Radiol 1989; 24: 794–804

29. Yousem D M, Patrone P M, Grossman R I. Leptomeningeal metastases: M R evaluation. J Comput Assist Tomogr 1990; 14: 255–261

30. Bansal S, Brady L W, Olsen A et al. The treatment of metastatic spinal cord tumours. J Am Med Assoc 1967; 202: 686–688

31. Hildebrand J. Lesions of the nervous system in cancer patients. Monograph series of the European Organisation for Research on Treatment of Cancer (Vol. 5) New York: Raven Press, 1978

32. Klein S L, Sanford R A, Muhlbauer M S. Paediatric spinal epidural metastases. J Neurosurg 1991; 74: 70–75

33. Barron K D, Hirano A, Araski S et al. Experiences with metastatic neoplasms involving the spinal cord. Neurology 1959; 9: 91–106

34. Jones A L, Williams M P, Powles T J et al. Magnetic resonance imaging in the detection of skeletal metastases in patients with breast cancer. Br J Cancer 1990; 62: 296–298

35. Murphy W T, Bilge N. Compression of the spinal cord in patients with malignant lymphoma. Radiology 1964; 82: 495–501

36. MacVicar D, Williams M P. CT scanning in epidural lymphoma. Clin Radiol 1991; 43: 95–102

37. Moore N R, Dixon A K, Wheeler T K. Axillary fibrosis or recurrent tumour. An MRI study in breast cancer. Clin Radiol 1990; 42: 42–46

38. Posniak H V, Olson M C, Dudiak C M. MR imaging of the brachial plexus. Am J Roentgenol 1993; 161: 373–379

39. Iyer R B, Fenstermacher M J, Libshitz H I. MR Imaging of the treated brachial plexus. Am J Roentgenol 1996; 167: 225–229

40. Sumi S M, Farrell D F, Knauss T A. Lymphoma and leukaemia manifested by steroid responsive polyneuropathy. Arch Neurol 1983; 40: 577–582

41. McLeod J G. Peripheral neuropathy associated with lymphomas, leukaemias and polycythaemia vera. In: Dyck P J and Thomas P K (eds) Peripheral neuropathy (Vol 2, 3rd ed.) Philadelphia: W B Saunders, 1993; 1591–1598

Chapter 40

Adrenal glands

Delia Peppercorn and Rodney Reznek

INTRODUCTION

The routine use of cross-sectional imaging in the staging of intra-abdominal and extra-abdominal malignancy has shown that the adrenal gland is a frequent site of unexpected metastatic disease. Although modern computed tomography (CT) and magnetic resonance imaging (MRI) can be expected to detect nodules exceeding 8–10 mm, and despite the clear demonstration of the normal adrenals on CT and MRI, autopsy studies show that many adrenal metastases go undetected due to their small size.

Demonstration of such metastases will almost always markedly influence the patient's management by indicating that the patient has Stage-IV disease. However, a major problem exists in the radiological demonstration of metastases; benign cortical adenomas are common and always have to be distinguished from metastases before assuming that the patient has metastatic disease.

INCIDENCE

The adrenal glands are the fourth most common site in the body for metastases after the lungs, liver and bone. Common sites of origin of adrenal metastases are listed in Table 40.1. At autopsy adrenal metastases are found in up to 27% of patients dying of cancer.[1] Certain tumours show a higher incidence; around 30–40% of patients with breast, and lung cancer have adrenal metastases.[2,3] Fifty percent of melanomas spread to the adrenal.[4] Adrenal metastases are found in gastro-intestinal tumours and renal tumours in between 10 and 20% of cases.[5,6]

Infiltration is usually within the normal cortex and/or medulla, but spread to adenomas has been reported.[7,8] Metastases are asymptomatic as a rule, but occasional cases of hypoadrenalism have been observed.[9]

Table 40.1. *Common sites of origin of adrenal metastases*

• Breast	• Melanoma	• Kidney
• Lung	• Gastro-intestinal	

Imaging, by any technique, will only detect metastases if there is a focal mass or distortion of the contour of the adrenal gland, but a normal-appearing gland does not exclude microscopic tumour infiltration.[10] One study of patients with small cell lung cancer and morphologically normal adrenal glands on CT found that 17% of the glands were positive for metastases on fine needle aspiration.[11]

THE NORMAL ADRENAL GLAND

An appreciation of the normal appearances of the adrenal gland is important if small abnormalities are to be observed. The adrenals are usually well-visualized as an inverted Y or V shape against the surrounding retroperitoneal fat on both CT and MRI. On ultrasound identification of the normal adrenal gland is technically difficult; the gland is very small and its echotexture is similar to that of the surrounding tissues. Bowel gas can often obscure the gland, particularly on the left.

To date, normal measurements have referred almost entirely to the body of the adrenal gland. However, in view of the predominance of cortical tissue within the limbs, measurement of their size is important.[12] The maximum width of the body measured perpendicular to the long axis, at the junction of the adrenal body and limb, is 0.79 mm (SD 0.21) on the left and 0.6 mm (SD 0.2) on the right.[12] The thickness of the limbs of the right adrenal are slightly less than the left, measuring 0.14–0.49 mm, compared with 0.13–0.52 mm on the left. In practice, the normal adrenal limb should not measure over 5 mm.[12]

IMAGING APPEARANCES OF ADRENAL METASTASES

The radiological appearances of adrenal metastases are not specific. They can be large or small, unilateral or bilateral.

Small adrenal metastases (less than 2 cm) are difficult to detect on ultrasound; however, large adrenal masses should be readily identifiable. Metastases are usually rounded or oval and poorly reflective. Ultrasound imaging will not differentiate between metastases and a benign adenoma.

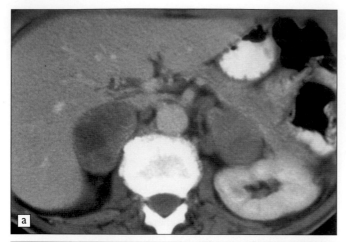

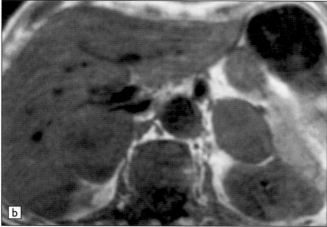

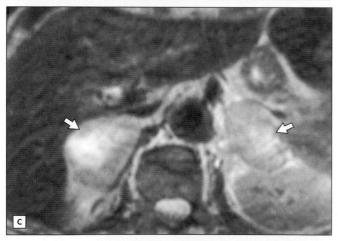

Figure 40.1. *Bilateral adrenal metastases in a patient with oat cell lung cancer. (a) CT scan performed after intravenous injection of contrast medium showing large bilateral adrenal masses enhancing only partially and inhomogeneously; (b) T1-weighted MR image showing masses of intermediate signal intensity; (c) T2-weighted image on the same patient showing typical inhomogeneous appearance of metastases with areas of very high signal intensity interspersed with areas of low signal intensity within large bilateral adrenal masses (arrows).*

On CT, metastases less than 3 cm in diameter are usually homogeneous. Larger lesions may show central necrosis or areas of haemorrhage (Fig. 40.1a). They tend to be of inhomogeneous density and occasionally have a thick enhancing rim after intravenous contrast medium.[13]

On MR they are typically hypointense compared to liver on T1-weighted images and relatively hyperintense on T2-weighted images (Figs 40.1b and c). Some adrenal metastases are atypical and either isointense or hypointense relative to liver on T2-weighted images.[14,15]

In addition, some metastases have very long T2 relaxation times and can mimic phaeochromocytomas although, phaeochromocytomas can usually be differentiated on clinical grounds (Fig. 40.2 a–c). Thus an adrenal metastases cannot be distinguished clearly from benign lesions such as an adenoma, haematoma, pseudocysts or inflammatory masses on the basis of morphology (Figs 40.3 a and b). As discussed below, CT attenuation and chemical-shift MR imaging can be helpful in distinguishing between adenomas and metastases.

DIFFERENTIAL DIAGNOSIS OF AN ADRENAL MASS (TABLE 40.2)

The differential diagnosis of a non-hyperfunctioning adrenal mass includes a benign cortical adenoma, adrenal cyst, adrenal carcinoma and a myelolipoma. Functioning adrenal masses such as phaeochromocytomas should also be considered, especially if there is an underlying syndrome such as von Hippel–Lindau, or multiple endocrine neoplasia (Fig. 40.4 a–c). Some of these masses have specific imaging features which help in the diagnosis (Table 40.2).

Adrenal cysts are rare and occur more commonly in women than men.[16] They have a similar appearance on imaging to cysts elsewhere in the body, although the presence of proteinaceous fluid, infectious debris or haemorrhage within a cyst will alter its appearance. Primary adrenal carcinomas are rare, highly malignant tumours. They are usually large (>6 cm) and are heterogeneous where there is necrosis and calcification.[17] However, 16% of tumours are less than 6 cm and on imaging are homogeneous, morphologically resembling a non-hyperfunctioning adenoma.[18]

Myelolipomas are composed of mature fat and haemopoietic tissue in varying proportions. The diagnosis is made by demonstrating the presence of fat within an adrenal mass. This can be accomplished with either CT or MRI although the presence of haemorrhage or infection can complicate the diagnosis.[19] Nevertheless, the use of narrow collimation on CT will usually allow demonstration of any fat that is present. On MR the presence of fat is best demonstrated on T1-weighted images with and without fat suppression. The fat-containing area in a myelolipoma should be equal in signal intensity to that of subcutaneous and retroperitoneal fat on all pulse sequences.[20]

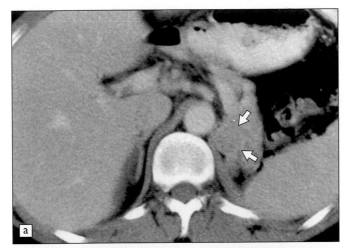

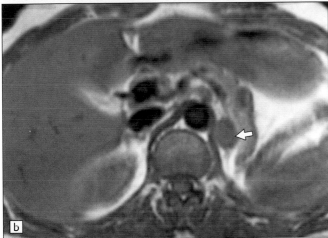

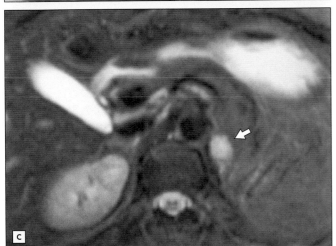

Figure 40.2. *Adrenal metastasis in a patient with carcinoma of the kidney. (a) Contrast-enhanced CT scan showing normal right adrenal and left adrenal metastasis (arrows); (b) T1-weighted MR image showing the mass to be of intermediate signal intensity (arrow); (c) T2-weighted MR image of the same mass showing signal mimicking a phaeochromocytoma (arrow).*

Table 40.2. *Differential diagnosis of adrenal metastases*

Unilateral	Bilateral
Adrenal adenoma	Bilateral adenoma
Adrenal cyst	Bilateral phaeochromocytoma
Adrenal carcinoma	Tuberculosis
Myelolipoma	
Phaeochromocytoma	

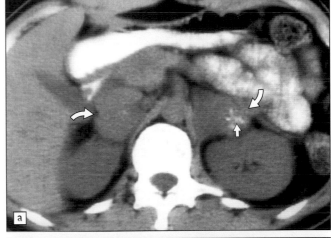

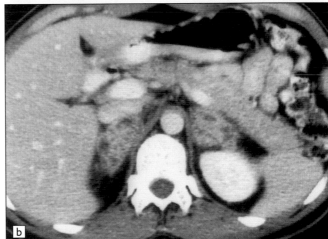

Figure 40.3. *Adrenal tuberculosis. (a) CT scan prior to intravenous injection of contrast medium showing bilateral adrenal masses (curved arrows). Typical punctate calcification is demonstrated in the left adrenal gland (small arrow). (b) Appearance following intravenous injection of contrast medium showing typical non-enhancing areas within the gland corresponding to multiple small caseating granulomata.*

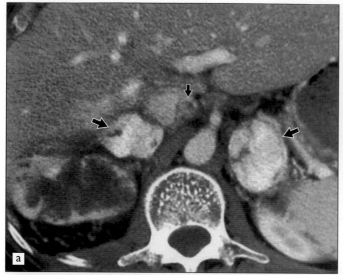

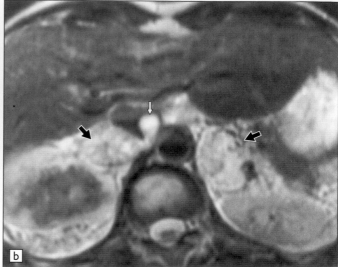

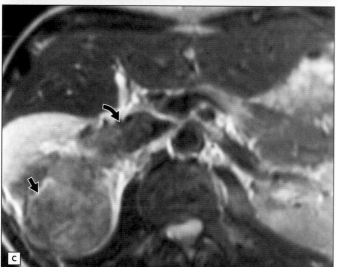

Figure 40.4. *Bilateral phaeochromocytomas and small paraganglionoma in association with a right renal cancer in a patient with von Hippel–Lindau disease. (a) CT scan taken after injection of intravenous contrast medium showing large bilateral adrenal masses enhancing intensely (large arrows). A third smaller mass consistent with a paraganglionoma can be seen lying just medial to the inferior vena cava (small arrow); (b) T2-weighted FSE MR sequence corresponding to CT scan showing the typical high signal intensity of the phaeochromocytomas bilaterally (black arrows) and the high signal intensity of the small paraganglioma (white arrow); (c) T2-weighted MR image of the large right renal carcinoma (arrow) infiltrating the right renal vein (curved arrow).*

EVALUATION OF THE ADRENAL MASSES IN ONCOLOGICAL PATIENTS

Influence on staging

In most cancers the presence of adrenal metastases, even if the sole site of distant spread, will render the tumour Stage IV (i.e. distant metastases). The exception is in renal cell carcinoma when the demonstration of ipsilateral adrenal involvement does not increase the stage of the disease from Robson Stage II, but involvement of the contralateral gland upgrades the staging to IVB.

However, not all adrenal masses are metastases, even in patients with known malignancy.[21] When an adrenal mass is the only finding suspicious of metastatic disease in an oncological patient, confirmation of its nature may be crucial in determining whether curative therapy of the primary tumour is warranted. This dilemma occurs most commonly in patients with carcinoma of the lung, because confirmation of an isolated adrenal metastasis will preclude a thoracotomy or curative radiotherapy. However, non-functioning adrenal adenomas are very common, with a prevalence at autopsy in the general population of approximately 3%.[22] Benign adrenal masses of at least 1 cm are found in 0.6–1.5% of the population during abdominal CT.[23,24] The number and size of these nodules increase with age,[25] and they occur with increased frequency in obese, diabetic patients, and elderly women.[26] Even in patients with lung cancer, an adrenal mass is more likely to be an adenoma than a metastasis.[21]

Key points: adrenal metastases

- At autopsy more than 25% of all patients dying of a cancer have adrenal metastases

- Metastases are usually asymptomatic

- In almost all cancers, demonstration of an adrenal secondary renders the tumour Stage IV (except in renal cell cancer where only a deposit in the contralateral adrenal gland upgrades the staging to IV)

- As benign adrenal cancers are found in 0.6–1.5% of the population on CT, even in patients with lung cancer, an adrenal mass is more like to be an adenoma than metastasis

When characterizing adrenal masses by non-invasive imaging the consequences of incorrectly characterizing a mass must be considered. In a patient with an extra-adrenal primary neoplasm it is unlikely that potentially curative treatment of the primary tumour would be withheld without biopsy confirmation of an adrenal lesion thought to be the sole site of metastatic spread. Non-invasive characterization of the adrenal mass as an adenoma, however, could result in a decrease in the number of percutaneous biopsies. Thus, the specificity for diagnosis of an adenoma needs to be very high, to ensure that a patient with adrenal metastases does not unnecessarily undergo curative resection of the primary tumour because of misdiagnosis of the adrenal lesion as an adenoma. The sensitivity is much less critical as the only consequences of a false-negative diagnosis is that a percutaneous biopsy will be necessary to establish the diagnosis.

Key point

- The specificity for diagnosis of an adenoma on non-invasive imaging needs to be very high to ensure that a patient with adrenal metastases does not undergo unnecessary curative resection of the primary tumour

Adrenal masses greater than 3 cm are malignant in 90–95% of cases and 78–87% of lesions less than 3 cm are benign.[27,28] However, several studies have shown that the size alone is poor at discriminating between adenomas and non-adenomas.[29–31] Lee, using a threshold of 1.5 cm, found the specificity for the diagnosis of adenoma to be reasonably high (93%), but the sensitivity only 16%.[30] In the same series, using 2.5 cm as the size cut-off, the specificity was 79% and the sensitivity 84%.

Computed tomography

Computed tomography attenuation is more discriminatory than assessment of size. In a large study by Korobkin et al.,[29] all adrenal masses with a CT attenuation value of less than 18 Hounsfield units on a non-enhanced scan were adenomas (specificity 100%, sensitivity 85%). At attenuation values of less than 10 Hounsfield units the specificity was 100% and the sensitivity 68%. This supported earlier studies by Lee et al. who reported a specificity of 96% and sensitivity of 79% using a threshold of 10 Hounsfield units.[30] A much greater overlap was seen in attenuation value on enhanced CT. However, recent work suggests that if CT densitometry is performed on delayed images obtained between 15 minutes and 1 hour after enhancement with intravenously injected contrast medium, a threshold of between 24 and 37 Hounsfield units may be useful in characterizing an adrenal mass as an adenoma.[32–34]

The presence of bilateral masses does not support a diagnosis of metastases. Katz et al. showed that bilateral adrenal adenomas were almost as common as bilateral metastases even in patients with known malignant disease.[35] Other causes of bilateral masses such as phaeochromocytoma and tuberculosis also result in confusion (Figs 40.3 and 40.4).

Magnetic resonance imaging

A variety of MRI protocols using different pulse sequences have been advocated in an attempt to distinguish between benign and metastatic lesions. Techniques include conventional spin-echo imaging, gadolinium-enhanced imaging, chemical-shift and fat-saturation imaging.

Conventional spin-echo imaging

Early reports were enthusiastic that MR imaging would allow differentiation of benign from malignant adrenal masses on the basis of signal intensity differences on T2-weighted spin-echo images. Several studies performed on middle-field strength magnets reported that adrenal-to-liver and adrenal-to-fat signal intensity ratios could distinguish benign from malignant masses. However, considerable overlap was seen in most of these studies with up to 31% of lesions being indeterminate, based on their signal intensity characteristics.[14,36–38] The hepatic signal intensity may not be a reliable universal standard at high-field strengths; because of this some investigators have recommended the use of adrenal mass T2 calculations for differential diagnosis.[15,39] However, even with this method there is still overlap between benign and malignant masses. In addition, T2 measurements are prone to numerous machine-related errors and may vary on different MR machines. Thus, neither of these techniques have proved useful clinically.

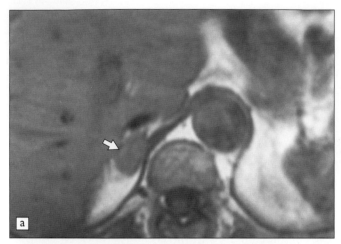

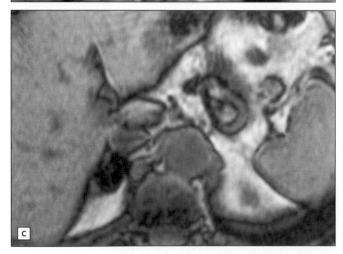

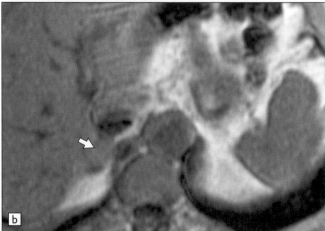

Figure 40.5. *Adrenal adenoma in a patient with lung cancer. (a) T1-weighted MR image showing right adrenal mass of intermediate signal intensity (arrow). (b) In-phase chemical shift imaging (90° flip angle, TR = 150, TE = 4.2) showing the resultant signal intensity (arrow). (c) Out-of-phase chemical shift imaging (90° flip angle, TR = 150, TE = 2.3) showing marked loss of signal intensity indicating the presence of intracellular lipid.*

Gadolinium-enhanced MRI

The accuracy of MRI in differentiating benign from malignant masses can be improved by using intravenous gadolinium injection with gradient-echo imaging.[40–42] On MR images obtained after administration of gadolinium, adenomas show mild enhancement with quick washout, whereas malignant tumours and phaeochromocytomas show strong enhancement and slower washout. However, again there is considerable overlap in the characteristics of benign and malignant masses, limiting its clinical applicability in distinguishing adenomatous from non-adenomatous masses.

Chemical-shift imaging

More recent attempts have been made to characterize adrenal masses with MR on the basis of fat content.[43–48] Benign, non-functioning adenomas generally contain large lipid-laden cells, in contrast to malignant lesions which contain little or none. Chemical-shift imaging relies on the fact that protons in water molecules process at a slightly different rate to the protons in lipid molecules in a magnetic field. As a result, water and fat protons cycle in and out of phase with respect to one another. By selecting an appropriate TE, one can acquire an in and an out-of-phase image. The signal intensity of a pixel on an in-phase image is derived from the signal of water plus fat protons. On out-of-phase images the signal intensity is derived from the difference of the signal of water and fat protons. Therefore, adenomas lose signal intensity on out-of-phase images compared with in-phase images, whereas metastases remain unchanged (Figs. 40.5 and 40.6).

There are several ways of assessing the degree of loss of signal intensity. Quantitative analysis can be made using a variety of ratios, essentially comparing the loss of signal in the adrenal with that of liver, paraspinal muscle or spleen on in-phase and opposed-phase images. Fatty infiltration of the liver (particularly in oncology patients receiving chemotherapy) and iron overload make the liver an unreliable internal standard. Fatty infiltration may also affect skeletal muscle to a lesser extent. The spleen has been shown to be the most reliable internal standard.[46]

Simple visual assessment of relative signal intensity loss, in comparison with the reference organ, is just as accurate as quantitative methods, but quantitative methods may be useful in equivocal cases.[46,47] When loss of signal is demonstrated in an adrenal mass on chemical-shift imaging, an adrenal adenoma can be diagnosed with a high degree of certainty. However, although specificities of 100% are reported, metastatic lesions from hepatocellular carcinomas, renal cell carcinoma and liposarcomas can contain lipid, and two cases of adrenocortical carcinomas containing microscopic amounts of fat showing areas of loss of signal intensity on chemical shift imaging were recently reported.[49]

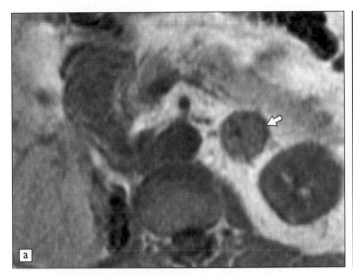 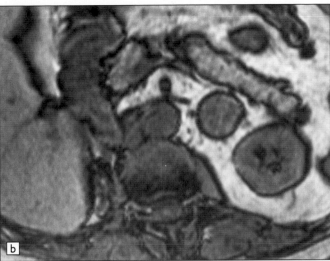

Figure 40.6. *Chemical-shift imaging to evaluate adrenal masses in patients with carcinoma. Adrenal metastases from a lung cancer. (a) In-phase chemical shift imaging (90° flip angle, TR = 150, TE = 4.2) shows a left adrenal mass of intermediate signal intensity (arrow). (b) Out-of-phase imaging (90° flip angle, TR = 150, TE = 2.3) showing that there has been no loss of signal intensity and that the presence of intercellular fat has not been demonstrated.*

However, in these cases signal loss was heterogeneous and not uniform. Conversely, it is probable that some functioning adenomas may contain insufficient lipid to result in loss of signal on out-of-phase imaging.[50] However, these would presumably be identified biochemically.

Nuclear scintigraphy

Nuclear scintigraphy using iodine-131-6-iodomethyl-19-nor-cholesterol (NP-59) has shown some potential in separating benign from malignant masses.[19,51] Benign adenomas take up cholesterol analogues such as NP-59, whereas metastases do not. However, haemorrhage or inflammatory masses do not take up NP-59 either, resulting in considerable overlap between benign and malignant processes.

Another promising technique for differentiating benign from malignant adrenal masses, is 2-[F-18]-fluoro-2-deoxy-D-glucose, (18-FDG) PET scanning. In a study of 20 patients 18-FDG PET scanning correctly differentiated all patients with benign non-hyperfunctioning adenomas from patients with metastases.[52] However, this technique may prove prohibitively expensive for routine use.

Percutaneous adrenal biopsy

Even with improved imaging and new techniques, such as chemical-shift MRI, a small percentage of adrenal masses, cannot be accurately characterized and require percutaneous biopsy for diagnosis. In a study of 33 patients with known malignancy, 48% were characterized as benign on CT and chemical-shift MRI. Forty-six percent were thought to be malignant. Only 5% were considered indeterminate on MRI and CT and required biopsy for diagnosis.[53] Minor complications of adrenal biopsy include abdominal pain, haematuria, nausea and small pneumothoraces. Major complications, generally regarded as those requiring treatment, occur in 2.8–3.6% of cases and include pneumothoraces requiring intervention, and haemorrhage, with isolated reports of adrenal abscesses, pancreatitis and seeding of metastases along the needle track.[54–57] The type of complication varies with the approach used, but does not appear to be related to needle size.[56,57] The reported accuracy ranges from 90–96%. One study showed accuracy was increased with the use of larger needles.[56]

Key points: adenoma versus metastases

- Size alone is poor at distinguishing between adenoma and a deposit (it is highly specific but insensitive)

- Bilateral adenomas are as common as bilateral metastases

- On CT, measurement of the attenuation value can identify adenomas with high specificity

- Chemical shift imaging can achieve 100% specificity in identifying adenomas

- CT/MRI reduces the need for biopsy of the adrenal gland, but as sensitivity in these techniques is lower than their specificity, biopsy or aspiration may still be necessary

NON-METASTATIC ADRENAL ENLARGEMENT

Diffuse adrenal enlargement without metastatic adrenal involvement has been demonstrated in patients with malignant disease, including lymphoma, not known to produce ectopic adrenocorticotrophic hormone (ACTH) (Figs 40.7a and b). The glands enlarge uniformly with preservation of the normal shape of the adrenal gland and without CT evidence of focal or multifocal masses. It is thought to be due to adrenal hyperplasia and is not related either to the site of primary disease or the stage of disease.[58] These patients can be shown not to suppress serum cortisol levels on a low dose dexamethasone-suppression test, indicating that they are biochemically Cushingoid. Nevertheless, the ACTH levels are low indicating that this phenomenon is not due to ectopic ACTH but is mediated through some other factor.

Summary

- The adrenal glands are a relatively frequent site of metastatic disease.

- Demonstration of adrenal metastases almost always indicates Stage-IV disease.

- Adrenal metastases have a variable appearance on CT and MRI.

- Adrenal metastases often have to be distinguished from other causes of adrenal masses, particularly benign cortical adenomas.

- Currently, non-invasive techniques (CT/MRI/scintigraphy) have a high specificity in confirming the presence of a benign adenoma.

- When an adrenal mass cannot be characterized as an adenoma, further more invasive investigation may be required.

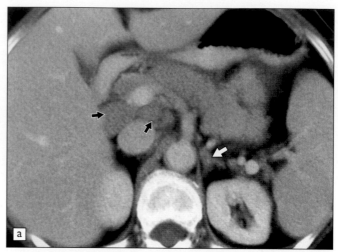

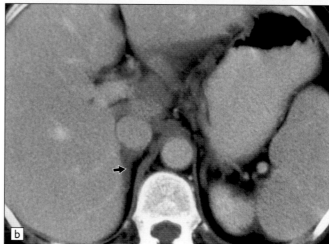

Figure 40.7. *Lymphadenopathy (black arrows in a) due to lymphoma with bilateral adrenal hyperplasia: (a) of the left (white arrow) and (b) of the right adrenal gland (black arrow). This patient failed to suppress on a low dose dexamethasone-suppression test but the ACTH level was undetectable indicating that the patient was biochemically Cushingoid and that this was not due to ectopic ACTH production.* .

REFERENCES

1. Abrahams H L, Spiro R, Goldstein N. Metastases in carcinoma. Cancer 1950; 3: 74–85

2. Cho S Y, Choi H Y. Causes of death and metastatic patterns in patients with mammary cancer. Am J Clin Pathol 1986; 73: 232–234

3. Sahagian-Edwards A, Holland J F. Metastatic carcinoma of the adrenal glands with cortical hypofunction. Cancer 1954; 7: 1242–1245

4. Das Gupta T, Brasfield R. Metastatic melanoma. A clinicopathological study. Cancer 1964; 17: 1323–1339

5. Cedermark B J, Blumenson L E, Pickren J W et al. The significance of metastases to the adrenal glands in adenocarcinoma of the colon and rectum. Surg Gynaecol Obstet 1977; 144: 537–546

6. Campbell C M, Middleton R G, Rigby O F. Adrenal metastases in renal cell carcinoma. Urology 1983; 21: 403–405

7. Moriya T, Manabe T, Yamashita K, Arita S. Lung cancer metastases to adrenocortical adenomas. A chance occurrence or a predilected phenomenon? Arch Pathol Lab Med 1988; 112: 286–289

8. McMahon R F. Tumour to tumour metastases: Bladder carcinoma metastasising to an adrenocortical adenoma. Br J Urol 1991; 67: 216–217

9. Travis W D, Oertel J E, Lack E E. Miscellaneous tumours and tumefaction lesions of the adrenal gland. In: Lack E E (ed) Pathology of the adrenal glands. New York: Churchill Livingstone 1990; 351 378

10. Allard P, Yankaskas B C, Fletcher R H, Parker L A, Halvorsen R A. Sensitivity and specificity of CT for the detection of adrenal metastatic lesions among 91 autopsied lung cancer patients. Cancer 1990; 66: 457–462

11. Pagani J J. Normal adrenal glands in small cell lung carcinoma: CT-guided biopsy. AJR 1983; 140: 949–951

12. Vincent J M, Morrison I D, Armstrong P, Reznek R H. The size of normal adrenal glands on computed tomography. Clin Radiol 1994; 49: 453–455

13. Gillams A, Roberts C M, Shaw P, Spiro S G, Goldstraw P. The value of CT scanning and percutaneous fine needle aspiration of adrenal masses in biopsy-proven lung cancer. Clin Radiol 1992; 46: 18–22

14. Reinig J W, Doppman J L, Dwyer A J, Johnson A R, Knop R H Adrenal masses differentiated by M R. Radiology 1986; 158: 81–84

15. Kier R, McCarthy S. M R characterization of adrenal masses: Field strength and pulse sequence considerations. Radiology 1989; 171: 671–674

16. Ghandur-Mnaymneh L, Slim M, Muakassa K. Adrenal cysts: Pathogenesis and histological identification with a report of 6 cases. J Urol 1979; 122: 87–91

17. Dunnick N R, Heaston D, Halvorsen R, Moore A V, Korobkin M. CT appearance of adrenal cortical carcinoma. J Comput Assist Tomogr 1982; 6: 978–982

18. Fishman E K, Deutch B M, Hartman D S et al. Primary adrenocortical carcinoma. CT evaluation with clinical correlation. Am J Roentgenol 1987; 148: 531–535

19. Manger W M, Gifford R W, Hoffman B B. Phaeochromocytoma: A clinical and experimental overview. Curr Probl Cancer 1985; 9: 1–89

20. Cyran K M, Kenney P J, Mernel D S, Yacoub I. Adrenal myelolipoma. Am J Roentgenol 1996; 166: 395–400

21. Oliver T W Jr, Bernardino M E, Miller J I et al. Isolated adrenal masses in nonsmall-cell bronchogenic carcinoma. Radiology 1984; 153, 217–218

22. Commons R R, Callaway C P. Adenomas of the adrenal cortex. Arch Intern Med 1984; 81: 37–41

23. Glazer H S, Weyman P J, Sagel S S, Levitt R S, McLennan B. Non-functioning adrenal masses: incidental discovery on computed tomography. Am J Roentgenol 1982; 139: 81–85

24. Ambos M A, Bosniak M A, Lefleur R S, Mitty H A Adrenal adenoma associated with renal cell carcinoma. Am J Roentgenol 1981; 136: 81–84

25. Doppman J L, Travis W D, Nieman L et al. Cushing syndrome due to primary pigmented nodular adreno-cortical disease: findings at CT and MR imaging. Radiology 1989; 172: 415–420

26. Gross M D, Wilton G P, Shapiro B et al. Functional and scintigraphic evaluation of the silent adrenal mass. J Nucl Med 1987; 28: 1401–1407

27. Candel A G, Gattuso P, Reyes C V, Prinz R A, Castelli M J Fine needle aspiration of adrenal masses in patients with extraadrenal malignancy. Surgery 1993; 114: 1132–1137

28. McGahan J P. Adrenal gland: MR imaging. Radiology 1988; 166: 284–285

29. Korobkin M, Brodeur F J, Yutzy G G et al. Differ-entiation of adrenal adenomas from nonadenomas using CT attenuation values. Am J Roentgenol 1996; 166: 531–536

30. Lee M J, Hahn P F, Papanicolaou N et al. Benign and malignant adrenal masses: CT distinction with attenuation coefficients, size, and observer analysis. Radiology 1991; 179: 415–418

31. van Erkel A R, van Gils A P G, Lequin M et al. CT and MR distinction of adenomas and nonadenomas of the adrenal gland. J Comput Assist Tomogr 1994; 18: 432–438

32. Korobkin M, Brodeur F J, Francis I R et al. Delayed enhanced CT for differentiation of benign from malignant adrenal masses. Radiology 1996; 200: 737–742

33. Boland G W, Hahn P F, Pena C, Mueller P R. Adrenal masses: Characterisation with delayed contrast-enhanced CT. Radiology 1997; 202: 693–696

34. Szolar P H, Kammerhuber F. Quantitative CT evaluation of adrenal gland masses: A step forward in the differentiation of adenomas and nonadenomas? Radiology 1997; 202: 517–521

35. Katz R L, Shirkhoda A Diagnostic approach to incidental adrenal nodules in the cancer patient. Cancer 1985; 55: 1995–2000

36. Chang A, Glazer H C, Lee J K T, Heiken J P. Adrenal gland M R imaging. Radiology 1987; 163: 123–128

37. Remer E M, Weinfeld R M, Glazer G M et al. Bookstein F L Hyperfunctioning and nonhyperfunctioning benign adrenal cortical lesions: characterization and comparison with MR imaging. Radiology 1989; 171: 681–685

38. Glazer G M, Woolsey E J, Borrello J et al. Adrenal tissue characterization using MR imaging. Radiology 1986; 158: 73–79

39. Baker M E, Spritzer C, Blinder R et al. Benign adrenal lesions mimicking malignancy on MR imaging: report of 2 cases. Radiology 1987; 163: 669–671

40. Krestin G P, Steinbrich W, Friedman G. Adrenal masses: Evaluation with fast gradient-echo MR imaging and Gd DTPA-enhanced dynamic studies. Radiology 1989; 171: 675–680

41. Krestin G P, Friedman G, Fischbach R, Neufang K F R, Allolio B. Evaluation of adrenal masses in oncologic patients: dynamic contrast-enhanced MR vs CT. J Comput Assist Tomogr 1991; 15: 104–110

42. Semelka R C, Shoenut J P, Lawrence P H et al. Evaluation of adrenal masses with gadolinium enhancement and fat-suppressed MR imaging. J Mag Res Imag 1993; 3: 332–343

43. Mitchell D G, Crovello M, Matteucci T, Petersen R O, Miettinen M M. Benign adrenocortical masses: diagnosis with chemical shift MR imaging. Radiology 1992; 185: 345–351

44. Tsushima Y, Ishizaka H, Matsumoto M. Adrenal masses: differentiation with chemical shift, fast low-angle shot MR imaging. Radiology 1993; 186: 705–709

45. Bilbey J H, McLoughlin R F, Kurkjian P S et al. MR imaging of adrenal masses: value of chemical-shift imaging for distinguishing adenomas from other tumors. Am J Roentgenol 1995; 164: 637–642

46. Mayo-Smith W W, Lee M J, McNicholas M M J et al. Characterization of adrenal masses (<5 cm) by use of chemical shift MR imaging: observer performance versus quantitative measures. Am J Roentgenol 1995; 165: 91–95

47. Korobkin M, Lombardi T J, Aisen A M et al. Characterization of adrenal masses with chemical shift and gadolinium-enhanced MR imaging. Radiology 1995; 197: 411–418

48. Schwartz L H, Panicek D M, Koutcher J A et al. Adrenal masses in patients with malignancy: Prospective comparison of echo-planar, fast spin-echo, and chemical shift MR imaging. Radiology 1995; 197: 421–425

49. Schlund J F, Kenney P J, Brown E D et al. Adrenocortical carcinoma: MR imaging appearance with current techniques. J MRI 1995; 5: 171–174

50. Tsushima Y. Different lipid contents between aldosterone-producing and nonhyperfunctioning adrenocortical adenomas: In vivo measurement using chemical shift MRI. J Clin Endo Metab 1994; 79: 1759–1762

51. Francis I R, Smid A, Gross M D et al. Adrenal masses in oncologic patients: Functional and morphological evaluation. Radiology 1988; 166: 353–356

52. Boland G W, Goldberg M A, Lee M J et al. The inde-terminate adrenal mass in patients with cancer: evaluation with fluorodeoxyglucose PET imaging. Radiology 1995; 194: 131–134

53. Nicholas M M J, Lee M J, Mayo-Smith W W et al. An imaging algorithm for the differential diagnosis of adrenal adenomas and metastases. Am J Roentgenol 1995; 165: 1453–1459

54. Habscheid W, Pfeiffer M, Demmrich J, Muller H A Metastases to the needle puncture track after ultrasound-guided fine needle adrenal biopsy. A rare complication? Dtsch Med Wochenschr 1990; 115: 212–215

55. Silverman S G, Mueler P R, Pinkney L P, Koenker R M, Seltzer S E Predictive value of image-guided adrenal biopsy: analysis of results of 101 biopsies. Radiology 1993; 187: 715–718

56. Welch T J, Sheedy P F, Stephens D H, Johnson C M, Swensen S J. Percutaneous adrenal biopsy: review of a 10-year experience. Radiology 1994; 193: 341–344

57. Mody M K, Kazerooni E A, Korobkin M. Percutaneous CT-guided biopsy of adrenal masses: immediate and delayed complications. J Comput Assist Tomogr 1995; 19: 434–439

58. Vincent J M, Morrison I D, Armstrong P, Reznek R H. Computed tomography of diffuse, non-metastatic enlargement of the adrenal glands in patients with malignant disease. Clin Radiol 1994; 49: 456–460

Chapter 41

Peritoneum

Jeremiah Healy and Rodney Reznek

INTRODUCTION

The peritoneal cavity is the potential space between the visceral and parietal layers of the peritoneum, which consists of a main region, termed the greater sac, and a diverticulum, the omental bursa or lesser sac, situated behind the stomach. In early foetal life as the abdominal cavity divides into the retroperitoneum and peritoneum, the parietal peritoneum is reflected over the peritoneal organs to form a series of supporting ligaments, mesenteries and omenta. These peritoneal reflections act as a natural connecting pathway for the dissemination of intra-abdominal disease within the peritoneum, but also for extension of disease from the retroperitoneum to structures enveloped by peritoneum, via the subperitoneal space.[1]

The anatomy of the peritoneum can therefore be considered as a system of spaces and peritoneal reflections that can be used as conduits for spread of metastatic disease, which is the most common malignant process involving the peritoneum (Fig. 41.1). Metastases are usually from intra-abdominal primary neoplasms, such as carcinoma of the stomach, colon, ovary and pancreas, or from intra-abdominal lymphoma.

Prior to the advent of CT, peritoneal metastases were not radiographically detectable until late in the disease, when they displaced adjacent organs, caused intestinal obstruction, or produced radiological signs due to massive ascites on plain films. Computed tomography can identify peritoneal metastases as small as a few millimetres in size and also identify very small volumes of ascites. This information is essential in staging tumours, assessing resectability, monitoring response, and identifying recurrence.

IMAGING TECHNIQUES

Computed tomography

Computed tomography is the best imaging procedure for the evaluation of patients with known or suspected peritoneal metastases. The use of intraperitoneal positive contrast and pneumoperitoneum with CT has been suggested to improve the detection of small peritoneal metastases but these techniques do not routinely opacify all the peritoneal recesses.[2–4] These methods are more interventional and time consuming and consequently are not used widely.

Barium studies

Barium studies provide only indirect signs of peritoneal and mesenteric disease and thus are not used initially. However, a barium study will occasionally reveal abnormalities related to peritoneal metastases not clearly demonstrated on CT.

Magnetic resonance imaging

Recent reports describe the use of MR imaging in identifying peritoneal implants.[5,6] Magnetic resonance imaging of the peritoneum has been most successfully achieved using fat-saturated T1-weighted sequences following intravenous gadolinium.[7] However, at present, the inferior spatial resolution, the problems of motion artefact related to respiration and bowel peristalsis, and the lack of an effective bowel opacification agent makes MR imaging a much less accurate test than CT for the identification of peritoneal metastases.

Ultrasound

Ultrasound will demonstrate superficial peritoneal and omental metastases as small as 2–3 mm in the presence of ascites. However, centrally located deposits, for example in the small bowel mesentery, will not be visualized because of the acoustic impedance of bowel gas and fat.[8,9]

Scintigraphy

Scintigraphy has also been used to identify peritoneal metastases but is not very sensitive or specific and needs CT for anatomical location.[10]

Key points: imaging techniques

- Although the sensitivity of CT in detecting peritoneal metastases is less than 50%, the specificity exceeds 85%

- At present, MR is less sensitive than CT for the detection of peritoneal metastases

- Although ultrasound can detect extremely small peritoneal deposits in the presence of ascites, centrally located deposits (e.g. in the small bowel mesentery) will usually be obscured

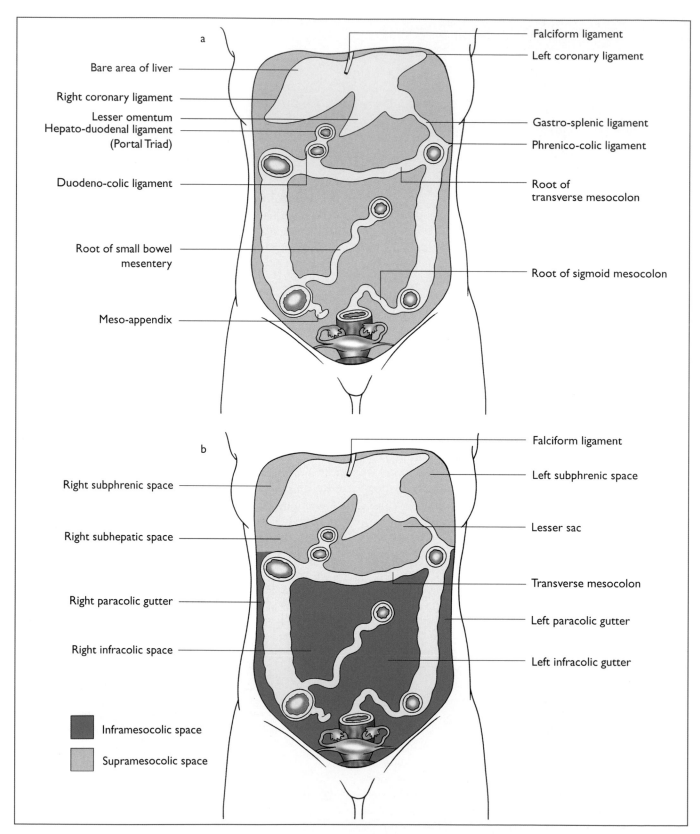

Figure 41.1. *Diagrammatic representation of the peritoneal anatomy. (a) Coronal view of the peritoneal attachments to the abdominal wall. (b) Coronal view of the posterior peritoneal spaces.*

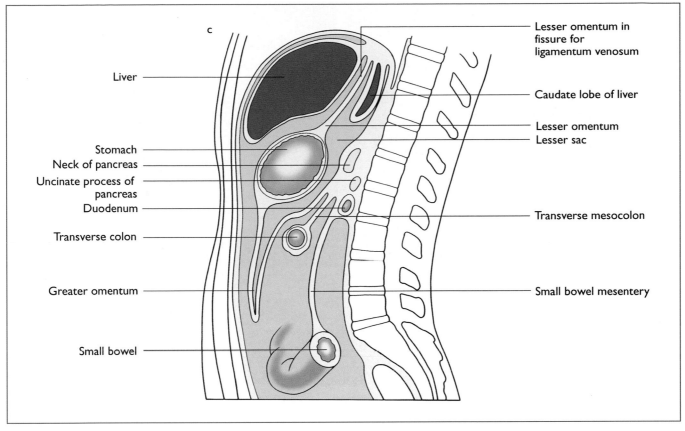

Liver

Stomach
Neck of pancreas
Uncinate process of pancreas
Duodenum

Transverse colon

Greater omentum

Small bowel

Lesser omentum in fissure for ligamentum venosum

Caudate lobe of liver

Lesser omentum
Lesser sac

Transverse mesocolon

Small bowel mesentery

Figure 41.1. *(cont.) (c) Midsagittal section through the upper abdomen to show the peritoneal spaces and mesenteries.*

MODES OF SPREAD AND IMAGING APPEARANCES

Metastases spread throughout the peritoneum in four ways:

- Directly along peritoneal ligaments, mesenteries and omenta to non-contiguous structures
- Intraperitoneal seeding via the flow of ascitic fluid
- Lymphatic extension
- Embolic haematogenous spread[11]

Direct spread
Direct invasion from primary tumours to non-contiguous organs occurs along the peritoneal reflections (Figs. 41.1b and c). These include:

- Eight ligaments — the right and left coronary, falciform, hepatoduodenal, duodenocolic, gastrosplenic, splenorenal and phrenicocolic ligaments
- Four mesenteries — the small bowel mesentery, the transverse mesocolon, the sigmoid mesocolon, and the meso-appendix
- Two omenta — the lesser and greater omentum[11,12]

Spread along these peritoneal reflections is commonly seen with malignant neoplasms of the stomach, colon, pancreas and ovary.

Appearances on CT
Carcinoma of the stomach often spreads directly into the left lobe of the liver via the lesser omentum, extending between the lesser curvature of the stomach and the liver (Figs. 41.1b and c and Fig. 41.2a).[13] Computed tomography shows loss of the fat plane between these two organs.[14] Direct spread from retroperitoneal tumours, such as carcinoma of the pancreas, into the liver can occur along the hepatoduodenal ligament, which is the free edge of the lesser omentum, extending from the junction of the first and second parts of the duodenum to the porta hepatis. The portal vein, hepatic artery and common bile duct are found within this ligament (Fig. 41.1b).[15,16] Biliary and hepatic malignancies can also spread in the reverse direction to the stomach and pancreas via the lesser omentum and hepatoduodenal ligaments. On CT these masses are often hypervascular and may have low attenuation centrally due to central necrosis.[17,18]

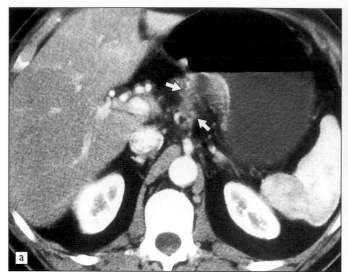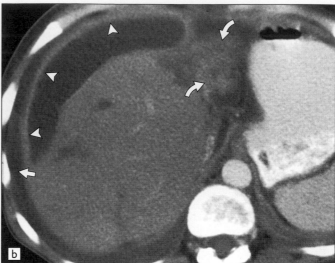

Figure 41.2. *Metastatic deposits in the lesser omentum. (a) Axial postcontrast CT scan in a 59-year-old male with gastric cancer showing extension of gastric cancer into the lesser omental fat (arrows); (b) axial postcontrast CT scan in a 41-* *year-old female with carcinoma of the ovary showing a large metastatic deposit in the lesser omentum (curved arrows). Note also ascites with marked uniform peritoneal thickening (arrowheads) and a right pleural effusion (straight arrow).*

Neoplasms of the colon, stomach, and pancreas often use the transverse mesocolon and greater omentum as conduits for spread (Figs. 41.1b and c).

The transverse mesocolon suspends the transverse colon within the peritoneal cavity, passing anterior to the descending duodenum and pancreas (Figs. 41.1b and c). It is continuous in the left upper quadrant with the splenorenal and phrenicocolic ligaments (Fig. 41.1b). Direct invasion is well demonstrated on CT as increased density or discrete soft tissue masses in the fat of the transverse mesocolon. The right hand margin of the transverse mesocolon is thickened as the duodenocolic ligament providing a direct route for extension of colonic cancer from the hepatic flexure to the duodenum.[19,20]

The greater omentum extends from the greater curve of the stomach and suspends the transverse colon (Fig. 41.1c). On CT early involvement of the greater omentum produces increased density within the fat adjacent to the primary neoplasm (Fig. 41.3a). Subsequently, masses contiguous with the primary neoplasm may be seen extending into the greater omentum, producing 'omental caking', which separates the colon from the anterior abdominal wall (Figs. 41.3c and d). Spread of metastatic disease along the left hand margin of the greater omentum stops abruptly at the phrenicocolic ligament, extending from the splenic flexure to the diaphragm. It marks the point at which the mesenteric transverse colon becomes the extraperitoneal descending colon.

In the left upper quadrant the gastrosplenic ligament (Fig. 41.1b), continuous with the greater omentum, extends from the greater curve of the stomach to the spleen. It can be involved by extramural spread from gastric cancer and explains the association of splenic abscess with this tumour, often seen on CT.[21]

Direct involvement of the small bowel mesentery is commonly seen in carcinoid (Figs. 41.4a and b), lymphoma, pancreatic, breast and colonic metastases.

The root of the small bowel mesentery is approximately 15 cm long extending from the pancreas to the right iliac fossa (Figs. 41.1b and c). Spread from the retroperitoneum, via the subperitoneal space, to the small bowel is frequently seen in lymphoma. On CT, this produces soft tissue thickening within the mesenteric fat, perivascular encasement, and tethering of the bowel.

Appearances on barium studies

Direct invasion along the transverse mesocolon from pancreatic cancer produces tethering and pseudosacculation of the posterior–inferior margin of the colon on barium studies. This is because the transverse mesocolon inserts into the taenia mesocolica on the inferior margin of the colon. Direct spread of gastric cancer along the greater omentum causes similar appearances along the superior haustral margin of the transverse colon, as the greater omentum inserts superiorly into the taenia omentalis.[22]

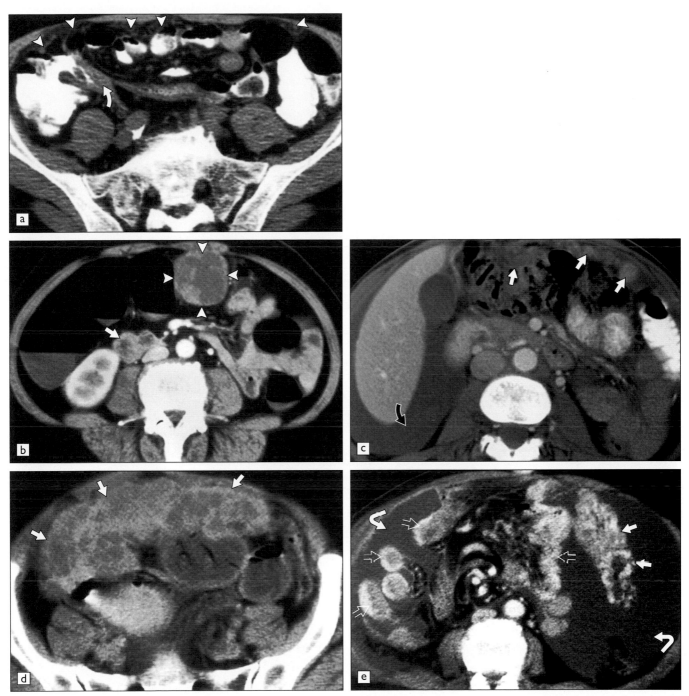

Figure 41.3. *Metastatic deposits in the greater omentum. (a) Axial CT scan in a 42-year-old male with a carcinoid tumour of the terminal ileum (curved arrow) showing minimal nodular and linear deposits in the greater omental fat (arrowheads); (b) postcontrast axial CT scan in a 65-year-old female with carcinoma of the ovary showing a well-defined, round mass in the greater omentum, with fluid attenuation centrally (arrowheads). Note also precaval enlarged lymphadenopathy (arrow); (c) postcontrast axial CT scan in a 49-year-old female with carcinoma of the ovary showing several nodular, ill-defined masses in the greater omentum anterior to the colon (white arrows). Note also the ascites surrounding the right lobe of the liver (black arrow); (d) axial postcontrast CT scan in a 66-year-old female with adenocarcinoma of the bowel showing a bulky, 'cake-like', enhancing omental deposit (arrows); (e) axial postcontrast CT scan in a 65-year-old male patient with renal carcinoma showing markedly enhancing deposits within the greater omentum (straight white arrows) surrounded by ascites (curved arrows). Note also the enhancing serosal deposits on the surface of the bowel (open arrows).*

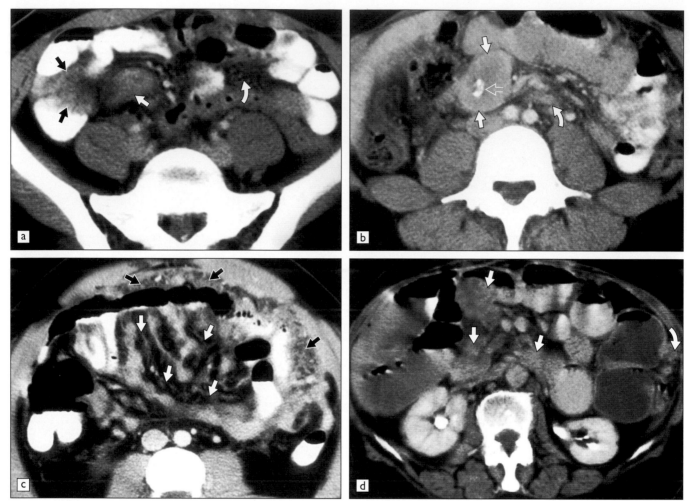

Figure 41.4. *Small bowel mesenteric deposits. (a) Postcontrast axial CT scan in a 28-year-old female with carcinoid tumour of the terminal ileum (straight black arrows). Note the large mesenteric mass at the root of the small bowel mesentery (straight white arrow) and linear soft tissue stranding in the small bowel mesenteric fat elsewhere (curved white arrow); (b) the same patient as in (a) demonstrating a mesenteric deposit (straight arrows) containing calcification (open arrow). There are also ill-defined masses elsewhere within the mesenteric fat (curved arrow); (c) axial postcontrast CT scan in a 70-year-old male with adenocarcinoma of the colon showing soft tissue thickening around the perivascular bundles (white arrows). In addition note the ill-defined omental 'cake' in the greater omentum (black arrows); (d) axial postcontrast CT scan in a 62-year-old female with ovarian cancer showing multiple ill-defined deposits within the small bowel mesentery (straight arrows). Note also ill-defined deposits in the left paracolic gutter (curved arrow).*

Intraperitoneal seeding

Intraperitoneal fluid is constantly circulating throughout the abdomen influenced by gravity and negative intra-abdominal pressure, produced beneath the diaphragm during respiration. It allows transcoelomic dissemination of malignant cells, their deposition, fixation and growth are encouraged in particular sites due to relative stasis of ascitic fluid.[23]

The most common tumours to spread in this fashion include ovarian cancer in females and malignancies of the gastro-intestinal tract in males, especially cancer of the stomach, colon, and pancreas.

The sites most commonly involved by peritoneal seeding are (Fig. 41.1a):

- The pelvis, especially the pouch of Douglas
- The right lower quadrant at the inferior junction of the small bowel mesentery
- The superior aspect of the sigmoid mesocolon
- The right paracolic gutter[23]

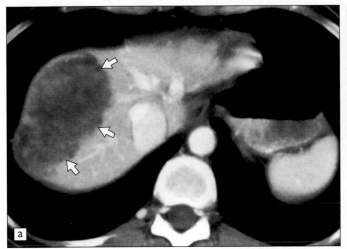 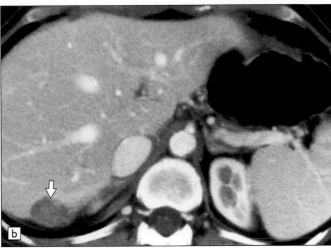

Figure 41.5. *Intraperitoneal seeding producing metastatic deposits on the surface of the liver in a 52-year-old female with carcinoma of the ovary. (a) Postcontrast CT scan shows a large low density ill-defined deposit on the superior surface of the liver (arrows); (b) this is associated with a low density cystic deposit in Morison's pouch (arrow).*

Spread of deposits to the right subhepatic and subphrenic spaces is also frequently seen, especially in ovarian cancer. Almost 90% of patients with ovarian cancer have peritoneal implants at postmortem and 60–70% have ascites.[24,25]

CT appearances

On CT, seeded metastases appear as nodular or plaque-like soft tissue masses in association with ascites. Intraperitoneal deposits as small as 5 mm can be identified, even in the presence of small amounts of ascites.[26–28] Rounded or oval low-density deposits on the surface of the liver are frequently seen on CT in ovarian cancer (Figs. 41.5a and b).[29] These are generally of 0.5–1 cm diameter located on the dorsomedial and dorsolateral parts of the right lobe of the liver and often associated with deposits in Morison's pouch (Fig. 41.5b). It is presumed that these deposits infiltrate the liver capsule following their deposition on the liver surface. The parietal peritoneum may be diffusely involved producing smooth (Fig. 41.2b) or nodular thickening (Fig. 41.6a) on CT which often enhances (Fig. 41.6b).[30] Peritoneal calcification is also frequently seen on CT with serous cystadenocarcinoma of the ovary (Fig. 41.6c), carcinoid tumour, and rarely with gastric carcinoma.[31–33]

A distinctive CT appearance is produced by pseudomyxoma peritonei, resulting from the rupture of a mucinous cystadenocarcinoma or cystadenoma of the ovary or appendix (Figs. 41.7a and b). The gelatinous nature of the deposits produces a mantle of low-density material over the surface of the liver, causing scalloping of its margin, in association with cystic peritoneal collections (Fig. 41.7a). The walls of the cystic collections may contain calcification. The pressure of the gelatinous material prevents the bowel loops floating up towards the anterior abdominal wall, which may be a useful sign in differentiating pseudomyxoma peritonei from ascites (Fig. 41.7b).[34]

The small bowel mesentery and greater omentum are frequently involved by intraperitoneal seeding of metastases. Four patterns of involvement are described on CT: round masses (Fig. 41.3b), 'cake-like' masses (Figs. 41.3c and d), ill-defined masses (Figs. 41.4c and d), and stellate masses.[35]

Irregular, 'cake-like' masses are seen most often with ovarian cancer.[36] Densely calcified omental 'cake' has been reported in metastatic serous cystadenocarcinoma.[37] The stellate pattern of mesenteric or omental mass is seen with pancreatic, colonic and breast cancer and results from diffuse infiltration, causing thickening and rigidity of the perivascular bundles (Fig. 41.4c). Widespread peritoneal metastases, including omental infiltration is a rare consequence of retroperitoneal malignancy, such as renal cell carcinoma (Figs. 41.3e and 41.6b).[38]

Metastatic deposits to the ovaries from gastric or colonic primary tumours in association with ascites and other peritoneal deposits are a well-recognized entity. These tumours, known as 'Krukenberg' tumours, are presumed to be a consequence of transcoelomic spread and are clearly visualized on CT.[39]

Appearances on barium studies

Metastatic seeding in the pouch of Douglas produces a characteristic nodular mucosal impression on barium enema, with associated mucosal tethering on the ventral aspect of the rectosigmoid junction.

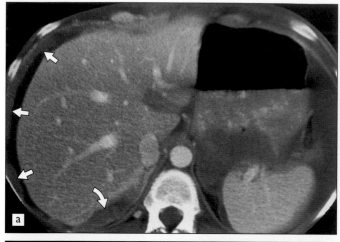

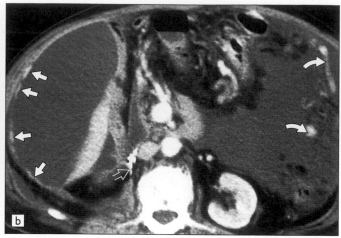

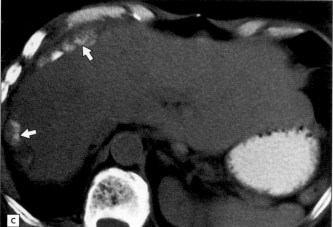

Figure 41.6. *Peritoneal metastases. (a) Postcontrast CT scan in a 49-year-old female with carcinoma of the ovary demonstrating nodular parietal peritoneal thickening (straight arrows), in association with a deposit in Morison's pouch (curved arrow), and ascites; (b) postcontrast CT scan in the same patient as in Figure 41.3e. Note the clips from previous renal surgery (open arrow). Multiple enhancing peritoneal metastases are outlined by ascites (straight arrows). Note also enhancing deposits in the greater omental fat (curved arrows); (c) CT scan in a 66-year-old female with carcinoma of the ovary showing calcified peritoneal metastases (arrows).*

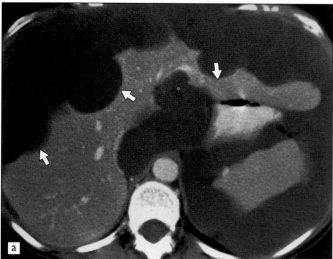

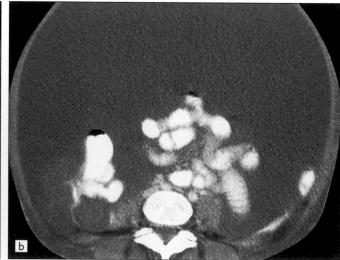

Figure 41.7. *Pseudomyxoma peritonei in mucinous cystadenocarcinoma of the appendix in a 44-year-old female. (a) Axial postcontrast CT scan shows low-density deposits producing scalloping of the liver margin (arrows). (b) The pressure of the gelatinous material prevents bowel loops floating up towards the anterior abdominal wall.*

Metastatic seeding in the small bowel mesentery, especially in the right infracolic space can produce separation of small bowel loops in a parallel configuration, known as 'pallisading', on barium follow-through studies. Marked bowel angulation and mucosal tethering is also seen if the deposits stimulate a desmoplastic response, which is commonly seen with pancreatic carcinoma and mucin secreting gastric carcinoma.

Lymphatic metastases

Lymphatic metastases play a minor role in the intraperitoneal dissemination of metastatic carcinoma, but is very important in the spread of lymphoma to mesenteric lymph nodes. Almost 50% of patients with non-Hodgkin's lymphoma will have mesenteric nodes at presentation, compared to only 5% of patients with Hodgkin's disease.[40] On CT, mesenteric lymph node involvement in lymphoma produces round or oval masses in the mesenteric fat, which may displace adjacent loops of bowel.[35] Large conglomerations of lymph nodes may surround the superior mesenteric artery and vein on CT and demonstrate the so-called sandwich sign where lymphomatous mesenteric masses are separated from retroperitoneal lymphadenopathy by an intact anterior pararenal fat plane.[41]

Embolic metastases

The abdomen is a common site for haematogenous metastases from both intra-abdominal and extra-abdominal primary tumours. The tumour emboli spread via the mesenteric arteries to deposit on the antimesenteric border of the bowel in the smallest arterial branches, where they grow into mural nodules.

The most common tumours that metastasize embolically to bowel and the peritoneal reflections are melanoma, breast and lung cancer. These metastases often occur several years after treatment of the primary neoplasm. Occasionally bowel obstruction or intussusception, as a consequence of embolic metastases, may be the first manifestation of an occult malignancy.

CT appearances

On CT, embolic metastases may produce thickening of the bowel wall, which is often asymmetric with associated ulceration, and thickening of the adjacent bowel wall.[42] They may also appear as well-defined round masses within the peritoneal fat (Fig. 41.8). Embolic metastases to the stomach from breast cancer, produce marked gastric wall thickening with almost complete obliteration of its lumen, an appearance that is indistinguishable from primary schirrous gastric carcinoma or lymphoma.[43]

Appearances on barium studies

On barium studies embolic metastases produce a 'bull's-eye' appearance due to their submucosal site. Their borders are usually well-defined with central ulceration and sometimes linear fissuring gives a 'spokewheel' pattern. They grow eccentrically with bulky extension into the lumen of the bowel. Larger lesions may undergo necrosis to produce apparent aneurysmal dilatation of the bowel.[44] Embolic metastases to the stomach from breast produce a 'linitis plastica' appearance, with thickened and angulated gastric folds and diminished or absent peristalsis.

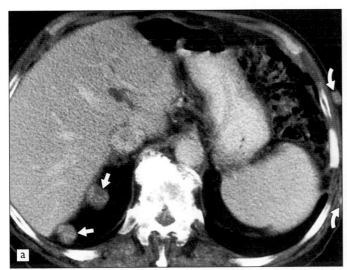

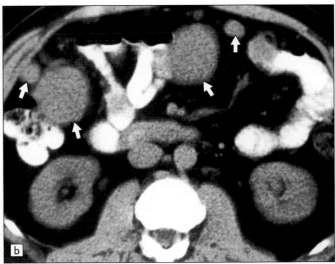

Figure 41.8. *Embolic metastases. (a) Postcontrast CT scan in a 60-year-old male with malignant melanoma showing well-defined embolic deposits in Morison's pouch (straight arrows). Note the subcutaneous melanomatous deposits in the left flank (curved arrow); (b) CT scan in a 40-year-old male with leiomyosarcoma of the retroperitoneum showing multiple well-defined soft tissue masses adjacent to the bowel in the mesenteric fat (arrows).*

Key points: methods of spread

- Malignant spread to the peritoneum occurs directly along peritoneal ligaments, mesenteries and omenta, through seeding via the flow of ascitic fluid, via lymphatic extension and haematogenously

- Seeding of cells most commonly occurs in the pelvis (especially the pouch of Douglas), at the inferior junction of the small bowel mesentery, the superior aspect of the sigmoid mesocolon and the right paracolic gutter

- Embolic metastases to bowel and peritoneal reflections occur most commonly in tumours arising in the breast and lung and in malignant melanoma

- Lymphatic spread plays only a small role in spread of malignant disease to the peritoneum and its reflections

Accuracy of CT in identifying peritoneal metastases

The CT identification of peritoneal metastases has been correlated with second-look laparotomy. The specificity of CT for the diagnosis of peritoneal metastases is high ranging from 85–87%; however, its sensitivity is low, ranging from 42 to 47%.[45,46] Laparoscopy has also demonstrated a significant incidence of peritoneal metastases in patients with a negative CT scan. Notably if ascites is present but no peritoneal deposits are seen on CT, laparoscopy demonstrated deposits in 75% of cases.[47]

Summary

- Dynamic factors affect the flow of peritoneal fluid determining the eventual site of peritoneal metastases.

- A clear understanding of the peritoneal anatomy is necessary for the identification of peritoneal metastatic disease and will aid identification of the primary tumour.

- Metastases disseminate throughout the peritoneum in four ways: (1) direct spread along peritoneal ligaments, mesenteries and omenta; (2) intraperitoneal seeding via the flow of ascitic fluid; (3) lymphatic extension, and (4) embolic haematogenous spread.

- Peritoneal metastases are usually from intra-abdominal primary neoplasms, such as carcinoma of the stomach, colon, ovary and pancreas, or from intra-abdominal lymphoma. The site and nature of the primary tumour facilitate a particular direction and method of spread.

- Although CT is quite specific in identifying peritoneal metastases it is not very sensitive.

- Despite its limitations CT is the imaging procedure of choice for evaluating patients known to have, or suspected of having peritoneal metastases. It is essential in staging tumours, assessing resectability, monitoring response and identifying recurrence.

REFERENCES

1. Oliphant M, Berne A S, Meyers M A. The subperitoneal space of the abdomen and pelvis: Planes of continuity. Am J Radiol 1996; 167: 1433–1439

2. Halvorsen R A, Panushka C, Oakley G J et al. Intraperitoneal contrast material improves the CT detection of peritoneal metastases. Am J Radiol 1991; 157: 37–40

3. Nelson R C, Chezmar J L, Hoel M J, Buck D R, Sugarbaker P H. Peritoneal carcinomatosis: Preoperative CT with intraperitoneal contrast material. Radiology 1992; 182: 133–138

4. Caseiro-Alves F, Goncalo M, Abraul E et al. Induced pneumoperitoneum in CT evaluation of peritoneal carcinomatosis. Abdom Imaging 1995; 20: 52–55

5. Chou C K, Liu G C, Chen L T et al. MRI manifestations of peritoneal carcinomatosis. Gastrointest Radiol 1992; 17: 336–338

6. Chou C-K, Liu G-C, Su J-H et al. MRI demonstration of peritoneal implants. Abdominal Imaging 1994; 19: 95

7. Semelka R C, Lawrence P H, Shoenut J P et al. Primary ovarian cancer: Prospective comparison of contrast enhanced CT and pre and post contrast, fat suppressed MR imaging, with histologic correlation. J Mag Res Imaging 1993; 3: 99–106

8. Derchi L E, Solbiati L, Rizziatto G et al. Normal anatomy and pathologic changes of the small bowel mesentery: US appearance. Radiology 1987; 164: 649–652

9. Goerg C, Schwerk W-B. Malignant ascites: Sonographic signs of peritoneal carcinomatosis. Eur J Cancer 1991; 27: 720–723

10. Carrasquillo J A, Sugarbaker P, Colcher D et al. Peritoneal carcinomatosis: Imaging with intraperitoneal injection of I-131-labelled B72.3 monoclonal antibody. Radiology 1988; 167: 35–40

11. Meyers M A, Oliphant M, Berne M S et al. The peritoneal ligaments and mesenteries: Pathways of intra-abdominal spread of disease. Annual oration. Radiology 1987; 163: 593–604

12. Oliphant M, Berne A, Meyers M A. Subperitoneal spread of intra-abdominal disease. In: Myers M A (ed) Computed tomography of the gastrointestinal tract including the peritoneal cavity and mesentery. New York: Springer Verlag, 1986; 95–137

13. Balfe D M, Mauro M A, Kooehler R E et al. Gastrohepatic ligament: Normal and pathologic CT anatomy. Radiology 1984; 150: 485–490

14. Dehn C B, Reznek R H, Nockler B et al. The preoperative assessment of advanced gastric cancer by computed tomography. Br J Surg 1984; 71: 413–417

15. Weinstein J B, Heiken J P, Lee J K T et al. High resolution CT of the porta hepatis and hepatoduodenal ligament. Radiographics 1986; 6(1): 55–73

16. Baker M E, Silverman P M, Halvorsen R A et al. Computed tomography of masses in periportal/hepatoduodenal ligament. J Comput Assist Tomogr 1987; 11: 258–263

17. Kim T K, Han J K, Chung J W et al. Intraperitoneal drop metastases from hepatocellular carcinoma: CT and angiographic findings. J Comput Assist Tomogr 1996; 20(4): 638–642

18. Ohtani T, Shirai Y, Tsukada K, Muto T, Hatakeyama K. Spread of gallbladder carcinoma: CT evaluation with pathologic correlation. Abdom Imaging 1996; 21(3): 195–201

19. Diamond R T, Greenberg H M, Boult I F. Direct metastatic spread of right colonic adenocarcinoma to duodenum: Barium and computed tomography findings. Gastrointest Radiol 1981; 6: 339–341

20. Mc Daniel K P, Charnsangavej C, Du Brow R A et al. Pathways of nodal metasases in carcinomas of the cecum, ascending colon, and transverse colon. CT demonstration. Am J Radiol 1993; 160: 49–52

21. Chun C H, Raff M F, Conteras L et al. Splenic abscess. Medicine (Baltimore) 1980; 59: 50–65

22. Meyers M A, Volberg F, Katzen B et al. Haustral anatomy and physiology: A new look II. Roentgen interpretation of pathologic alterations. Radiology 1973; 108: 505–512

23. Meyers M A. Distribution of intraabdominal malignant seeding: Dependency on dynamics of flow of ascitic fluid. Am J Radiol 1973; 119: 198–206

24. Bergman F. Carcinoma of the ovary: A clinicopathological study of 86 autopsied cases with special reference to mode of spread. Acta Obstet Gynaecol 1966; 45: 211–231

25. Dagnini G, Marin G, Caldironin M W et al. Laparoscopy in staging, follow-up, and re-staging ovarian carcinoma. Gastrointest Endoscop 1987; 33: 80–83

26. Jeffrey R B Jr. CT demonstration of peritoneal implants. Am J Radiol 1980; 135: 323–326

27. Buy J-N, Moss A A, Ghossain M A et al. Peritoneal implants from ovarian tumours: CT findings. Radiology 1988; 169: 691–694

28. Megibow A J, Bosniak M A, Ho A G et al. Accuracy CT in detection of persistent or recurrent ovarian carcinoma: Correlation with second look laparotomy. Radiology 1988; 166: 341–354

29. Triller J, Goldnirsch A, Reinhard J-P. Subscapular liver metastases in ovarian cancer: Computed tomography and surgical staging. Eur J Radiol 1985; 5: 261–266

30. Walkey MM, Friedman AC, Sohotra P et al. CT manifestations of peritoneal carcinomatosis. Am J Radiol 1988; 150: 1035–1041

31. Mitchell D G, Hill M C, Hill S et al. Serous carcinoma of the ovary: CT identification of metastatic calcified implants. Radiology 1986; 158: 649–652

32. Matsuoka K, Okuhira M, Nonaka T et al. Calcification of peritoneal carcinomatosis from gastric carcinoma: A CT demonstration. Eur J Radiol 1991; 13: 207–208

33. Woodard P K, Feldman J M, Paine S S, Baker M E. Midgut carcinoid tumours: CT findings and biochemical profiles. J Comput Assist Tomogr 1995; 19: 400–405

34. Seshul M B, Coulam C M. Pseudomyxoma peritonei: Computed tomography and sonography. Am J Radiol 1981; 136: 803–806

35. Whitley N O, Bohlman M E, Baker L P. CT patterns of mesenteric disease. J Comput Assist Tomogr 1982; 6: 490–496

36. Cooper C, Jeffrey R B, Silverman P M et al. Computed tomography of omental pathology. J Comput Assist Tomogr 1986; 10: 62–66

37. Pandolfo I, Blandino A, Gaeta M et al. Calcified peritoneal metastases from papillary cystadenocarcinoma of the ovary: CT features. J Comput Assist Tomogr 1986; 10: 545–546

38. Tartar V M, Heiken J P, McClellan B L. Renal cell carcinoma presenting with diffuse peritoneal metastases: CT findings. J Comput Assist Tomogr 1991; 15(3): 450–453

39. Cho K C, Gold B M. Computed Tomography of Krukenberg tumours. Am J Radiol 1985; 145: 285–288

40. Goffinet D R, Castellino R A, Kim H et al. Staging laparotomies in unselected patients with non-Hodgkin's lymphoma. Cancer 1973; 32: 672–681

41. Mueller P R, Ferrucci J T Jr, Harbin W P et al. Appearance of lymphomatous involvement of the mesentery by ultrasonography and body computed tomography: the 'sandwich sign'. Radiology 1980; 134: 467–473

42. Kawashima A, Fishman E K, Kuhlman J E et al. CT of malignant melanoma: Patterns of small bowel and mesenteric involvement. J Comput Assist Tomogr 1991; 15(4): 570–574

43. Caskey C I, Scatarige J C, Fishman E K. Distribution of metastases in breast carcinoma. CT evaluation of the abdomen. Clin Imaging 1991; 15: 166–171

44. Oddson T A, Rice R R P, Seiler H F et al. The spectrum of small bowel melanoma. Gastrointest Radiol 1978; 3: 419–423

45. Pectasides D, Kayianni H, Facou A et al. Correlation of abdominal computed tomography scanning and second look operation findings in ovarian cancer patients. Am J Clin Oncol 1991; 14: 457–462

46. De-Rosa V, Mangoni-di-Stefano M L, Brunetti A et al. Computed tomography and second-look surgery in ovarian cancer patients. Correlation, actual role and limitations of CT scan. Eur J Gynaecol Oncol 1995; 16: 123–129

47. Brady P G, Peebles M, Goldschmid S. Role of laparoscopy in the evaluation of patients with suspected hepatic or peritoneal malignancy. Gastointest Endosc 1991; 37: 27–30

Chapter 42

Radiological investigation of carcinoma of unknown primary site

Christopher Gallagher, Rodney Reznek and Janet Husband

INTRODUCTION

Cancer of unknown primary site is a common referral problem accounting for between 3–9% of all patients seen in most tertiary treatment centres.[1–3] In the population as a whole, as estimated by the SEER (Surveillance Epidemiology and End Results) statistics, in the US 2% of cancers were registered as cancer of unknown primary site. Of these, adenocarcinoma comprised 55%, squamous carcinoma 14%, cancer undifferentiated 21% and 10% other specific diagnoses such as sarcoma, neuro-endocrine cancer and melanoma.[4]

Patients present with the symptoms of their metastases without a clinically apparent primary site. The frequency of the site of presentation of the metastases vary, in part due to differences in patient selection in the reported series. However, the most common sites of presentation (excluding head and neck) are as shown in Table 42.1.[1,2]

The *definition* of what constitutes a (metastatic) cancer of unknown primary site has shifted over the years with the changes in histological and radiological investigations. Thus in the earlier clinical series most will have simply had a careful history, physical examination and chest X-ray. However,

in one recent series[5] one-third of the patients had already had a chest computed tomography (CT) scan, one-half an abdominal CT scan, one-third a pelvic CT scan and 15% a mammogram before referral for investigation of the unknown primary site. Even after postmortem examination the primary site will remain unknown in approximately 15–20% of patients diagnosed as having cancer of unknown primary site in life.[6,7]

HISTOLOGY

The most critical step in the assessment of any patient with cancer of unknown primary site is a review of the histological findings from which three main groups can be derived:[8]

- Adenocarcinoma (50–60%)
- Squamous (5%)
- Poorly differentiated (35%)
    Lymphoma (6%)
    Germ cell (1%)
    Melanoma, sarcoma, neuro-endocrine (1%)

The most common histological type is that of adenocarcinoma comprising 50–60% of patients in all series. Squamous carcinomas are present in 5% although perhaps under represented by the exclusion of head and neck cancers from some series. Poorly differentiated cancers comprise the final 35% of patients and are an important group containing those patients with the most highly treatable cancers. Careful histological and immunocytochemical review can identify chemotherapy-curable lymphoma in 6% and atypical germ cell tumours in 1%. Other specific histologies such as melanoma, sarcoma and poorly differentiated neuro-endocrine tumours[9] are identified in a further 1%. It is not proposed in this chapter to discuss further the investigation of patients with specific histological types but rather to concentrate on patients with squamous and adenocarcinoma.

Table 42.1. *Common sites of presentation of metastases (%)*

Lymph nodes	14–37
Thorax	28–30
Lung	28
Pleura	2–12
Abdomen/pelvis	
Liver	19–31
Adrenal	6
Other	15
Bone	16–28
CNS	8
Skin	2

SQUAMOUS CARCINOMA OF UNKNOWN ORIGIN

Most patients with squamous carcinoma of unknown primary present with cervical lymphadenopathy although rare inguinal presentations may also occur in relation to disease originating in the vulva or penis. Most malignant lymph node masses in the neck are metastatic and the majority (85%) arise from primary head and neck tumours.[10] The majority (>50%) of primary sites are identified at routine clinical examination, with a further 16%, at panendoscopy and 4% by radiological investigation. The latter mainly related to the finding of lung primaries in patients with nodes in the lower cervical region. Nevertheless, between 3 and 9% have no identifiable primary site after such a programme of investigation. Those identified as having a head and neck primary tumour following investigation and treatment have a 20–30% five-year survival rate, whereas those in whom the primary is never discovered have a median survival of 1 year.[10]

Radiological examination including CT may be required for examination of:

- Paranasal sinuses
- Staging of the extent of nodal enlargement
- Detection of mediastinal or lung disease prior to treatment

Patients without an identifiable primary and N1 disease (lymph nodes <3 cm on one side of the neck) have a better prognosis than those with N2 or N3 disease. However, a series reporting the results of surgical resection alone have found that up to 40% of patients subsequently develop a primary site in the head and neck region. Therefore, most authors would now recommend the inclusion of radiotherapy in the primary treatment to include the naso-, hypo- and oropharynx plus the contralateral neck where there is a 15% likelihood of developing further deposits.

ADENOCARCINOMA OF UNKNOWN ORIGIN

Adenocarcinoma is the most frequent histology in cancers of unknown origin. In defining the plan of investigation, the likely incidence of the various primary diagnoses and the treatment options available following diagnosis need to be considered. Exhaustive investigation of patients with cancers of unknown primary is often counterproductive, because of the diminishing likelihood of identifying a primary site, and the increasing expense and discomfort to the patient with limited life expectancy.[2,3,7,11] Treatment options for this group of patients are also limited except in certain special circumstances (see below).

In series such as those of Le Chavalier (1988) and Nystrom (1979) patients with adenocarcinoma of unknown primary site were subjected to postmortem examination and a primary site was identified in 82–84%.[6,7] The most common sites were:

- Lung (17–28%)
- Pancreas (11–27%)
- Liver (3–6%)
- Colorectal (4–6%)
- Gastric (3–5%)
- Renal (3–7%)
- Ovary (2%)
- Prostate (2–3%)
- Thyroid (1–3%)
- Adrenal (1–3%)
- Breast (1%)
- Parotid (<1%)

The authors compared postmortem findings with the investigations prior to death to define the investigational yield and found that the proportion of primary sites that had been identified was:[6,7]

- Chest radiography (12–24%)
- IVU (6–9%)
- Barium enema (5–9%)
- Barium meal (4–6%)
- Thyroid scan (8%)

By contrast, in their patients who did not undergo a postmortem, the primary site was identified in only 16% during life although in more recent series, following the advent of CT scanning, a primary cancer was found in 20–31%.[1,2]

Clinical series have revealed a similar distribution of frequency of primary sites of cancer.[1,5] Overall, body CT has proved most successful in identifying the primary site, showing up to 35–40% of all primaries discovered.[2,12] In the chest particularly, it can show over 70% of all primary tumours. Abdominopelvic CT will also be successful and in one series has shown 86% of all pancreatic cancers, 67% of ovarian primaries and 56% of renal primaries. At other sites, the investigational yield was considerably less with 36% of colorectal primaries, 33% of hepatobiliary primaries and 20% of oesophageal primaries detected by CT scan. In addition, CT scan will detect other clinically unsuspected sites of

Table 42.2. *Test performance compared with postmortem findings*[7]

Test	Number performed	Sensitivity (%)	Specificity (%)	Positive predictive value (%)
Chest X-ray	302	69	63	38
Barium meal	150	75	92	30
Barium enema	105	71	96	55
Thyroid radio-iodine scan	45	57	76	31

metastasis in two-thirds of patients examined.[12] It is not possible to estimate the sensitivity and specificity of the findings in most studies, except in one postmortem series by Le Chavalier in 1988, in which conventional radiological investigations are shown to have a low sensitivity and positive predictive value and variable specificity (Table 42.2).

Key points: clinical presentation

■ 3–9% of all referrals to an oncology unit are for investigation of a cancer of unknown primary site

■ Adenocarcinoma is the most common histological type in this group of patients

■ Poorly differentiated cancers (35%) are an extremely important group as it contains those patients with the most treatable cancers

■ Most patients with squamous carcinoma of unknown origin present with cervical lymphadenopathy and 85% arise from head and neck tumours

■ In patients presenting with adenocarcinoma of unknown origin, postmortem studies show that the primary tumour most commonly arises in the lung or pancreas

TREATMENT OPPORTUNITIES AND RADIOLOGICAL STRATEGY

The investigational strategy for patients presenting with metastatic adenocarcinoma should aim to identify those primaries with the greatest treatment potential. At present there are a relatively limited number of cancers that are likely to present in this manner and have a high likelihood of response, if not cure, following treatment. These include:

• Breast
• Ovary
• Prostate

The breast and ovary represent a small proportion of cases, approximately 5–26%[1–3] of the adenocarcinomas of unknown primary, but their treatment potential makes it important for them to be identified with a high degree of sensitivity. Overall, in patients presenting with cancer of unknown primary site, only 11–14% of radiologically identified primary tumours are considered treatable.[1,2,5,11] The overall median survival for the group for all cancers of unknown primary site varies from 12 weeks[5] to 22 weeks.[1,7,11] In general, those patients with only limited nodal sites involved, a performance status of 0–2 and weight loss of <10% represent a better prognostic group with a median survival up to 11–14 months, irrespective of the primary site.[5,7,11] Those in whom a primary site is found at initial investigation may have a better prognosis than those in whom a primary is not found. In some series, however, this is almost entirely due to the identification of those patients with breast and ovarian primaries. Against this, the cost of investigating such patients has always to be considered. In one series, the estimated cost of a limited evaluation was U$3,350 per patient, 70% of which was accounted for by the cost of CT scanning.

A selective policy of investigating and identifying the primary site of origin in patients with adenocarcinoma of unknown primary will avoid over-investigation of patients with a poor prognosis while allowing the clinician to apply established tumour guidelines or experimental treatment protocols to palliate disease where appropriate. Finding the primary site often provides much psychological relief for patient and physician although the practical benefit may be relatively small. Bearing these points in mind, a radiological strategy should be agreed by clinician and radiologist to reflect locally available diagnostic facilities amd treatment strategies. There are special clinical situations in which well-defined guidelines for investigation can be recommended:

• In women presenting with isolated axillary lymph node metastases, a primary breast cancer may be found in 40–70% of cases. In one series, only half of these were mammographically detectable, the remainder being found on pathological examination of the mastectomy specimen.[13] Recently, MRI has been found to be a valuable adjunct to mammography and ultrasound in examination of these patients. The prognosis for the group as a whole with breast cancer type treatment is similar to that of other women with Stage-II breast cancer with a median survival of 5 years.[13]

On considering these statistics, it is clear that a thorough search for a primary breast cancer is justified. Ultrasound, mammography and MRI, if available, should be performed in this group of patients. If a primary tumour is found, then a thorough staging should be carried out as for patients presenting with a clinically diagnosed primary breast cancer.

- Women presenting with peritoneal carcinomatosis are another example of potentially treatable adenocarcinomas of unknown primary site in particular those with papillary serious carcinoma on histological examination but no primary tumour within the ovary. These patients may either have primary peritoneal carcinomatosis,[14,15] or spread from a preinvasive ovarian primary and respond to platinum-based chemotherapy. The prognosis is similar to that in other women with Stage-III ovarian carcinoma with a median survival of 17–23 months.

In these patients CT scanning is the investigation of choice, which should include the chest, abdomen and pelvis. The information provided by CT gives an excellent baseline for monitoring response to platinum-based chemotherapy.

- Men with adenocarcinoma of unknown primary and an elevated serum or tumour biopsy prostate specific antigen (PSA) level are usually found to have an unsuspected primary prostatic cancer and form another readily treatable group with a clinical course similar to those presenting with prostatic cancer. Response to androgen deprivation is approximately 70% and median survival 18–24 months.

In such patients transrectal ultrasound or MRI of the prostate gland should be performed in an attempt to identify the primary tumour. If a tumour is shown, then a biopsy may be helpful in patients with only minimal elevation of PSA in the serum. In patients suspected of harbouring an occult prostatic tumour, then full staging with a plain chest radiograph, CT of the abdomen and pelvis, to identify nodal disease, and a technetium bone scan is recommended.

- Occasionally patients present with liver metastases, which are discovered incidentally, or as a result of symptoms due to increasing abdominal discomfort and/or weight loss. In such patients the nature of the liver metastases may occasionally point to the site of origin. For example, calcification with metastases is seen most commonly in gastro-intestinal and ovarian tumours. In patients with bowel symptoms suspected of harbouring a gastro-intestinal tumour, barium studies are warranted, since the primary tumour may be excised to avoid obstruction either before or after chemotherapy with 5-fluorouracil.

- Other treatable patients include those with multiple small-volume lung metastases due to thyroid carcinoma. This is a rare clinical situation, but response to treatment with radio-iodine, if the tumour is shown to be metabolically active, can be achieved in a high proportion of patients.

In conclusion, patients presenting with cancers of unknown origin represent a heterogeneous group in which the detection of the primary site is becoming increasingly relevant to clinical oncological practice. There are now several tumours that present with metastatic disease and which are treatable with specific drugs, provided the organ of origin is known. Although the cost of investigation is high, there are certain situations in which a thorough search for the primary site is justified. In the future it is likely that these special situations, in which the primary tumour is treatable, will be expanded to a much wider range of malignancies.

Key points: imaging investigation

- Currently, in patients presenting with cancer of unknown primary site, only about 11–14% of radiologically identified primary tumours are considered treatable, and these include predominantly those arising in the breast, ovary and prostate

- The imaging strategy should always take into account the likelihood of identifying those tumours that are treatable

- Special situations that warrant thorough imaging studies include a search for breast cancer in women with isolated axillary lymph node metastases, ovarian carcinoma in women with peritoneal carcinomatosis, and prostate cancer in men with elevated serum PSA

Summary

■ The radiological investigation of patients with cancer of unknown primary site should be tailored to provide information that is relevant to prognosis and treatment.

■ To this end, all patients should have a chest X-ray and for women bilateral mammography and examination of the pelvic organs by ultrasound, whilst men should be screened for a prostatic primary by transrectal ultrasound if the PSA is elevated.

■ Further investigation, for example for thyroid carcinoma, by ultrasound or radio-iodine scanning can be reserved for those cases with the appropriate histology and or metastatic pattern.

■ Investigation by chest CT scan and bronchoscopy to identify primary large cell lung carcinoma does not seem to be generally warranted.

■ In the absence of gastro-intestinal tract symptoms, barium studies have a low diagnostic yield and a paucity of therapeutic options.

■ The application of much of the information, which can already be obtained by our increasingly sensitive imaging techniques, is not matched by improvements in the treatment of the most commonly discovered primary sites in the lung and pancreas.

REFERENCES

1. Kirsten F, Chi C H, Leary J A et al. Metastatic adeno or undifferentiated carcinoma from an unknown primary site — natural history and guidelines for identification of treatable subsets. Q J Med 1987; 62: 143–161

2. Abbruzzese J L, Abbruzzese M C, Lenzi R et al. Analysis of a diagnostic strategy for patients with suspected tumors of unknown origin. J Clin Oncol 1995; 13: 2094–2103

3. Hamilton C S, Langlands A O. ACUPS (Adenocarcinoma of unknown primary sites): A clinical and cost benefit analysis. Int J Radiat Oncol Biol Phys 1987; 13: 1497–1503

4. Muir C. Cancer of unknown primary site. Cancer 1995; 75: 353–356

5. Abbruzzese J L, Abbruzzese M C, Hess K R et al. Unknown primary carcinoma: Natural history and prognostic factors in 657 consecutive patients. J Clin Oncol 1994; 12: 1272–1280

6. Nystrom J S, Weiner J M, Wolf R M et al. Identifying the primary site in metastatic cancer of unknown origin. JAMA 1979; 241: 381–383

7. Le Chevalier T, Cvitkovic E, Caille P et al. Early metastatic cancer of unknown primary origin at presentation. A clinical study of 302 consecutive autopsied patients. Arch Intern Med 1988; 148: 2035–2039

8. Hainsworth J D, Greco F A. Treatment of patients with cancer of an unknown primary site. N Engl J Med 1993; 329: 257–263

9. Moertel C G, Kvols L K, O'Connell M J, Rubin J. Treatment of neuroendocrine carcinomas with combined etoposide and cisplatin. Cancer 1991; 68: 227–232

10. Jones A S, Cook J A, Phillips D E, Roland N R. Squamous carcinoma presenting as an enlarged cervical lymph node. Cancer 1993; 72: 1756–1761

11. Stewart J F, Tattersall M H N, Woods R L, Fox R M. Unknown primary adenocarcinoma: incidence of over-investigation and natural history. Br Med J 1979; 1: 1530–1533

12. McMillan J H, Levine E, Stephens R. Computed tomography in the evaluation of metastatic adenocarcinoma from an unknown primary site. Radiology 1982; 143: 143–146

13. Rosen P. Axillary lymph node metastases in patients with occult noninvasive breast carcinoma. Cancer 1980; 46: 1298–1306

14. Strand C M, Grosh W W, Baxter J et al. Peritoneal carcinomatosis of unknown primary site in women. Ann Int Med 1989; 111: 213–217

15. Ransom D T, Patel S R, Keeney G L et al. Papillary serous carcinoma of the peritoneum. Cancer 1990; 66: 1091–1094

TREATMENT EVALUATION

Chapter 43

Radiological intervention in oncology

Anthony Lopez

INTRODUCTION

Over the past 20 years huge advances have been made in oncological management, no more so than in the development of new interventional techniques in radiology. These changes have had important implications for both the diagnosis and therapeutic management of a wide range of malignancies. Many of the developments reflect advances in technology, including the development of digital imaging, major progress in image guidance techniques such as computed tomography (CT), ultrasound and endoscopy, and an increase in the wide range of needles, guidewires, catheters and stents. It seems likely that in the near future magnetic resonance imaging (MRI) will play an increasing role in interventional management with the development of open-plan magnet configurations, MRI-compatible equipment for biopsy, ablation and endovascular intervention, and MRI-compatible endoscopes.

THORACIC INTERVENTION

Biopsy techniques

Almost any part of the thorax is now accessible to biopsy using percutaneous, endoscopic or open techniques and radiologists are already involved in all such procedures. Generally speaking, fine needle aspiration biopsy (FNAB) is usually sufficient for diagnosis provided adequate cellular material has been aspirated, especially with new cytological techniques, e.g. DNA cytofluorometry, immunocytochemistry, tumour markers and chemosensitivity. In primary lymphoreticular malignancies, however, larger pieces of tissue are usually desirable for diagnosis, subclassification and immunotyping[1] necessitating the use of larger cutting needles to obtain a good tissue core (Fig. 43.1). Localization of superficial lesions can often be achieved with palpation or ultrasound guidance using a free-hand technique. Imaging guidance has a more significant effect on results

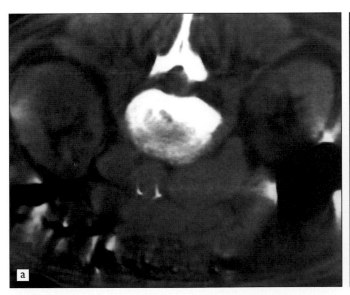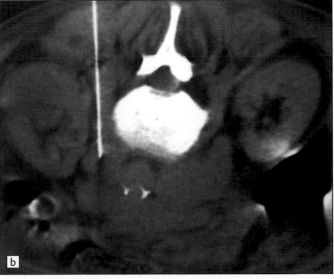

Figure 43.1. *CT guided biopsy of lymph node in a patient with treated non-Hodgkin's lymphoma. (a) Bulky para-aortic lymphadenopathy (patient prone); (b) tip of 18-gauge cutting needle in discrete left lateral para-aortic lymph node. Note presence of 'photon starvation artefact' confirming actual tip of needle.*

than sampling techniques.[2] The most likely indications for ultrasound guidance include pleural biopsy, rib lesions, subcutaneous deposits and peripheral lung lesions reaching a pleural surface. For deeper and particularly for poorly accessible lesions, e.g. pulmonary apices (Fig. 43.2), near the hila or diaphragms, either fluoroscopy or CT guidance is recommended,[3] especially when trying to obtain a tissue core where a co-axial technique may be useful.[4] For central and hilar lung lesions, bronchoscopy and transbronchial biopsy is usually safer and more appropriate, providing good tissue cores. Similarly, for oesophageal lesions, endoscopic biopsy is usually desirable unless the lesion is predominantly-exophytic and not visible with the endoscope, a situation in which a percutaneous image-guided approach would be more suitable. Some complications of thoracic biopsy are suitably managed in the interventional suite, e.g. lung aspiration for pneumothorax and embolization for haemoptysis.

Image guidance has also been used for needle localization in the preoperative location of chest wall lesions as well as intrapulmonary nodules prior to thorascopic resection.[5] The latter has been particularly useful with the use of hooked wire markers similar to those used for breast localization procedures.

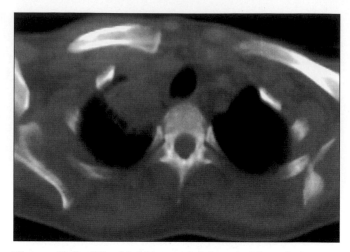

Figure 43.2. *CT-guided biopsy of right apical lung lesion. Small apical lesion with prominent adjacent bony structures limiting access for transaxial biopsy. Note tip of 21-gauge needle (scanned in short axis) within mass later confirmed as squamous cell carcinoma.*

- Empyemas
- Parapneumonic collections
- Pulmonary and mediastinal abscesses

Percutaneous drainage can often be achieved using image guidance, particularly CT and ultrasound (Fig. 43.3). For pleural effusions 7 French gauge (Fr) drainage catheters are usually effective except where the collection has become more organized and catheters up to 24 Fr (sometimes with intrapleural fibrinolysis) may be required. Ultrasound guidance is particularly well suited to the drainage of malignant pericardial effusions using real-time. Sclerotherapy of both pleural and pericardial collections in the absence of associated infection has been attempted with variable results. The most commonly used agents are Corynebacterium parvum, tetracycline, talc and bleomycin.

Key points: thoracic biopsy

■ Fine-needle aspiration cytology is usually sufficient for diagnosis of malignancy if adequate cellular material has been obtained

■ Larger tissue cores are required to accurately classify primary lymphoreticular malignancies

■ Imaging guidance has a more significant effect on results than sampling techniques

■ CT-guided biopsy is recommended for lesions with poor accessibility

■ Transbronchial biopsy is safer and more appropriate for central and hilar lung lesions

Key point: ultrasound

■ Ultrasound guidance is particularly well suited to the drainage of malignant pleural and pericardial effusions

Thoracic drainage procedures

Thoracic collections may occur as a complication of the malignancy (and include malignant pleural and pericardial effusions), and following diagnostic or therapeutic interventional procedures. Examples are haemothorax following lung biopsy and biliary effusion following transpleural hepatic drainage procedures. Thoracic collections may also occur directly as a complication of treatment and include:

Venous access and related intervention

The rapid development of new chemotherapeutic agents and more intensive regimes for treatment has been accompanied by an increase in requirements for central venous catheters providing long-term venous access for chemotherapy, fluids, blood and related products as well as a portal for the aspiration of blood samples. A wide range of

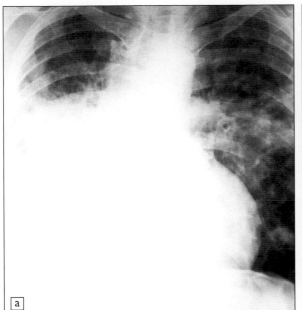
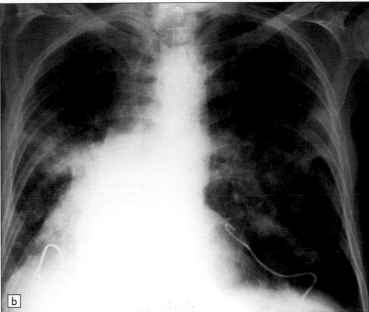

Figure 43.3. *Percutaneous drainage of malignant pleural and pericardial effusions in recurrent breast carcinoma: (a) chest radiograph demonstrating massive pericardial and large right pleural effusions. Note also infective consolidation in left lung;*

(b) two 7 Fr pig-tail drainage catheters have been inserted using ultrasound-guidance with satisfactory post-drainage appearances. The acute pneumonia also responded to antibiotics with marked clinical improvement.

catheters has been developed over the last 10 years, usually made of either silicone or polyurethane with one or more lumens, that usually require subcutaneous tunnelling or even implantation in the case of port systems. Traditionally, such venous access devices were inserted in theatre by surgical cutdown but it has become increasingly recognized that radiologists trained in interventional techniques are ideally suited for percutaneous insertion of such devices using their expertise in image guidance, guidewire and catheter manipulation with shorter procedure times, fewer complications and improved success rate compared with the surgical approach.[6] Furthermore, with such high demands for catheter insertion, the angiography suite has been shown to provide more flexibility than the rigid time-tabling of theatre sessions while at the same time providing the necessary aseptic environment that is desirable.[7,8] There is, however, some debate on these issues and not all cancer centres utilize the services of radiology for central line insertion.

The preferred access routes are typically the internal jugular or subclavian veins, although in cases of difficulty the common femoral vein has been used. Translumbar and transhepatic vena caval puncture have also been described.[9] Even dilated intercostal veins may be used if there is associated central venous obstruction.[10]

The role of the radiologist in this field is expanding beyond that of insertion of central venous catheters so that in many centres there are now requirements for radiologists to manage the complications associated with these central venous access catheters. Assessment of such complications frequently requires diagnostic techniques such as direct catheter venograms, duplex sonography of in situ catheters and related veins as well as peripheral venography (Fig. 43.4). Furthermore, where appropriate, thrombolysis of occluded catheters and veins can be performed as well as repositioning of misplaced or displaced catheters.

One of the commonest longer term complications associated with venous access systems is the development of catheter-related stenosis and thrombosis often requiring peripheral or central venous thrombolysis with or without venous angioplasty and endovascular stenting.

Central venous obstruction

Central venous obstruction may occur secondary to catheter-related stenosis or fibrosing mediastinitis in the treatment of malignant disease. A more sinister finding, however, is malignant venous obstruction typically in the superior vena cava (SVC), either by direct tumour invasion e.g. bronchial neoplasms or by extrinsic compression from perihilar or paratracheal lymphadenopathy. Interventional techniques have been developed to provide palliation in these circumstances and self-expanding metallic stents are usually inserted following chemical or mechanical thrombolysis and angioplasty. When successful, this procedure is followed by almost immediate relief of the distressing symptoms (Fig. 43.5). In

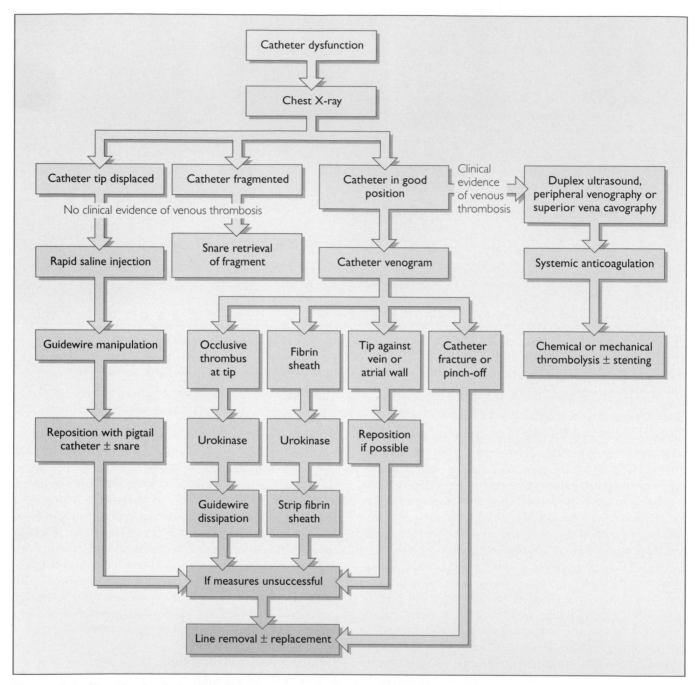

Figure 43.4. *Algorithm for the investigation of venous access device malfunction.*

cases where there is obstruction of the central neck veins bilaterally, as well as the SVC, relief of obstruction on one side alone often provides adequate palliation.[11] A metallic stent also provides an excellent visible localizer to optimize the target volume for palliative radiotherapy.

Recently, similar techniques have been applied to the inferior vena cava (IVC) when obstructed secondary to large hepatic tumours or retroperitoneal nodal masses with encouraging results.[12]

Fluoroscopic and bronchoscopic tracheobronchial stenting

One of the commonest malignancies in the western world is bronchial carcinoma which is often associated with obstruction of the major airways. Significant developments in stent technology and close working relationships between radiologists, thoracic surgeons and physicians have led to the introduction of self-expanding metallic stents of similar design to the venous stents already described (Fig. 43.6).[13]

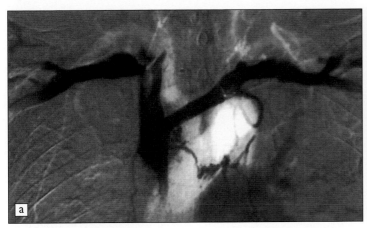

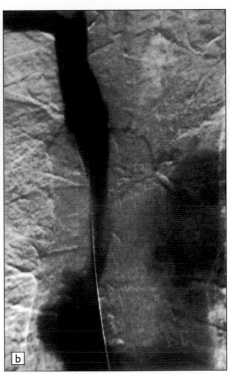

Figure 43.5. *Self-expanding metallic wall stent insertion (Schneider A G, Bülach, Switzerland) in superior vena caval obstruction (SVCO) preceding palliative radiotherapy in bronchial carcinoma. (a) Superior vena cavagram demonstrating extrinsic compression of superior vena cava by tracheobronchial lymph nodes; (b) repeat study following endovascular venoplasty and metallic stenting confirmed relief of SVCO with good filling of right atrium and less prominent collaterals. There was immediate clinical improvement and further stent expansion occurred over the following week.*

The stents are usually inserted under general anaesthesia using combined fluoroscopic and bronchoscopic guidance with stent insertion following balloon dilatation of the stricture (Fig. 43.7). This development has resulted in a reduction in morbidity associated with major airway obstruction from malignant disease.

Key points: central line insertion

◼ The interventional suite is a suitable environment for the percutaneous insertion of central venous catheters and the management of catheter-related complications

◼ In the absence of conventional venous access sites, the transhepatic and translumbar routes may be useful

◼ In central venous obstruction, relief of obstruction on one side alone may provide adequate palliation

Techniques for management of haemoptysis

Major haemoptysis in oncological patients is associated typically with bronchial malignancy, although it may also result from percutaneous and transbronchial biopsy techniques. Less frequently, haemoptysis occurs due to complications of treatment. For example, in immunosuppressed patients haemoptysis may be due to tuberculosis or other

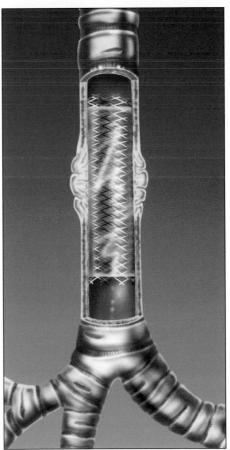

Figure 43.6. *Diagrammatic representation of a self-expanding uncovered metallic stent in situ across a malignant tracheal stricture.*

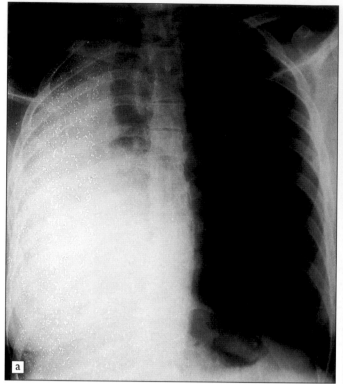

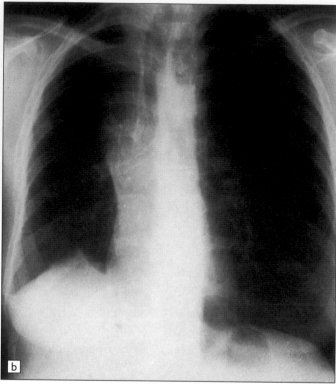

Figure 43.7. *Tracheobronchial stenting in a woman with recurrent squamous cell carcinoma (Reproduced from ref 13 with permission). (a) Chest radiograph immediately prior to stenting with complete collapse of right lung and ipsilateral mediastinal shift; (b) chest radiograph 1 week after deployment* *of a 49 mm long, 8 mm diameter wall stent endoprosthesis (Schneider AG, Bülach, Switzerland) in the right main and intermediate bronchi showing complete expansion of remaining right lung (note patient has had a previous right upper lobectomy for a large cell carcinoma).*

pulmonary infections or may be seen in pneumonitis induced by radiotherapy.

Bronchial arteriography and embolization are well recognized techniques used in the management of recurrent and significant haemoptysis (Fig. 43.8). The technique requires exquisite, preferably digital, imaging because anterior and posterior spinal arteries sometimes originate from the intercostal arteries and bronchial to coronary artery communications are also well described. If such vessels are not appreciated, severe or even fatal consequences may ensue.

Key points: thoracic intervention

■ Tracheobronchial stenting can palliate major airway obstruction

■ Bronchial artery embolization may be required to palliate haemoptysis

GASTRO-INTESTINAL INTERVENTION

Biopsy techniques

Biopsy techniques have already been described in some detail in the previous section and the same general principles apply to the gastro-intestinal tract. Image guidance is particularly useful for obtaining large tissue cores which are required for lymph node histopathological examination to ensure accurate diagnosis, particularly if lymphoma is suspected (Fig. 43.1). Empirically, enlarged para-aortic nodes should be biopsied in preference to paracaval nodes because haemorrhage from inadvertent injury of the IVC is much less likely to stop without intervention than haemorrhage from aortic injury.

Formerly, fluoroscopy was used from guidance of many procedures such as the biopsy of lymph nodes opacified at lymphography,[14] as well as biopsy of lesions in the opacified biliary tree (Fig. 43.9), gastro-intestinal tract and urinary tract. However, today CT and ultrasound have superseded fluoroscopy as the standard methods for percutaneous image guidance.[15]

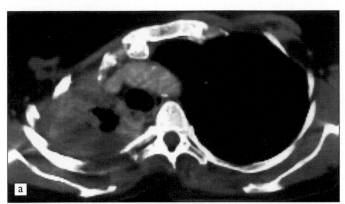

Figure 43.8. *Bronchial arteriography and embolization in a man with recurrent significant haemoptysis secondary to an apical adenocarcinoma arising in an old tuberculous scar and resistant to radiotherapy. (a) CT scan showing slightly necrotic and moderately enhancing right apical mass. Note lytic involvement of posterior end of adjacent rib; (b) right bronchial arteriogram demonstrating hypervascular apical mass; (c) following successful embolization with polyvinyl alcohol and gelfoam, only staining of the embolized tumour (arrow) is demonstrated. Note preservation of the right superior intercostal artery with intercostal branches shown not to supply the tumour.*

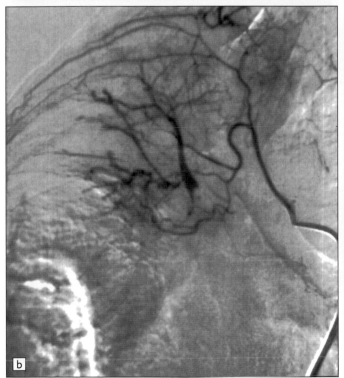

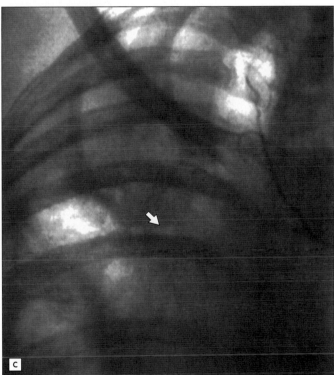

Remarkable developments have been made in endoluminal ultrasound and some lesions deep in the pelvis can now be biopsied using transrectal or transvaginal ultrasound guidance (Fig. 43.10). Certainly the transvaginal approach is the best method for the diagnostic aspiration of small ovarian cysts and the transrectal approach is now more commonly used for prostatic biopsy than the transperineal and transurethral methods. These endoluminal approaches may replace the transgluteal route for biopsy or abscess drainage.

Endoscopic ultrasound (EUS) has been particularly useful for assessing the depth of tumour invasion in primary oesophageal carcinoma.[16] Regional lymph node metastases may also be detected but the specificity of the technique is limited since inflammatory nodes may mimic malignant lymphadenopathy. Endoscopic ultrasound-guided lymph node biopsy will help to overcome this constraint of endoscopic ultrasound. Similarly, endoscopic ultrasound-guided biopsy can be used to diagnose and stage gastric and colorectal cancer as well as for localizing small pancreatic lesions.[17–19]

Radiologists are increasingly being requested to perform image-guided liver biopsy which is clearly most appropriate when there is one or more focal hepatic lesions rather than diffuse disease. Standard percutaneous liver biopsy, however, may be contraindicated in patients with a significant or uncorrectable coagulopathy. In such cases morbidity and mortality can be reduced by using the transjugular approach for liver biopsy or by performing a plugged liver biopsy with embolization of the biopsy tract after removing the biopsy needle from the sheath. A similar technique may be used to obtain a splenic core, advisable even when the bleeding and coagulation times are not prolonged (Fig. 43.11). A modification of

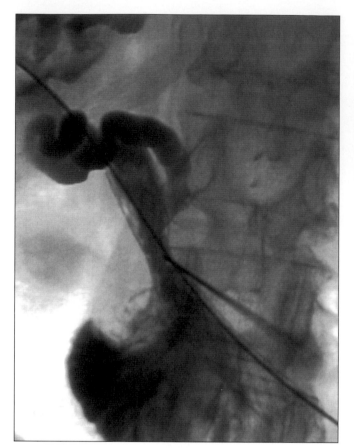

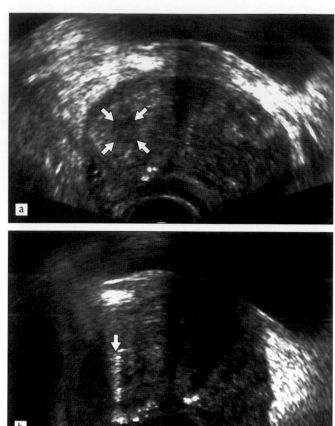

Figure 43.9. *Fluoroscopic biopsy of obstructive lesion subsequently shown to be cholangiocarcinoma. An 8.5 Fr metallic endoprosthesis has been inserted (Memotherm, Angiomed, Europe) via PTC to relieve the obstruction and the 21-gauge needle inserted into the tumour at the site of waisting.*

Figure 43.10. *Transrectal ultrasound (TRUS)-guided biopsy of prostatic lesion subsequently shown to be prostatic adenocarcinoma: (a) 1.5 cm hypoechoic nodule (short arrows) in peripheral zone of right midgland (prostatic capsule intact); (b) tip of 18-gauge needle within nodule (long arrow) inserted using TRUS-guidance.*

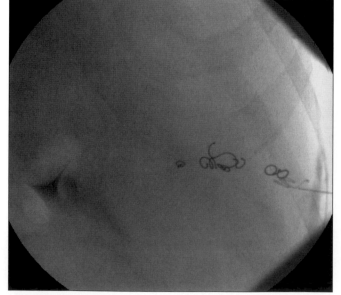

Figure 43.11. *Plugged splenic biopsy in a patient with 'massive splenomegaly' and 'B' symptoms but no other abnormal appearances on CT. An 18-gauge biopsy needle was introduced through a sheath into the spleen. Following core biopsy (revealing diffuse lymphomatous infiltration), the track (shown not to communicate with a large vessel) has been plugged with alternating spongistan pledgets and 5 mm stainless steel coils. Note small linear area of contrast at splenic capsule to show splenic edge ensuring coils within splenic parenchyma.*

the former technique is the use of the bioptome for percutaneous transcaval biopsy of tumours which have invaded the IVC,[20] such as primary or secondary liver tumours and renal tumours. Such techniques should be reserved for those situations when conventional methods are contraindicated or inappropriate.

Percutaneous drainage procedures

Abdominal ascites is a common finding in many gastrointestinal and pelvic malignancies, particularly where there is peritoneal and/or omental seeding. Malignant ascites is most distressing for the patient and can usually be drained using a percutaneous technique without image guidance. In cases of difficulty, however, or loculation, ultrasound guidance using a free-hand technique is extremely useful for achieving complete drainage prior to consideration of sclerotherapy.

Key points: gastro-intestinal biopsy

- ■ Transrectal and transvaginal ultrasound are commonly employed for pelvic biopsy and drainage procedures

- ■ Endoscopic ultrasound with biopsy is useful in the staging of oesophageal, gastric and colorectal malignancy

- ■ If direct liver biopsy is contraindicated, a transjugular or percutaneous plugged approach should be considered

Abdominal fluid collections and abscesses may develop as a complication of treatment and in the postoperative patient subphrenic and pelvic collections are not uncommon. They are easily drained using ultrasound or CT for guidance. Pelvic abscess drainage is safer using the transrectal or transvaginal approach compared with the transgluteal route and is also considerably less painful for the patient.

Management of oesophageal and upper gastro-intestinal strictures

Malignant oesophageal strictures are typically due to primary oesophageal carcinoma and less frequently due to metastatic oesophageal lesions, nodal disease or local tumour invasion from bronchial neoplasms. Benign oesophageal strictures may also follow radiotherapy to the mediastinum, as a late complication. All these lesions can be managed using either fluoroscopic or endoscopic techniques.

Traditionally, oesophageal strictures have been dilated using either rubber bougies (such as the Savary–Guillard type) or rigid metal dilators (Eder–Puestow). Optimally, such dilatation, which can be up to 60 Fr is performed endoscopically under fluoroscopic control, to reduce the risk of perforation and other complications. The endoscopic route also affords the possibility of performing diagnostic biopsy imme-

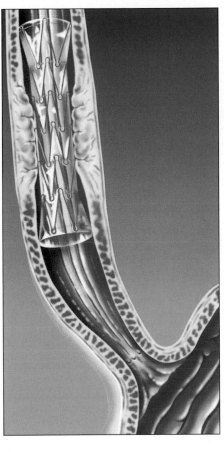

Figure 43.12.
Diagrammatic representation of a self-expanding covered metallic stent in situ across a distal malignant oesophageal stricture.

diately after rigid or balloon dilatation, although this is better avoided. Alternatively, dilatation can be performed entirely fluoroscopically using a large balloon over the guidewire.

For malignant strictures, where staging using EUS or CT has indicated that primary surgical resection is impossible, stenting is advisable either using a self-expanding metallic stent (Figs. 43.12 and 43.13) or a rigid device (Fig. 43.14) both of which can be inserted directly under screening control or via endoscopy using fluoroscopic guidance.

In cases of tracheo-oesophageal fistula, similar techniques have been applied using a covered self-expanding metallic stent (uncovered for a short interval at either end to reduce migration). These can be applied to the oesophagus up to just below the level of the cricopharyngeus muscle (Fig. 43.15). For higher lesions, covered stents have been inserted into the trachea, thereby successfully occluding the fistula.

One of the advantages of the expandable metallic stent is that it expands to a diameter of between 18 and 22 mm although it is delivered to the site on a relatively small delivery device. In cases of tumour overgrowth, laser therapy can be performed directly through the stent or even bougie of the stent can be performed using a balloon to shear off tumour from the mesh. Covered stents have been used in an attempt to reduce tumour ingrowth and newer stents are

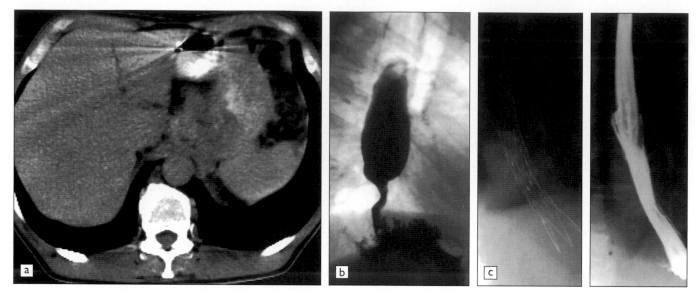

Figure 43.13. *Endoscopic insertion of self-expanding metallic endoprosthesis for unresectable adenocarcinoma of distal oesophagus involving cardia. (a) CT scan demonstrating bulky nodal disease along lesser curve and around coeliac axis; (b) barium swallow showing tight malignant distal oesophageal stricture with 'shouldering' involving cardia; (c) a 12 cm long, 22 cm diameter Gianturco–Rösch covered metallic endoprosthesis (William Cook, Europe) has been inserted endoscopically across stricture ensuring distal 'funnel' end lies just within the stomach but adequately below the tumour margin. Note minor residual waisting which subsequently disappeared without further dilatation; (d) barium swallow (one day postinsertion) demonstrating widely patent stent with immediate relief of dysphagia.*

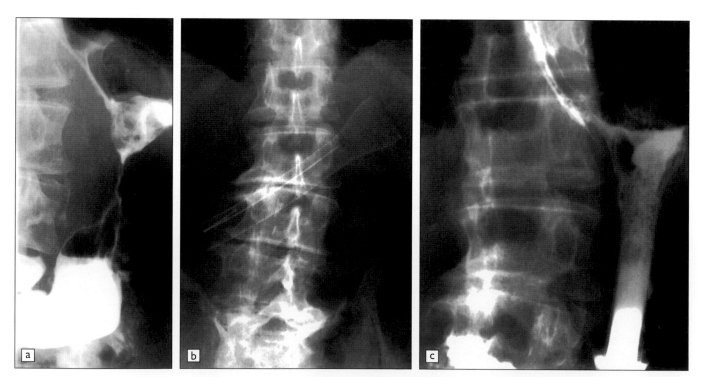

Figure 43.14. *Endoscopic insertion of Medoc tube for annular stenosing adenocarcinoma of stomach to palliate intractable emesis. (Reproduced with kind permission of Dr. R A Frost.). (a) Spot film from upper gastro-intestinal series demonstrating tight gastric stricture; (b) a Medoc tube has been inserted endoscopically across stricture; (c) relief of gastric obstruction demonstrated on barium meal.*

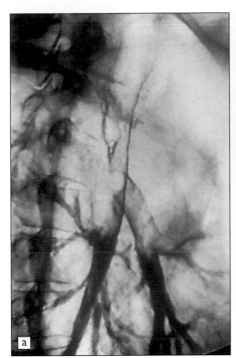 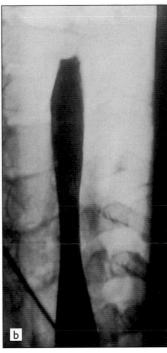

Figure 43.15. *Fluoroscopic insertion of covered metallic wall stent (Schneider AG, Bülach, Switzerland) for malignant tracheo-oesophageal fistula. (Reproduced with kind permission of Professor A. Adam). (a) Immediately following a contrast swallow, a bronchogram is demonstrated distal to a malignant tracheo-oesophageal fistula; (b) following endoprosthesis insertion, the stented oesophagus is widely patent with minor residual waisting only, but complete exclusion of the malignant fistula.*

being developed which are made of metal alloys, with metals of differing electrochemical potentials, which create a current inhibiting tumour ingrowth (personal communication). It is also relatively simple to insert a further stent within the 'in situ' stent. This is a useful manoeuvre if there is focal extrinsic compression or narrowing of the upper or lower ends either due to tumour recurrence or stent migration. An advantage of rigid stents over metallic stents is that they may be exchanged endoscopically as necessary.

Gastric outlet obstruction may occur as a complication of pyloric surgery, such as palliative bypass for pancreatic carcinoma, and is usually due to postoperative ischaemia. Other causes include local tumour recurrence, invasive pancreatic malignancy and stomal malignancy following previous peptic ulcer surgery. The techniques of dilatation and stenting have been applied to the gastric outlet for malignant strictures with good palliation in some cases.[21] Although longer per-oral delivery systems are being developed, gastrostomy may be required for stent insert-ion (Fig. 43.16). If stenting is unsuccessful, a double lumen gastroenterostomy tube may be inserted with the distal lumen (for feeding) in the jejunum and the proximal lumen (for gastric drainage) in the gastric antrum.

Dilatation and stenting of lower gastro-intestinal tract strictures

Lower gastro-intestinal tract strictures can be managed in a similar manner to other gastro-intestinal lesions, either endoscopically, fluoroscopically or using a combined approach. In cases of benign postoperative stricture follow-ing resection of a malignant lesion, dilatation is usually sufficient to achieve a good faecal passage with alleviation of obstruction. In the setting of acute large bowel obstruction secondary to a stenosing malignancy, the stricture may be crossed, dilated and stented accurately with metallic self-expanding stents to provide immediate relief of large bowel obstruction (Fig. 43.17). This may be a temporizing measure before proceeding to definitive surgery when the tumour and stent are removed, often with primary anastomosis rather than defunctioning colostomy.[22] Alternatively, where patients are not considered surgical candidates, the stent may provide adequate palliation. Any subsequent tumour overgrowth can be treated using endoscopic laser therapy.[23]

Insertion of gastrostomy and gastro-enterostomy feeding tubes

Nutritional support is essential in the overall management of patients with malignant disease, particularly those who are severely debilitated or unable to swallow. Tunnelled central venous catheters have been widely used for this purpose, especially when there is a need for coexistent administration of intravenous chemotherapy, blood and related products. The use of central venous lines for this purpose, however, is associated with significant morbidity and considerable expense. It is therefore desirable that enteric feeding support should be established via a naso-gastric tube in the early stages and subsequently via a gastrostomy when appropriate. Gastrostomy feeding tubes can be inserted using a percutaneous/endoscopic approach or entirely percutaneously

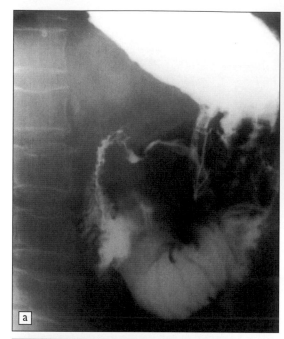

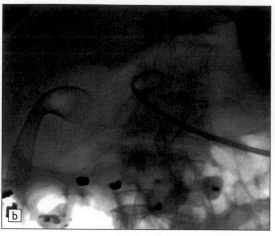

Figure 43.16. *Palliative stenting of malignant gastric outflow obstruction in advanced local pancreatic carcinoma. (a) Spot film from upper gastro-intestinal series demonstrating tight irregular stricture involving proximal duodenum; (b) following percutaneous gastrostomy and gastropexy, a 10 cm long, 20 mm diameter wall stent (Schneider AG, Bülach, Switzerland) has been deployed ensuring coverage of stricture and the proximal end lies across the pylorus 'flared' just within the stomach; (c) spot film from upper gastro-intestinal series demonstrating widely patent stent in good position with immediate relief of gastric outflow obstruction.*

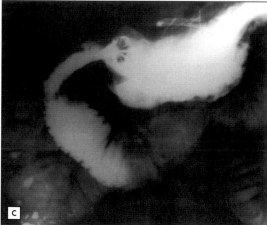

(with or without gastropexy) under fluoroscopic guidance which has a reduced cost, as well as lower morbidity and mortality. Gastrostomy may also be performed for gastric drainage in patients with gastric outlet obstruction due to retroperitoneal or mesenteric malignancy.

In cases of gastric outlet obstruction or problems associated with the gastrostomy tube, including gastro-oesophageal reflux, aspiration or reflux along the stomal tract, the gastrostomy can be converted to a gastro-enterostomy. This should be performed under fluoroscopic guidance to position the tube distal to the ligament of Treitz. In several institutions primary transgastric jejunostomy has been adopted (Fig. 43.18). Surgical or laparoscopic gastrostomy usually requires general anaesthesia which carries the risk of postoperative ileus whereas radiological tube insertion is performed under light sedation using local anaesthesia. A

further advantage of the percutaneous radiological approach is that success is not dependent upon the presence or absence of pharyngeal/ oesophageal strictures which can make the endoscopic approach extremely difficult. Several studies have shown that the percutaneous approach is less expensive and is associated with fewer minor and major complications than endoscopic or surgical gastrostomy.[24]

Management of obstructive jaundice

Obstructive jaundice with dilated extrahepatic and intrahepatic biliary ducts is easily demonstrated using either ultrasound, CT or MRI. The level of obstruction can often be determined as well as an indication of the likely nature of the underlying cause. In some cases, however, the obstructing lesion is not fully demonstrated using non-invasive techniques. Endoscopic retrograde cholangiopancreatography (ERCP)

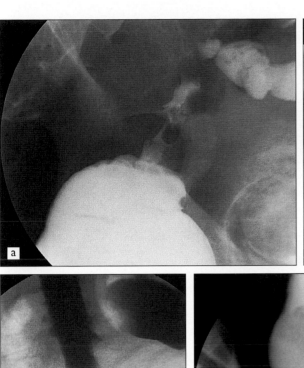
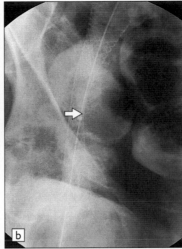
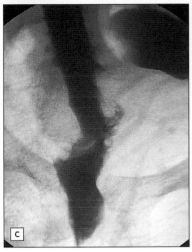
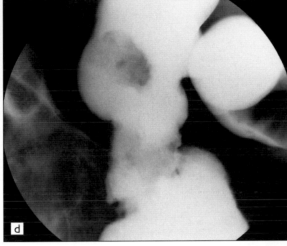

Figure 43.17. *Palliative stenting of malignant annular stenosing adenocarcinoma of rectosigmoid junction. (a) Oblique spot film from barium enema series demonstrating tight irregular stricture at rectosigmoid junction. (b) After crossing the stricture using fluoroscopic guidance, a 10 cm long 20 mm diameter Wall-stent (Schneider) has been deployed with evidence of residual 'waisting' in mid-stent (arrow). (c) Frontal spot film from barium enema series demonstrating a widely patent stent with immediate relief of large bowel obstruction following stent deployment. (d) Five months following stent insertion and local palliative radiotherapy (patient refused surgery), the stricture was almost completely relieved and the stent passed with excellent luminal patency on contrast enema.*

and percutaneous transhepatic cholangiography (PTC) have been particularly useful in the further investigation of obstructive lesions as well as in their interventional management (Fig. 43.19). The endoscopic method (ERCP) is preferred for low common bile duct lesions, while PTC is considered to have a high success and low complication rate for liver hilar lesions.

Percutaneous transhepatic cholangiography is now a readily available low-cost technique which is able to demonstrate the proximal level of obstruction (Fig. 43.19). With modern catheters and guidewires the obstructive lesion can often be traversed and either an internal/external biliary drainage catheter left in situ or the obstruction can be stented using plastic endoprostheses or self-expanding metallic stents (Fig. 43.20). Self-expanding metallic stents require a smaller transhepatic track for insertion yet provide a larger luminal diameter on full expansion compared to the plastic endoprosthesis (Fig. 43.21). Although they are considerably more expensive than plastic stents, these metallic stents have lower complication rates of haemorrhage, cholangitis and occlusion which lead to re-intervention.[25]

Key points: gastro-intestinal strictures

■ Oesophageal strictures are dilated endoscopically and/or fluoroscopically with rigid bougies or balloons

■ Stents provide excellent palliation for malignant oesophageal strictures and/or fistulae

■ Metal stents may provide palliation for malignant gastric outflow obstruction and acute large bowel obstruction

■ External feeding should be established where appropriate if the gastro-intestinal tract is 'intact'

Although PTC and stenting can be performed as a primary one-step procedure, ERCP has become the procedure of choice in the initial invasive investigation of obstructive jaundice in our department as well as in many others. This strategy is adopted because strictures or occlusions are often traversed more easily using the retrograde approach and

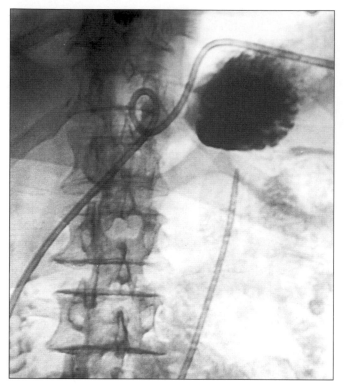

Figure 43.18. *Percutaneous transgastric jejunostomy feeding tube inserted for patient with advanced laryngeal malignancy where percutaneous endoscopic gastrostomy was precluded. Note the tip of the feeding tube at the duodenojejunal flexure and a self-retaining locking pig-tail in the gastric antrum.*

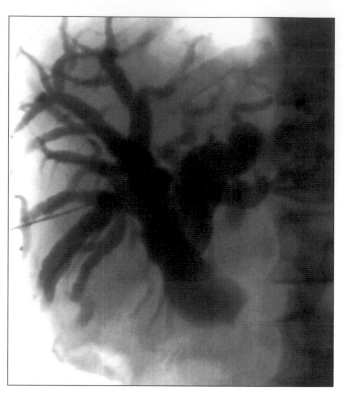

Figure 43.19. *Percutaneous transhepatic cholangiography demonstrating marked intra- and extrahepatic bile duct dilatation with malignant occlusion of common hepatic duct by cholangiocarcinoma.*

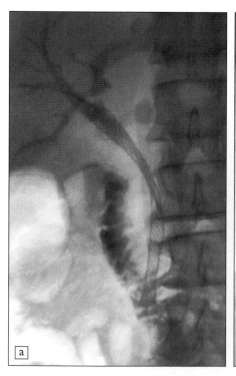

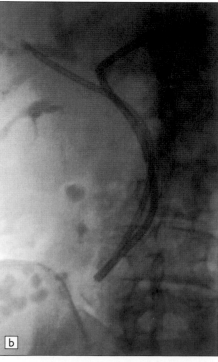

Figure 43.20. *Palliative stenting to relieve malignant obstructive jaundice. (a) Self-expanding metallic endoprosthesis (Memotherm, Angiomed, Europe) has been inserted following PTC and biliary drainage (same patient as Figure 43.19.) Note a little residual 'waisting' but complete relief of biliary obstruction; (b) 'kissing' plastic endoprostheses have been included to relieve malignant jaundice secondary to a Klatskin tumour. The right duct system was drained endoscopically with a 10.5 Fr Cotton–Leung stent and the left subsequently with a 12.5 Fr Carey–Coons stent following percutaneous left duct puncture.*

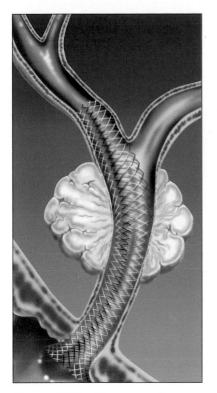

Figure 43.21. *Diagrammatic representation of a self-expanding uncovered metallic stent in situ across a malignant hilar biliary stricture.*

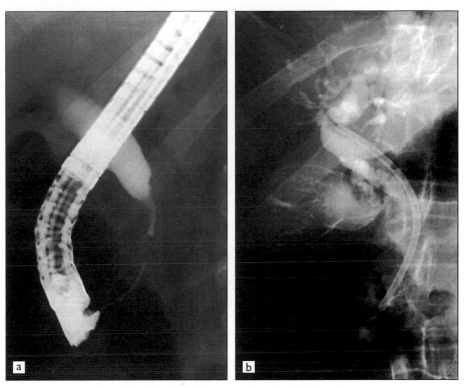

Figure 43.22. *Endoscopic relief of malignant obstructive jaundice secondary to carcinoma of head and pancreas. (a) ERCP demonstrating distal common bile duct stricture; (b) a 10.5 Fr Cotton–Leung plastic endoprosthesis has been inserted retrogradely to relieve biliary obstruction.*

primary stenting (plastic or metallic) can be performed without the requirement for external drainage (Fig. 43.22).

Both techniques allow bile to be aspirated for cytological examination and brushings taken from a lesion suspected to be cholangiocarcinoma. However, the yield from the brush technique is often disappointing. Endoscopic retrograde cholangiopancreatography has the advantage that tissue biopsy of lesions in the common bile duct, pancreatic duct and from the periampullary region can be performed.

Endoscopic ultrasound, using the retrograde approach, is an excellent technique for imaging the distal common bile duct (and other upper gastro-intestinal lesions) and the development of new methods utilizing endobiliary probes, with or without cholangioscopy for diagnosis and staging of biliary tumours, may offer considerable potential in the evaluation of biliary tract tumours.

Biliary metallic stents can be redilated, restented or unblocked using the percutaneous transhepatic approach (Fig. 43.23). The retrograde approach by ERCP is probably the most desirable, where possible, with removal of the occluded plastic biliary stent and exchange for a new stent as a one-stage procedure.

Iridium seeds have been implanted with good palliation in small cholangiocarcinomas using the nasobiliary, transhepatic and endoscopic routes for insertion.[26] In addition, in certain institutions, a superficial Roux loop is used routinely for recurrent access to the biliary tree across a biliary–enteric anastomosis.[27]

Visceral arteriography and related intervention

Visceral arteriography has been shown to have an important role in the diagnostic and therapeutic management of patients with malignant disease. The coeliac axis, superior and inferior mesenteric arteries are usually catheterized via a femoral artery approach. This technique is used for:

- Assessing the hepatic arterial supply to malignant lesions
- Detecting vascular involvement by infiltrative visceral malignancy (particularly pancreatic carcinoma)
- Identifying the site of bleeding in upper and lower gastro-intestinal malignancies prior to embolization

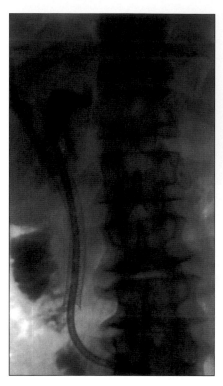

Figure 43.23. *A metallic endoprosthesis had been inserted 6 months previously to relieve obstruction secondary to cholangiocarcinoma. Following recurrent jaundice, a plastic stent was inserted at PTC as the patient had more advanced metastatic liver disease than at the time of primary stenting.*

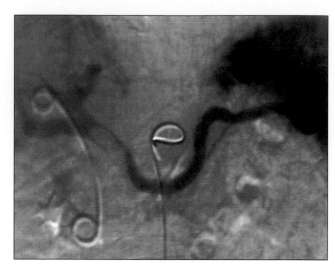

Figure 43.24. *Indirect splenoportogram demonstrating portal venous thrombosis secondary to malignant invasion. Note tip of Sidewinder II arterial catheter in proximal splenic artery and double pig-tail ended plastic endoprosthesis in situ. The latter had been inserted endoscopically for temporary relief of malignant jaundice from pancreatic carcinoma thought to be resectable.*

Although portal vein patency can be assessed using duplex sonography and CT (particularly spiral CT), elegant images of the superior mesenteric, splenic and portal vein and its branches can be imaged in real time using indirect portography with the tip of the arterial catheter either in the superior mesenteric artery distal to any replaced hepatic arteries or in the splenic artery (Fig. 43.24). This principle is also used in the assessment of the portal venous supply to hepatic metastases using CT arterial portography (CTAP),[28] which has been shown to be one of the most sensitive methods for assessing small hepatic metastases (Fig. 43.25). Dual-phase scanning (arterial and portal) should be used with both conventional and spiral CT to differentiate hepatic lesions from perfusion anomalies.

Key points: obstructive jaundice

■ Ultrasound, CT and MR cholangiopancreatography are most useful for the initial non-invasive evaluation of biliary obstruction

■ Endoscopic retrograde cholangiopancreatography is the procedure of choice for low bile duct lesions

■ Endoscopic retrograde cholangiopancreatography enables stenting and biliary drainage to be performed as a one-step procedure

■ Percutaneous transhepatic cholangiography has a higher success and lower complication rate for hilar lesions than ERCP

■ Metal stents have lower rates of haemorrhage, cholangitis, occlusion and re-intervention than plastic stents

Visceral arteriography may be combined with a number of ingenious biochemical methods to localize small gastrointestinal tumours, particularly in the body and tail of the pancreas, avoiding direct transhepatic portal venous sampling. For example, calcium stimulation hepatic venous sampling has been used for the detection of occult insulinomas and other apudomas.[29]

For malignant hepatic metastases, with a predominantly hepatic arterial supply and for primary hepatocellular carcinoma, visceral arteriography can be followed by hepatic chemo-embolization using chemotherapeutic agents (e.g. 5-fluorouracil and epirubicin) combined with radio-opaque material, such as lipiodol which has been shown to be taken up preferentially by the capillary circulation of hepatic tumours.[30] As well as providing high doses of chemotherapy locally, the lipiodol component of the preparation retained in the lesions is utilized as a marker of the tumour on subsequent CT examinations (Fig. 43.26). However, embolization of hepatocellular carcinoma should be avoided in patients with underlying cirrhosis where further hepatic failure may

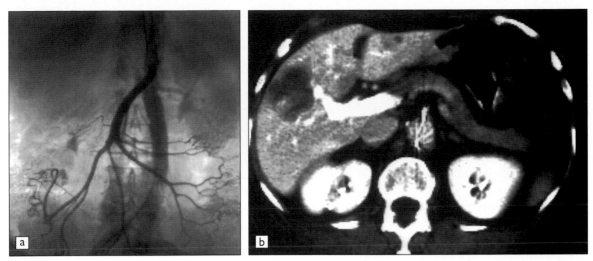

Figure 43.25. *CT arterial portography demonstrating large metastasis in right lobe of liver and smaller lesions in left lobe. (a) Superior mesenteric arteriogram confirming conventional visceral arterial anatomy; (b) dynamic CTAP image using conventional CT scanner showing excellent enhancement of portal vein with 'splaying' of vessels around large hepatic metastasis. The smaller lesions in the left lobe were confirmed as simple cysts on intra-operative ultrasound with aspiration and immediate cytology.*

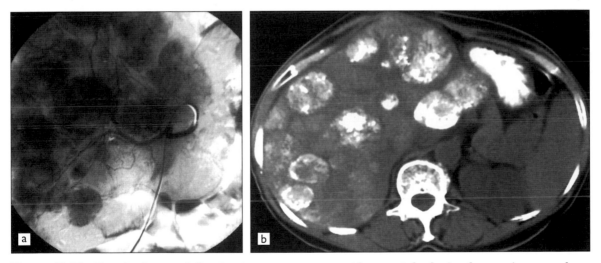

Figure 43.26. *Hepatic chemo-embolization in a young woman with a resected colonic adenocarcinoma and multiple hepatic metastases. (a) Selective catheterization of common hepatic artery allows a mixture of lipiodol and 5-fluorouracil to be continually injected; (b) a subsequent CT scan utilizes the retained lipiodol to help follow the progress of marker lesions.*

be precipitated. The principle of hepatic chemo-embolization has been extended to percutaneous insertion of selectively placed catheters attached to implantable ports:[31] Unfortunately, the response to treatment of hepatic metastases is less than for primary hepatocellular carcinoma.

Other indications for gastro-intestinal embolization in malignancy are for inoperable tumours and for bleeding caused by tumour or chemotherapeutic agents; for example, bleeding is a well-recognized complication of chemotherapy

for gastric lymphoma. The technique is particularly suitable when endoscopic procedures have failed or are impractical.

The pancreas has a multiple arterial supply which therefore limits the effects of embolotherapy and for this reason the technique is rarely used for the treatment of pancreatic malignancy. In some cases, such as hypervascular apudomas superselective embolization has been used for symptomatic control of intractable pain, haemorrhage and hormone production. Splenic embolization is now rarely performed, although it has been recommended in the past for malignancies associated with marked splenomegaly, such as lymphoma, the objective being to improve platelet function and achieve preoperative splenic devascularization prior to elective surgical splenectomy.[32]

Similarly, adrenal embolization is rarely performed but may help to palliate tumours or control hormone secretion. Either the three arteries supplying the adrenal or the single draining vein can be embolized. Deliberate obstruction of the adrenal veins has been used to obliterate adrenal function as an alternative to bilateral surgical adrenalectomy in patients with advanced malignant disease.[33] In addition, wedged retrograde injection of contrast medium mixed with sclerosant liquids such as hypertonic dextrose and alcohol, has been used in the treatment of Cushing's syndrome and primary hyperaldosteronism due to an adrenal adenoma.

Percutaneous insertion of inferior vena cava, filters and stents

A well recognized indication of inferior vena caval filtration is recurrent pulmonary embolism despite optimal anticoagulation, or where there is significant risk of pulmonary embolism in patients who cannot be anticoagulated. Another indication is deep pelvic vein and iliofemoral venous thrombosis due to local pelvic malignancy.

Contraindications to anticoagulant therapy in the oncology setting include:

- Gastro-intestinal bleeding
- Recent major surgery
- Widespread metastatic disease
- Malignancy of the central nervous system (CNS)

A wide range of IVC filters have been designed including both permanent and temporary filters, the latter not usually being appropriate in patients with advanced local malignant disease unless they are inserted for a short period prior to surgical resection of the tumour (Fig. 43.27). Although filters are usually inserted into the IVC in an infrarenal position, in patients with renal vein tumour invasion who are at risk of tumour emboli, the IVC filter may be placed in an infrahepatic suprarenal position in the IVC.

Brief mention has been given above to the use of IVC stents which remain an uncommon procedure but may relieve inferior venal caval obstruction secondary to extrinsic compression, for example from paracaval nodal disease.[12]

Percutaneous neurolysis

An extensive network of neural tissue around the upper abdominal aorta constitutes the coeliac plexus. Direct invasion of the coeliac plexus and surrounding tissues results in considerable pain and in some cases of visceral maligancy

the pain becomes intractable and unresponsive to conventional analgesia. Neurolytic coeliac plexus blockade is performed by injecting alcohol into the retroperitoneum near the coeliac plexus using a fine needle. The anterior, posterior translumbar and transaortic approaches under fluoroscopic or CT guidance may be used. The anterior approach is less commonly performed, contraindications including the presence of ascites, which introduces the risk of peritonitis, and an uncorrectable coagulopathy.

Key points: visceral arteriography

- Visceral arteriography is used as a vehicle for indirect portography, CTAP, venous sampling and hepatic chemoembolization

- Computed tomography arterial portography is one of the most sensitive methods for assessing small hepatic metastases

- Hepatocellular carcinomas show a greater response to hepatic chemoembolization than metastases

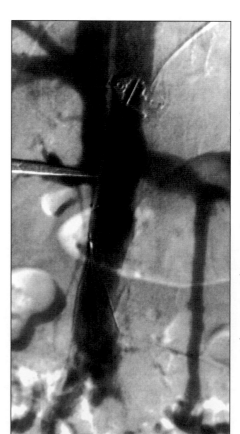

Figure 43.27. *Transjugular insertion of modified Günther Tulip IVC filter for temporary filtration prior to removal of large pelvic tumour. Note presence of thrombosis in iliac veins and preferential filling of left ascending lumbar vein. The filter was removed via the transjugular route 7 days following tumour excision.*

Tumour ablation techniques

Most percutaneous ablation techniques have been directed towards isolated hepatic metastases using a wide range of destructive agents including:

- Absolute alcohol
- Cryotherapy
- Thermoablation
- Radiofrequency pulses

Ultrasound-guided percutaneous alcohol injection was first described by Sugiura et al. in 1983.[34] Similar techniques have been extended for use in renal, rectal and parathyroid tumours. Proponents of the technique have suggested that it is particularly suitable for lesions which lack hypervascularity and therefore are unlikely to respond to transarterial chemoembolization. These tumours include adenomatous hyperplasia and atypical adenomatous hyperplasia which are precursors of hepatocellular carcinoma. Both ultrasound and MRI have been used to guide fine needles for such interstitial therapy. One of the problems with liquid agents is the possibility of ethanol or microbubbles entering vessels (or bile ducts) or refluxing back along the needle track. More recently, this has been obviated by the use of methods such as cryo- and thermo-ablation, high intensity focused ultrasound and interstitial laser and radiofrequency pulses. Computed tomography guidance is used primarily for smaller lesions, either undetected by ultrasound or in those sites difficult for access such as under a diaphragmatic dome.

Honda et al. have pioneered a technique of percutaneous hot saline injections which produce local heat-induced coagulation necrosis of the tumour with the liquid returning to physiological saline on cooling.[35] Tabuse et al. reported the use of microwave tissue coagulation to prevent malignant seeding, bleeding and biliary leakage along the needle track following liver biopsy.[36] More recently, Murakami et al. have applied these techniques to the treatment of hepatocellular carcinoma greater than 3 cm in diameter.[37] Microwaves produce larger volumes of coagulation necrosis than laser therapy during a shorter duration and the depth of microwave penetration can be limited.

Key point: inferior vena caval filtration

■ Inferior vena caval filtration is indicated for recurrent pulmonary embolism despite optimal anticoagulation

URINARY TRACT INTERVENTION

Percutaneous nephrostomy and ureteric stent insertion

Percutaneous nephrostomy is one of the commonest procedures performed in oncological intervention. There are several indications in cancer management which include:

- Relief of urinary tract obstruction prior to ureteric stent insertion
- Provision of urinary diversion in cases of chemotherapy-related haemorrhagic cystitis
- Treatment of upper urinary tract fistulae prior to occlusion of the fistula whether with an embolic agent or by direct closure using a metal clip under percutaneous fluoroscopic guidance[38]

Variants to this procedure include percutaneous placement of large bore rubber tubes to block the distal ureter accompanied by external drainage, and the use of endoluminal radiofrequency electric cautery to achieve permanent ureteral occlusion.[39,40] A modified occlusal nephro-ureteral catheter has been developed for severe haemorrhagic cystitis or bladder irritation from other causes such as tumour irradiation or chemotherapy.[41] More recently, radiologists have been asked to remove or exchange blocked indwelling ureteric stents and retrieve stent fragments which can also be performed fluoroscopically using a vascular snare (Fig. 43.28).

Following decompression of the dilated urinary tract with a percutaneous nephrostomy and diagnostic aspiration of urine for microbiological/cytological analysis, antegrade pyelography may demonstrate a ureteric stricture causing partial or complete obstruction (Fig. 43.29). It is usually possible to cross these lesions, even if the stricture is very tight, using appropriate guidewires and catheters. This sometimes necessitates dilatation prior to insertion of a double pigtail ureteric stent so that the proximal pigtail can be positioned in the renal pelvis and the distal pigtail in the bladder (Fig. 43.30). Ureteric stenting is not only suitable for ureteric malignancies but it is also helpful for alleviation of obstruction secondary to malignant retroperitoneal masses and pelvic cancers, e.g. lymphadenopathy, cervical, bladder and prostate cancers as well as postradiation retroperitoneal fibrosis.

A major dilemma is whether to perform percutaneous nephrostomy and related intervention in patients with disseminated malignancy in whom relief of urinary tract obstruction may prolong life only for the patient to die from advanced local disease, often with distressing symptoms. However, if chemotherapy, radiotherapy or hormonal manipulation may be expected to provide good palliation then ureteric stenting is appropriate and easily performed.

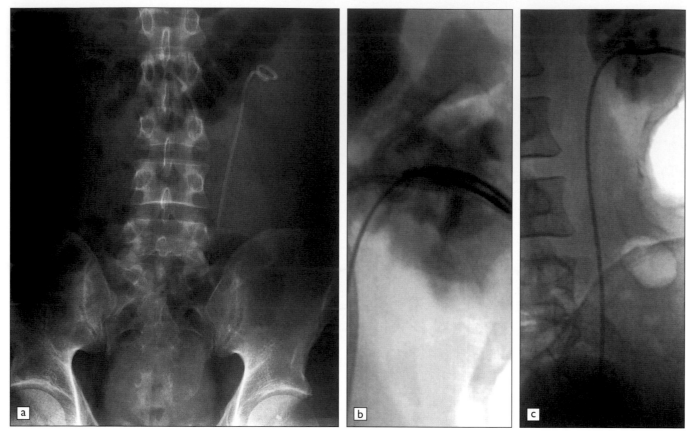

Figure 43.28. *Percutaneous retrieval of fragmented ureteric stent in patient with malignant distal ureteric stricture. (a) Plain abdominal radiograph demonstrating fragmented left ureteric stent following stent exchange at cystoscopy; (b) a percutaneous track has been created and the proximal end of the stent snared with a 'goose-neck' snare via an 8 Fr sheath (with the end cut at an angle to increase effective luminal diameter); (c) following fragment extraction, the stricture has been crossed and a multiple side-hole drainage catheter left in situ prior to further definitive stenting.*

Ureteric fistulae may result from radical pelvic surgery, pelvic malignancy or radiotherapy and in such cases ureteric stents may be inserted either retrogradely or antegradely. If a catheter and guidewire cannot be advanced across the fistula, consideration should be given to embolotherapy (vide supra). An alternative approach is medical nephrectomy by renal vascular embolization. Bilateral diversion of urinary flow may be required to assist healing to keep the patients dry for rectovesical or vesicovaginal fistulae.

Percutaneous and ureteroscopic tumour ablation

The traditional management of transitional cell carcinoma involving the upper urinary tract is nephro-ureterectomy with removal of a cuff of bladder surrounding the ipsilateral ureteral orifice. An alternative is endoscopic treatment of these tumours either by the antegrade approach via a percutaneous track to the renal pelvis or retrogradely at ureteroscopy. The indications for regional treatment using a minimally invasive approach are:

- Tumour involving a solitary kidney
- Bilateral synchronous tumours
- Renal insufficiency such that renal function will not be maintained by removal of one kidney
- Low-grade and low-stage lesions
- Transplanted kidneys when another organ is not available
- Benign upper-tract tumours including fibro-epithelial polyps
- Poor patient tolerance of a major surgical procedure

Working in close collaboration, the radiologist establishes a percutaneous approach, the urologist then removes the tumour with a resectoscope, cold-cup biopsy forceps with or without laser therapy, or by the placement of iridium (Ir-192) wires. Radiologists may also be asked to create percutaneous tracts to allow urologists to perform percutaneous cryotherapy to advanced renal cell carcinoma.

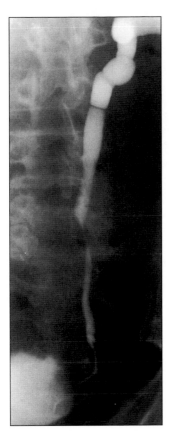

Figure 43.29.
Antegrade pyelography demonstrating tight irregular distal ureteric stricture. This examination was performed following percutaneous nephrostomy and drainage prior to ureteric stenting.

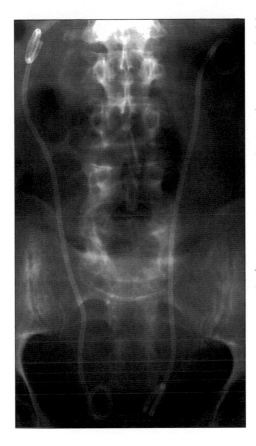

Figure 43.30.
Percutaneous insertion of bilateral double pig-tailed ureteric stents in a woman with extensive para-aortic lymphadenopathy (Hodgkin's disease). Following bilateral nephrostomy and drainage the stents were inserted to relieve obstruction during chemotherapy and were subsequently removed fluoroscopically using a perurethral approach.

Renal artery embolization

Renal cell carcinoma accounts for 3% of all malignancies. Surgical nephrectomy has been the conventional treatment for localized disease (Stages I–III). Tumours that are unresectable, due to a large tumour volume or evidence of local extension, can be downstaged to operable tumours by embolization. Embolization is not indicated for small tumours, oncocytomas or cancer of the renal pelvis. The aims of preoperative embolization are:

- Permanent blockage of capillary and precapillary arterioles by occlusion of the renal artery at or close to its division into segmental vessels but at a safe distance from the origin of the aorta (Fig. 43.31)
- Reduction of subsequent operative blood loss

An improved prognosis is noted in 3-year survival rates of Stage-T3 tumours which have been treated by preoperative arterial embolization. Reduced tumour cell dissemination during nephrectomy is assumed to be responsible for the increased survival rates. Embolization may also be used to palliate unresectable tumours and for managing complications associated with tumours, for example pain and haematuria.

Key points: urinary tract intervention

- Percutaneous nephrostomy enables stenting for urinary obstruction, allows urinary diversion and may help urinary fistulae to heal

- Medical nephrectomy may be required to aid healing of fistulae

- Radiologists can create percutaneous tracks thus enabling endourological procedures to be performed

- Renal and pelvic arterial embolization may be required as either a preoperative or palliative measure

Therapeutic pelvic embolization

The major indication for pelvic embolization is the treatment of pelvic malignancies, including bladder cancer, prostate cancer and gynaecological tumours. The commonest indications for therapeutic pelvic embolization include:

- Control of bleeding
- Palliation of pain
- Shrinkage of tumour
- Reduction of subsequent intra-operative blood loss in large vascular tumours

In addition, good palliation of intractable haemorrhage from the bladder, due to radiation cystitis, may be achieved by bilateral embolization of the anterior divisions of both internal iliac arteries.

MUSCULOSKELETAL INTERVENTION

Percutaneous skeletal biopsy

Percutaneous skeletal biopsy is a simple and safe procedure providing an effective alternative to open surgical biopsy. Needle biopsy is now much better accepted than previously as experience in interpretation of even small tissue samples has been gained.

Biopsy is usually performed using fluoroscopy or CT guidance with osteoblastic or sclerotic bone lesions biopsied using large-bore needles whilst osteolytic lesions can sometimes be managed with fine needles. If soft tissue masses are associated with destructive bone lesions, good cores can usually be obtained without the need to directly sample the associated destroyed bone (Fig. 43.32). Rib and extremity lesions are easily biopsied with either thin- or large-bore needles, according to the nature of the lesion. Thoracic and lumbar vertebral body lesions are best approached with the patient prone utilizing a posterolateral approach on the ipsilateral side of the lesion. Although fluoroscopic guidance alone can be used for biopsying the vertebral bodies of the lower cervical vertebrae (using a lateral approach), CT guidance is

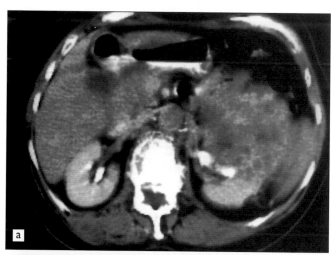

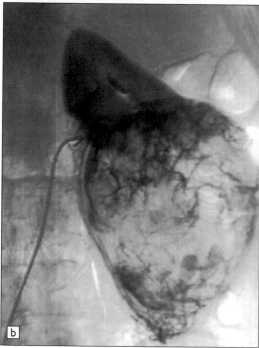

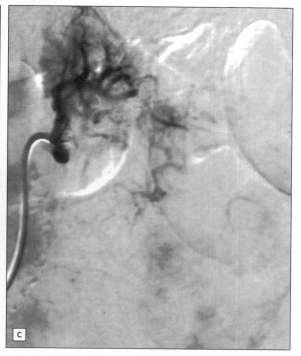

Figure 43.31. *Preoperative embolization of large renal cell carcinoma. (a) CT scan demonstrating a large tumour involving lower pole of left kidney and distorting left pelvicalyceal system. Note local invasion of perinephric fat; (b) selective left renal arteriogram demonstrates large hypervascular tumour with marked neovascularity and some central necrosis; (c) satisfactory appearances following selective embolization of tumour circulation with polyvinyl alcohol, gelfoam and two 4 mm platinum coils. Note residual staining of tumour capillary bed.*

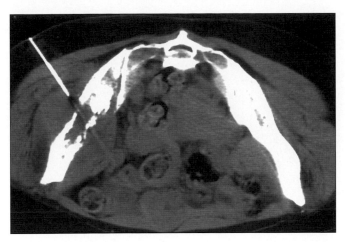

Figure 43.32. *CT-guided biopsy of lytic deposit in right ilium (patient prone). Note 'photon starvation artefact' demonstrating exact position of tip and confirming needle 'throw'. This technique will sample soft tissue masses as well as lytic bone deposits. Histology subsequently revealed metastatic renal cell adenocarcinoma.*

essential for biopsy of the upper cervical spine (using an anterior transpharyngeal approach) and the base of the skull and facial bones. Computed tomography guidance is also desirable for the posterolateral approach of thoracic lesions to avoid transgressing the pleural cavity. Bone biopsy is discussed further in Chapter 20.

Key points: musculoskeletal biopsy

■ Fine-needle aspiration biopsy of the soft tissue mass adjacent to a bone lesion often provides adequate material for diagnosis

■ Percutaneous vertebroplasty induces almost immediate pain relief

Percutaneous vertebroplasty

Percutaneous vertebroplasty, initially described for the treatment of vertebral haemangiomas, has also been used in the management of vertebral metastases.[42] It involves the injection of acrylic cement directly into the vertebral lesion to achieve consolidation and direct embolization of the vertebra. it provides almost immediate relief of pain compared to radiotherapy which may take several weeks and may be appropriate palliation when radiotherapy has been ineffective.

Therapeutic embolization of bone and soft tissue tumours

The initial use of vascular embolization in the management of skeletal tumours was as a preoperative measure to reduce intra-operative blood loss in hypervascular tumours. This treatment has now been extended to palliative embolization, particularly when the tumour is inoperable and has failed to respond to radiotherapy (Fig. 43.33).

The commonest hypervascular tumours treated with preoperative embolization are giant cell tumours (particularly around the knee and distal radius) and metastatic renal adenocarcinoma; nasopharyngeal tumours and paragangliomas may also be treated in this way. Following embolization it is advisable to transfer the patient from the interventional radiology suite to the operating theatre for immediate resection in order to minimize the 'postembolization syndrome'.

Giant cell tumours originating in the ilium are often advanced at presentation precluding primary surgical resection. These tumours are usually insensitive to chemotherapy and irradiation carries the risk of sarcomatous transformation. Therefore, vascular embolization has a place in the multimodality management of these tumours, for example in unresectable giant cell tumours and aneurysmal bone cysts after other therapeutic methods have failed or are considered inappropriate.

OTHER ONCOLOGICAL INTERVENTIONS

Breast intervention

Following improvements in mammography and ultrasound, as well s the development of specialized needles for localization and biopsy, breast intervention has become an integral part of breast cancer management. Such techniques are particularly important in the localization of mammographic abnormalities where reliable differentiation between benign and malignant lesions cannot be established with certainty. Biopsy and localization are also essential or possibly malignant yet non-palpable lesions.

Some cysts, for example, complex cysts, are quite reasonably treated with caution and aspiration biopsy should be considered regardless of patient symptomatology or mammographic appearance. Ultrasound is particularly useful for guidance using a free-hand technique to perform breast cyst aspiration and can characterize lesions as simple cysts, complex cysts, fibrosis, areas of fibrocystic disease or solid lesions. Patients with persistent nipple discharge in the absence of a palpable lesion or one that has been demonstrated on ultrasound or mammography may undergo galactography. This procedure outlines the involved duct unit and may be helpful in identifying small early intraductal carcinomas, benign papillomas, papillomatosis or papillary carcinomas. To facilitate surgical excision, the involved duct can be marked with a permanent dye, such as methylene blue.

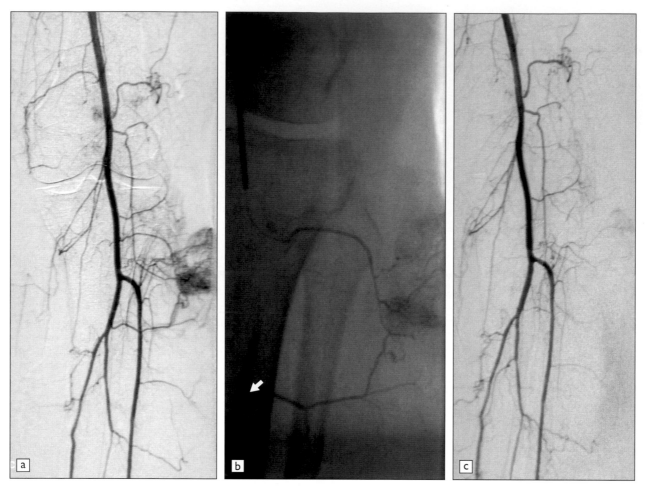

Figure 43.33. *Palliative embolization of recurrent soft tissue tumour mass (malignant melanoma): (a) selective arteriogram demonstrating hypervascular tumour with multiple feeding vessels; (b) superselective study revealing 'front' and 'back' door feeding supply. Note reflux into tibio-peroneal trunk (arrowed) requiring both 'doors' to be 'closed' to prevent reflex of embolic material; (c) tumour circulation has been excluded on final selective study with excellent palliation.*

Both fine-needle (22 gauge) and large-core breast biopsy (14–18 gauge with a 2 cm throw) can be performed using mammographic or ultrasound guidance under local anaesthesia. With ultrasound guidance a free-hand technique is usually used and FNAB alone may be sufficient if a cytologist is in attendance. Approximately 80% of impalpable breast lesions are visible on ultrasound. Biopsy and wire localization under ultrasound guidance avoids the discomfort of breast compression, waiting for films to be processed and repositioning of wires. The remaining 20% of lesions (mainly microcalcifications and some architectural distortions) require mammographic guidance. Traditionally, conventional mammography has been used for localization although more recently stereotactic mammography has provided exquisitely high pin-point accuracy. Some manufacturers provide stereotactic equipment which can accommodate both aspiration needles and automated biopsy guns for large-bore needles.

Needle localization of breast lesions has been used to reduce the amount of tissue excised at surgery. Hookwires have traditionally been used with either standard mammography units (with or without a fenestrated compression plate) or with stereotactic mammography. Once orthogonal or stereotactic views have confirmed that the tip of the needle is within the lesion (or close by), the hookwire can be deployed prior to transfer of the patient to theatre. Stereotactic mammography guidance for wire placement has a theoretical accuracy of within 1 mm. Ultrasound can also be used for accurate placement of wires using the free-hand technique in particular.

Tumour localization using venous sampling

The use of transhepatic portal venous sampling and hepatic venous sampling following stimulation has been described above in the detection of occult apudomas. In fact, venous sampling techniques can be applied to the detection of occult tumours in many other areas where perhaps cross-sectional imaging has failed to demonstrate the lesion adequately. This technique has been particularly useful in the detection of tumours causing increased hormone production, including parathyroid adenomas, Conn's tumours, phaeochromocytomas and pituitary tumours. The latter involves sampling the inferior petrosal venous sinuses and jugular veins, the sensitivity of the technique being increased by simultaneous stimulation of the appropriate releasing factor. Such intervention helps in the differentiation of pituitary-dependent Cushing's syndrome from ectopic adrenocorticotrophic hormone syndrome.

Parathyroid tumour ablation

In over 85% of cases, the cause for primary hyperparathyroidism is a solitary adenoma with the remaining cases being mainly due to parathyroid glandular hyperplasia. Less than 1% of cases are caused by parathyroid carcinoma. Surgical excision has a success rate of approximately 95% in experienced hands but where the risks of surgery are excessive or in cases of failed surgery, parathyroid venous sampling may be performed for tumour localization.

In view of the difficulties encountered in operating on a previously explored neck, which may be extensively scarred, parathyroid arteriography and angiographic ablation may be considered. Once the lesion has been identified on arteriography, a single end-holed catheter is wedged into the feeding vessel and multiple boluses of dense contrast material are injected to achieve intense parenchymal staining of the gland. This is followed by occlusion of the main feeding vessel with gelfoam or coils. In these difficult patients this technique has met with some considerable success with few complications.[43] Even if the procedure is unsuccessful, the technique will have localized the lesion elegantly for a further surgical attempt at excision.

Solbiati et al. performed parathyroid tumour ablation by percutaneous injection of absolute alcohol into the tumours under sonographic guidance.[44] Indications included high surgical risk, refusal of operation and recurrence after previous subtotal resection. The presence of all lesions was first confirmed on FNAB.

Percutaneous retrieval techniques

With the large number of intravascular catheters used for chemotherapy, the increasing usage of biliary and ureteric stents and the use of coils for palliative tumour embolization, there has been an increased requirements for the retrieval of displaced or misplaced fragments and a number of ingenious, yet well established, techniques have been developed which include:

- Wire-loop snares
- Fragment graspers
- Dormia baskets
- Deflector wires

Minimally invasive techniques to achieve such extraction are particularly important in patients with malignancy who are often extremely ill and may have coagulopathy. In such patients major surgery (for example, thoracotomy) is particularly undesirable.

Key points: other applications

- Galactography may help identify early intraductal carcinoma, papillomatosis or papillary carcinoma

- Stereotactic biopsy and localization provide pin-point accuracy for mammographically visible lesions

- Ultrasound guidance avoids uncomfortable breast compression, waiting for film processing and repositioning of wires

- Venous sampling techniques may help to localize occult tumours

- Parathyroid tumour ablation may be useful for the scarred, previously explored, neck

- Minimally invasive techniques may be employed to relieve misplaced or displaced fragments and coils

Intra-operative ultrasound

Intra-operative ultrasound has been used to biopsy a number of lesions, for example liver, pancreas, kidney, brain and spinal cord.[45] In our institution we routinely localize hepatic metastases to segmental level prior to resection, using a dedicated operative probe which not only demonstrates the lesions but allows accurate anatomical mapping. More recently, image-guided ablation of small hepatic lesions has been performed at the time of surgical resection of larger lesions.

Locoregional chemotherapy

Selective infusion of intra-arterial chemotherapy may reduce the side-effects of systemic chemotherapy while increasing the local concentration of drug in an attempt to achieve the best tumour response. The most common example is hepatic chemoembolization described above. Other examples of chemo-infusion therapy include locoregional intra-arterial chemotherapy of local chest wall recurrence in breast carcinoma via the internal mammary artery, isolated limb perfusion in malignant melanoma and chemo-infusion therapy of advanced primary transitional cell carcinoma of the bladder (T3 and T4 bladder carcinomas) with or without simultaneous radiotherapy, and infusion of sarcomas, bone and cerebral tumours.

Interventional imaging of neurological tumours

Interventional CT, MRI and positron emission tomography (PET) techniques have been used to provide stereotactic guidance for the biopsy of image-proven tumours.[46] The technique has been extended to both CT-guided stereotactic interstitial brachytherapy,[45] a technique in which radioactive sources have been implanted into unresectable brain tumours, and CT-guided stereotactic surgery when deep-seated intracerebral neoplasms can be vaporized using a stereotactically directed CO_2 laser.

Following presurgical evaluation of the vascular supply to intra- and extracranial vascular tumours, e.g. haemangiomas, meningiomas, glomus tumours and haemangioblastomas, pre-operative embolization may be performed using particulate emboli in patients of poor operative risk.

Summary

- Fine-needle aspiration biopsy (FNAB) is usually sufficient for diagnosis of malignancy provided adequate cellular material has been obtained.

- Tissue cores are required for the accurate classification of lymphoma.

- In the chest, ultrasound guidance is well suited for the drainage of malignant effusions and other collections.

- The interventional imaging suite is becoming increasingly used for percutaneous insertion of central venous catheters and for the management of ensuing complications.

- In lung cancer, interventional techniques, such as bronchoscopic tracheobronchial stenting and bronchial artery embolization, have a useful role in patient management.

- In the gastro-intestinal tract, endoscopic ultrasound (EUS) is becoming increasingly used for staging primary tumours, for biopsy of tumour and lymph nodes and for drainage of fluid collections and abscesses.

- Liver biopsy should be carried out using the transjugular approach or by performing a plugged liver biopsy in the presence of uncorrectable coagulopathy.

- Endoscopic and fluoroscopic techniques (dilatation/stents) provide palliation for oesophageal strictures, fistulae, gastric outlet obstruction and large bowel obstruction. Gastrostomy feeding tubes can also be inserted using the percutaneous/endoscopic approach.

- In the management of obstructive jaundice, both endoscopic retrograde cholangiopancreatography (ERCP) and percutaneous transhepatic cholangiography (PTC) are useful for diagnosis. Endoscopic retrograde cholangiopancreatography is the procedure of choice for low bile duct lesions whereas PTC has a higher success and lower complication rate for hilar lesions.

- Visceral arteriography is used as a vehicle for indirect portography, CT arterial portography (CTAP), venous sampling and hepatic chemo-embolization.

- Inferior vena caval infiltration is indicated for recurrent pulmonary embolism or in patients at high risk of pulmonary embolism who cannot be anticoagulated.

- Image-guided tumour ablation techniques are mostly used for hepatic malignant lesions and include cryo- and thermoablation, high intensity focused ultrasound and interstitial laser and radiofrequency pulses.

- Renal and urinary tract interventional procedures include nephrostomy, ureteric stenting, ureteroscopic tumour ablation and renal arterial embolization.

- Renal arterial embolization may be used for unresectable tumours in an attempt to downstage disease prior to surgery. It may also be used as a palliative procedure for pain and/or haematuria.

- Therapeutic embolization for pelvic and musculoskeletal tumours may be preoperative or palliative measures.

- Percutaneous vertebroplasty may be useful in the management of spinal metastatic pain.

- Venous sampling techniques are useful for localizing occult tumours which are biochemically active.

- Percutaneous retrieval techniques may be required for fragmented catheters, stents and misplaced coils.

- Interventional CT, MRI and PET scanning are being developed to provide stereotactic guidance for biopsy, interstitial brachytherapy and surgery.

REFERENCES

1. Husband J E, Golding S J. The role of computed tomography guided needle biopsy in an oncology service. Clin Radiol 1983; 34: 255–260

2. Anderson T, Eriksson B, Lindgren P G et al. Percutaneous ultrasonography-guided cutting biopsy from liver metastases of endocrine gastro-intestinal tumours. Ann Surg 1987; 206: 728–732

3. Van Sonnenberg E, Casola G, Ho M et al. Difficult thoracic lesions: CT guided biopsy experience in 150 cases. Radiology 1988; 167: 457–461

4. Haaga J R, Reich N E, Havrilla T R et al. Interventional CT scanning. Radiol Clin North Am 1977; 15: 449–456

5. Templeton P A, Krasna M. Needle/wire lung nodule localization for thorascopic resection. Chest 1993; 104: 953–958

6. Robertson L J, Mauro M A, Jacques P F. Radiologic placement of Hickman catheters. Radiology 1989; 170: 1007–1009

7. Page A C, Evans R A, Kaczmarshi R et al. The insertion of chronic indwelling central venous catheters (Hickman Lines) in interventional radiology suites. Clin Radiol 1990; 42: 105–109

8. Adam A. Insertion of long term central venous catheter: Time for a new look. Br Med J 1995; 311: 341–342

9. Azizkhan R G, Taylor L A, Jaques P F et al. Percutaneous translumbar and transhepatic inferior vena caval catheters for prolonged vascular access in children. J Pediat Surg 1992; 27: 165–169

10. Kaufman J A, Crenshaw W B, Kuter I et al. Percutaneous placement of a central venous access device. Am J Roentgenol 1995; 164: 459–460

11. Gaines P A, Belli A M, Anderson P B et al. Superior vena caval obstruction managed by the Gianturco Z Stent. Clin Radiol 1994; 49: 202–208

12. Furui S, Sawada, S, Kuramoto K et al. Gianturco stent placement in malignant caval obstruction: analysis of factors for predicting the outcome. Radiology 1995; 195: 147–152

13. Tan B S, Watkinson A F, Dussek J E et al. Metallic endoprosthesis for malignant tracheo-bronchial obstruction: Initial experience. Cardiovasc Intervent Radiol 1996; 19: 91–96

14. Gothlin J H. Post-lymphographic percutaneous fine needle aspiration biopsy of lymph nodes guided by fluoroscopy. Radiology 1976; 120: 205–207

15. Ho C S, McLoughlin M J, McHattie J D et al. Percutaneous fine needle aspiration biopsy of the pancreas following endoscopic retrograde cholangiography. Radiology 1977; 125: 351–353

16. Botet J F, Lightdale C J, Zauber A G et al. Pre-operative staging of oesophageal cancer. Radiology 1991; 181: 419–425

17. Ziegler K, Sanft C, Zimmer T et al. Comparison of computed tomography, endosonography and intra-operative assessment in TN staging of gastric carcinoma. Gut 1993; 34: 604–610

18. Tio T, Coene P, Van Delden O et al. Colorectal carcinoma: Pre-operative TNM classification with endosonography. Radiology 1991; 179: 165–170

19. Müller F, Meyenberger C, Bertschinger P et al. Pancreatic tumours: Evaluation with endoscopic US, CT and MR imaging. Radiology 1994; 190: 745–751

20. Jackson J E, Adam A. Percutaneous transcaval tumour biopsy using a 'road map' technique. Clin Radiol 1991; 44: 195–196

21. Iguchi H, Kimora Y, Yanada J et al. Treatment of a malignant stricture after oesophagojejunostomy by a self-expanding metallic stent. Cardiovasc Intervent Radiol 1993; 16: 102–104

22. Tejero E, Mainar A, Fernandez L et al. New procedure for the treatment of colorectal neoplastic obstructions. Dis Colon Rectum 1994; 37: 1158–1159

23. Rey J-F, Romancyk T, Grett M. Metal stents for palliation of rectal carcinoma: a preliminary report on 12 patients. Endoscopy 1995; 27: 501–504

24. Wollman B, D'Agostino H B, Walus-Wigle J R et al. Radiologic, endoscopic and surgical gastrostomy: An institutional evaluation and meta-analysis of the literature. Radiology 1995; 197: 699–704

25. Adam A, Chetty N, Roddie M et al. Self-expandable stainless steel endoprostheses for the treatment of malignant bile duct obstruction. Am J Roentgenol 1991; 156: 321–325

26. Fletcher M S, Brinkley D, Dawson J L et al Treatment of high bile duct carcinoma by internal radiotherapy with iridium-192 wires. Lancet 1981; ii: 172–174

27. Hutson D G, Russell E, Schiffe E et al. Balloon dilatation of biliary strictures through a choledochojejunocutaneous fistula. Ann Surg 1984; 199: 637–644

28. Reduanly R D, Chezmar J L. CT arterial portography: Technique, indications and applications. Clin Radiol 1997; 52: 256–268

29. O'Shea D, Rohrer-Theurs A W, Lym J A et al. Localization of insulinomas by selective intra-arterial calcium injection. J Clin Endocrinol Metab 1996; 81: 1623–1627

30. Raoul J L, Bourguet P, Bretagne J F et al. Hepatic artery injection of I-131-labelled Lipiodol: Part I Biodistribution study results in patients with hepatocellular carcinoma and liver metastases. Radiology 1988; 168: 541–545

31. Arai Y. Required basic procedures of hepatic arterial infusion chemotherapy for interventional radiologists. Jap J Clin Radiol 1993; 38: 1497–1508

32. Wholey M H, Chamorro H A, Rao G et al. Splenic infarction and spontaneous rupture after therapeutic embolization. Cardiovasc Radiol 1978; 1: 249–253

33. Jahlonski R D, Meaney T F, Schumacher C P. Transcatheter adrenal ablation for metastatic carcinoma of the breast. Cleveland Clin Quart 1977; 44: 57–63

34. Sugiura N, Takara K, Ohto M et al. Percutaneous intratumoral injection of ethanol under ultrasound imaging for treatment of small hepatocellular carcinoma. Acta Hepatol Japonica 1983; 24: 920–924

35. Honda N, Guo Q, Uchida H et al. Percutaneous hot saline injection therapy for hepatic tumours: An alternative to percutaneous ethanol injection therapy. Radiology 1994; 190: 53–57

36. Tabuse Y, Tabuse K, Mori K et al. Percutaneous microwave tissue coagulation in liver biopsy: Experimental and clinical studies. Arch Jpn Chit 1986; 55: 381–392

37. Murakami R, Yoshimatsu S, Yamashita Y et al. Treatment of hepatocellular carcinoma: Value of percutaneous microwave coagulation. Am J Roentgenol 1995; 164: 1159–1164

38. Lund A, Rysavy J A, Hunter D W et al. Percutaneous occlusion of the ureter: A new approach for relief of urinary tract fistulae. Semin Intervent Radiology 1984; 1: 92–98

39. Castaneda F, Moradian G P, Epstein D H et al. A new technique for complete temporary occlusion of the ureter. Am J Roentgenol 1989; 153: 81–82

40. Kopecky K U, Sutton G P, Bihrle R et al. Percutaneous transrenal endocureteral radio-frequency electrocautery for occlusion: Case report. Radiology 1989; 170: 1047–1048

41. Bush W, Mayo M. Catheter modification for transrenal temporary total ureteral obstruction: the 'occlusive' nephroureteral catheter. Urology 1994; 43: 729–733

42. Weill A, Chiras J, Simon J M et al. Spinal metastases: Indications for and results of percutaneous injection of acrylic surgical cement. Radiology 1996; 199: 241–247

43. Miller D L, Doppman J L, Change R et al. Angiographic ablation of parathyroid adenomas: Lessons from a 10 year experience. Radiology 1987; 165: 601–607

44. Solbiati L, Giangrande A, De Pra L et al. Percutaneous ethanol injection of parathyroid tumours under US guidance: Treatment for secondary hyperparathyroidism. Radiology 1985; 155: 607–610

45. Machi J, Sigel B, Kurohisi T et al. Operative ultrasound guidance for various surgical procedures. Ultrasound Med Biol 1990; 16: 37–42

46. Quinones-Molina R, Alaminos A, Molina H. Computer-assisted CT-guided stereotactic biopsy and brachytherapy of brain tumours. Stereotactic Functional Neurosurg 1994; 63: 52–55

Chapter 44

Imaging for radiotherapy treatment planning

Jane Dobbs and Ann Barrett

INTRODUCTION

The goal of curative radiotherapy is to focus the prescribed radiation dose to cover the tumour and to keep the dose to normal tissues to a minimum. Improved precision in localizing the exact site and extent of a tumour decreases the risk of missing the tumour with a radiation beam, and also makes it possible to treat smaller volumes of tissue to a higher radiation dose with a potential for increase in cure. Rapid advances in technology have made it possible to:

- Use complex beam configurations for radiotherapy treatment
- To visualize tumours and calculate dose distributions in three dimensions
- To conform fields more tightly to irregularly shaped tumours

These elements together constitute what is known as conformal therapy. However, achieving the potential for progress depends very much on having an excellent, dedicated multidisciplinary team which includes a committed diagnostic radiologist as well as an oncologist, physicist, planning technician and therapy radiographer to ensure that these technological advances are used accurately.

TARGET VOLUMES

'Target volumes' are used to describe volumes of tissue which are irradiated. The International Commission on Radiation Units and Measurements (ICRU) Report No. 50[1] has defined a series of target volumes (Fig. 44.1) which are used to describe where the treatment is given anatomically and enables comparisons to be made between treatments given in different cancer centres. Defining the clinical target volume (CTV), at which radiation beams will be aimed, remains the most difficult step in the planning process and because of its inherent variability, it is the weakest link in the chain of events which occur during the radiotherapy procedure (Fig. 44.2).

Figure 44.1. *ICRU target volumes (From ref. 1. with permission).*

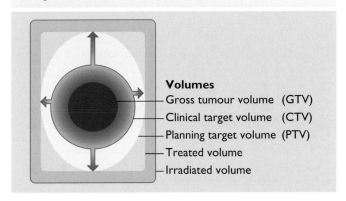

Volumes
Gross tumour volume (GTV)
Clinical target volume (CTV)
Planning target volume (PTV)
Treated volume
Irradiated volume

Figure 44.2. *Steps in planning radiotherapy treatment from ICRU 50 (From ref. 1. with permission).*

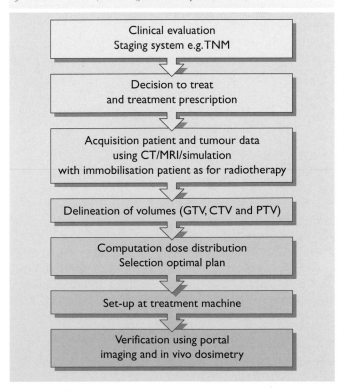

Clinical evaluation
Staging system e.g. TNM

Decision to treat
and treatment prescription

Acquisition patient and tumour data
using CT/MRI/simulation
with immobilisation patient as for radiotherapy

Delineation of volumes (GTV, CTV and PTV)

Computation dose distribution
Selection optimal plan

Set-up at treatment machine

Verification using portal
imaging and in vivo dosimetry

The first step in planning radiotherapy treatment is to define the extent of gross macroscopic tumour by clinical examination and optimum imaging. The ICRU Report 50, first defines the gross tumour volume (GTV) as the palpable or visible extent of tumour representing macroscopic disease. Delineation of the gross tumour volume is dependent on imaging modality and technique. It is of course impossible to define this volume when the tumour has already been removed and, where appropriate clinically, initial preoperative images will be used to define the preoperative GTV.

All tumours are classified according to recognized staging systems (discussed in Chapter 3) such as the TNM system which describes tumour, nodes and metastases, or for example the FIGO classification. However, these rarely give guidelines as to which imaging modality is best for defining the T stage for each primary site. The role of the radiologist here is vital in deciding, with the oncologist, which imaging modality should be used for each tumour site to map its local extent most precisely. The oncologist needs to know:

- The site of the tumour within the patient according to fixed coordinates
- Three-dimensional measurements of tumour size
- Details of the edge of the tumour where it forms a clear boundary with adjacent normal tissue
- Details of anatomy where no clear boundary exists

The GTV contains the maximum concentration of tumour cells, although there may be central necrosis where clonogenic cell numbers are reduced. Around the macroscopic or imaged tumour, there will probably be a zone of direct local microscopic spread. A margin, which must be added to encompass the spread, is chosen using histological parameters such as:

- Grade (which correlates with invasiveness and growth rate)
- Vascular and lymphatic permeation
- Histological type
- Knowledge of tumour-specific spread patterns

This zone around the GTV is assumed to have a decreasing malignant cell density toward the periphery and for many tumours may involve oedema (Fig. 44.3).

Currently studies are being performed on cerebral tumours, where, at the time of surgery, biopsies have been taken sequentially from the centre of the tumour out into normal brain tissue. The histological examination of these specimens is correlated with appearances of preoperative imaging to define more clearly what is happening at the apparent boundary between tumour and normal tissues. The finding of tumour cells in zones of oedema suggests that using tight margins around the enhancing tumour on computed

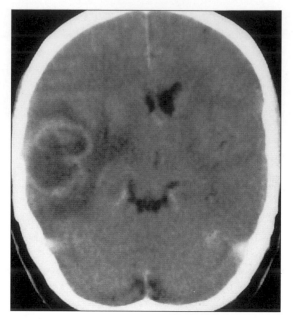

Figure 44.3. *CT scan of brain showing enhancing area of obvious tumour with surrounding oedema, probably containing single tumour cell spread.*

tomography (CT) or magnetic resonance imaging (MRI) may lead to decreased rather than greater tumour control.

For many other tumours, little research has been carried out with regard to the changes which occur at the edge of the tumour in response to therapy. Some tumours after chemotherapy appear to shrink down to their point of origin, whereas others may leave nests of cells within a fibrotic matrix (e.g. Ewing's sarcoma). These patterns of behaviour need to be clearly understood if appropriate margins for tumour spread are to be clearly defined.

The high degree of spatial resolution which can now be achieved with imaging, even with the improved utilization of intravenous contrast medium, still may not be adequate to give this information, but functional studies may provide more information about this tumour–normal tissue interface. More research using 'old-fashioned' meticulous pathological examination of tissue specimens could also be used to address these problems. This information is vital for defining the CTV which is the gross tumour volume with an added margin for subclinical spread.

The CTV may, however, be affected by organ movement caused by:

- Respiration
- Cardiac motion
- Swallowing
- Displacement of organs such as the prostate with bladder and rectal filling

For pelvic radiotherapy, patients with bladder tumours may be treated after micturition with the bladder 'empty' to minimize the bladder volume and help reduce toxicity. For treatment of prostate cancer, some centres treat patients with the bladder 'full' after maximum fluid intake in order to distend the bladder mucosa away from the prostate target volume and to displace the small bowel, thereby reducing normal tissue dosage.

Ten Haken[2] showed movement of the prostate gland of between 0–2 cm (mean of 0.5 cm) when the bladder or rectum were filled using catheters to simulate daily variations due to urine and stool contents. These data showed that displacement of the prostate out of the dosimetric zone led to failure to deliver the full radiation dose to the prostatic tumour. Organ movement such as this becomes particularly important in conformal therapy where margins are reduced and the dose is escalated.

The amount of organ movement varies in different parts of the body, being greatest in the lung and abdomen and least in the brain and head and neck region. For cerebral tumours, perspex shells (Fig. 44.4) used for immobilization of the patient can limit movement to 1–2 mm.[3] In the chest, greater excursions occur with respiration, and for breast radiotherapy Gagliardi et al.[4] has shown a 4 cm displacement of a skin tattoo in the axilla with movement of the arm. This is especially relevant if the arm is raised above the head for CT scanning of the breast, but then returned to a neutral position for treatment. Computed tomography scanning for radiotherapy treatment planning must be performed with the patient in exactly the same position as for treatment to avoid these errors. This information regarding organ movement and other measurements of variability of patient movement are used to define the planning target volume (PTV) which is the CTV plus a margin for movement.

Key points: target volumes

- The first step in planning radiotherapy is to define the gross macroscopic tumour volume (GTV)

- The zone around the GTV is assumed to have a decreasing malignant cell density towards the periphery

- The CTV is the GTV plus a margin for subclinical tumour spread

- The CTV may be affected by tumour/organ movement

- The PTV takes into account the CTV as well as information regarding organ movement and other measurements of variability

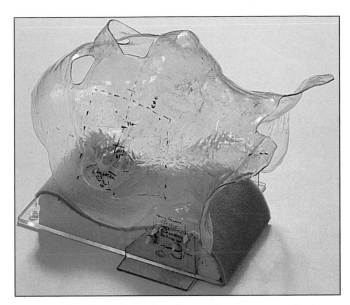

Figure 44.4. *Perspex shell used to restrict movement during treatment in the brain or head and neck region.*

Sources of error in determining target volumes

Denham et al.[5] reported a study in which different clinicians and radiologists were given CT scans and simulator films, depicting lung tumours for the same series of patients, and asked to construct target volumes. He showed that error in interpretation of CT data was one cause of inaccurate target volume construction by clinicians, who were particularly prone to misinterpret mediastinal vascular structures. Leunens et al.[6] performed a similar study using CT scans of cerebral tumours and showed that there was also a wide variation between radiologists and neurosurgeons, as well as oncologists, in the interpretation of CT data. Interpretation of diagnostic imaging by a radiologist is vital for obtaining maximum information about the tumour. Joint sessions with an oncologist are the best way to achieve this collaboration and produce excellence in target-volume definition for radiotherapy.

Variability between clinicians in choice of target volumes may, however, not just be due to incorrect interpretation of images, but, as indicated previously, may be due to a genuine ignorance of tumour behaviour at apparent boundaries as seen on imaging. This problem cannot be addressed by comparisons between clinicians, but only by further research on tumour behaviour at boundaries.[7]

CONFORMAL THERAPY

Conformal therapy has become possible with an explosion of technological advances.[8,9] Three dimensional image handling and algorithms for 3D dose distribution make it possible to produce sophisticated plans for treatment. Multileaf collimators (Fig. 44.5) can shape the beam to the tumour, and intensity modulation of the beam allows shaping of the dose distribution. Computerized verification systems are important to check the accuracy of treatment delivery. All these elements are used to match the volume of tissue irradiated as closely as possible with the target volume. Before these advances, 2D treatment planning was used and irradiation beams were square or rectangular, coplanar and static. Now target volumes can be any shape rather than being simple cubes, and radiation beams can be conformed to irregular target volumes and can deliver an even dose across the volume.

However, it has become increasingly clear that in order to deliver this high precision therapy, basic requirements such as the immobilization of the patient now assume prime importance. If the patient and the organ containing the tumour move from day to day during a fractionated course of radiotherapy treatment (e.g. 30 radiotherapy treatments), a geographical miss may occur and all the sophisticated technology will be wasted. Devices for immobilization include:

- Perspex shells (Fig. 44.4)
- Vacuum bags (Fig. 44.6a)
- Alpha cradles
- Poles and pads to secure limbs (Fig. 44.6b)

A system of skin tattoos and lasers (Fig. 44.7) has to be developed to ensure precise alignment of the patient.

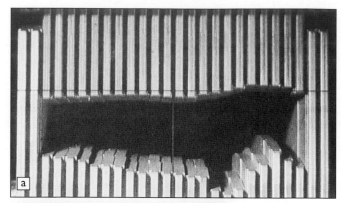

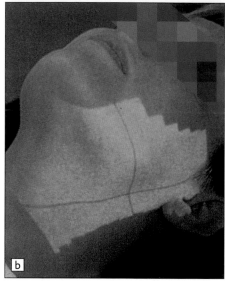

Figure 44.5. *(a) Multileaf collimator. Each individual leaf position may be varied to produce an irregularly shaped field. (b) Treatment field showing use of multileaf collimator.*

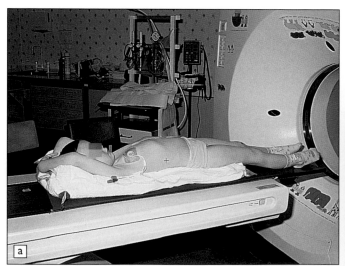

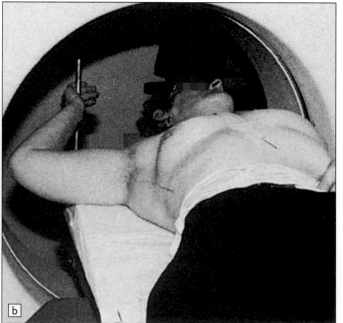

Figure 44.6. *Immobilization devices: (a) vacuum bag which can be moulded to patient shape and then fixed by creating a vacuum; (b) arm pole to reproduce position of arm accurately for breast radiotherapy.*

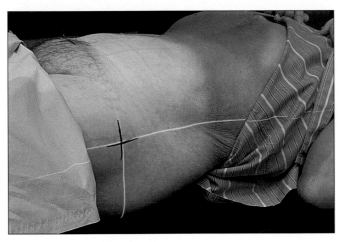

Figure 44.7. *Skin tattoos and laser lights used to ensure correct alignment of the patient.*

Key point: conformal radiotherapy

■ Conformal radiotherapy allows the radiation beam to be shaped according to the shape of the tumour and intensity modulation of the beam allows shaping of the dose distribution

CT-SCANNING TECHNIQUES FOR PLANNING

There are important differences between CT scans taken for radiotherapy treatment planning and those taken purely for diagnostic use, as the aim of the scan is different. A radiotherapy planning scan must define:

- The exact position of the tumour
- The extent of tumour in all directions
- The site of adjacent structures
- The relationship between normal organs, the tumour and external landmarks

External landmarks are used for setting up the patient on the therapy unit. Computed tomography scans for radiotherapy treatment planning must be taken under identical conditions to those for later radiotherapy treatment as Dutreix[10] has clearly shown that displacement of normal organs occurs with variation in the position of the patient. The exact set up of the position of the patient for radiotherapy can best be ensured by the presence of a therapy radiographer assisting the diagnostic team in the positioning of the patient on the CT couch. The CT scanner couch must be flat like the couch of the treatment machine. The same immobilization devices e.g. perspex shell, vacuum bag, or arm pole must be used on the CT scanner and treatment machine and a clear record must be made of these devices.

Any polystyrene head or knee pads or pillows used must also be the same. Midline and lateral lasers should be available in the CT scanning room to ensure that the patient is lying correctly and permanent skin markers or tattoos are made on the skin over the nearest immobile bony landmark to the site of the patient's tumour. Lateral tattoos are also made to ensure accurate alignment of the patient and prevent lateral rotation. Skin markers should then be covered with either radio-opaque catheters or barium paste so that their position is recorded on both the topogram and CT scan.

A topogram (scout view) with lines showing the positions of CT slices is useful but is not divergent in three dimensions as is a radiation beam, because there is no divergence in the craniocaudal plane. When the treatment fields are verified on the simulator or with portal imaging, the margins will therefore appear greater in the craniocaudal dimension due to divergence of the therapy beam in all planes. Measurements of the superior and inferior dimensions of the tumour rely on accurate CT couch movements, as these distances are used to measure the length of the tumour. Small slice thickness and interval (2–5 mm) are essential for 3-D reconstructions to provide sufficient data for visualization of the tumour and dose calculations on the planning computer. Spiral (helical) CT technology is a considerable advance with respect to acquiring accurate information on tumour volume.

As well as the use of oral contrast medium to outline small bowel, it may also be important to mark structures such as the introitus, anal margin and vagina using a tampon, and any palpable tumour masses or operative scars with barium or radio-opaque catheters so that they are visualized on both the CT image and topogram. Such procedures aid localization of normal structures to be used in planning the target volume. However, it should be remembered that an excessive volume of oral contrast medium, such as gastrografin (sodium meglumine diatrizoate), given as preparation for CT scanning when planning radiotherapy of bladder tumours, may cause a urinary diuresis with unnecessary enlargement of the bladder even after voluntary micturition. Figure 44.8 shows a comparison of a planning CT scan of a patient with bladder cancer after administration of oral contrast medium after micturition, and a scan taken immediately before radiotherapy treatment 1 week later with an empty bladder, with no oral preparation. The reduction in volume of the bladder when oral contrast is not given as preparation is clearly shown. The use of only 400 ml of oral contrast medium provides adequate bowel opacification without a false diuresis. Patients with bladder tumours are irradiated immediately after voluntary micturition to empty the bladder as much as possible and to minimize the target volume. If the bladder is overdistended, the CTV will be unnecessarily large and the side-effects of radiotherapy will increase.

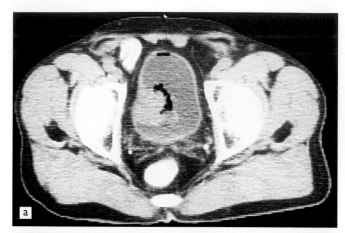

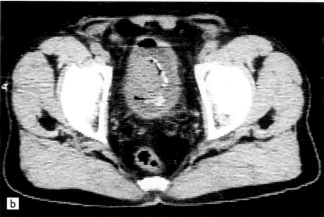

Figure 44.8. *Effect of bladder distension on CTV for bladder tumours: (a) after gastrografin planning CT; (b) first week on radiotherapy (smaller volume) CT scan.*

It is important that protocols for CT scanning of different anatomical areas for planning are drawn up jointly between the diagnostic radiologist and oncologist. For instance, using conventional CT, CT sections taken at 10 mm intervals may be adequate for the abdomen, but a 5 mm thickness and interval may be more appropriate for the prostate and bladder. If three-dimensional reconstruction and planning is to be used, 2–5 mm slice thickness may be required which can be achieved on a conventional scanner or using spiral equipment. Even when diagnostic CT scans have already been taken as part of the initial work-up, additional CT planning scans will be needed because the patient must be scanned in the treatment position with accurate external markers on the skin.

Studies by Goitein[11] and Dobbs et al.[12] compared conventional planning with CT planning used for localization of the target volume and showed that in approximately 30% of cases a change in the margins of the target volume was necessary to cover the tumour adequately. Two studies have addressed the issue of whether improvement in accuracy of targetting radiotherapy using CT translates into an improve-

ment in survival, but there is no randomized study which has investigated improvement in local tumour control. Rothwell et al.[13] made a retrospective comparison of the survival rate of patients whose bladder tumours were adequately treated within an 90% isodose with those who, by CT criteria, had a geographical miss. Overall, the study predicted a 4–5% increase in survival of the whole group of patients with bladder cancer at 3 years if all tumours were included within the target volume.

The advent of spiral CT has posed a new problem for radiotherapy planning. Treatments are delivered over 1 or 2 minutes during which normal breathing continues and several respiratory excursions will therefore occur during each treatment. Computed tomography scans of tumours in the chest can now be taken in a single breath-hold and therefore will not show the movement of the tumour, particularly in the craniocaudal direction, which will occur during treatment. If the target volume is designed on a snapshot image of the tumour, parts of the tumour may be excluded from therapy subsequently. Collaboration is needed between radiologist, physicist and oncologist to overcome this problem. Possible solutions are the use of slower CT scans for treatment planning in the chest so that the full breathing cycle is encompassed. Pulsed treatment could be gated to a particular phase of the respiratory cycle, such as full inspiration or expiration, and matched with stage of respiratory cycle during diagnostic CT scanning. Spiral CT images could possibly be compared with central and peripheral slices obtained with conventional CT on maximum inspiration and expiration to address this problem.

Key points: CT requirements for radiotherapy

■ Computed tomography scans for radiotherapy planning must be taken under identical conditions to those for later radiotherapy treatment (e.g. flat couch, immobilization devices)

■ Midline and lateral lasers should be available to ensure correct patient positioning

■ A topogram (scout view) is useful for defining the upper and lower limits of the tumour but 3D reconstructions are superior

■ Anatomical landmarks should be labelled with radio-opaque or other markers

■ A major problem with spiral CT is that scanning through the tumour is obtained in a single breath-hold, whereas therapy is given over several minutes during respiration. This may lead to a geographical miss

Image handling

Three-dimensional visualization of tumours is now available using a variety of imaging handling systems (Fig. 44.9). Coronal and sagittal images, as well as axial CT scans, can therefore be utilized to see the tumour in three dimensions. Most treatment planning computers are CT based and therefore currently CT scanning remains the main imaging modality for radiotherapy treatment planning. If the tumour has not been removed surgically, CT scans give directly relevant information. If the tumour has been resected, diagnostic imaging performed before surgery and referral for radiotherapy provides vital information about the site and size of the tumour. It is on this information that postoperative radiotherapy must be based. Integration of the postoperative planning CT scan with preoperative CT or MRI scans improves delineation of the CTV.

Image fusion

Computed tomography, MRI, transrectal or transvaginal ultrasound, single photon emission tomography (SPECT) or PET and isotopic images may all give information about a particular tumour. However, for this information to be useful to the radiotherapist in targeting treatment, it must be reformatted or coregistered with the CT-based planning image (Fig. 44.10).

The diagnostic quality of MRI can then be combined with the geometric accuracy and electron density information of the planning CT scan for delineation of the tumour and dosimetric calculation.

Coregistration of images has developed using semi-automated methods which need significant observer skills to identify point landmarks or interactively delineated contours.[14,15] These techniques are time consuming and prone to observer bias or error. Chamfer matching[16,17] depends on alignment of corresponding surfaces which require prior identification and segmentation of those surfaces, which may not correspond anatomically between different imaging modalities. Studholme et al.[18] report progress using voxel intensity similarity as a method of fully automating MR and PET-image registration in the head using the mutual information measure, which may speed up the process considerably.

Which tumour sites for CT planning?

The sites which are potentially best treated by conformal therapy are often those for which CT scanning is already used routinely and is most helpful. Most of these are tumours in the pelvis such as prostate, bladder and rectum where the organs are relatively easy to define. The patterns of local spread are clearly understood and the variability with organ movement has been most studied. The target volume is often confined to the primary tumour, rather than extended to the whole pelvis to include regional lymph nodes and hence small volume, accurately localized radical treatment is the aim.

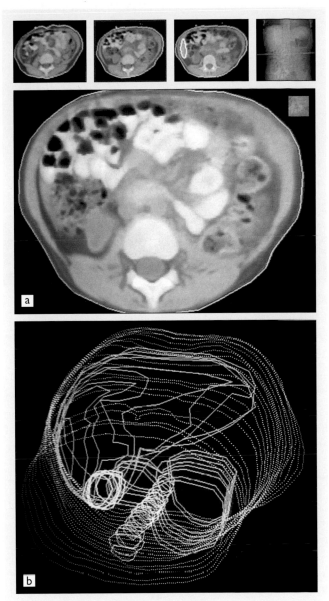

Figure 44.9. *(a) Postoperative CT scan in patient treated for neuroblastoma. (b) 3D target volume (blue) contralateral kidney (yellow).*

This is in contrast with tumours in the head and neck where, although CT scanning gives invaluable information about the extent of the tumour, the treatment policy of including potential areas of nodal spread means that in practice often large simple field arrangements are used for which three-dimensional conformal planning may be less appropriate. The role of conformal radiotherapy for these tumours therefore, may be in defining residual primary tumour for a final high-dose small-volume boost of irradiation, sparing vital adjacent organs, for example in treatment of tumours of the nasopharynx.

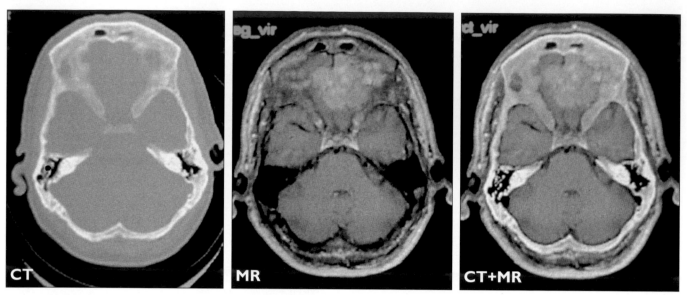

Figure 44.10. *Coregistration enables information from CT and MRI to be integrated to aid planning using diagnostic information. (Reproduced with kind permission of Dr David Hawkes, Dept of Radiological Sciences, Guy's & St Thomas' UMDS).*

In the brain, CT planning is extremely useful. However, this is at present limited by difficulties in coregistration of MRI and CT data. Use of MRI and SPECT scanning has indicated that tumour volumes may in fact need to be increased, rather than decreased, to encompass zones of oedema which may contain infiltrating tumour. The finding that SPECT positivity often correlates with the active part of the tumour may be helpful in targeting volumes more accurately or defining areas for 'boost' irradiation.

Computed tomography scanning for lung tumours is helpful for defining the primary tumour volume. Intravenous contrast is important for outlining mediastinal structures to determine whether nodal areas should be included in target volumes. It is not yet clear whether conformal therapy of lung tumours will produce substantial benefit because of the proximity of sensitive organs such as the spinal cord, adjacent normal lung tissue and the heart.

For breast tumours, CT scanning is useful for documenting the amount of lung and cardiac tissue irradiated in three dimensions and CT studies have added to our knowledge of the inhomogeneity of breast radiotherapy.[19] Improvement in the delivery of radiotherapy, including the use of intensity modulated beams, which will compensate for variations in thickness across an

organ, may be particularly useful in improving homogeneity of treatment of the breast. Hitherto, it has been difficult to treat the breast evenly because of irregularity of breast contour and the presence of lung with reduced attenuation deep to the chest wall.

MAGNETIC RESONANCE IMAGING IN RADIOTHERAPY TREATMENT PLANNING

Magnetic resonance imaging provides excellent soft tissue characterization of tumours, especially those of the central nervous system (CNS), head and neck, soft tissue sarcomas and some pelvic tumours.[20] Studies have shown that MR data supplements CT-based radiotherapy planning by increasing diagnostic confidence and for some sites, such as the CNS,[21] giving better definition. However, MR imaging is not in use yet for radiotherapy planning because of: (a) absence of signal in cortical bone, (b) geometric distortions intrinsic to the MR image, (c) lack of electron density information for dosimetry, and (d) lack of software in treatment planning systems. Currently, image fusion methods are being developed to match the improved tumour definition obtained with MRI and the geometric accuracy and electron density dosimetric capabilities of CT.

Summary

- CT planning has improved the accuracy of defining the tumour and target volumes and provided 3D visualization of the target and normal structures.

- CT provides potential for 3D dose calculations and conformal radiotherapy.

- To use the facility accurately, good communication between the members of the multidisciplinary team is essential.

- The role of the diagnostic radiologist is critical in ensuring optimum imaging modalities are used and that interpretation of data is correct.

- Accurate construction of the target volume is the first key step in attempting cure in a patient with a localized tumour treated with radiotherapy.

- Multimodality imaging and registration provide powerful tools for further improvements in the delivery of radiotherapy.

- MRI shows excellent soft tissue characterization of tumours and the technique is currently being developed to match the improved tumour definition of MRI with the geometric accuracy and electron density dosimetric capabilities of CT.

REFERENCES

1. Landberg T, Chavaudra J, Dobbs H J et al. International Commission on Radiation Units and Measurements (ICRU) Report 50. Prescribing, Recording and Reporting Photon Beam Therapy. Bethesda, Maryland: ICRU, 1993. ISBN: 091 339 4483

2. Ten Haken R K, Forman J D, Heimburger D K et al. Treatment planning issues related to prostate movement in response to differential filling of the rectum and bladder. Int J Radiat Oncol Biol Phys 1991; 20: 1317–24

3. Graham J D, Warrington A P, Gill S S et al. A non-invasive, relocatable stereotactic frame for fractionated radiotherapy and multiple imaging. Radiother Oncol 1991; 21: 60–2

4. Gagliardi G, Lax I, Rutqvist L E. Radiation therapy of Stage I breast cancer: Analysis of treatment technique accuracy using three-dimensional treatment planning tools. Radiother Oncol 1992; 24: 94–101

5. Denham J W, Hamilton C S, Joseph D J et al. The use of simulator and CT information in the planning of radiotherapy for non-small cell lung cancer: An Australasian pattern of practice study. Lung Cancer 1993; 8: 275–284

6. Leunens G, Menten J, Weltens C et al. Quality assessment of medical decision making in radiation oncology: Variability in target volume delineation in brain tumours. Radiother Oncol 1993; 29: 169–175

7. Austin-Seymour M, Chen G T Y, Rosenman J et al. Tumour and target delineation: Current research and future challenges. Int J Radiat Oncol Biol Phys 1995; 33 (5): 1041–1052

8. Leibel S A, Ling C C, Kutcher G J et al. The biological basis for conformal three dimensional radiation therapy. Int J Radiat Oncol Biol Phys 1991; 21: 805–811

9. Perez C A, Purdy J A, Harms W et al. Three dimensional treatment planning and conformal radiation therapy: Preliminary evaluation. Radiother Oncol 1995; 36: 32–43

10. Dutreix A. When and how can we improve precision in radiotherapy? Radiother Oncol 1984; 2: 275–292

11. Goitein M. Applications of computed tomography in radiotherapy treatment planning. In: Orton C G (ed) Progress in medical radiation physics. New York, Plenum Press. 1982; 195–287

12. Dobbs H J, Parker R P, Hodson N J et al. The use of CT in radiotherapy treatment planning. Radiother Oncol 1983; 1: 133–141

13. Rothwell R I, Ash D V, Thorogood J. An analysis of the contribution of computed tomography to the treatment outcome in bladder cancer. Clin Radiol 1985; 36: 369–372

14. Kessler M L, Pitluck S, Petti P et al. Integration of multimodality imaging data for radiotherapy treatment planning. Int J Radiat Oncol Biol Phys 1991; 21: 1653–1667

15. Hill D L G, Hawkes D J, Crossman J E et al. Registration of MR and CT images for skull base surgery using point like anatomical features. Br J Radiol 1991; 64: 1030–1035

16. Borgefors G. Hierarchical chamfer matching: A parametrical edge matching algorithm. IEEE transactions on pattern recognition and machine intelligence 1988; 10: 849–865

17. Van Herk M, Kooy H M. Automatic three-dimensional correlation of CT–CT, CT–MRI, and CT–SPECT using chamfer matching. Med Phys 1994; 21: 1163–1178

18. Studholme C, Hill D L G, Hawkes D J. Automated 3D registration of MR and PET brain images by multi-resolution optimisation of voxel similarity measures. Med Phys 1997; 24: 1

19. Neal A J, Mayles W P, Yarnold J R. Invited review: Tangential breast irradiation — rationale and methods for improving dosimetry. Br J Radiol 1994; 67: 1149–1154

20. Pötter R, Heil B, Schneider L et al. Sagittal and coronal planes from MRI for treatment planning in tumours of brain, head and neck: MRI assisted simulation. Radiother Oncol 1992; 23: 127–130

21. Shumman W P, Griffin B R, Haynor D R et al. MR Imaging in radiation therapy planning. Radiology 1985; 156: 146–147

Chapter 45

Assessment of response to treatment and detection of relapse

Janet Husband and David MacVicar

INTRODUCTION

Cancer imaging is increasingly identified as a specialist field within radiology, reflecting a growing need to evaluate disease status, not just at the time of diagnosis and staging, but also at regular intervals during follow-up. These changing attitudes largely result from the increasing incidence of many cancers as well as an aggressive approach to therapy which places huge demands on imaging resources. Thus today, imaging of treated cancer is one of the major expanding areas of radiology in departments where cancer patients are imaged and at the Royal Marsden Hospital, a dedicated cancer centre, over 50% of computed tomography (CT) examinations are performed during cancer follow-up to assess therapeutic response, to identify progressive disease or to detect relapse. Although the overall 5-year survival rate for cancer remains at approximately 40% in the western world (see Chapter 2),[1,2] many patients are achieving a sustained remission with multimodality therapy in many different tumours, and in some cancers such as testicular cancer and Hodgkin's disease, dramatic improvements in survival have been achieved.[1,2] Furthermore the information which can be provided regarding the presence and extent of tumour, as well as information on the changes which occur during therapy, has been expanded beyond all recognition due to the highly sophisticated developments in technology. As a result, the clinician and radiologist are faced with many choices regarding the most appropriate technique for a given clinical situation and the optimum timing of follow-up studies. Such decisions are complex and must take into account the availability of equipment, local expertise and the workload of a particular imaging device. For example, a patient with a primary brain tumour such as a high-grade glioma may be adequately imaged both on computed tomography and magnetic resonance imaging (MRI). Thus even though MRI may provide more precise information in terms of defining the extent of oedema and tumour edge on contrast-enhanced scans (due to superior contrast resolution and its multiplanar capability), CT will also demonstrate a reduction or increase in overall tumour volume as well as changes in mass effect due to increasing or decreasing oedema.

One of the most important principles for the use of imaging in follow-up is that the same technique should be used for monitoring response as for staging the initial study, but if this is not possible a baseline examination immediately after initial therapy, for example surgery, should be performed with the imaging modality which has been chosen to evaluate the patient's clinical course. Such decisions should be made by close collaboration between clinician and radiologist and once protocols are agreed, they should be adhered to as rigidly as possible.

Decisions on the use of a particular imaging modality are influenced by progress in imaging evaluation and education as well as developments in technology. For example, advances in MRI which have taken place over the last 5 years include the evaluation of the use of intravenous contrast agents in different tumours, and today it is clear that intravenous contrast enhancement is helpful for staging certain tumours but in others it has no benefit. Technical developments now allow the radiologist to consider the use of abdominal MRI for the evaluation of the liver as a highly sensitive method of detecting metastases. As yet, however, there is little, if any, experience in the use of MRI in the follow-up of liver metastases but the oncological radiologist must keep abreast of all these advances and be ready to take advantage of new information regarding tumour detection, delineation and monitoring response to cancer which is now bombarding the radiological literature.

Against this background of an ever expanding demand for cancer imaging, it is essential to consider a strategic approach so that imaging is used to the best advantage for patient care and in the most efficacious manner to contain finite resources. Furthermore such an approach should be designed to limit the waste in resources which to some extent is inevitable in departments where large numbers of patients with cancer are being followed. Inappropriate use of imaging occurs in the following circumstances:

- Duplication of information from the use of more than one imaging technique usually arises from lack of in-depth knowledge of: (a) the patient's

clinical condition, (b) the clinical question posed, or (c) the likelihood that additional information would be obtained by performing a further test
- The chosen imaging technique may be unsuitable for answering the question posed

Even if the appropriate imaging modality is chosen to answer a specific question, strict protocols are mandatory for examination of a particular malignancy with a particular imaging device. Such protocols are especially important with highly flexible technology such as MRI. Thus, the choice of sequences and imaging planes is so wide that it is quite feasible to undertake an examination of a patient during follow-up which bears no relation to the initial study and comparison of the two studies is therefore subject to considerable error in the assessment of therapeutic response. Needless to say, one of the hallmarks of good practice in the follow-up of malignancy is to define imaging protocols for the follow-up of each and every tumour likely to be examined and to ensure that all previous imaging studies are available for review at the time of follow-up.

Key points: rationalization of imaging

■ Imaging for cancer follow-up is of equal importance to imaging for diagnosis and staging of malignancy

■ The same imaging technique should be used for follow-up throughout the course of disease and ideally this should be the same technique as used for staging

■ A strategic approach to follow-up should be devised so that the most appropriate technique is used and the timing of follow-up studies is optimized

■ Examination protocols for a particular technique should be set up for each tumour and adhered to as rigidly as possible

RATIONALIZATION OF RADIOLOGICAL ASSESSMENT IMAGING STRATEGIES

Strategies for imaging during follow-up are closely linked to the clinical circumstances, to the type of therapy given, the timing of therapy and the likelihood of a successful outcome. The strategies adopted are therefore clinically based and fall into three major categories.

- Strategies for individual patient management
- Strategies to assess curable disease
- Strategies to support clinical research

In the first group, a radiological investigation is requested to resolve a specific clinical problem in an individual patient which is often related to an unusual event during a planned course of treatment. Such an event may represent a complication of therapy, such as infection, haemorrhage or the onset of symptoms suggestive of progressive disease or relapse.

Strategies required for the assessment of patients with treatable or curable disease are easy to establish by close collaboration between clinical and radiological colleagues; strategies for supporting clinical research are usually restricted to those centres which specialize in cancer treatment and research. In such centres, imaging studies are increasingly seen as the core of a clinical trial and as more complex therapeutic approaches are investigated, this use of imaging may be difficult to contain within a routine clinical department.

Strategies for individual patient management
In this clinical setting guidelines are difficult to define because imaging is usually tailored to answer a specific question. Cancer patients are frequently debilitated as a result of their disease and also the toxicity of therapy, so it may be impossible on clinical grounds to determine whether the patient's deterioration is a result of intercurrent complications during successful treatment or whether it is due to progression of malignant disease. In order to achieve the optimum results from imaging studies, the radiologist needs to know:

- The initial stage of tumour at presentation
- The details of previous treatment
- The timing of the previous treatment
- The clinical question posed

There are many examples in clinical practice in which the lack of appropriate information traps the radiologist into giving an erroneous report, and although both the clinician and radiologist are responsible for such misinterpretation, it is incumbent on the radiologist to ensure that he/she completely understands the details of the clinical question posed and all relevant background clinical information. For example, following anterior resection for colonic cancer, postoperative granulation tissue at the anastomotic site may be indistinguishable from persistent or recurrent tumour based solely on the CT findings (Fig. 45.1).[3] However, knowledge of the time interval between surgery and imaging, as well as detailed information about the operative findings, frequently permit correct interpretation of the CT study. A follow-up study is also helpful; postoperative granulation tissue usually remains stable or may regress on follow-up studies (Fig. 45.2). Another example where errors are easily made is in the assessment of an anterior mediastinal mass which develops following chemotherapy. In patients with lymphoma, such a mass may represent recurrent tumour or thymic

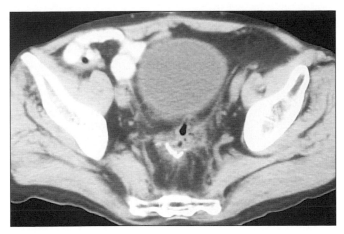

Figure 45.1. *CT scan 4 weeks following anterior resection for carcinoma of the sigmoid colon. There is thickening of the wall of the colon with extension of abnormal tissue into the pericolic fat. This abnormal tissue represents postsurgical change but is indistinguishable from persistent or recurrent tumour.*

rebound hyperplasia. Careful consideration of the patient's stage of disease at presentation, status of disease in relation to therapy at other sites, the clinical well being of the patient and timing of completion of chemotherapy frequently allow the distinction between relapsed lymphoma and thymic rebound hyperplasia to be made (Fig. 45.3).[4]

Strategies for assessment of curable disease

Strategies for assessment of curable disease are based on initial staging information obtained at imaging. Computed tomography is the major staging modality for most of the

solid cancers and lymphoma. At the time of staging all disease sites are documented and a strategic plan of follow-up studies should be instigated. This plan for follow up will vary depending upon the stage of disease which in turn will dictate therapeutic choice. The timing of imaging is also dependent upon the type of therapy. Thus, in patients who have received radiotherapy or undergone surgical resection of a primary tumour, imaging should be delayed until at least 3 months after treatment to allow the effects of radiotherapy or surgery to stabilize. In general, imaging is carried out immediately after chemotherapy has been completed as the reaction to treatment locally in the region of the tumour is usually insignificant.

The need for further imaging is then determined by the tumour type, the presence of residual abnormal tissue and the likelihood that this tissue represents active tumour. Continued follow-up also depends upon the overall chance of relapse which varies not only with the individual tumour type but also depends on the grade of malignancy and other prognostic factors such as tumour volume.

Strategies for curable disease

Excellent examples of a strategic approach for curable disease is provided by patients with non-seminomatous germ cell tumours (NSGCT) and by patients with Hodgkin's disease.

Non-seminomatous germ cell tumours

In patients with NSGCT, CT examination of the chest, abdomen and pelvis is performed for staging purposes following orchidectomy. If there is evidence of metastatic disease in the retroperitoneal lymph nodes, four courses of cisplatin-based chemotherapy are given. CT is then repeated immediately after chemotherapy to evaluate ther-

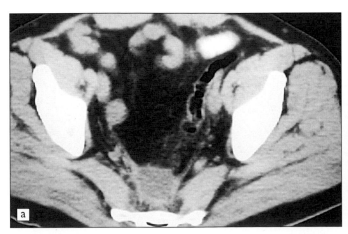

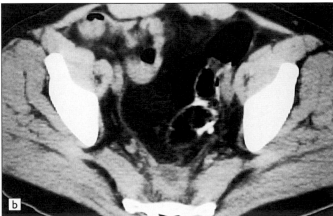

Figure 45.2. *A male patient who had undergone abdominoperineal resection for carcinoma of the rectum; (a) 6 weeks after surgery there is a mass in the sacral hollow of approximately 4 cm in diameter which has a relatively low central density on*

CT; (b) a follow-up scan 3 months later shows reduction in size of the mass indicating that this represents postoperative haematoma/granulation tissue.

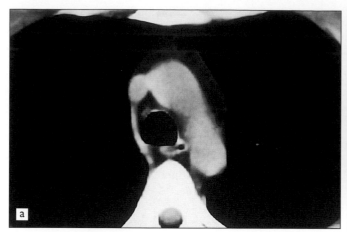
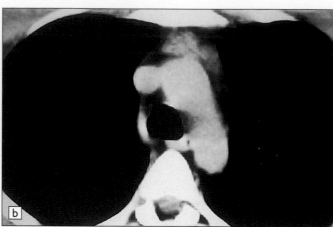

Figure 45.3. *Thymic rebound hyperplasia: (a) CT scan before chemotherapy for a Stage-II NSGCT of the testis; (b) CT scan taken 6 months after the completion of chemotherapy shows 'a soft tissue mass' in the anterior mediastinum. There was no evidence of disease elsewhere and the patient has remained well for over 1 year. (From ref. 78, with permission.)*

apeutic response (Fig. 45.4). Any residual detectable masses which may contain differentiated or undifferentiated teratoma should be considered for resection. The site and size of the mass is critical to the decision-making process as to whether lymphadenectomy should be performed and CT is therefore central to management at this time.[5–7] In general, retroperitoneal masses greater than 1 cm in diameter are resected (Fig. 45.5) but residual masses less than 1 cm are followed by a further CT examination after an interval of 6 months to make sure there has been no subsequent growth.[7]

In patients who are deemed to be Stage I following orchidectomy, and in whom serum marker levels are falling normally, a surveillance policy may be employed. Again, CT is an integral part of the surveillance policy, being undertaken at 3-monthly intervals during the first year and at 6-monthly intervals during the second year after diagnosis. This rationale is based on the fact that approximately 70% of patients who are deemed to be Stage I after orchidectomy do not have metastatic disease and therefore require no further treatment.[8,9] Of the individuals who do relapse, 80% will do so during the first 12 months and 95% of relapses occur during the first 2 years.[8,9] This strategic approach in testicular cancer requires careful forward planning to adhere to the CT schedule but in addition, the radiologist needs to be alert to small changes in the size of lymph nodes, particularly in the retroperitoneum, which may be the first sign of relapse.

Hodgkin's disease
In patients presenting with Hodgkin's disease, imaging studies vary with the stage and histological subtype. For example, in patients presenting with enlarged lymph nodes in the neck due to nodular sclerosing Hodgkin's disease, CT of the chest, abdomen and pelvis is routinely performed and if no other sites of disease are detected radiotherapy is the standard treatment.[10,11] In patients with enlarged lymph nodes in the mediastinum, however, radiotherapy or chemotherapy may be given, the choice depending upon the bulk of disease and the presence or absence of disease elsewhere.[12] As in testicular cancer, this example illustrates the central role that CT plays in a multimodality strategic approach.

Strategies for imaging to support clinical research
Imaging studies are now pivotal to the assessment of new chemotherapeutic regimes. Many clinical trials are carried out in patients with advanced local disease or with widespread disseminated malignancy while others are performed in the adjuvant setting (in patients who have undergone primary treatment and in whom there is no evidence of metastatic disease) and in the neo-adjuvant setting (in patients in whom chemotherapy is given to down-stage the primary tumour before surgery). In such studies imaging is usually required more frequently than for the evaluation of established therapy (Fig. 45.6).

Figure 45.4. *A strategy for imaging (I_1, I_2, I_3) with CT in patients with NSGCT Stage-II disease (abdominal nodal metastases).*

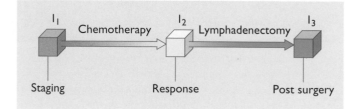

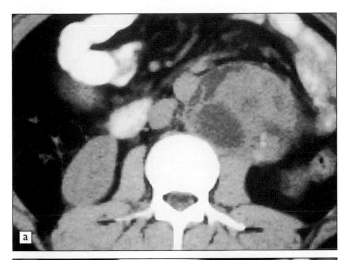

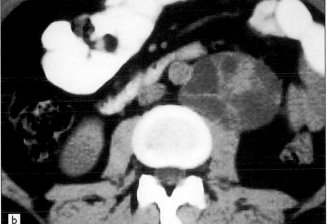

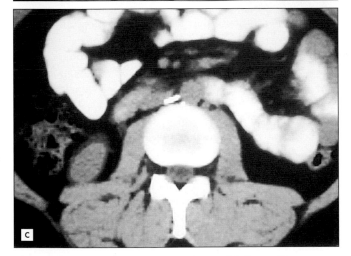

Figure 45.5. *CT scans in a patient with Stage-II NSGCT. (a) Before chemotherapy, and (b) following chemotherapy. Note significant reduction in size of the mass which is partially cystic and partially solid. This patient proceeded to surgery for removal of the residual mass and a follow-up scan (c) 6 months later shows no evidence of recurrence.*

Figure 45.6. *Strategy for imaging for support of clinical trials.*

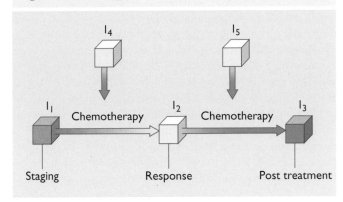

Table 45.1. *Definitions of objective response. (from ref. 13)*

Complete response (CR)	Disappearance of all known disease
Partial response (PR)	50% or more decrease in total tumour load (single or multiple lesions, bidimensional or unidimensional measurement)
No change (NC)	50% decrease or 25% increase not established
Progressive disease (PD)	25% or more increase in the size of measurable lesion or appearance of new lesions

Novel chemotherapeutic agents are assessed in Phase II trials where the aim is to demonstrate an objective response; in Phase-III trials different drug regimens are compared.

The objectives of all such studies are to assess:

- Sites of response
- Timing of response
- Rate of response
- Differential response
- Clinical remission rate

Well-defined criteria for measuring therapeutic response are essential and those currently used were proposed by Miller et al. in 1981 (Table 45.1) under the auspices of the World Health Organisation.[13] These criteria allow description of response ranging from complete remission to progressive disease.

These criteria have been adopted worldwide and remain the standard method of reporting tumour response to treatment and permit studies between different centres to be compared. The original article states that 'objective response can be determined clinically, radiologically, biochemically or by surgicopathological restaging'. The method of determining response should therefore always be 'specified'. These authors recommend that a partial response may be designated by bidimensional measurement of a single lesion where decrease in tumour area of greater than 50% is observed. This is calculated by multiplication of the longest diameter of the tumour by the greatest perpendicular diameter; partial response may also be denoted in multiple lesions if there is 'a 50% decrease in the sum of the product of the perpendicular diameters of the multiple lesions'. There are also separate categories for unidimensional measurements of measurable disease, bone metastases and 'non-measurable' disease. No consideration is given to calculation of tumour volume.

Although these criteria have been the mainstay of evaluating new therapies for the last two decades, review of the criteria is now necessary because the technological advances in imaging permit more accurate assessment of tumour response than is required by Miller's criteria. Thus:

- Tumour volume can be calculated from reformatted axial CT slices or by outlining the tumour on three-dimensional datasets using spiral (helical) CT
- Tumour volume may also be calculated from MR images obtained in multiple planes or by direct threedimensional imaging
- Several imaging techniques now provide information which reflect changes in tumour composition as well as size. Image fusion allows areas of tumour 'activity' to be superimposed on anatomical images of tumour morphology

As further information on the accuracy of new imaging techniques to define tumour volume and to assess changes in tumour composition is accrued by imaging research, it is hoped that such information will be incorporated into standard tumour assessment, thereby providing more accurate information and additional indicators of tumour response.

Even so, although relatively crude, Miller's currently used criteria do allow for errors of measurement on imaging which may be significant, particularly when evaluating tumours which are irregular in shape and those which infiltrate into adjacent tissues with no obvious boundary. Furthermore, in patients with multiple sites of disease, most radiologists currently measure one marker lesion and assess the remaining lesions subjectively. However, if more stringent criteria are instigated to assign partial response then it may be necessary for the radiologist to measure all lesions accurately and the whole process would be cumbersome and time consuming. A further difficulty is that tumour deposits may show a differential response, e.g. a liver metastasis in the right lobe of the liver may enlarge whereas other lesions within the same lobe may regress. In such situations an overall judgement is easier using Miller's criteria than if small

percentages of change are applied. Further difficulties are envisaged if changes in composition are incorporated into the criteria as one lesion may become mainly necrotic without changing size, whereas another lesion may shrink considerably with no obvious change in composition. These latter considerations highlight the need for vigorous research, not only to demonstrate changes in composition which occur within tumours, but also to develop methods of measuring their significance.

Recently, we have reported the results of a Phase-II clinical trial conducted at the Royal Marsden Hospital in which Miller's criteria were used to measure the chemotherapeutic response in patients with advanced metastatic gastric cancer.[14] In this study CT was performed on six occasions in each patient who completed therapy (prior to treatment, following 3 cycles of chemotherapy, following 6 cycles of chemotherapy and finally after a further 2 cycles of therapy) (Fig. 45.6). A total of 91 patients were studied and each patient was also assessed by endoscopy at the time of each CT study. The primary tumour in all sites of metastatic disease was evaluated and the results showed an overall objective response in 71% of patients with complete remission in 12%. However, in this study, the primary tumour was only measurable in 60 of the 91 patients because in the remaining one-third the tumour was either difficult to delineate with certainty or diffuse and infiltrating involving the stomach wall circumferentially. Other difficulties encountered were that the marker lesions chosen in the initial study for measurement did not always reflect changes seen in other lesions so that re-evaluation of all the examinations was sometimes required (Fig. 45.7).

With regard to tumour composition, a parameter not currently used within the criteria for monitoring response, an important database of posttreatment findings is now being accrued and in the longer term, these data may provide information on the significance of post-treatment changes with respect to outcome. Several studies have already demonstrated the potential role of MRI in the evaluation of residual masses following treatment of lymphoma, following cryosurgery for prostate cancer.[15–18] The detection of residual active cancer is also currently being explored with functional imaging techniques which include dynamic MRI scanning with contrast enhancement and studies of positron emission tomography (PET) using 2[F-18] fluoro-2-deoxy-D-glucose (18-FDG-PET).[19–22] Each of these methods of evaluation in different tumours has identified particular problems associated with tumour measurement; nevertheless, as imaging continues to advance it is likely, in the longer term that both morphological and functional imaging methods will be applied to clinical trials.

Cross-sectional imaging is now extensively employed in clinical research projects and although the criteria currently used do not specify which imaging modality is to be employed

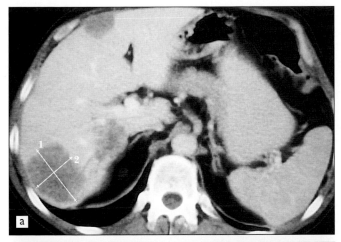

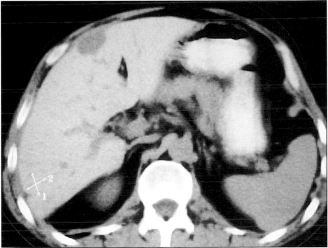

Figure 45.7. *CT scans of a patient with hepatic metastases from colon cancer treated with infusional 5-fluorouracil. (a) Before treatment; (b) after four courses of chemotherapy. Note the metastasis in the posterior aspect of the right lobe of the liver shows a partial response whereas the metastasis lying adjacent to the falciform ligament is stable.*

most chemotherapeutic trials rely on CT and ultrasound. Magnetic resonance imaging is also likely to be incorporated into such trials as the technique becomes more widely available, for example, for assessment of liver metastases. Any radiologist participating in research projects must be aware of the standard criteria, but nevertheless alert to the difficulties inherent in measuring and sensitive to the fact that some subjectivity will inevitably creep into the results. Many pharmaceutical companies involved with therapeutic trials now use a system of an 'independent radiological review panel' and the authors' experience of participating in such independent review indicates that there is considerable variation in the quality of scanners used, the expertise of the observers and in protocols for examination.

The information derived from imaging in the assessment of tumour response ranges from a change in the silhouette of a tumour on a plain chest radiograph to variations in molecular structure on highly complex functional imaging. For the radiologist working in an oncology practice, the information derived from imaging throughout this broad spectrum is all important and his/her expertise lies in the appropriate deployment of this wealth of information to promote further understanding of cancer treatment.

Key points: imaging strategies

- ■ A strategy for assessment of curable disease is based mainly on clinical stage at presentation

- ■ Imaging plays a pivotal role in the support of clinical trials for new chemotherapeutic agents

- ■ Well-defined criteria for measuring therapeutic response are essential

INFORMATION DERIVED FROM IMAGING IN THE ASSESSMENT OF TUMOUR RESPONSE

Radiological techniques employed in the assessment of tumour response are able to provide information on:

- Changes in size
- Changes in tumour composition

Although conventional radiology, ultrasound, CT, MRI and radionuclide studies all have a place in evaluating treatment, CT is the most frequently used technique in the follow-up of cancer. MRI is just beginning to evolve as an important method of cancer monitoring but as yet is not used widely for this purpose in routine practice. It must be emphasized that conventional plain radiographs continue to play a critical role in the assessment of many tumours. For example, in patients with mediastinal lymphoma with large bulky disease plain chest radiographs are entirely satisfactory for evaluating initial tumour regression. However, once the tumour has resolved to the extent that the mediastinum has resumed its normal contour, plain chest radiographs are inadequate for evaluating the presence and volume of residual disease. Plain chest radiographs are also an excellent method of determining chemotherapeutic response to treatment of primary lung cancer and pulmonary metastases. In addition the high spatial resolution of conventional radiography gives exquisite detail of changes in calcification and ossification of both primary and secondary bone tumours and X-ray mammography can demonstrate changes in microcalcification and size of primary breast cancers treated with neo-adjuvant chemotherapy (Fig. 45.8).[23]

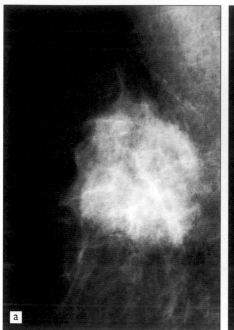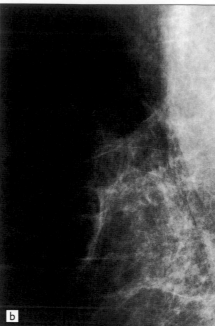

Figure 45.8. *Primary breast cancer: (a) before treatment; (b) following neo-adjuvant chemotherapy. Mammography demonstrates an excellent response to treatment. No invasive cancer was demonstrated in the resected specimen.*

Ultrasound, although less reproducible than CT, is now highly sophisticated with the development of endoscopic methods,[24] enhanced colour Doppler techniques[25] and the introduction of intravenous contrast agents.[26] Such advances render ultrasound an increasingly important method of evaluating tumours both at diagnosis and during follow-up. Advances in radionuclide scanning such as 18-FDG-PET and MR spectroscopy are exciting new areas in which to explore the mechanisms and results of new drug therapy.[27,28]

Tumour volume

The clinical significance of measuring changes in tumour volume and thus assessing the growth of human tumours was first recognized as early as the 1950s, much of this early work being pioneered by Collins and co-workers using serial measurements of pulmonary metastases to determine tumour growth rates.[29,30] These investigators introduced the concept of tumour doubling time, hypothesizing that a single cell of 10 μm in diameter would grow to a nodule of 1 mm in 10 doublings and to a lesion of 1 cm in 20 doublings. At 40 doublings the mass would weigh 1 kg and the patient would be near to death. This concept assumed pure exponential tumour growth and that pulmonary metastases were spherical and therefore able to grow equally in all directions. These early data revealed that certain tumours grew rapidly whereas others grew more slowly, information which opened the way to the further understanding of tumour behaviour, highlighting the fact that cancer was not a single disease entity but comprises a group of widely diverse neoplasms (see Chapter 1).

Conventional radiography

As indicated above, plain chest radiographs continue to play a pivotal role in the evaluation of primary and metastatic thoracic malignancy as well as lymphoma, because accurate volume measurements are seldom required for management decisions. In the evaluation of pulmonary metastases using Miller's criteria,[13] reduction in tumour volume can usually be evaluated with reasonable accuracy on bidimensional measurement.

Although plain radiographs are used to evaluate changes in primary and metastatic bone cancer, accurate changes in volume of tumour involving bone and soft tissues are seldom appreciated on plain films. This is largely because the extent of bone marrow disease cannot be appreciated on plain films and the soft tissue component is often obscured by overlying tissues.

Cross-sectional imaging

Ultrasound, CT and MRI all have the major advantage over conventional radiology in that tumours can be imaged directly in the cross-sectional plane. Based on inherent characteristics of echo pattern, soft tissue density and signal intensity, tissue boundaries and tumour contours can be depicted, thus allowing tumour volume measurements to be made.

Ultrasound

Although ultrasound may be used for assessing tumour volume in superficial tumours such as primary breast tumours (Fig. 45.9), difficulties are often encountered in the serial evaluation of intra-abdominal tumours due to the presence of bowel gas which may obscure tumour visibility. Another problem is that

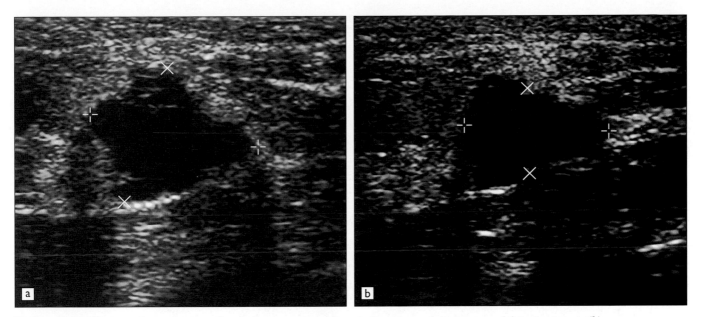

Figure 45.9. *Ultrasound examination showing response to treatment of a primary breast cancer: (a) pretreatment; (b) following 1 month of combination chemotherapy a reduction in tumour volume is readily appreciated.*

ultrasound is sufficiently operator dependent that if the follow-up examination is carried out by a different ultrasonographer it may be impossible to reproduce the same imaging plane previously used for measurement.

Computed tomography

When computed tomography was first introduced in the 1970s there was considerable enthusiasm regarding the possibility of providing accurate tumour volume measurements. At the Royal Marsden Hospital we investigated the accuracy of CT for measuring tumour volume by scanning potatoes in a water bath and then compared the measurements made by CT on contiguous 1 cm slices with potato volumes calculated using the water displacement technique. The difference between the true and measured potato volumes ranged from −0.4 to +2%, thus demonstrating that CT was indeed an accurate method of determining the volume of a tumour provided the mass had a different density from the surrounding structures and therefore the boundary could be delineated.[31] Following this initial study, we then measured the volume of residual masses in vivo applying the technique to patients with abdominal nodal metastases from testicular cancer following chemotherapy. These patients underwent resection of the residual mass and the volume of the excised specimens were then compared with the CT volumes obtained prior to surgery.[32] There was excellent correlation between CT volume and the volume of the excised surgical masses, the error being considerably less than 10% in the majority of patients.[32] Thus the technique appeared to be robust and had potential value for studying tumour

regression of intra-abdominal masses in a way which has previously been impossible; the regression rates of testicular seminoma nodal metastases were shown to be greater than the regression rates of NSGCT (Figs 45.10 and 45.11) illustrating the exquisite sensitivity of seminoma to chemotherapy and radiotherapy.[33] This study also revealed that residual masses following treatment continued to regress for

Figure 45.10. *Regression rates of seminomatous abdominal masses plotted as the mean percentage of initial maximum diameter (+/- one standard deviation).*

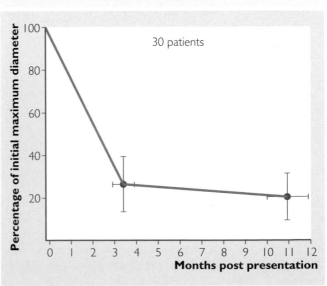

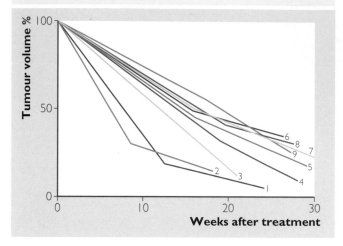

Figure 45.11. *Tumour volume-regression rates in 9 patients with abdominal nodal metastases from NSGCT treated with chemotherapy.*

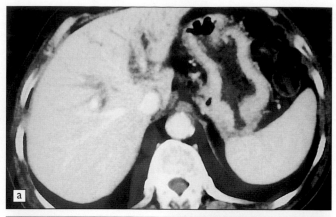

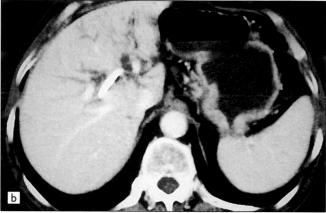

a period of up to 2 years after completion of treatment. Such studies thus provided new information on the appearances of treated tumours by demonstrating the presence and size of residual masses in tumours such as seminoma, NSGCT and lymphoma. In seminoma, histological data has revealed that these residual masses are almost invariably benign, representing fibrosis due to a severe desmoplastic reaction, necrosis and occasionally calcification.[34]

Several limitations apply to the measurement of tumour volume using cross-sectional imaging. Factors which render measurement difficult include:

- An irregular tumour contour even if the mass is well-defined
- Diffuse and infiltrating tumours (Fig. 45.12)
- Artefacts which obscure the tumour edge (e.g. due to movement)
- Contiguity of a tumour with adjacent soft tissue structures and organs of similar density
- Tumour of hollow viscera, for example, the oesophagus and colon in which reliable measurement is difficult due to the concentric growth of a tumour (Fig. 45.12)
- The degree of distension of a hollow viscera is variable and may lead to errors due to over- or underestimation of tumour extent

In some tumours such difficulties may be overcome to some extent by the use of dynamic contrast-enhanced techniques which frequently show tumour as a heterogeneous enhancing mass with significantly different characteristics to the homogeneous enhancement of normal tissues (Fig. 45.13), but even so, precise delineation of tumour margin may be

Figure 45.12. *A diffuse and infiltrating carcinoma of the stomach illustrating the limitations of imaging in assessing tumour volume. (a) Before treatment diffuse concentric thickening of the stomach is noted. (b) Following neo-adjuvant chemotherapy persistent stomach wall thickening is observed in some areas but precise evaluation of response is impossible. (From ref. 78, with permission.)*

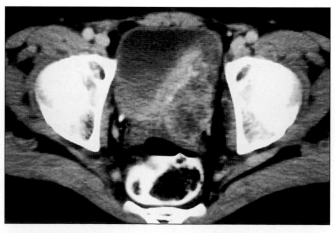

Figure 45.13. *CT scan of a patient with bladder cancer showing heterogeneous enhancement of the mass. This pattern of enhancement in contiguity with the main tumour mass helps to identify invasion of the vagina.*

impossible. The advent of spiral CT provides the opportunity to assess tumour volume in multiple imaging planes by reformatting or by producing a direct 3D image display. These advances permit more accurate tumour volume measurements, particularly of irregularly shaped tumours, but their application in assessing response is as yet limited to research protocols. This is largely because the procedure is time consuming and quantitative measurements rarely influence patient management decisions on an individual basis. However, on occasion reformatting and 3D display may provide superior demonstration of the full extent of disease (Fig. 45.14).

As technology advances, the ease and speed of obtaining 3D volume measurements with CT will improve and it is hoped that such measurements will be applied to the measurement of therapeutic response in the not too distant future.

Magnetic resonance imaging

Magnetic resonance imaging is well suited to the evaluation of tumour volume changes partly due to its multiplanar capability but also due to the increased contrast resolution compared with CT which may help to delineate tumour edge. This is particularly relevant in tumours which directly invade adjacent tissues, such as muscle, because differentiation between tumour and muscle is obvious on MRI whereas distinction between tumour and muscle may be extremely difficult on CT (Figs. 45.15). Due to the improved inherent contrast resolution of MRI, the technique has become the

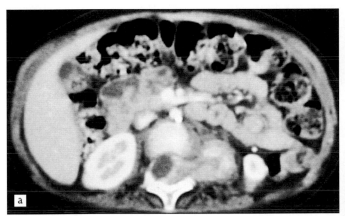

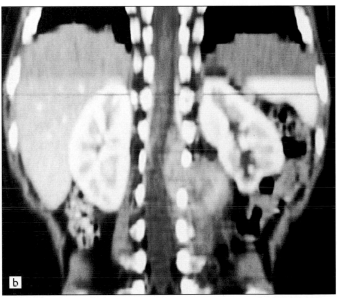

Figure 45.14. *(a and b) CT scans of a child with neuroblastoma. Enhancing tumour extends through the intervertebral foramina into the spinal canal. The full extent of intraspinal invasion is elegantly demonstrated on the reformatted image.*

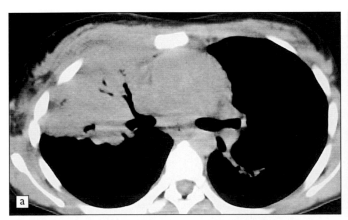

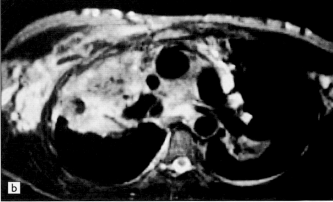

Figure 45.15. *(a) CT scan (b) T2-weighted MR image (TR/TE 2100/90 ms) in a patient with advanced mediastinal Hodgkin's disease. The T2-weighted MR image is superior to* CT *in definition of tumour spread into the anterior chest wall. Note displacement of the pectoralis major muscle on the right. Tumour and muscle cannot be differentiated on CT.*

best method of evaluating tumour volume changes of soft tissue sarcomas (Fig. 45.16) as well as the soft tissue component of primary bone tumours which are usually treated with neo-adjuvant chemotherapy prior to surgery. Lymphomatous masses are also well documented with MRI but it should be appreciated that tumour volume on MRI, particularly in the mediastinum, often appears greater than on CT. This is probably due to:

- Magnetic resonance imaging scans have usually been performed during quiet respiration whereas CT is performed during a single breath-hold.[35] (Breath-hold MRI techniques are now widely available and the problem should be overcome)

- The inherent signal intensity of tumour allows better delineation of lymphomatous masses in such sites as the subcarinal area and aortopulmonary window and therefore tumours appear more extensive
- The improved contrast resolution of MRI permits the delineation of strands of tumour within normal mediastinal fat, whereas on CT this delicate infiltration of normal tissues is frequently invisible

In a recent retrospective review we compared the post-treatment appearances of thymic lymphoma on MRI with those of CT.[35] In 20 of the 25 patients studied, the dimensions of the residual mass were considerably larger on MRI than those demonstrated on CT (Fig. 45.17).

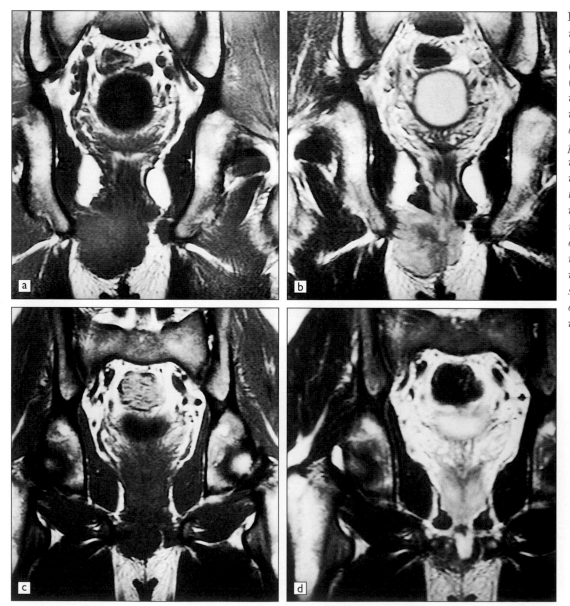

Figure 45.16. *Patient with a malignant soft tissue sarcoma (rhabdomyosarcoma): (a) coronal T1-weighted and (b) T2-weighted MR images before treatment; (c) post-treatment T1-weighted; and (d) T2-weighted images. Both the T1- and the T2-weighted images are useful for demonstrating reduction in tumour volume. Reduction in signal intensity is observed on the T2-weighted image (d).*

Figure 45.17. *Histogram showing post-treatment bidimensional measurements of residual thymic masses following chemotherapy on MRI and CT. In 20 patients the bidimensional measurements on MRI are larger than those measured on CT. (From ref.35, with permission.)*

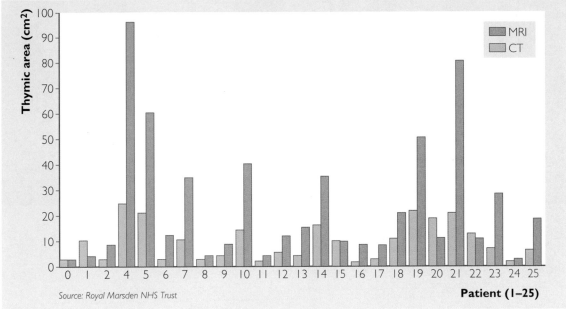

Source: Royal Marsden NHS Trust

As with CT, 3D techniques can be applied for more accurate tumour volume measurement but these are seldom undertaken on a routine clinical basis for body imaging and furthermore are currently not yet incorporated into research protocols to evaluate therapeutic response.

Key points: radiological assessment

■ Plain radiographs remain central to the evaluation of tumour response in intrathoracic malignancy, primary breast cancer and bone tumours

■ Computed tomography is the mainstay of measuring changes in tumour volume with imaging

■ Regression rates are different for different histological types of tumour

■ Measurement of tumour volume changes is difficult in irregular and diffuse tumours as well as those involving hollow viscera

■ On MRI, intrathoracic tumours appear larger than on CT

Tumour composition

Although tumour shrinkage is generally recognized as the major indicator of tumour response, it is important to appreciate that some tumours show only moderate reduction in volume, even with successful treatment, because active cancer may be transformed into 'benign' tissues such as differentiated tumour, fibrosis and necrosis. Thus, an accurate statement on changes in tumour composition, as well as changes in tumour volume, would be a significant breakthrough in the assessment of therapeutic response. However, even using all the sophisticated imaging technology available, it is not yet possible to characterize tumour composition reliably. Ultrasound, CT, MRI, MR spectroscopy and radionuclide studies all have a place in evaluating tumour composition by providing both anatomical and functional analysis.

Ultrasound
Ultrasound may show changes in tumour echogenicity in response to therapy but, as in tumour volume measurement, such changes are difficult to quantify and compare on follow-up studies. Colour Doppler techniques and intravenous contrast agents may permit an assessment of changes in tumour vascularity and encouraging results have been reported in the assessment of primary medical therapy for breast cancer.[36]

Computed tomography
On CT, the majority of tumours appear as soft tissue density masses but may contain areas of low attenuation within the mass representing necrosis or cystic change or areas of high attenuation reflecting calcification or haemorrhage. On follow-up CT examination, areas of low attenuation within a mass may increase or may appear during therapy,

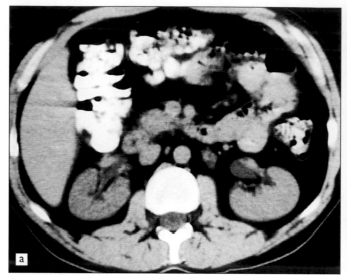 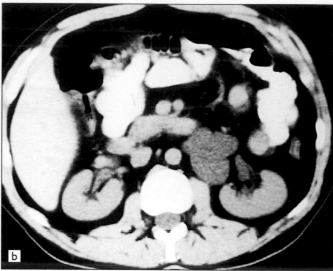

Figure 45.18. *CT scan of a patient with an abdominal nodal metastasis from NSGCT: (a) prechemotherapy, (b) postchemotherapy. On the pretreatment scan a small soft tissue density nodal metastasis is seen in the left para-aortic region. Following chemotherapy this nodal metastasis has enlarged and now measures 5 × 5 cm in diameter. The mass is of homogeneous water density and at surgery represented a cyst. The wall of the cyst contained differentiated teratoma with no evidence of active malignancy.*

presumably representing the development of necrosis in response to treatment. In patients with NSCGT, abdominal nodal metastases may become 'cystic' during follow-up and may also enlarge on treatment.[32,37] These changes may be seen in retroperitoneal lymph node masses, in mediastinal and supr-aclavicular nodal metastases and cystic change also probably occurs in lung metastases. In NSGCT these changes usually represent a favourable response to treatment, 'cysts' usually showing 'differentiated tumour' in the wall of the cyst histo-logically without evidence of undifferentiated malignancy (Fig. 45.18).[37] However, it should be emphasized that a small soft tissue nodule within the wall of a 'cyst' may represent active cancer and indeed all residual masses in NSGCT which are par-tially cystic or partially solid should be regarded as potentially malignant. In the lung, metastases may cavitate on treatment leaving a rim of irregular soft tissue around an air-containing central space (Fig. 45.19). The precise event leading to cavita-tion is not clear but it is interesting to speculate that a cystic lung metastasis could rupture, emptying its contents into the adjacent bronchus thus leaving a cavity within a treated deposit.

The development, increase or reduction in calcification within a tumour may also be seen on follow-up. Such a phe-nomenon is seen in neuroblastoma and in liver metastases from colorectal, ovary and breast cancer (Fig. 45.20).[38,39] In a recent study of 264 patients with hepatic metastases from colorectal cancer we found an incidence of calcification in 14%. These patients were followed during chemotherapy and the presence, character and changes in calcification were correlated with clinical outcome. Our results showed that the presence of calcification in hepatic metastases from colorectal cancer carries no prognostic significance but it may influence change in tumour volume measurement due to the inability of the lesion to regress in the presence of conglomerated lumps of calcium.

Intravenous contrast medium adds another dimension in the CT evaluation of changes in tumour composition, as tumour perfusion can be measured,[40] but as yet this para-meter has been little explored. The advent of spiral CT opens the way to rapid multislice studies of the patterns of tumour contrast enhancement which could be evaluated using a three-dimensional image display.

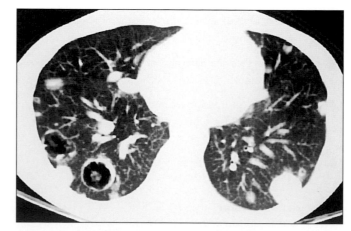

Figure 45.19. *CT scan showing cavitated lung metastases in a patient treated with chemotherapy for NSGCT.*

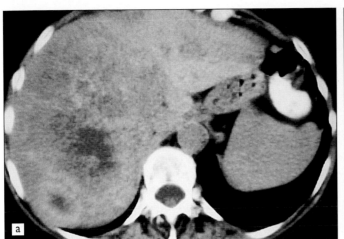 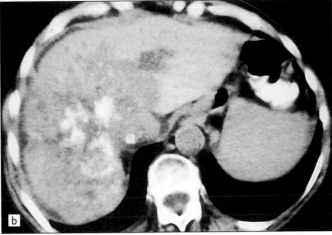

Figure 45.20. *CT scan showing increasing calcification in multiple liver metastases from colorectal cancer: (a) prechemotherapy; (b) 6 months after commencement of treatment.*

Magnetic resonance imaging

Magnetic resonance imaging (MRI) demonstrates tumours as relatively low signal intensity masses on T1 weighting and as intermediate to high signal intensity masses on T2-weighted spin-echo sequences reflecting the longer T1 and T2 relaxation times of tumours compared with adjacent normal tissues (Figs. 45.15 and 45.16). The signal intensity of a tumour reflects its free water content and if surrounded by tissue, which has a higher water content than that of the tumour, it will appear as a relatively low signal intensity lesion. For example, in prostate cancer a tumour in the peripheral zone of the gland will appear as a relatively low signal intensity mass but an untreated soft tissue sarcoma in muscle will have a high signal intensity compared to the surrounding normal tissue (Fig. 45.16). The signal intensity of a malignant lesion is usually heterogeneous due to the different components of the tumour; thus areas of relatively high and relatively low signal intensity on different sequences are seen due to the presence of fresh haemorrhage, haemosiderin, cysts, necrosis, calcification and active cancer (Fig. 45.21).

Magnetic resonance imaging can undoubtedly demonstrate changes in these complex signal characteristics on various pulse sequences following therapy; in general, tumours which respond to treatment show a reduction in signal intensity on T2-weighted spin-echo sequences, due at least in part to a reduction in the amount of free water within the mass. Fibrosis, with deposition of collagen macromolecules, may also contribute to a reduction of proton relaxation times, resulting in lower signal intensity. The resultant signal intensity of the mass often remains heterogeneous as it represents areas of active tumour, inflammation, cystic change, necrosis and haemorrhage which all have a high signal intensity on

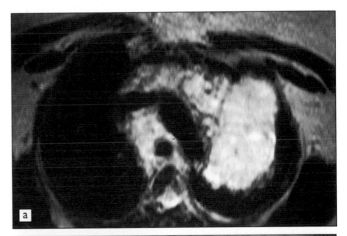

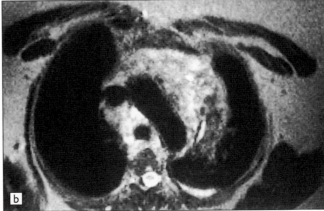

Figure 45.21. *T2-weighted spin-echo MR images in a patient with non-Hodgkin's lymphoma: (a) prechemotherapy; (b) postchemotherapy. Note persistent areas of high signal intensity within the residual mass. The mass is heterogeneous both before and after treatment. (From ref. 16, with permission.)*

913

T2 weighting as well as areas of fibrosis, calcification and haemosiderin which have a low signal intensity on T2 weighting[15–17,41–45] Conventional spin-echo sequences are preferable to fast (turbo spin-echo) sequences for evaluating these changes in signal intensity on T2 weighting because conventional spin-echo sequences are a more reliable reflection of T2 relaxation times.[46]

In the early days of clinical MRI it was anticipated that the technique might be an accurate method of distinguishing persistent tumour from fibrosis and indeed early reports were encouraging. One of the first of these was a study reported by Glazer and colleagues[41] which showed a reduction in signal intensity on T2 weighting following irradiation of primary lung cancers and further reports on carcinoma of the cervix, bone tumours and lymphoma also showed reduction in signal intensity following both chemotherapy and radiotherapy.[15,16,43–45] However, while reduction in signal intensity may be regarded as a favourable sign of tumour response, it has now been clearly established that small foci of persistent tumour within low signal intensity regions cannot be identified reliably on T2-weighted images alone.[44] In a study of 34 patients with mediastinal masses due to lymphoma,[16] we showed that MRI had a sensitivity of only 45% but a specificity of 90% in detecting persistent active cancer within the residual mass following chemotherapy. The positive predictive value was 71%, and the negative predictive value was 75%, these results comparing favourable with those of Ga-67 citrate scanning and the erythrocyte sedimentation rate (ESR). Other studies evaluating residual masses in lymphoma have also shown reduction in signal intensity in response to treatment, but as yet MRI is not used widely to direct the further management of residual lymphomatous masses.

Thymic infiltration occurs in up to 50% of patients with lymphoma and is almost invariably associated with nodal disease.[35,47] In a study comparing the results of MRI and CT in treated lymphoma we have shown that the gland has a heterogeneous or homogeneous low signal intensity in the majority of patients who have been successfully treated. In those patients who relapsed within 1 year of the posttreatment MRI scan, the majority (4 out of 6) had large volume residual masses of heterogeneous high signal intensity[35] (Fig. 45.21). Thymic cysts may also be observed following chemotherapy within residual thymic masses and should not be confused with persistent active malignant residua (Fig. 45.22). Radiotherapy induces a fibrotic reaction both in tumour and surrounding normal tissues. In the prostate the zonal anatomy is lost following radiotherapy which makes evaluation of response difficult as the primary lesion cannot be clearly delineated (Fig. 45.23).

In the assessment of tumour response complete reliance on signal intensity change is clearly impossible, but such signal intensity changes can provide a guide as to the likelihood of persistent active tumour, particularly if a large heterogeneous high signal intensity mass persists.[16,35] However, it should be remembered that residual tumour may be purely microscopic and thus beyond the resolution of contemporary imaging methods. In a prospective study of children with Ewing's sarcoma in which the primary tumour was resected following neo-adjuvant chemotherapy, clusters of active malignant cells were found in areas of high signal intensity within the bone marrow cavity and also in nests of 50–100 cells surrounded by dense sclerotic cortical bone which returned very low signal intensity on all pulse sequences.[44] Such studies highlight the need for exploiting other characteristics of MRI, in particular the effects of paramagnetic contrast medium uptake.

Over many years considerable attention has been focused on neovascularity of tumours and factors have been isolated which promote and suppress tumour angiogenesis.[48,49] In parallel to these advances, imaging techniques, such as CT and MRI, are now able to explore the effects of neovascularity in tumours through the exploitation of intravenous contrast agents. New tumour blood vessels are

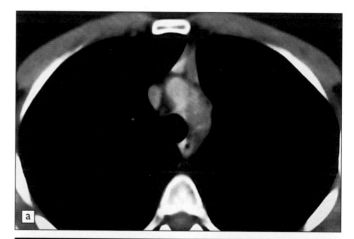

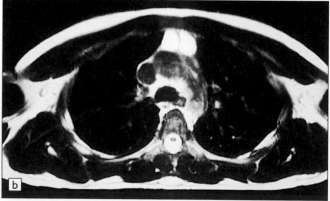

Figure 45.22. (a) CT scan; (b) T2-weighted MR image showing a residual thymic mass following chemotherapy for Hodgkin's disease. The mass has a homogeneous high signal intensity on MRI representing cysts. On the CT scan taken on the same day as MRI, the residual mass appears smaller. (From ref. 35, with permission.)

abnormal morphologically and are also more numerous than in normal tissue. The basement membrane of these new capillaries is incomplete which leads to increased perfusion and increased permeability allowing leakage of fluid and other substances into the expanded extravascular space.[48] By evaluation of the pattern of uptake of contrast medium into a tumour on MRI, signal intensity–time curves can be obtained which show significantly different patterns of uptake in malignant lesions compared with benign lesions and normal tissues.[50–54] Measurement of the onset of enhancement, slope of enhancement, maximum amplitude and washout phase following injection of intravenous gadolinium-DTPA on T1-weighted gradient-echo images can provide quantitative information which reflects tumour capillary permeability and the extracellular tumour leakage space.[53,54] In general there is good separation between benign and malignant lesions but overlap of signal intensity characteristics does occur which may lead to false-positive diagnoses of malignancy. Functional studies in MRI are

likely to be further enhanced by the development of echoplanar imaging which allows extremely rapid data acquisition of volumetric changes in signal intensity–time ratios over a short time scale.[55]

Current research in the measurement of neovascularity and changes in these parameters which occur in response to treatment is a challenging area of oncological imaging. Such studies may permit the distinction between tumour boundaries and surrounding tissues as well as the identification of viable foci of tumour within a mass following treatment. In a recent study Verstraete and colleagues[20] were able to identify residual active tumour using dynamic contrast-enhanced MRI with analysis of parametric 'first pass' images to depict tumour vascularization and perfusion. These authors were able to show a reduction in the slope and maximum amplitude of signal intensity curves following one course of chemotherapy and suggest that this may be a valuable method of demonstrating early tumour response before morphological change. Similar studies in breast and prostate cancer have revealed changes in the characteristics of signal intensity–time curves in response to neo-adjuvant chemotherapy (Fig. 45.24).

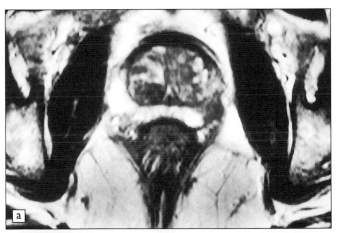

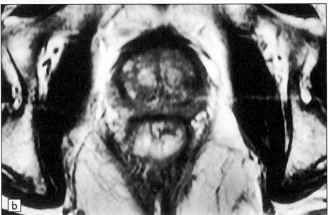

Figure 45.23. *MR images of prostate cancer: (a) pre-radiotherapy; (b) post-radiotherapy. There is loss of signal throughout the peripheral zone and the primary tumour is no longer distinguishable from adjacent normal tissue.*

Key points: tumour composition

- Changes in tumour composition, such as necrosis, do not necessarily parallel changes in tumour volume

- Information provided by ultrasound and CT is limited but necrosis, cystic change and calcification can be demonstrated

- Enlarging cysts in NSGCT indicate a favourable treatment response

- The development of calcification in liver metastases has no prognostic significance in colorectal cancer

- On MRI, reduction of signal intensity of T2-weighted images reflects a reduction in the free water content of a tumour

- Signal intensity changes on MRI are helpful for predicting persistent malignancy but are not totally reliable

- Contrast-enhanced imaging with MRI and CT provides information on tumour perfusion

- Analysis of signal intensity time curves is helpful and appear to be a valuable method of measuring therapeutic response and distinguishing active tumour from benign tissue, but overlap does occur

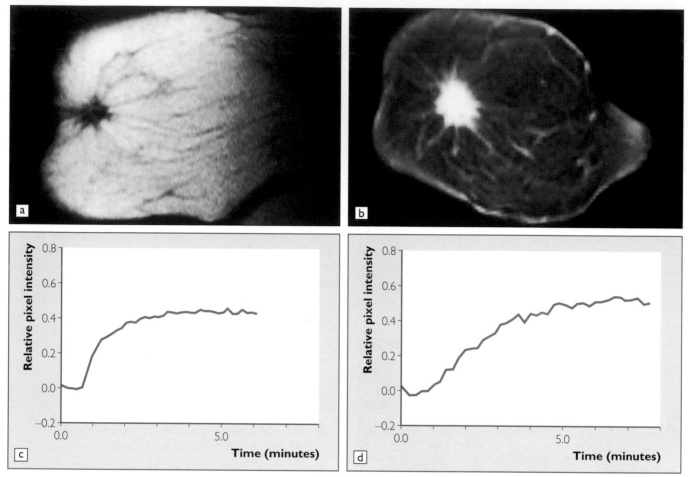

Figure 45.24. *MR images of a patient with primary breast cancer: (a) a T1-weighted 3D flash image showing the low signal intensity tumour prior to chemotherapy; (b) a contrast-enhanced T1-weighted fat-suppressed image in the coronal plane also before treatment; (c) time/signal intensity curve showing pattern of contrast enhancement of the carcinoma before chemotherapy; (d) time/signal intensity curve showing* *contrast enhancement pattern of the carcinoma after four courses of chemotherapy. The 'slope' of the enhancement curve has been reduced following chemotherapy, indicating a reduction in tumour capillary permeability. Histological examination of the excised residual mass showed extensive fibrosis containing small foci of residual cancer. (From ref. 78, with permission.)*

Functional imaging research (whether with MRI, CT or ultrasound) to evaluate changes in neovascularity has important implications for the future assessment of treatment response because using such techniques will make it possible to combine morphological and functional information to address the complex issues of tumour response. Currently such methods are limited to the examination of only a single slice or at most three to five slices through the tumour and most techniques utilize a selected 'region of interest' which therefore only provides a 'sample'. Pixel-by-pixel analysis and multislice techniques are currently being investigated.

Radionuclide studies
Proliferating tumour cells have a rapid cell turnover and using radio-isotope techniques, tumour metabolism can be quantified. One of the most exciting advances in nuclear medicine during recent years has been the development of clinical appraisal of PET using various radiopharmaceuticals such 2-[F-18] fluoro-2-deoxy-D-glucose (18-FDG).[21,22,27,56] Indeed, this agent has been the most widely used in oncology although other agents, such as amino acids labelled with carbon-11, are currently under investigation.[22,35] Using positron emitting agents, tumour metabolism, tumour perfusion, protein synthesis, oxygen metabolism and glucose metabolism can be studied.

Most of the studies in oncology have been carried out with 18-FDG-PET which has already been shown to have enormous potential in detecting foci of malignancy,[57] that are difficult or impossible to demonstrate by morphological anatomical techniques. Initial studies which have been reported indicate that

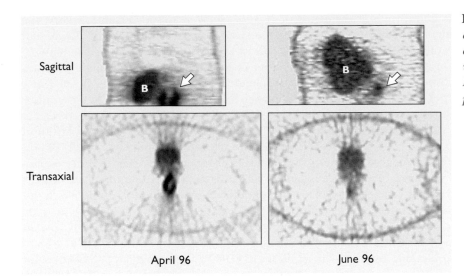

Sagittal		
Transaxial		
April 96	June 96

Figure 45.25. *18-FDG-PET scan showing an inoperable rectal cancer before and after chemotherapy (arrows). Note reduction in uptake of 18-FDG following chemotherapy. B = bladder. (Reproduced with kind permission from Professor M Maisey.)*

18-FDG-PET is an accurate method of follow-up in patients with brain tumours, head and neck tumours, breast cancer, rectal cancer (Fig. 45.25) and particularly lymphoma.[58–62] However, even at this early stage of the clinical evaluation of PET several limitations have been highlighted which include the relative non-specificity of 18-FDG-PET in that inflammatory tissue, which frequently co-exists with active cancer or may be induced by treatment, also shows high uptake of 18-FDG.[22,56] Furthermore, the spatial resolution of PET is such that anatomical images provided by cross-sectional morphological imaging techniques are required to pinpoint the location of a lesion detected on PET scanning. Such correlation is best obtained by multimodality image registration, another focus of current technological development in imaging.[63]

Other radioisotope techniques such as immunoscintigraphy are also under evaluation having potential not only for monitoring response to treatment but also for the detection of relapse.[64]

Key point: positron emission tomography

■ 18-FDG-PET scanning has enormous clinical potential for the measurement of therapeutic response in oncology

Magnetic resonance spectroscopy
Magnetic resonance spectroscopy remains a clinical research tool, but has enormous clinical potential in the longer term.[65,66,67,68] It is another field where imaging plays a central role by providing anatomical maps on which metabolic changes can be displayed and with MR spectroscopy, tumour metabolism, phospholipid metabolism and drug metabolism can be investigated. Current research in many areas is focusing on the ability of MR spectroscopy to track the uptake of drugs within a tumour and to measure the changes in tumour metabolites in response to treatment.[67]

DETECTION OF RELAPSE

The diagnosis of tumour relapse should be made as quickly and accurately as possible if further therapy is to be effective. For many patients, once relapse has been diagnosed, curative treatment will not be an option but even in this situation imaging plays a key role in defining the presence and extent of recurrence so that palliative treatment may be given appropriately.

Disease relapse is usually evident by:

• Clinical symptoms and signs suggestive of recurrence
• A rise in tumour marker estimations
• Imaging features suggestive or diagnostic of relapse on regular follow-up

The role of imaging and the diagnosis of recurrent disease depends upon the way in which it presents; in patients with clinical symptoms and signs suggestive of relapse, imaging will be tailored to evaluate the local area where relapse is suspected as well as other sites which are determined by the known pattern of disease spread. For example, in a patient with prostate cancer and a raised prostate specific antigen level (PSA), it is important to image the prostate either with transrectal ultrasound (TRUS) or MRI, to evaluate the pelvic lymph nodes, retroperitoneal lymph nodes and the bone. These sites may all be assessed with MRI, but radionuclide scanning is usually performed to detect bone metastases. A plain chest radiograph will also identify pulmonary metastases and mediastinal lymphadenopathy. In patients who have been treated with previous radiotherapy to the whole pelvis, lymph node metastases usually recur in the retroperitoneum because the pelvic nodes have been 'sterilized'.[65] This emphasizes the importance of a full knowledge of the patient's previous treatment and the predicted pattern of tumour spread when searching for sites of relapse.

Imaging itself may be the first technique to suggest relapse. This is commonly seen in patients who undergo routine imaging during follow-up after treatment, for example in patients with lymphoma, testicular cancer or rectal cancer. In such patients a slight increase in size of a soft tissue residuum may herald disease progression, but according to Miller's criteria the enlargement is considerably less than 25% and therefore cannot be classified as progressive disease. Thus although such a patient cannot be diagnosed as having relapsed, it is prudent to document such small changes in tumour size and to repeat the study after a short interval of say 6–8 weeks.

One of the major problems in the detection of relapse is the distinction of post-treatment residual abnormalities from tumour. Baseline studies following treatment are helpful in distinguishing these entities since enlargement and change in shape of a residual mass suggests recurrence. A classic example is the distinction of postoperative fibrosis from tumour in patients with residual masses in the sacral hollow following surgery for colorectal cancer.[3,70–73] Follow-up CT examinations may show a change in the residual mass indicative of recurrence (Fig. 45.26) but in the absence of previous studies for comparison and other

evidence of relapse, such as raised serum markers, the diagnosis of relapse may be impossible.[73] Recurrent tumour may coexist with infection, abscess or haematoma. In this situation, further imaging with dynamic contrast-enhanced MRI, immunoscintigraphy and 18-FDG-PET may help, but biopsy is often required to reach a definitive diagnosis (Fig. 45.27).[62,64,74–76] However, these new techniques, such as fast dynamic contrast-enhanced MRI and FDG-PET studies are likely to become increasingly important in the diagnosis of recurrent disease as more experience is gained. Thus, dynamic contrast-enhanced MRI is a useful method of detecting recurrence in patients with suspected relapse of prostate cancer due to a rising prostate specific antigen level, who have been previously treated with radiotherapy (Fig. 45.28).

In addition, 18-FDG-PET scanning has also been found useful in the assessment of patients with suspected relapse from NSGCTs of the testis in whom CT has failed to reveal evidence of disease progression. (Fig. 45.29).

CONCLUSION

Imaging has a critical and expanding role in the measurement of therapeutic response which is one of the most exciting and scientifically challenging areas in oncology. Established imaging techniques provide useful information for patient management but at the same time vigorous research is being conducted to explore the potential of new imaging modalities and to combine morphological and functional information to evaluate the tumour as a whole.

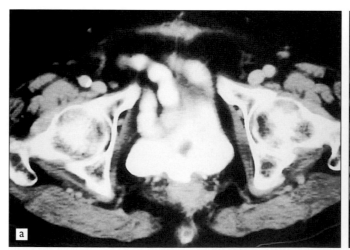
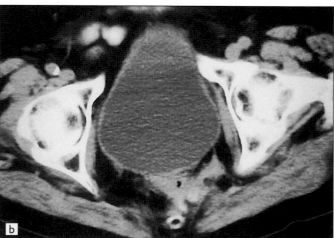

Figure 45.26. *(a) CT scan showing a mass in the sacral hollow following abdominoperineal resection for rectal cancer. (b) Six months later the soft tissue mass in the sacral hollow has increased in size and become more irregular, indicating recurrent tumour.*

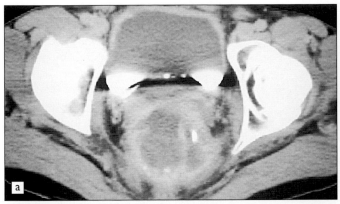

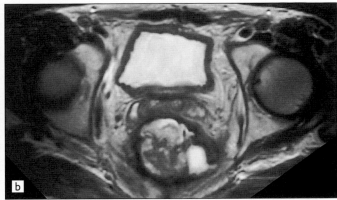

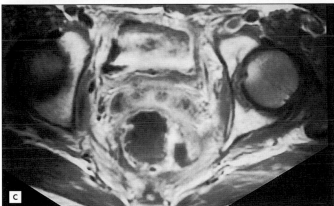

Figure 45.27. *Large mass in the sacral hollow. This female patient had undergone abdominoperineal resection for carcinoma of the rectum followed by radiotherapy for recurrent disease: (a) CT shows a large mass with a thick ragged wall and a low-density centre; (b) A T2-weighted MR image shows that the mass has a heterogeneous signal intensity with areas of high and low signal centrally and a thick low signal intensity wall; (c) T1-weighted image following intravenous gadolinium-DTPA. The wall of the mass enhances. The central component of the mass is a low signal intensity showing little if any enhancement. The appearances on CT and MRI are comparable. Recurrent tumour cannot be distinguished from an abscess on imaging.*

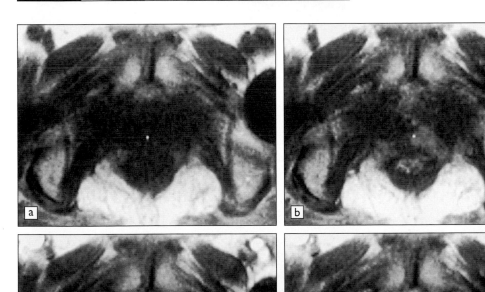

Figure 45.28. *MR images images of a patient previously treated with radiotherapy for prostate cancer with an elevated prostate specific antigen (PSA) level (60 ng/ml): (a) before injection of contrast medium; (b) at 30 seconds after injection; (c) at 1 minute per injection; (d) at 3 minutes after injection. There is an area of intense enhancement indicating recurrent disease.*

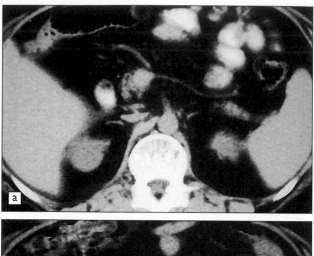

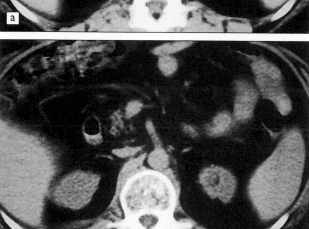

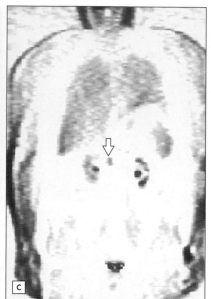

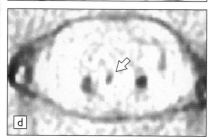

Figure 45.29. *A patient with an NSGCT of the testis. The patient was initially treated for Stage-IIb disease. A CT examination was performed 2 years later at the time of rising markers (alpha-foetoprotein): (a) CT scan following initial treatment; (b) CT scan at the time of raised serum markers. There is abnormal soft tissue deep to the right crus of the diaphragm on (b) which could represent the site of recurrence; (c and d) 18-FDG-PET scan: (c) coronal image; (d) axial imaging showing high uptake of 18-FDG in a lesion in the same anatomical position as the abnormal tissue seen deep to the right crus of the diaphragm. [(c and d) Reproduced with kind permission from Professor M Maisey.]*

Summary

■ The increasing incidence of cancer and an aggressive approach to therapy has led to the imaging of treated cancer becoming a major expanding area in oncological imaging.

■ Imaging permits evaluation of therapeutic response by measuring changes in tumour volume and tumour composition.

■ The same technique should be used for monitoring response throughout the clinical course of disease. Ideally, this should be the same technique as used for pretreatment tumour staging.

■ The radiologist plays a central role in the multidisciplinary team which allows a strategic approach to be adopted for the most appropriate use of imaging resources.

■ Strategies for imaging include those for the evaluation of individual patient management, strategies to assess curable disease and strategies to support clinical research.

■ Currently, Miller's criteria provides the standard for evaluating therapeutic response in terms of changes in tumour size, but no consideration is given to the calculation of tumour volume.

■ Miller's criteria do not take into account changes in tumour composition.

■ While current imaging modalities reflect changes in tumour volume, accurate assessment is not possible in all tumours due to poor definition.

■ Evaluation of changes in tumour composition are limited with ultrasound and CT.

■ Contrast-enhanced MRI techniques may provide information which reflects changes in tumour neovascularity.

■ 18-FDG-PET scanning is likely to have a critical role in the clinical evaluation of therapeutic response when the technique becomes more widely available.

REFERENCES

1. Cancer Facts and Figures 1997. American Cancer Society, 1997

2. Cancer in South East England 1992. Thames Cancer Registry, 1995

3. Kelvin F M, Koreobkin M, Heaston D K et al. The pelvis after surgery for rectal carcinoma: Serial CT observations with emphasis on non-neoplastic features. Am J Roentgenol 1993; 141: 959

4. Kissin C M, Husband J E, Nicholas D et al. Benign thymic enlargement in adults after chemotherapy: CT demonstration. Radiology 1987; 163: 67

5. Einhorn L H, Williams S D, Loehrer P J et al. Evaluation of optimal duration of chemotherapy in favourable-prognosis disseminated germ cell tumors: a Southeastern Cancer Study Group protocol. J Clin Oncology 1989; 7: 387

6. Horwich A, Dearnaley D P, Nicholls J et al. Effectiveness of carboplatin, etoposide, bleomycin (CEB) combination chemotherapy in good prognosis metastatic testicular non-seminomatous germ cell tumours. J Clin Oncol 1991; 9: 62

7. Hendry W F, Goldstraw P, Horwich A et al. Paraaortic lymphadenopathy after chemotherapy for testicular tumour. Br J Urol 1988; 62: 470

8. Read G, Stenning S, Cullen M et al. Medical Research Council prospective study of surveillance for Stage I testicular teratoma. J Clin Oncol 1992; 10: 1762

9. Nicolai N, Pizzocaro G. A surveillance study of clinical stage I nonseminomatous germ cell tumours of the testis: 10-year follow-up. J Urol 1995; 154: 1045

10. Tubiana M, Henry-Amar M, Carde P et al. Toward comprehensive management tailored to prognostic factors of patients with clinical stages I and II in Hodgkin's disease. The RORTC Lymphoma Group controlled clinical trials 1964–1987. Blood 1989; 73: 47–56

11. Verger E, Easton D, Brada M et al. Radiotherapy results in laparotomy staged early Hodgkin's disease. Radiology 1988; 39: 428–431

12. Canellos G P, Anderson J R, Propert K J et al. Chemotherapy of advanced Hodgkin's disease with MOPP, ABVD or MOPP alternating with ABVD. New Engl J Med 1992; 327: 1478–1484

13. Miller A, Hoogstraten B, Staqut M et al. Reporting results of cancer treatment. Cancer 1981; 47: 207

14. Ng V W K, Husband J E S, Nicolson V M C et al. CT evaluation of treatment response in advanced gastric cancer. Clin Radiol 1996; 51: 214

15. Rahmouni A, Tempany C, Jones R et al. Lymphoma: Monitoring tumor size and signal intensity with MR imaging. Radiology 1993; 188: 445

16. Hill M, Cunningham D, MacVicar D et al. Role of magnetic resonance imaging in predicting relapse in residual masses after treatment of lymphoma. J Clin Oncol 1993; 11: 2273

17. Nyman R S, Rehn S M, Glimelius B L G et al. Residual mediastinal masses in Hodgkin disease: Prediction of size with MR imaging. Radiology 1989; 170: 435–440

18. Kalbhen C L, Hricak H, Shinohara K et al. Prostate carcinoma: MR imaging findings after cryosurgery. Radiology 1996; 198: 807

19. Padhani A R, Parker G J M, Tanner S F et al. Evaluation of the response of breast carcinoma to chemotherapy using dynamic MR mammography: Preliminary observations (Abstract). Proceedings of Society of Magnetic Resonance Fourth Scientific Meeting, New York, April 1996

20. Verstraete K L, de Deene Y, Roels H et al. Benign and malignant musculoskeletal lesions: Dynamic contrast-enhanced MR imaging: parametric first-pass images depict tissue vascularization and perfusion. Radiology 1994; 192: 835

21. Okada J, Yoshikawa K, Imazeki K et al. The use of FDG-PET in the detection and management of malignant lymphoma: Correlation of uptake and prognosis. J Nucl Med 1991; 32: 686

22. Cook G J R, Maisey M N. Review: The current status of clinical PET imaging. Clin Radiol 1996; 51: 603–613

23. Vinnicombe S J, MacVicar A D, Guy R L et al. Primary breast cancer: mammographic changes after neoadjuvant chemotherapy with pathologic correlation. Radiology 1996; 198: 333–340

24. Muller M F, Meyenberger C, Bertschinger P et al. Pancreatic tumors: evaluation with endoscopic US, CT and MR imaging. Radiology 1994; 190: 745

25. van der Woude H-J, Bloem J L, Schipper J et al. Changes in tumor perfusion induced by chemotherapy in bone sarcomas: Color Doppler flow imaging compared with contrast-enhanced MR imaging and three-phase bone scintigraphy. Radiology 1994; 191: 421

26. Balen F G, Allen C M, Lees W R. Review: Ultrasound contrast agents. Clin Radiol 1994; 49: 77

27. Minn H, Paul R. Cancer treatment monitoring with fluorine-18 2-fluoro-2-deoxy-D-glucose and positron emission tomography: Frustration or future? Eur J Nucl Med 1992; 19: 921–924

28. Findlay M P N, Leach M O, Cunningham D et al. The non-invasive monitoring of low dose, infusional 5-fluorouracil and its modulation by interferon using in vivo ^{19}F magnetic resonance spectroscopy in patients with colorectal cancer: A pilot study. Ann Oncol 1993; 4: 597

29. Collins V P, Loeffler R K, Tivey H. Observations on growth rates of human tumours. Am J Roentgenol 1956; 76: 988

30. Spratt J S, Spratt T L. Rates of growth of pulmonary metastases and host survival. Ann Surg 1964; 159: 161

31. Husband J E. Diagnostic techniques: Their strengths and weaknesses. Br J Cancer 1980; 41: 21

32. Husband J E, Hawkes B S, Peckham M J. CT estimations of mean attenuation values and volume in testicular tumours: A comparison with surgical and histologic findings. Radiology 1982; 144: 553

33. Williams M P, Naik G, Heron C W et al. Com-puted tomography of the abdomen in advanced semi-noma: Response to treatment. Clin Radiol 1987; 38: 629

34. Peckham M, Horwich A, Hendry W. Advanced seminoma treatment with cisplatinum based combination chemotherapy or carboplatin. Br J Cancer 1985; 52: 7

35. Spiers A S D, Husband J E S, MacVicar D. Treated thymic lymphoma: Comparison of MR imaging with CT. Radiology 1997; 203: 369–376

36. Kedar R P, Cosgrove D O, Smith I E et al. Breast carcinoma: Measurement of tumour response to primary medical therapy with colour Doppler flow imaging. Radiology 1994; 190: 825–830

37. Stomper P C, Jochelson M S, Barnick M B et al. Residual abdominal masses after chemotherapy for non-seminomatous testicular cancer: Correlation of CT and histology. Am J Roentgenol 1985; 145: 743

38. Gossios K, Tsianos E V, Nicolson V et al. CT evaluation of the resectability of gastric cancer postchemotherapy. Abdom Imag 1996; 21: 293–298

39. Hale H L, Husband J E, Gossios K et al. Calcified liver metastases in colorectal carcinoma (Submitted)

40. Miles K A, Hayball M P, Dixon A K. Functional images of hepatic perfusion obtained with dynamic CT. Radiology 1993; 188: 405

41. Glazer H S, Lee J K T, Levitt R G et al. Radiation fibrosis: Differentiation from recurrent tumour by MR imaging. Radiology 1985; 156: 721

42. Lemmi M A, Fletcher B D, Marina N M et al. Use of MR imaging to assess results of chemotherapy for Ewing's sarcoma. Am J Roentgenol 1990 155: 343

43. Flueckiger F, Ener F, Poschauko H et al. Cervical cancer: Serial M R imaging before and after primary radiation therapy: A 2-year follow-up study. Radiology 1992; 184: 89

44. MacVicar A D, Olliff J C, Pringle J et al. Ewing sarcoma: MR imaging of chemotherapy-induced changes with histologic correlation. Radiology 1992; 184: 859

45. Kim K H, Lee B H, Do Y S et al. Stage 1B cervical carcinoma: M R evaluation of effect of intraarterial chemotherapy. Radiology 1994; 192: 61

46. Baudouin C J, Ward J, Ridgway J P et al. A comparison of fast and conventional T2 weighted spin echo sequences in the detection of focal liver lesions at 1.0 T. Clin Radiol 1996; 51: 769–774

47. Wernecke K, Vassallo P, Rutsch F et al. Thymic involvement in Hodgkin's disease: CT and sonographic findings. Radiology 1992; 181: 375–383

48. Folkman J. Angiogenesis in cancer, vascular, rheumatoid and other disease. Nature Med 1995; 1: 27

49. Auerbach W, Auerbach R. Angiogenesis inhibition: A review. Pharmacology Therapeutics 1994; 63: 265

50. van der Woude H, Bloem J L, Verstraete K L et al. Osteosarcoma and Ewing's sarcoma after neoadjuvant chemotherapy: Value of dynamic MR imaging in detecting viable tumour before surgery. Am J Roentgenol 1995; 165: 593

51. Boetes C, Barentsz J O, Mus R D et al. MR characteris-ation of suspicious breast lesions with a gadolinium-enhanced TurboFLASH subtraction technique. Radiology 1994; 193: 777

52. Barentsz J O, Jager G J, Witjes J A et al. Primary staging urinary bladder cancer after transurethral biopsy: Value of fast dynamic contrast-enhanced MR imaging. Radiology 1996; 201: 185

53. Parker G J M, Padhani A R, Suckling J et al. Probing tumour microvascularity by measurement, analysis and display of contrast agent uptake kinetics. J Mag Res Imag (in press)

54. Böck J C, Henrikson O, Götze A H G et al. Magnetic resonance perfusion imaging with gadolinium-DTPA: Quantitative approach for the kinetic analysis of first-pass residue curves. Invest Radiol 1995; 30: 693

55. Kwong K K, Chesler D A, Wiesskoff R M et al. MR perfusion studies with T1-weighted echo planar imaging. Mag Res Med 1995; 34: 878

56. Strauss L G, Conti P S. The applications of PET in clinical oncology. J Nucl Med 1991; 32: 623

57. Koh W-J, Griffin T W, Rasey S J et al. Positron emission tomography: New tool for characterization of malignant disease and selection of therapy. Acta Oncol 1994; 33: 323

58. Coleman R E, Hoffman J M, Hanson M W et al. Clinical application of PET for the evaluation of brain tumours. J Nucl Med 1991; 32: 616–622

59. Haberkorn U, Strauss L G, Dimitrakapolou A et al. Fluorodeoxyglucose imaging of advanced head and neck cancer after chemotherapy. J Nucl Med 1993; 34: 12

60. Wahl R L, Zasadny K R, Hutchins G D et al. Metabolic monitoring of breast cancer chemohormonotherapy using positron emission tomography (PET): Initial evaluation. J Clin Oncol 1993; 11: 2101

61. Goldberg M A, Lee M J, Fischman A J et al. Fluorodeoxyglucose PET and abdominal and pelvic neoplasms: Potential role in oncologic imaging. Radiographics 1993; 13: 1047–1062

62. Haberkorn U, Strauss L G, Dimitrakopoulou A et al. PET studies of fluorodeoxyglucose metabolism in patients with recurrent colorectal tumours receiving radiotherapy. J Nucl Med 1991; 32: 1485–1490

63. Hill D L G, Hawkes D J, Gleeson M J et al. Accurate frameless registration of MR and CT images of the head: Applications in planning surgery and radiation therapy. Radiology 1994; 67: 1

64. Stomper P C, D'Souza D J, Bakshi S P et al. Detection of pelvic recurrence of colorectal carcinoma: Prospective, blinded comparison of Tc-99m-IMMU-4 monoclonal antibody scanning and CT. Radiology 1995; 197: 688

65. Castellio M, Kwock L, Mukherji S K. Clinical applications of proton MR spectroscopy. Am J Neuroradiol 1996; 17: 1

66. Cousins J P. Clinical M R spectroscopy: Fundamentals, current applications, and future potential. Am J Roentgenol 1995; 164: 1337

67. Presant C A, Wolf W, Albright M J et al. Human tumour fluorouracil trapping: Clinical correlations of in vivo ^{19}F nuclear magnetic resonance spectroscopy pharmacokinetics. J Clin Oncol 1990; 8: 1868

68. Sostman H D, Prescott D M, Dewhirst M W et al. MR imaging and spectroscopy for prognostic evaluation in soft-tissue sarcomas. Radiology 1994; 190: 269

69. Spencer J A, Golding S J. Patterns of lymphatic metastases at recurrence of prostate cancer: CT findings. Clin Radiol 1994; 49: 404

70. Husband J E, Hodson N H, Parsons C A. The role of computed tomography in recurrent rectal tumours. Radiology 1980; 4: 1–16

71. Reznek R H, White F E, Young J W R. The appearances on computed tomography after abdomino-perineal resection for carcinoma of the rectum: A comparison between the normal appearances and those of recurrence. Br J Radiol 1983; 56: 237–240

72. Méndez R J, Rodrígue R, Kovacevich T et al. CT in local recurrence of rectal carcinoma. J Comput Assist Tomogr 1993; 17: 741–744

73. Sugarbaker P H, Gianola F J, Dwyer A et al. A simplified plan for follow-up of patients with colon and rectal cancer supported by prospective studies of laboratory and radiological test results. Surgery 1987; 102: 79–87

74. Pema P J, Bennett W F, Bova J G, Warman P. CT vs MRI in diagnosis of recurrent rectosigmoid carcinoma. J Comput Assist Tomogr 1994; 18: 256–261

75. Beets G, Penninckx F, Schiepers C et al. Clinical value of whole-body positron emission tomography with [18F]fluorodeoxyglucose in recurrent colorectal cancer. Br J Surg 1994; 1666–1670

76. Kissin C M, Husband J E, Nicholas D et al. Benign thymic enlargement in adults after chemotherapy: CT demonstration. Radiology 1987; 163: 67

77. Muller-Schimpfle M, Brix G, Layer G et al. Recurrent rectal cancer: diagnosis with dynamic MR imaging. Radiology 1993; 189: 881

78. J E Husband. Monitoring tumour response. In: J E S Husband, R H Reznek (eds). Oncology Imaging. Mini Categorical Course Syllabus, European Congress of Radiology, Vienna, March 2–7, 1997; 81–91. (From Eur Radiol, Volume 6, 1996)

Chapter 46

Radiological manifestations of acute complications of treatment

Louise Wilkinson, David MacVicar and Janet Husband

INTRODUCTION

There are many complications of treatment in the cancer patient which include acute treatment-related events and longer term late effects. These complications result from surgery, chemotherapy and radiotherapy. In this chapter the acute complications, mainly related to chemotherapy, will be discussed focusing on those pathological processes which are relevant to imaging. The complications associated with radiotherapy have been covered in detail elsewhere (see Chapters 48, 49 and 50) and the late complications related to chemotherapy are mentioned in other chapters as appropriate.

ACUTE COMPLICATIONS OF TREATMENT: THE THORAX

Catheters

Long-term intravenous catheters are frequently used in oncological practice for infusion of chemotherapy. The nature of the device (external catheter, implanted port, single or multilumen) and the route of insertion (into the subclavian vein or a more peripheral site) depends on local practice and the needs of the individual patient.[1] The complications of indwelling catheters include:

- Malposition
- Occlusion
- Sepsis

Complications at the time of insertion: malposition

The optimal position of the tip of the catheter is in a large vessel that can accommodate high flow rates.[2] The distal catheter should be parallel to the vessel wall to avoid erosion by local pressure effects. A curve at the tip of the catheter may indicate that the catheter tip is abutting the wall of the vessel.[3] At the time of insertion, the catheter may be misdirected into any of the central veins, most commonly the internal jugular vein.[4] The potential positions of a misplaced catheter are listed below:[5]

- Internal jugular vein
- Contralateral brachiocephalic vein
- Right atrium
- Right ventricle
- Inferior vena cava
- Hepatic veins
- Azygos vein
- Right superior intercostal vein
- Internal thoracic artery
- Pericardiophrenic vein
- Left superior intercostal vein
- Inferior thyroid vein
- Coronary sinus (via right atrium)
- Persistent left superior vena cava

Familiarity with the venous anatomy of the thorax on both the posteroanterior (PA) and lateral chest radiographs will help to identify the location of a misplaced catheter (Figs. 46.1–46.4).

The right subclavian vein is the favoured route of access, because left-sided catheters are associated more commonly with erosion of the superior vena cava (SVC). This is manifested by mediastinal widening and pleural effusion within 1–7 days of catheter placement.[5] A cadaver study has shown that percutaneous subclavian venepuncture frequently penetrates the internal jugular or brachiocephalic vein via the subclavius muscle or costoclavicular ligament rather than directly entering the subclavian vein.[6] This may lead to impingement of the catheter during arm abduction.[7]

Local trauma at the time of insertion may result in pneumothorax or, rarely, brachial plexus or phrenic nerve injury. Catheters can be placed in the pleural space and drugs or fluid infused intrapleurally (Fig. 46.5). Inadvertent arterial puncture causes local bleeding which may result in an apical extrapleural or mediastinal collection. It is particularly important to be aware of failed attempts at central venous catheterization even when there is no line *in situ*. Fragmentation of the catheter may be caused at the time of insertion, resulting in embolic fragments. These can be removed by percutaneous techniques.[1] Occasionally the postinsertion radiograph may reveal an unsuspected lost guidewire or fragment.

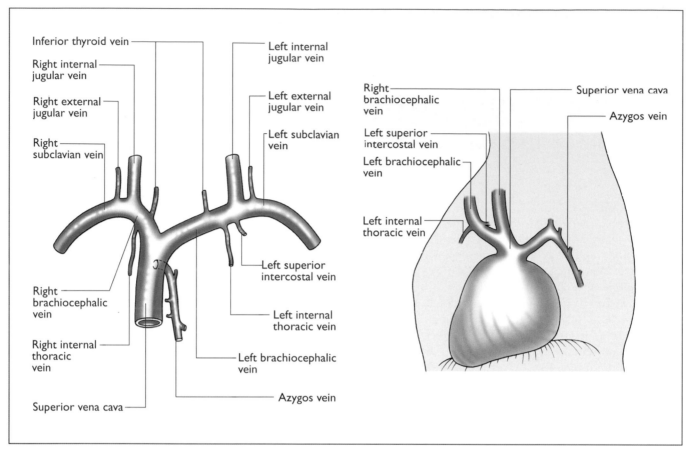

Figure 46.1. *Anatomy of the thoracic veins on the frontal and lateral radiographs.*

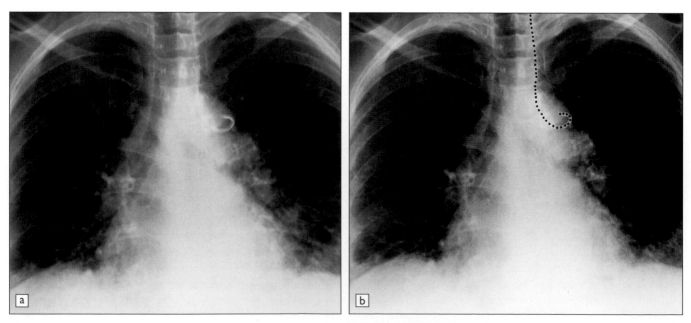

Figure 46.2. *Catheter in the left superior intercostal vein (a). Position of catheter is shown by dotted line (b).*

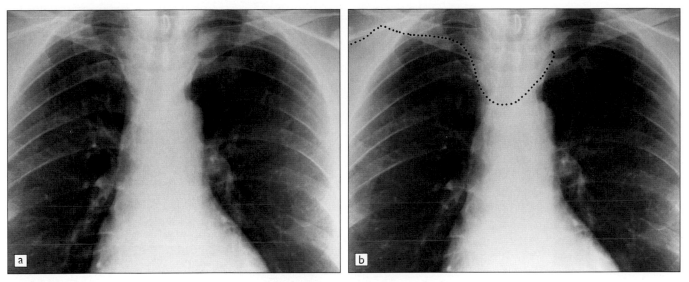

Figure 46.3. *Catheter in the left brachiocephalic vein (a). Position of catheter is shown by dotted line (b).*

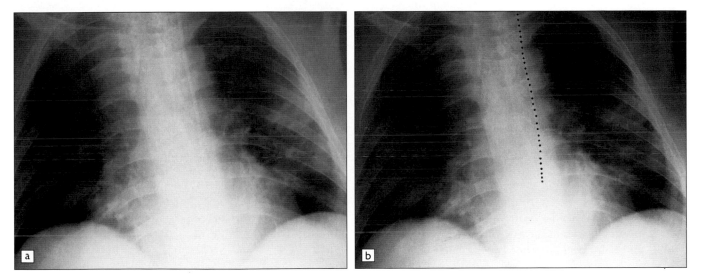

Figure 46.4. *Catheter in the persistent left superior vena cava (a). Position of catheter is shown by the dotted line (b).*

Key points: catheter insertion

■ The right subclavian vein is the favoured route of access because left-sided catheters more commonly erode the superior vena cava

■ Local trauma at the time of insertion include pneumothorax and rarely brachial plexopathy or phrenic nerve injury

■ Fragmentation of the catheter may occur at the time of insertion

Complications of the established catheter: catheter occlusion

Care of the indwelling catheter includes regular flushing with heparinized saline (unless the catheter has a two-way valve). It may be impossible either to aspirate blood or to infuse fluid if the catheter is occluded. Occlusion may be due to kinking of the catheter, malposition of the tip, fibrin sheaths, or mural thrombosis. An initial chest radiograph should be obtained following line placement, and follow-up films obtained in the event of malfunction to establish any change in position.

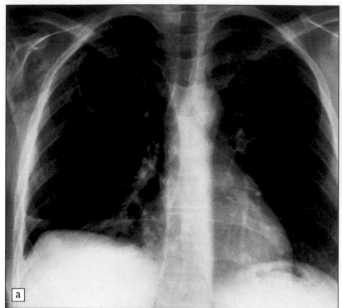

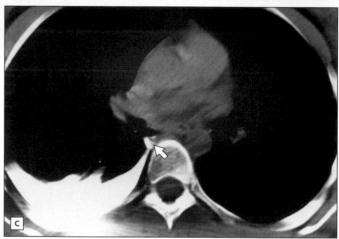

Figure 46.5. *Chest radiograph shows a Hickman line in an apparently satisfactory position (a). Position of catheter is shown by the dotted line (b). However, a hydropneumothorax and surgical emphysema suggest that the pleura has been breached. There is a subpulmonic effusion following administration of fluids through the catheter. (c) Following administration of contrast (for a staging CT investigation) contrast has entered the pleural space. The catheter position (arrow) is shown behind the right main stem bronchus, presumably within the pleural space.*

Catheter tip malposition

A catheter tip in the mid-SVC may slip into the azygos vein. It then appears looped in the SVC on the frontal chest radiograph, and is directed posteriorly on the lateral film. There may be an associated right pleural effusion (Fig. 46.6). The catheter should be removed or resited before further infusions. The catheter tip may be against the vessel wall in which case only minimal adjustment is required.

Fibrin sheaths

Fibrin sheaths form around the tip of up to 80% of indwelling catheters and this complication should be considered if the catheter may be flushed but not aspirated.[8] They are usually otherwise asymptomatic but may detach and cause pulmonary embolism when the catheter is removed.[9] Fibrin sheaths may be demonstrated by venography, or by a linogram (Fig. 46.7).

Occasionally, the line may be occluded by crystallization of the infusion fluid. Occlusion by calcium carbonite crystals, during infusion of 5-fluorouracil and leucovorin through a single lumen has been described.[10]

Mural thrombosis

The reported incidence of mural thrombosis varies widely.[11–13] It is related to the duration of catheter placement, sepsis, low cardiac output, and hypercoagulability associated with carcinoma.[14] It may be asymptomatic, and detected only on routine investigation (e.g. staging computed tomography) or it may result in catheter malfunction. Some patients experience arm and neck pain.

Thrombosis of the subclavian, axillary and jugular veins may be demonstrated on Doppler ultrasound scanning. Echogenic thrombus is seen partially or totally occluding the vessel which may be distended. There is a lack of flow demonstrated on colour Doppler scanning, and damping of the normal response to respiration is seen in veins distal to the thrombus. There may be an impaired augmentation of flow in more central veins during compression of the arm (Fig. 46.8). Doppler scanning cannot reliably exclude subclavian vein thrombosis, and is unsuitable for assessing the superior vena cava.[15]

Venography will demonstrate partial or complete venous obstruction in those patients in whom there is clinical doubt

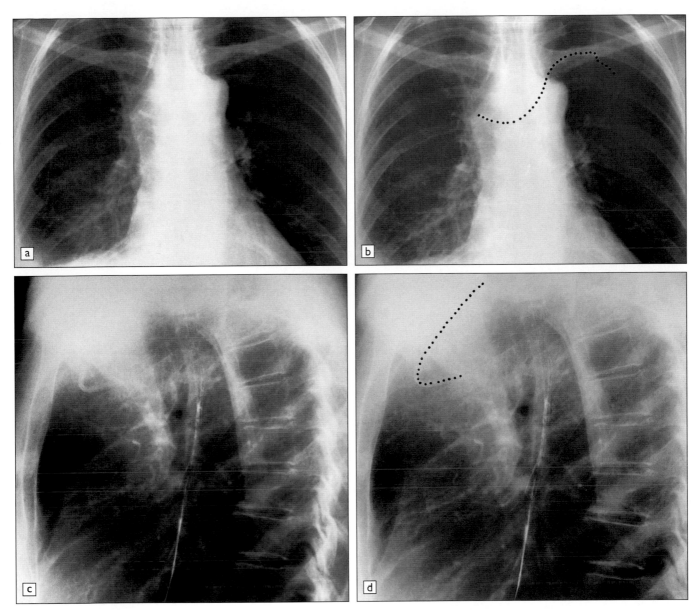

Figure 46.6. *This patient with known oesophageal carcinoma undergoing chemotherapy presented with chest pain and a right-sided pleural effusion clinically. The PA film (a) shows the pleural effusion and a Hickman line entering the left subclavian vein, with the tip in the azygos vein. The position of the catheter is shown by the dotted line (b). The lateral film (c) shows residual barium from a study performed to exclude oesophageal perforation. The tip of the Hickman line is directed posteriorly into the azygos vein. The position of the catheter is shown by the dotted line (d).*

following ultrasonography. It will also demonstrate the presence of collateral vessels and extrinsic compression of the vein. Bilateral simultaneous upper limb venography is necessary to demonstrate the central veins.

Occlusion of the superior vena cava (superior vena cava syndrome) is characterized by congestion and oedema of the upper extremities and head with engorged superficial veins. The plain film shows superior mediastinal widening and prominence of the left superior intercostal vein (aortic

nipple) and azygos arch.[7,16] Computed tomography with intravenous contrast medium demonstrates:

- The presence of occlusion
- The site of occlusion
- The extent of thrombus (Fig. 46.9)
- The presence of multiple collateral vessels
- Increased density of the mediastinal fat[17]

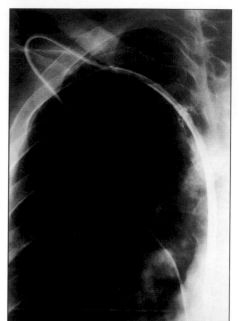

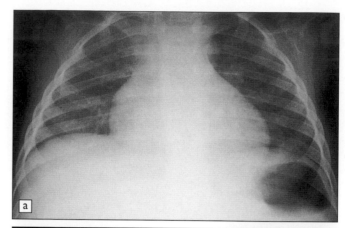

Figure 46.7. *Contrast injected through the catheter demonstrates a fibrin sheath around the intravascular component of the catheter.*

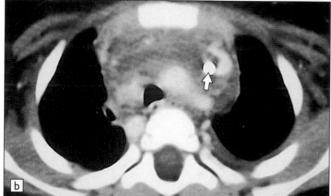

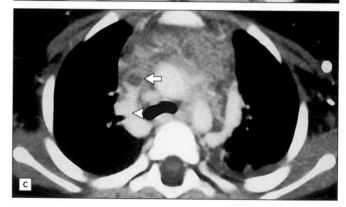

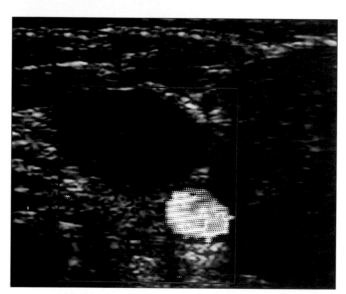

Figure 46.8. *Jugular vein thrombosis. Colour Doppler ultrasound demonstrates a distended jugular vein which is non-compressible. No flow is demonstrated, and sparse echos are returned from the intraluminal thrombus. Brisk flow is demonstrated in the adjacent carotid artery.*

Figure 46.9. *Chest radiograph (a) showing widened mediastinum in a 2-year-old child; (b) axial CT scan demonstrating the tip of the catheter (arrow) adjacent to a distended superior intercostal vein and no contrast in the left brachiocephalic vein; (c) axial CT scan showing the superior vena cava with central thrombus (arrow) and peripheral contrast enhancement via a distended azygos vein (arrowhead).*

Although some authors state that CT may not show small non-occlusive thrombi or the fine detail seen at veno-graphy[18] we have found that spiral (helical) CT is the most effective means of defining the extent and location of smaller thromboses, although Doppler ultrasound is recommended as the initial examination. Magnetic resonance imaging (MRI) using flow-sensitive sequences can assess patency of the larger thoracic veins,[19,20] but pitfalls include the misinterpretation of flow artefact, partial venous occlusion and the presence of metallic foreign bodies which degrade image quality.[20] Other disadvantages include the high cost of MRI and difficulties related to imaging critically ill patients.[21]

Pulmonary embolism as a consequence of central venous thrombosis associated with indwelling central venous catheters is probably under-reported.[22] A high level of suspicion is needed to identify this potentially lethal complication.[23]

Key points: catheter complications

- Occlusion of an established catheter may be due to malposition, fibrin sheaths or the development of thrombosis

- Fibrin sheaths develop in up to 80% of indwelling catheters and may detach producing pulmonary emboli

- Thrombosis of the subclavian, axillary and jugular veins may be demonstrated on Doppler ultrasonography

- Superior vena caval occlusion is best shown by venography or CT but may be suggested on plain radiographs by mediastinal widening

- Computed tomography demonstrates the presence, site and extent of occlusion, as well as presence of collaterals, and increased density in the mediastinal fat may also be observed.[17]

- Magnetic resonance imaging using flow sensitive sequences can assess patency of large intrathoracic vessels

- Catheter related sepsis occurs in 1% of patients

Complications of the established catheter: sepsis

Catheter related septicaemia is relatively uncommon; it occurs in approximately 1% of patients.[24] Infection may also occur at the exit site of an external catheter, or in the subcutaneous tunnel. It is more common in neutropenic patients, in patients less than 2 years old, and in patients with external catheters rather than implanted ports.[25]

Exit site infections in the absence of septicaemia require local wound care only. Tunnel or pocket infections with local cellulitis and pus formation are often only satisfactorily treated by removal of the catheter.[26]

Infection of the catheter does not always result in septicaemia, and a concurrent septicaemia is not necessarily related to catheter infection. Catheter infection may be diagnosed by culture of the catheter tip. This is considered positive when more than 15 colony-forming units are cultured.[27] Catheter related septicaemia may be diagnosed without removing the device when line cultures have a 10-fold increase in colony counts compared with peripheral blood samples obtained at the same time.[28]

Evidence of multifocal septic emboli on the chest radiograph may be the first indication of line infection. Areas of confluent air-space shadowing, often cavitating, suggest staphylococcal infection. Cross-sectional imaging may also show induration around the catheter, thickening of the vessel wall, intraluminal air and thrombosis.[4]

Drug reactions

Many drugs used in chemotherapy are toxic, and their dosage is limited by adverse effects. There are various mechanisms of pulmonary toxicity, which may be sporadic or dose related. The combination of chemotherapeutic agents with other therapy, for example bleomycin and cyclosporin or radiotherapy, may be synergistic. The vinca alkaloids (vincristine and vinblastine) do not cause pulmonary complications when used alone, but are associated with pulmonary oedema, occasionally progressing to fibrosis, when used in combination with mitomycin C.[25] Pulmonary fibrosis associated with cytotoxic drugs is usually irreversible and may be fatal; it is therefore important to recognize drug-related changes as early as possible.

The plain chest radiograph is the simplest method of identifying pulmonary disease in symptomatic and asymptomatic patients, but other imaging modalities, such as high resolution CT, may also be necessary for accurate assessment of the pulmonary changes. Drug related pulmonary change is most easily classified according to the radiological patterns of:[25,29]

Diffuse air-space shadowing
 Cytosine arabinoside
 Interleukin-2
 Vincristine
 Fluid loading prior to high dose melphalan
 Fluid loading during treatment for leukaemia

Diffuse interstitial disease
 Methotrexate
 Carmustine
 Bleomycin
 Busulphan
 Cyclophosphamide
 Procarbazine
 Mitomycin

Multiple pulmonary nodules
 Bleomycin
 Cyclosporin[25,29]

Diffuse air-space shadowing

In the context of chemotherapy-related pulmonary diseases, diffuse air-space shadowing is due to pulmonary oedema most commonly as a consequence of increased capillary permeability.

Pulmonary oedema caused by cytosine arabinoside (Ara-C) was presumed to be the cause of death of 28 out of 51 patients who had received Ara-C within 30 days of autopsy.[30] Symptoms of dyspnoea occur within the first month after the onset of treatment. The chest radiograph initially shows a diffuse (occasionally basal) interstitial and alveolar pattern. This resolves following withdrawal of the drug.

Interleukin-2 (IL-2) may cause a capillary-leak syndrome within the first week of treatment, which resolves after the drug is withdrawn. Radiographic signs of pulmonary oedema range from mild interstitial change to widespread confluent air-space shadowing.[31] A more aggressive, potentially fatal reaction causes symptoms of shock within 24 hours of administration of the drug.[29] Many chemotherapy regimens involve prehydration which may cause transient fluid overload and pulmonary oedema.

Diffuse interstitial opacities

Diffuse interstitial disease is the pattern most commonly associated with chemotherapy drug reactions. Bleomycin, carmustine (BCNU) and methotrexate are the drugs that most commonly cause interstitial lung disease. It usually results from severe alveolar wall damage which progresses to pulmonary fibrosis, but is occasionally due to a hypersensitivity reaction (e.g. methotrexate).[29] The main differential diagnoses are infection and progression of the under-lying disease (for example lymphangitis carcinomatosis).

Bleomycin: Pulmonary fibrosis secondary to bleomycin toxicity occurs in 2–3% of patients receiving bleomycin, and is fatal in approximately 1%.[32,33] Lung disease may be exacerbated by concomitant treatment with radiotherapy or oxygen.[17] Initially the effects are reversible if the drug is withdrawn, and patients should be monitored regularly with pulmonary function tests and chest radiographs.[33] The radiographic features of bleomycin toxicity include a diffuse bibasal infiltrate which may be linear or nodular, and which appears 6–12 weeks after treatment is commenced (Fig. 46.10).[34] Small pleural effusions may be present. High-resolution CT will identify these changes when the chest radiograph is apparently normal. In the early stages, pleurally based nodules are seen predominantly posteriorly at the lung bases. This progresses to coarse reticular shadowing extending towards the hila. In advanced disease, confluent irregular opacities are seen throughout the lung with relative sparing of the apices.[35] Recently we have observed pneumomediastinum in two patients with interstitial lung disease following bleomycin

therapy, a previously unreported phenomenon in the absence of pneumothorax (Fig. 46.10). Pneumothorax alone, however, has been reported as a complication of bleomycin toxicity[36].

Carmustine (BCNU): Pulmonary toxicity occurs in 20–30% of patients treated with BCNU. Combination of the drug with cyclophosphamide is synergistic and the effect is dose-related.[37] The risk is also increased by pre-existing lung disease and smoking.[38] The radiograph shows bibasal reticular infiltrates which occur relatively late in the disease. Pulmonary fibrosis, pleural effusion and pulmonary oedema are reported.[39] Spontaneous pneumothorax has also been described.[40]

Methotrexate: The incidence of pulmonary toxicity in patients receiving methotrexate is approximately 7%.[33] Symptoms occur within a few weeks of commencing therapy. The chest radiograph shows interstitial infiltrates and there may also be mediastinal and hilar lymphadenopathy and small pleural effusions. The pattern may be predominantly nodular, and rarely the chest radiograph is normal. Acute pleurisy has been described following methotrexate.[41] The radiographic changes usually regress after cessation of the drug, although the toxic changes can progress to irreversible pulmonary fibrosis.[42] The pneumonitis may regress despite continued administration of the drug.

Cyclophosphamide: Cyclophosphamide rarely causes pulmonary toxicity when used alone, but toxicity occurs more frequently when the drug is used in combination with other drugs and radiotherapy; its true incidence is therefore difficult to determine. The onset of symptoms may develop within only a few weeks of commencing the drug, or may be delayed for many years and in one report an interval of 13 years before the onset of toxicity has been reported.[37] The chest radiograph usually shows bibasal interstitial shadowing, although pulmonary oedema has been described.

Busulphan: The onset of busulphan related lung disease may be insidious occurring from 8 months to 10 years following administration of the drug. The chest radiograph shows a bibasal reticular pattern, rarely with pleural effusions. Ossific nodules may develop.[25]

Mitomycin: The incidence of pulmonary toxicity is approximately 10%[43] and is increased when mitomycin is used in combination with other agents. The chest radiograph shows bilateral reticular shadowing and occasionally fine nodules. A form of haemolytic uraemic syndrome with non-cardiogenic pulmonary oedema has been reported in association with mitomycin therapy.[44]

Procarbazine: This is a rare hypersensitivity reaction occurring within hours of administration of the drug. Radiographic findings include interstitial opacities, pleural effusion and alveolar infiltrates.

Other drugs: Other chemotherapy agents causing interstitial shadowing include *chlorambucil*, *melphalan*, *azathioprine* and *6-mercaptopurine*.

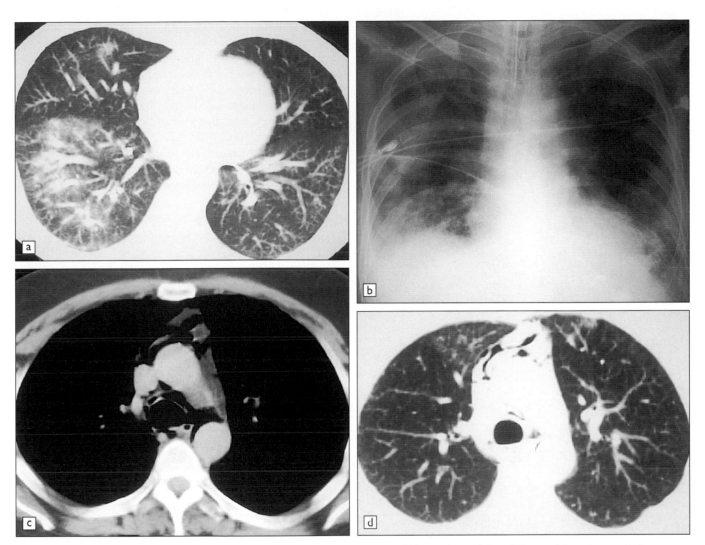

Figure 46.10. *High resolution axial CT scan (a) of the lungs in early bleomycin toxicity showing a peripheral, bibasal interstitial infiltrate extending towards the hila. (b) Chest radiograph showing extensive pulmonary fibrosis in the late stages of bleomycin toxicity. CT scan (c) on lung window settings showing bleomycin toxicity. A more cranial section (d) in the same patient demonstrating a pneumomediastinum.*

Pulmonary nodules

Bleomycin: Rarely bleomycin toxicity may cause multiple discrete nodules simulating metastases.[45]

Cyclosporin toxicity may also produce an abnormal nodular pulmonary pattern on plain chest radiography.

Opportunistic infections of the lung

Patients with haematological malignancies such as lymphoma and leukaemia, patients who have had bone marrow transplantation and those receiving chemotherapy for malignancy are all frequently severely immunocompromised. The lung is a prime site for potentially lethal infection. The recognized community-acquired infections are less often seen in this group of patients, and opportunistic infective agents should be actively sought in symptomatic patients. The plain chest radiograph is often the first investigation of a pyrexia, and may identify infection in asymptomatic patients. The infections are most easily classified by the radiographic pattern, although there may be some overlap in appearances. The differential diagnosis of infection on an abnormal radiograph includes:

- Progression of the underlying disease
- Drug reaction
- Radiation changes
- Non-specific interstitial pneumonitis

Plain chest film patterns of opportunistic infection are detailed below:[47]

Lobar consolidation:
Bacterial
    Gram-negative organisms
    Gram-positive organisms
    Legionella pneumophila
Mycobacterial disease

Multiple nodules: +/– consolidation
Bacterial
    Septic infarcts (Staphylococcus aureus)
    Nocardia
    Legionella micdedii
Fungal
    Cryptococcus
    Aspergillus
    Mucor
    Candida

Diffuse lung disease:
    Pneumocystis carinii
    Cytomegalovirus
    Herpes virus

Key points: drug-related pulmonary toxicity

- Radiological patterns of drug-related pulmonary toxicity are diffuse air-space shadowing, diffuse interstitial disease and multiple pulmonary nodules

- Diffuse air-space shadowing is most commonly caused by pulmonary oedema due to increased capillary permeability

- Diffuse interstitial infiltration results from severe alveolar damage which progresses to pulmonary fibrosis

- Bleomycin is the classic example of a drug causing pulmonary fibrosis

- Pulmonary nodules may be seen as a result of bleomycin and cyclosporine toxicity

Lobar or segmental consolidation

Bacterial pneumonia: The infecting organisms are often Gram-negative bacteria (Klebsiella, Enterobacter, Pseudomonas, Escherichia coli, Proteus and Serratia).[45] Gram-positive organisms include staphylococci. Radiological changes are similar to those in the non-immunocompromised patient with focal or patchy consolidation which may be lobar or segmental. Cavitation may occur, for example in staphylococcal

and Klebsiella infections. There may be small pleural effusions but empyema is rare.

Tuberculous mycobacterial infection is relatively uncommon compared with bacterial infection and usually represents reactivation of disease.[47] The radiograph shows apical disease with or without cavitation[47] (Fig. 46.11).

Non-tuberculous infection with atypical mycobacteria such as Mycobacterium avium-intracellulare complex, M. kansasii and M. chelonae[48] should also be considered. Radiographic signs suggesting atypical mycobacteria include an increased extent of cavitation with thinner walls and less dense surrounding con-

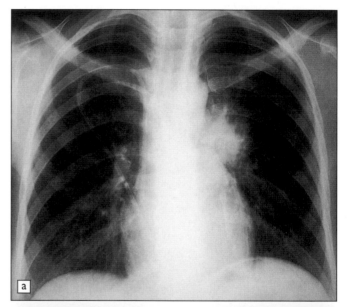

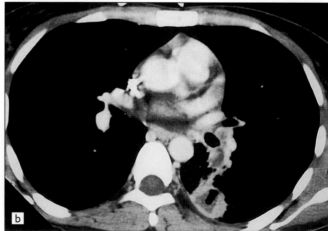

Figure 46.11. *Intercurrent infection with Mycobacterium tuberculosis in a patient on chemotherapy for acute lymphoblastic leukaemia. Chest radiograph shows a left hilar mass (a). CT scan demonstrates a cavitating lesion in the apical segment of the left lower lobe which was associated with left hilar and subcarinal lymphadenopathy (b).*

solidation than seen in tuberculous infection, anterior/apical segment disease rather than apico/posterior disease and marked pleural reaction over the involved lung.[49] An association between disseminated non-tuberculous mycobacterial infection and hairy cell leukaemia has been described.[50]

Pulmonary nodules

Bacterial infections

Multiple, rapidly developing pulmonary nodules, with or without cavitation are frequently seen in immuno-suppressed patients. The infecting organisms are usually fungal, although Nocardia can also give this appearance. Tuberculosis, Staphylococcus aureus infection and toxoplasmosis should also be considered in the differential diagnosis. Septic embolization related to long-term catheters may produce multiple nodules with cavitation.

Fungal infections

Aspergillosis: Invasive aspergillosis causes a severe necrotizing pneumonia. The chest radiograph shows multiple areas of consolidation which are usually peripheral and may contain an 'air-crescent' sign. Computed tomo-graphy- scanning shows single or multiple masses which have a blurred edge due to peripheral infarction (Fig. 46.12).[46] These features are also seen in patients with mucormycosis.[51]

Candida: Candida causes a non-specific picture of nodules, or a focal area of consolidation.

Cryptococcus: Cryptococcus causes single or multiple nodules, with or without cavitation, and occasionally well-defined lobar/segmental consolidation.[51]

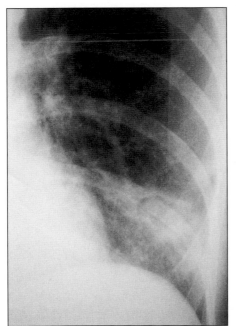

Figure 46.12. *Chest radiograph showing invasive aspergillosis in the left lower lobe. The cavitating nodule has a hazy edge and demonstrates the 'air-crescent' sign.*

Key points: pulmonary infections

- ■ The lung is the prime site for potentially lethal infection in immunocompromised patients

- ■ Lobar or segmental consolidation is frequently seen in bacterial infection as well as tuberculous and non-tuberculous microbacterial infections

- ■ Pulmonary nodules are frequently seen in fungal infection, particularly aspergillosis

- ■ Diffuse infective lung disease is often non-specific and may be seen in Pneumocystis carinii, cytomegalovirus pneumonia and other viral infections such as herpes simplex

Other infections

Nocardia: Nocardia is an opportunistic, higher transitional bacterium causing nodules, with or without cavitation, which may extend to the pleural surface, causing effusions and chest wall invasion.

Diffuse infective lung disease

Pneumocystis carinii

In most patients the initial radiographic appearance of Pneumocystis carinii pneumonia (PCP) is of diffuse, bilateral, symmetrical perihilar infiltrates that may represent interstitial or air-space shadowing.[52] In patients receiving prophylactic pentamidine aerosol treatment, the distribution may be predominantly in the upper lobes. Pleural effusions and lymphadenopathy are rare. Atypical patterns occur in 5% of cases and include:

- Lobar consolidation
- Multiple nodules
- Miliary patterns
- Endobronchial lesions
- Pleural effusions[53]

Pneumocystis carinii pneumonia may spare the irradiation port in irradiated lung.[54] Rarely the cystic changes, that are well described in AIDS patients, are seen in patients immuno-compromised for other reasons. The cystic lesions tend to be subpleural and predominantly of upper-lobe distribution.[55]

Computed tomography is useful in the symptomatic patient with an apparently normal chest radiograph. The CT findings cover a spectrum of abnormalities, from diffuse to patchy ground glass shadowing and there may be thickening of the interlobular septa. Interstitial fibrosis and cystic lesions are also well demonstrated.[52]

Cytomegalovirus pneumonia is difficult to distinguish radiologically from other infective agents and gives a wide variety of radiographic appearances. The appearances on plain film include consolidation, linear interstitial infiltrate and ground glass shadowing. This is predominantly in the lower zone, and usually bilateral (Fig. 46.13). Small nodules have also been described, and there may be associated pleural effusions, pneumothorax and pneumomediastinum.[56] Other viral pneumonias in the immunocompromised patient include herpes simplex virus, respiratory syncytial virus and measles. The radiographic appearances are non-specific.

Other causes of pulmonary disease in the immunocompromised patient

Non-specific interstitial pneumonitis
Occasionally even following lung biopsy it is impossible to isolate an organism in some immunocompromised patients with an interstitial pneumonia. Histology is most likely to show non-specific interstitial pneumonitis.[57] The chest radiograph usually shows an interstitial pattern, but occasionally an alveolar or mixed alveolar/interstitial pattern is seen. Rarely the plain chest radiograph is normal.[56]

Pulmonary haemorrhage
Pulmonary haemorrhage occurs most commonly in patients with leukaemia. Diffuse, patchy air-space shadowing that tends to be perihilar and basal in location and of rapid onset is seen in the acute phase. Computed tomography shows ground-glass opacification and sometimes frank consolidation.[58] If pulmonary haemorrhage is recurrent, then chest radiography in the later stages may also show interstitial changes and CT demonstrates a fine reticulonodular pattern.

Graft versus host disease
The pathological findings of pulmonary graft versus host disease are non-specific. Other disease entities such as cryptogenic organizing pneumonia and non-specific interstitial pneumonitis may coexist. The radiograph shows interstitial changes which may progress to fibrosis.[59]

Effects of treatment on the heart
The effects of anthracyclines on the myocardium have been discussed in Chapter 48. Cyclophosphamide may cause an acute haemorrhagic pancarditis when the dose exceeds 100 mg/kg per week. This results in pericardial effusion, mural thickening, and endocardial, myocardial and epicardial haemorrhage. Echocardiography demonstrates abnormal diastolic function, small pericardial effusions and occasionally a restrictive cardiomyopathy.[25]

ACUTE COMPLICATIONS OF TREATMENT: THE ABDOMEN AND PELVIS

Complications of treatment in the abdomen and pelvis relate to surgery, drug therapy and infection in the immunocompromised patient. Postoperative abdominal complications have been described in Chapter 50. Other entities include graft versus host disease following bone marrow transplantation, typhlitis and pneumatosis intestinalis.

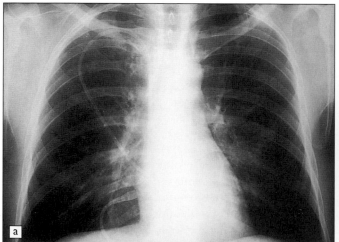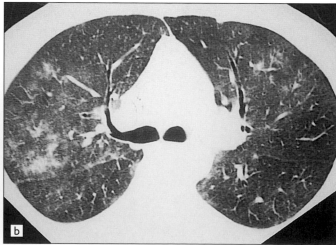

Figure 46.13. *Interstitial pneumonitis caused by cytomegalovirus infection: (a) Chest radiograph shows a subtle perihilar infiltrate; (b) high-resolution CT demonstrates soft tissue opacities and ground-glass opacification.*

Drug-related complications
Gastro-intestinal system

Although patients may have gastro-intestinal symptoms, there are few specific drug-related, radiologically-identifiable complications of treatment in the bowel. Complications are due to disordered motility, malabsorption and ischaemia.

Fluorouracil is the drug which causes gut toxicity most commonly; the clinical picture may mimic inflammatory bowel disease with diarrhoea that may be bloody; radiologically, colitic changes of bowel wall thickening and mucosal ulceration are seen. Ischaemic colitis has been described with cisplatin and fluorouracil.[60] Vincristine causes a neuropathy which may result in a chronic ileus, with dilated, air-filled small bowel loops on the plain film.[61] Cytosine arabinoside may cause gut ulcer-ation, pneumatosis intestinalis and gastro-intestinal haemorrhage.

Liver

Although many chemotherapeutic agents are hepatotoxic, few cause radiographic abnormality. Fatty infiltration, with increased echogenicity on ultrasonography and decreased attenuation on CT may be due to methotrexate and corticosteroids and occasionally occurs with a variety of combination chemotherapy regimens.[62] Several drugs cause hepatic veno-occlusive disease resulting in a clinical Budd–Chiari syndrome characterized by hepatomegaly and ascites. These include:

- Azathioprine
- Dacarbazine
- Thioguanine
- Adriamycin
- Vincristine
- Mitomycin
- Combination of cyclosporin and cyclophosphamide[62]

Ultrasound and CT findings show hepatomegaly and there may be a mosaic pattern of heterogeneous attenuation of the liver on both pre- and postcontrast CT.

Pancreas

Acute pancreatitis may occur secondary to high-dose steroid therapy. It has also been described in patients receiving chemotherapy notably L-asparaginase.[63] This is usually diagnosed on clinical and biochemical features, but contrast-enhanced CT may be useful to assess the extent of the condition, demonstrating a swollen oedematous pancreas, areas of necrosis, fluid collections and oedema of the adjacent fat.

Urinary tract

Patients may present with acute renal failure due to nephrotoxic chemotherapy agents but urinary tract obstruction must be excluded. Drugs causing nephrotoxicity[25] include:

- Azacitidine
- Cisplatin
- Diaziquone
- Gallium nitrate
- Ifosfamide
- Interleukin-2
- Methotrexate
- Mitomycin
- Pentostatin
- Plicamycin
- Streptozocin

Ultrasonography may demonstrate increased corticomedullary differentiation in parenchymal disease, or dilatation of the collecting system in the obstructed kidney. Cytotoxic agents may cause non-opaque renal calculi and treatment of myeloproliferative disorders can result in a uric acid nephropathy. Haemorrhagic cystitis during treatment with cyclophosphamide is described in Chapter 50.

Infectious complications of chemotherapy
Candida albicans

Disseminated candidiasis may be seen in the severely immunocompromised patient. This has few specific radiological features, although candidal infection of the gastrointestinal tract may cause mucosal erosion and ulceration. Hepatic abscesses due to Candida are rarely seen and may not be visible on imaging but larger lesions cause a typical bull's eye appearance.[64]

Cytomegalovirus

Abdominal radiographs in patients with known cytomegalovirus infection reveal bowel wall thickening, dilated bowel and fluid levels. Pneumatosis intestinalis may also occur, although this may be related to treatment such as whole body irradiation.[56] Cytomegalovirus may be difficult to distinguish from graft versus host disease in patients following bone marrow transplant.

Pseudomembranous colitis

Pseudomembranous colitis is associated with antibiotic use and is due to infection with Clostridium difficile. Plain films show thumb printing and segmental ileus. Barium enema is also non-specific with mucosal thickening, and plaque-like lesions. Computed tomography shows bowel wall thickening which may spare the rectum, with marked thickening of the haustral folds.[65]

Other abdominopelvic complications of treatment
Graft versus host disease

Graft versus host disease (GVHD) is described in patients following bone marrow transplantation (BMT). Acute graft versus host disease occurs within the first 100 days after transplant, causing a skin rash, severe mucosal inflammation and diarrhoea. Chronic graft versus host disease may occur within 45–50 days of transplantation. The skin rash resembles scleroderma, and the major gastro-intestinal organ affected is the oesophagus. Severe mucosal inflammation is followed by fibrosis and stricture formation. Similar changes occur less frequently in the small bowel.[66]

Abnormal features on the plain abdominal radiograph are non-specific and include air-fluid levels, bowel wall and mucosal fold thickening, a gasless abdomen, dilatation of bowel loops and ascites.[67] Barium studies confirm the mucosal thickening and flattening, causing 'ribbon bowel', rapid transit time, and in severe cases prolonged coating of the bowel wall.[68] Abnormalities on CT include:

- Bowel wall thickening
- Luminal narrowing
- Prolonged mucosal coating
- A halo of decreased attenuation within the thickened wall
- Increased density of the mesenteric fat[69]

A report of graft versus host disease in children showed that there was striking enhancement of the bowel wall, but mucosal thickening was patchy, and limited to the small bowel.[70]

In summary, the radiology of graft versus host disease is non-specific; the plain film characteristics are insufficient to differentiate between patients with and without acute graft versus host disease. In addition it may be difficult to discriminate radiologically between graft versus host disease and cytomegalovirus.

Typhlitis

Typhlitis (neutropenic colitis) is an inflammatory process causing transmural thickening of the bowel wall around the caecum and terminal ileum. It occurs in patients with leukaemia complicated by severe neutropenia and in patients with lymphoma, aplastic anaemia and AIDS.[66] It presents with right iliac fossa pain and if untreated may progress rapidly to transmural necrosis. The CT findings include:

- Diffuse wall thickening
- Pericolic fluid

The increased frequency of pneumatosis intestinalis may help to discriminate typhlitis from the important differential diagnosis of pseudomembranous colitis.[71]

Pneumatosis intestinalis

Pneumatosis intestinalis occurs following bone marrow transplantation and may be of no clinical significance, but may indicate sinister pathology such as graft versus host disease, cytomegalovirus or other infections and typhlitis.[66] It is predominately right-sided and should be considered a poor prognostic indicator in the context of systemic infection or shock (Fig. 46.14).[72]

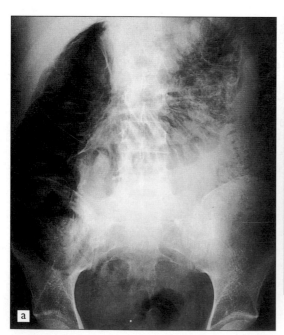
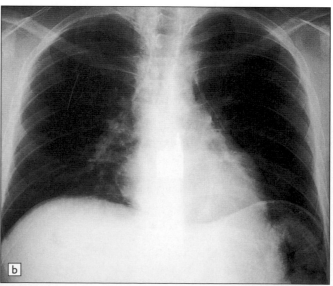

Figure 46.14. *(a) Abdominal film showing pneumatosis coli and (b) with pneumomediastinum on the chest radiograph.*

Other complications of treatment

Other abdominal complications seen in the oncology patient include faecal impaction which is seen in patients treated with opiates and other drugs which cause disordered gut motility. Faecal loading may be seen on the abdominal radiograph. This rarely causes further complications. Bowel wall haemorrhage and perforation may also occur.

Abdominal pain may also be caused by soft tissue abscesses in neutropenic patients. Infecting organisms include Staphylococcus aureus and Gram-negative bacteria.

Key points: gastro-intestinal complications

- Gastro-intestinal complications of chemotherapy include disordered motility, malabsorption and ischaemia

- Radiological signs are usually non-specific

- The liver may show fatty infiltration

- Acute pancreatitis has been described with L-asparaginase therapy and high dose steroids

- Urinary tract complications of drug treatment include acute renal failure, renal calculi and haemorrhagic, cystitis

- Immunocompromised patients are susceptible to gut infection with Candida, cytomegalovirus and Clostridium difficile (pseudomembranous colitis)

- GVHD produces non-specific but well recognized features on abdominal plain films, barium studies and CT

- Typhlitis is an inflammatory transmural process causing thickening of the bowel wall around the caecum and terminal ileum. It is seen in immunocompromised patients

ACUTE COMPLICATIONS OF TREATMENT: THE CENTRAL NERVOUS SYSTEM

Drug-related complications

A variety of drugs may be neurotoxic but the majority of these do not cause changes that can be identified radiologically (Table 46.1).

The most sensitive imaging modality is MRI,[73] which is used to identify white matter change in the brain that is not evident on CT. The white matter effect of chemotherapy is

Table 46.1. *Drugs causing neurotoxicity*

Drug	Toxicity
Vincristine	Peripheral neuropathy
Cisplatin	Peripheral neuropathy
Cytarabine	Cerebellar dysfunction
Ifosfamide	Personality change, cerebellar dysfunction, cranial nerve lesions
5-fluorouracil	Cerebellar dysfunction
Methotrexate	Focal neurological defects

often potentiated by radiotherapy.[74] Drugs which are known to cause leucoencephalopathy include methotrexate, 5-fluorouracil, cytarabine and cyclosporin A.[75] The probable mechanism of chemotherapeutic toxicity is vascular injury, causing endothelial thickening, with eventual infarction and necrosis.[75]

Intravenous methotrexate may cause white matter change that is of low density on CT and enhances with intravenous contrast media.[76] Magnetic resonance imaging also demonstrates transient, multifocal white matter lesions, within the first few days of initiating treatment. The patient may be asymptomatic.[77] A more aggressive focal or diffuse necrotizing leucoencephalopathy with associated demyelination and necrosis is described as a later complication occurring after weeks or months of treatment. This is more common with combinations of intravenous and intrathecal methotrexate and radiotherapy but may reverse if intrathecal infusion of methotrexate is discontinued.[78] Magnetic resonance imaging reveals patchy involvement of the periventricular white matter and centrum semiovale, which becomes confluent. The deep white matter tracts, brainstem and cerebellum are spared. Enhancement and mass effect are only seen in the most severe cases. Children treated with chemotherapy and radiotherapy for leukaemia may develop widespread perivascular calcification (mineralizing angiopathy).[74,79]

Treatment of colonic cancer with 5-fluorouracil and levamisole may cause acute demyelination with multifocal enhancing white matter lesions on MRI.[80] It may preferentially affect the cerebellum causing ataxia.

Patients with thrombocytopenia as a consequence of treatment may develop intracranial haemorrhage which may be epidural, subdural, subarachnoid or intracerebral.

Infectious complications

Neutropenic patients are predisposed to many infections of the central nervous system (CNS) including fungal infections, particularly aspergillosis and Cryptococcus. Infection of the meninges and brain may result from direct spread of aggressive infection in the paranasal sinuses. Computed tomography may show large soft tissue masses involving the sinuses with bone destruction and extension of disease into the underlying structures such as the orbit, meninges and brain parenchyma. Viral encephalitis is often due to cytomegalovirus. Other infections to consider are Listeria monocytogenes meningitis and tuberculous meningitis.[81] Bacterial meningitis with Haemophilus influenzae and S. pneumoniae may occur in splenectomized patients.[82] Reactivation of papovavirus is implicated in progressive multifocal leucoencephalopathy.

Aspergillosis

Central nervous system aspergillosis is invariably associated with pulmonary involvement. It invades the vessels, causing cerebral infarction and aneurysm formation. The mortality approaches 90%.[82] Computed tomography and MRI may demonstrate enhancing or non-enhancing low-attenuation masses within the brain in addition to the cerebral infarcts.

Cryptococcus neoformans

Hyperintense lesions are seen on T2-weighted images in the basal ganglia and midbrain, which enhance to a varying extent following intravenous gadolinium. (Gd-DTPA) Meningeal infection is difficult to detect on CT or MRI.[77]

Cytomegalovirus encephalitis

This usually represents reactivation of latent virus. Computed tomography and MRI show a thick, nodular periventricular rim, and subependymal enhancement is sometimes seen.

Herpes simplex encephalitis

This is less common than CMV and classical signs of temporal lobe encephalitis and perivascular inflammatory[77] change may not be seen on CT in the early stages of the disease.[75] Magnetic resonance imaging is the most sensitive investigation and reveals asymmetrical bilateral abnormal signal intensity in the temporal lobes.

Listeria meningitis

Computed tomography is often normal. Magnetic resonance imaging shows obliteration of the cisterns and the meninges may enhance strongly with intravenous contrast medium, gadolinium-DTPA. There may be some ventricular dilatation.[75]

Key points: CNS complications

- Magnetic resonance imaging is the most sensitive imaging modality to identify the neurotoxic effects of cancer treatment

- Intravenous methotrexate may produce acute white matter change as well as aggressive focal or diffuse necrotising leucoencephalopathy

- Necrotizing leucoencephalopathy is usually seen in combination therapy with intravenous or intrathrecal methotrexate and radiotherapy for the treatment of leukaemia

- Acute demyelination may be seen following treatment with other drugs such as 5-fluorouracil

- Immunocompromised patients are susceptible to CNS infection producing meningitis and encephalitis

- Progressive multifocal leucoencephalopathy is most commonly associated with AIDS and is associated with papovavirus infection

Tuberculosis

This most commonly causes hydrocephalus and meningeal enhancement. Parenchymal involvement occurs less frequently.[75]

Progressive multifocal leucoencephalopathy

Progressive multifocal leucoencephalopathy has been described in patients treated with immunosuppressive agents, although recently it has been more commonly associated with AIDS. It is a demyelinating disease that results from reactivation of latent papovavirus. Magnetic resonance imaging shows asymmetric, patchy, nonenhancing lesions of the peripheral white matter which progress to large confluent lesions involving the deep white matter. The brain stem and cerebellum are affected in approximately one-third of patients. Haemorrhage and peripheral enhancement occur rarely.[77]

Summary

■ Intravenous catheter related complications include malposition, occlusion and sepsis.

■ Pneumothorax is the most common complication of malpositioning of an indwelling catheter.

■ Computed tomography is currently the method of choice for demonstrating superior vena caval thrombosis.

■ Doppler ultrasonography may show thrombus within the subclavian, internal jugular and axillary veins.

■ Catheter-related sepsis occurs in 1% of patients.

■ Pulmonary fibrosis is the most common manifestation of lung toxicity due to chemotherapy and is seen most frequently with bleomycin.

■ Opportunistic infection of the lungs in immunocompromised patients is an important potentially fatal condition.

■ Abdominal complications of drug treatment include gut toxicity, fatty infiltration of the liver, pancreatitis, acute renal failure, renal calculi and haemorrhagic cystitis.

■ GVHD following BMT affects the oesophagus and small bowel. The typical findings of thickened bowel loops and luminal narrowing are non-specific on plain films, barium studies and CT.

■ Typhlitis represents an inflammatory process involving the caecum and is seen in immunocompromised patients.

■ Pneumatosis intestinalis is seen in GVHD, cytomegalovirus infection and typhlitis.

■ A variety of drugs are neurotoxic but the majority do not produce changes visible on imaging.

■ Magnetic resonance imaging is the most sensitive technique for identifying white matter abnormalities in the brain related to treatment.

■ The white matter effects of chemotherapy are often potentiated by radiotherapy, e.g. intravenous methotrexate and radiotherapy for treatment of acute leukaemia.

■ Diffuse necrotizing leucoencephalopathy is associated with methotrexate therapy and radiotherapy. This is a later effect of treatment and is usually irreversible.

■ Central nervous system infection is an important complication of treatment in immunocompromised patients.

■ Reactivation of papovavirus is implicated in the development of progressive multifocal leucoencephalopathy. This is particularly common in AIDS.

REFERENCES

1. Denny D F Jr. Placement and management of long-term central venous access catheters and ports. Am J Roentgenol 1993; 161: 385–393
2. Aronchick J M, Miller W T Jr. Tubes and lines in the intensive care setting. Semin Roentgenol 1997; XXXII(2): 102–116
3. Tocino I M and Watanabe A. Impending catheter perforation of superior vena cava: Radiographic recognition. Am J Roentgenol 1986; 160: 467–471
4. Wechsler R J, Steiner R M, Kinori I. Monitoring the monitors: The radiology of thoracic catheters, wires and tubes. Semin Roentgenol 1988; 23: 61–84
5. Duntley P, Siever J, Korwes M L et al. Vascular erosion by central venous catheters: Clinical features and outcome. Chest 1992; 101: 1633–1638
6. Magney J E, Flynn D M, Parsons J A et al. Anatomical mechanisms explaining damage to pacemaker leads, defibrillator leads, and failure of central venous

catheters adjacent to the sternoclavicular joint. Pacing Clin Electrophysiol 1993; 16: 445–457

7. Krutchen A E, Bjarnason H, Stackhouse D J et al. The mechanisms of positional dysfunction of subclavian venous catheters. Radiology 1996; 200: 159–163

8. Ahmed N and Payne R F. Thrombosis after central venous catheterisation. Med J Aust 1976; 1: 217–220

9. Brismar B, Hardstadt C, Jacobson S. Diagnosis of thrombosis by catheter phlebography after prolonged central venous catheterisation. Ann Surg 1981; 194: 779–783

10. Ardalan B, Flores M R. A new complication of chemotherapy administered by a permanent indwelling catheter. Cancer 1995; 75: 2165–2168

11. Moss J F, Wagman L D, Rihimaki D U et al. Central venous thrombosis related to the silastic Hickman–Broviac catheters in an oncological population. J Parenteral Enteral Nutr 1989; 13: 397–400

12. Gray W J and Bell W R. Fibrinolytic agents in the treatment of thrombotic disorders. Semin Oncol 1990; 17: 228–237

13. Ladefoged A, Efsen F, Cristofferson J K, Jarnum S. Long-term parenteral nutrition: ii. Catheter-related complications. Scand J Gastroenterol 1981; 16: 913–919

14. Hill S L and Berry R E. Subclavian vein thrombosis: A continuing challenge. Surgery 1993; 104: 561–567

15. Needlemen L, Nack T L, Feld R et al. Upper extremity venous disease: Sonographic–venographic comparison (Abstract). Radiology 1981; 181(P): 125–126

16. Carter M M, Tarr R W, Mazer M J, and Carroll F E. The 'aortic nipple' as a sign of impending superior vena caval syndrome. Chest 1985; 87: 775–777

17. Brown G, Husband J E. Mediastinal widening — a valuable radiographic sign of superior vena cava thrombosis. Clin Radiol 1993; 47: 415–420

18. Wechsler R J, Spirn P W, Conant E F et al. Thrombosis and infection caused by thoracic venous catheters: Pathogenesis and imaging findings. Am J Roentgenol 1993; 160: 467–471

19. Weinreb J C, Mootz A, Cohen J M. MRI evaluation of mediastinal and thoracic inlet venous obstruction. Am J Roentgenol 1986; 146: 679–684

20. Hansen M E, Spritzer C E, Sostmann H D. Assessing the patency of mediastinal and thoracic inlet veins: Value of MR imaging. Am J Roentgenol 1990; 155: 1177–1182

21. Haire W D, Lynch T G, Lunt G V et al. Limitation of magnetic resonance imaging and ultrasound-directed (duplex) scanning in the diagnosis of subclavian vein thrombosis. J Vasc Surg 1991; 13: 391–397

22. Horattas M C, Wright D J, Fenton A J et al. Changing concepts of deep venous thrombosis of upper extremity: Report of a series and review of the literature. Surgery 1988; 104: 561–567

23. Derish M T, Smith D W, Frankel L R. Venous catheter thrombus formation and pulmonary embolism in children. Paediatr Pulmonol 1995; 20(6): 347–348

24. Hampton A A and Sherertz R J. Vascular access infection in hospitalized patients. Surg Clin North Am 1988; 68: 57–71

25. Stoker D E. Pulmonary toxicity. In: Devita V T, Hellmann S, Rosenberg S A (eds). Cancer: Principles and Practice of Oncology (4th ed). Philadelphia: J B Lippincott, 1993

26. Press O W, Ramsey P G, Larson E B et al. Hickman catheter infections in patients with malignancies. Medicine (Baltimore) 1984; 63: 189–200

27. Maki D G, Weise C E, Saraffin H W. A semiquantitative culture method for identifying intravenous catheter-related infection. N Engl J Med 1977; 296: 1305–1309

28. Weightman N C, Simpson E N, Speller D C E et al. Bacteremia related to indwelling central venous catheters: Prevention, diagnosis and treatment. Eur J Clin Microbiol Infect Dis 1988; 7: 125–129

29. Aronchick J M and Gefter W B. Drug-induced pulmonary disorders. Semin Roentgenol 1995; XXX(1): 18–34

30. Haupt H M, Hutchins G M, Moore G W. Ara-C lung: Noncardiogenic pulmonary edema complicating cytosine arabinoside therapy of leukemia. Am J Med 1981; 70: 256–261

31. Conant E F, Fox K R, Miller W T. Pulmonary edema as a complication of interleukin-2 therapy. Am J Roentgenol 1989; 152: 749–752

32. Comis R L. Bleomycin: Current status and new developments. In: Carter S K, Umezawa H, Crooke S T (eds) Bleomycin Pulmonary Toxicity. New York: Academic Press, 1978

33. Mills P and Husband J E. Computed tomography of pulmonary bleomycin toxicity. Semin Ultrasound CT MR 1990; 11(5): 417–422

34. Horowitz A L, Freidman M, Smith J et al. The pulmonary changes of bleomycin toxicity. Radiology 1973; 106: 65–68

35. Bellamy E A, Husband J E, Blaquiere R M et al. Bleomycin-related lung damage: CT evidence. Radiology 1985; 156: 155–158

36. Doll D C. Fatal pneumothorax associated with bleomycin-induced pulmonary fibrosis. Cancer Chemother Pharmacol 1986; 17: 294–295

37. Twohig K J, Matthay R A. Pulmonary effects of cytotoxic agents other than bleomycin. Clin Chest Med 1990; 11: 32–54

38. Kreisman H, Wolkove N. Pulmonary toxicity of antineoplastic therapy. Semin Oncol 1992; 19: 508–512

39. Rubio C, Hill M E, O'Brien M E R, Cunningham D. Idiopathic pneumonia syndrome after high-dose chemotherapy for relapsed Hodgkin's disease. Br J Cancer 1997; 75(7): 1044–1048

40. Holoye P, Jenkins D E, Greenberg S D. Pulmonary toxicity in long-term administration of BCNU. Can Treat Rep 1976; 60: 1691–1694

41. Walden P A M, Mitchell-Heggs P F, Coppin C et al. Pleurisy and methotrexate treatment. Br Med J 1977; 2: 867

42. Sostman H D, Matthay R A, Putman C E. Methotrexate-induced pneumonitis. Medicine 1976; 55: 371–388

43. Verweij J, van Zanten T, Souren T et al. Prospective study on the dose relationship of mitomycin-C induced interstitial pneumonitis. Cancer 1987; 60: 756–761

44. Kris M G, Pablo D, Gralla R J et al. Dyspnea following vinblastine or vindesine administration in patients receiving mitomycin plus vinca alkaloid combination therapy. Cancer Treat Rep 1984; 68: 1029–1031

45. Glasier C M and Siegel M J. Multiple pulmonary nodules: An unusual manifestation of bleomycin toxicity. Am J Roentgenol 1981; 137: 155–156

46. Hruban R H, Mercieve M A, Zerhouni E A et al. Radiologic–pathologic correlation of the CT halo sign in invasive aspergillosis. J Comput Assist Tomogr 1987; 11: 534

47. Davis S D, Yankelevitz D F, Williams T, Henschke C I. Pulmonary tuberculosis in immunocompromised hosts: Epidemiological, clinical and radiological assessment. Semin Roentgenol 1993; XXVIII(2): 119–130

48. Wallace R J, Svenson J M, Silcox V A et al. Spectrum of disease due to rapidly growing mycobacteria. Rev Infect Dis 1983; 5: 657–679

49. McLoud T C. Pulmonary infections in the immunocompromised host. Radiol Clin North Am 1989; 27: 1059–1066

50. Bennett C, Vardiman J, Golomb H. Disseminated, atypical mycobacterial infection in patients with hairy cell leukaemia. Am J Med 1986; 80: 891–896

51. McLoud T C, Naidich D P. Thoracic disease in the immunocompromised patient. Radiol Clin North Am 1992; 30: 525–554

52. Kuhlman J E. Pneumocystis infections: The radiologist's perspective. Radiology 1996; 198: 623–635

53. Kennedy C A and Goetz M B. Atypical roentgenographic manifestations of Pneumocystis carinii pneumonia. Arch Inter Med 1992; 152: 1390–1398

54. Panicek D M, Groskin S A, Cheung C T, Heitzman E R, Sagerman R H. Atypical distribution of Pneumocystis carinii infiltrates during radiation therapy. Radiology 1987; 163: 689–690

55. Ferre C, Baguena F, Podzamczer D et al. Lung cavitation associated with Pneumocystis carinii in the acquired immune deficiency syndrome: A report of six cases and review of the literature. Eur Resp J 1994; 7: 134–139

56. Olliff J F C and Williams M P. Radiological appearances of cytomegalovirus infections. Clin Radiol 1989; 40: 463–467

57. Park J S, Lee K S, Kim J S et al. Nonspecific interstitial pneumonia with fibrosis: Radiographic and C T findings in seven patients. Radiology 1995; 195: 645–648

58. Cheah F K, Sheppard M N, Hansell D M. Computed tomography of diffuse pulmonary haemorrhage with pathological correlation. Clin Radiol 1993; 48: 89–93

59. Winer-Muram H T, Gurney J W, Bozeman P M, Krance R A. Pulmonary complications after bone marrow transplantation. Radiol Clin North Am 1996; 34: 97–117

60. Zilling T L and Ahren B. Ischaemic pancolitis. A serious complication of chemotherapy in a previously irradiated patient. Acta Chirurgica Scand 1989; 155: 77–79

61. Mannies P, Derriks R, Moens R et al. Multidisciplinary curative treatment for disseminated carcinoma of the breast. Cancer Treat Rep 1976; 60: 85–89

62. Gatenby R A. The radiology of drug-induced disorders in the gastrointestinal tract. Sem Roentgenol 1995; XXX: 62–76

63. Puckett J B, Butler W M, McFarland J L. Pancreatitis and cancer chemotherapy (letter). Ann Intern Med 1982; 97: 453

64. Haron E, Feld R, Tuffnell P et al. Hepatic candidiasis: an increasing problem in immunocompromised patients. Am J Med 1987; 83: 17–26

65. Fishman E K, Kavuru M, Jones B et al. Pseudo-membranous colitis: CT evaluation of 26 cases. Radiology 1991; 180: 57–60

66. Jones B and Wall S D. Gastrointestinal disease in the immunocompromised host. Radiologic Clin North Am 1992; 30: 555–577

67. Jones B, Cramer S S, Saral R et al. Gastrointestinal inflammation after bone marrow transplantation: Graft-versus-host disease or opportunistic infection? Am J Roentgenol 1988; 150: 277–281

68. Belli A M and Williams M P. Graft versus host disease: findings on plain abdominal radiography. Clin Radiol 1988; 39: 262–264

69. Jones B, Fishman E K, Cramer S S et al. Computed tomography of gastrointestinal inflammation after bone marrow transplantation. Am J Roentgenol 1986; 146: 691–695

70. Donnelly L F and Morris C L. Acute graft-versus-host disease in children: Abdominal CT findings. Radiology 1996; 199: 265–268

71. Merine D, Fishman E K, and Jones B. Pseudo-membranous colitis: CT evaluation. J Comput Assist Tomogr 1987; 11: 1017–1020

72. Day D L, Ramsey N K C, Letourneau J G. Pneumatosis intestinalis after bone marrow transplantation. Am J Roentgenol 1988; 151: 85–87

73. Packer R J, Zimmerman R A, Bilaniuc L T. Magnetic resonance imaging in the evaluation of treatment-related central nervous system damage. Cancer 1988; 61: 928–930

74. Paakko E, Vainionpaa L, Lanning M et al. White matter changes in children treated for acute lymphoblastic leukaemia. Cancer 1992; 70: 2728–2733

75. Osborn A G. Diagnostic neuroradiology. St Louis, Missouri: Mosby, 1994.

76. Pagani J J, Libshitz H I, Wallace S et al. Central nervous system leukaemia and lymphoma: Computed tomographic manifestations. Am J Roentgenol 1981; 137: 1195–1201

77. Hesselink J R. White matter disease. In: Edelman R R, Hesselink J R, Zlatkin M B (eds). Clinical Magnetic Resonance Imaging. (2nd edition). Philadelphia W B Saunders Co., 1996

78. Asato R, Akiyama Y, Ito M et al. Nuclear magnetic resonance abnormalities of the cerebral white matter in children with acute lymphoblastic leukaemia and malignant lymphoma during and after central nervous system prophylactic treatment with intrathecal methotrexate. Cancer 1992; 70: 1997–2004

79. Ebner F, Ranner G, Slavc I et al. MR findings in methotrexate-induced CNS abnormalities. Am J Neuroradiol 1989; 10: 959–964

80. Hook C C, Kimmel D W, Kvols L K et al. Multifocal inflammatory leukoencephalopathy with 5-fluorouracil and levamisole. Ann Neurol 1992; 31: 262–267

81. Patchell R A, White C, Clark A W et al. Neurologic complications of bone marrow transplantation. Neurology 1985; 35: 300–306

82. Davenport C, Dillon W P, Sze G. Neuroradiology of the immunosuppressed state. Radiol Clin North Am 1992; 30: 611–637

Chapter 47

Second malignancies

James Malpas

INTRODUCTION

There can be few more devastating events in the management of a patient with cancer than the discovery that the patient has a second malignancy. The finding of recurrence of primary cancer, or relapse (in leukaemia) has always been a recognized event, but it is only relatively recently, largely because of improved long-term survival, that the appearance of cancers apparently totally unrelated to the primary tumour has been seen.

Although reports of second malignant neoplasms (SMN) first appeared in the paediatric oncology literature, it was not until the late 1970s that the possibility that this might become a significant problem emerged. Li et al.[1] studied long-term survivors at the Sidney Farber Cancer Institute in Boston, and showed that in 425 children surviving cancer for 5 years, five developed SMN. An update from the Late Effects Study Group (LESG)[2] had found 292 SMN by 1985, and noted that the most common primary tumours were retinoblastoma, followed by Hodgkin's disease, soft tissue sarcoma and Wilms' tumour. Bone sarcomas and acute leukaemia were the most common SMN. Sarcomas occurred most commonly within the radiation field, while acute leukaemia was the commonest SMN not associated with radiation. It was also possible for these children to have more than one SMN — three cases were afflicted by four separate and different primary cancers. Numerous studies in the late 1980s recorded similar findings in Britain,[3] Nordic countries[4] and the USA.[5]

Britain and the Nordic countries, because of their sophisticated data retrieval, have been able to produce large population-based studies to supplement data from the LESG.[5] The percentages of children developing SMN after 25 years were 3.7, 3.5 and 12.1 respectively, which corresponds to a risk of 6, 4 and 15 times the risk in the normal population.[6]

Second malignant neoplasms are therefore a significant problem and will need to be prevented if optimal long-term survival is to be achieved. Great progress has been made in identifying the agents responsible, but a difficulty is that treatment modalities are changing, not only with regard to the drugs used, but to their dose intensity. There is also a change in the use of radiotherapy in paediatric oncology, a marked decline being noted recently.[7] Methods of prevention will, in a sense, be aiming at a moving target.

INCIDENCE

Death may occur in children treated with cancer for a variety of reasons — it may be due to recurrence of the original tumour, complications of the treatment programme used in the initial therapy, accidents (possibly related to the original treatment) which may result in long-term disability. The proportion will vary depending on the era in which the child was treated, and will also reflect the original diagnosis. Robertson et al.[8] put the importance of SMN into perspective in their study of 9080 5-year survivors of childhood cancer diagnosed between 1971 and 1985, and an earlier cohort diagnosed between 1940 and 1970. Causes of 793 deaths in 9080 subjects who survived 5 years after the diagnosis of neoplasm in 1971–85 are given as numbers and percentages in Table 47.1. This shows that 578 (75%) of deaths were due to recurrence of the primary tumour, while 52 (7%) were due to SMN. The commonest primary tumours to develop SMN were the lymphomas, soft tissue sarcomas and retinoblastoma (although the number of the latter is small). When the authors examined the influence of the era in which the children were treated, it was found that there was a small, but definite, increase in the risk of dying from a treatment-related cause in the more recent era, and they thought this could be attributed to intensification of therapy.

The differing risks of developing SMN after all types of childhood cancer are shown in the large population-based studies and treatment-centre data already referred to, and illustrated in Table 47.2.

The main conclusions were that bone cancer occurred with the highest frequency as an SMN, being three to four times as common as connective tissue cancers or thyroid carcinoma. These studies have helped to focus on the major risks, and are of great value in deciding priorities in follow-up clinics.

Table 47.1. *Causes of 793 deaths among 9080 subjects who had survived at least 5 years after diagnosis of childhood neoplasm in 1971–85. Values are numbers (percentages)* of deaths*

	Childhood neoplasm diagnosed											
Cause of death	Acute lymphoblastic leukaemia (n=2701)	Acute non-lymphoblastic leukaemia (n=138)	Hodgkin's disease (n=726)	Non-Hodgkin's lymphoma (n=450)	Tumour of central nervous system (n=908)	Neuro-blastoma (n=306)	Retino-blastoma (n=426)	Wilms' tumour (n=758)	Malignant bone (n=304)	Soft tissue sarcoma (n=543)	Other neoplasms (n=820)	All neo-plasms (n=9080)
Recurrent tumour	275 (78)	6 (67)	30 (61)	5 (31)	155 (78)	11 (61)	5 (63)	10 (50)	23 (79)	28 (76)	30 (71)	578 (74)
Medical condition related to treatment	62 (18)	3 (33)	9 (18)	5 (31)	23 (12)	4 (22)		5 (25)	4 (14)	1 (3)	5 (12)	121 (15)
Second primary tumour	13 (4)		7 (14)	6 (38)	9 (5)	2 (11)	2 (25)	1 (5)	2 (7)	5 (14)	5 (12)	52 (7)
Accident or homicide			2 (4)		5 (3)			2 (10)		1 (3)		10 (1)
Other medical cause (unrelated to tumour or its treatment)	3 (1)		1 (2)		8 (4)	1 (6)	1 (13)	2 (10)		2 (5)	2 (5)	20 (3)
Insufficient information	4				7	1						12
Total deaths	357	9	49	16	207	19	8	20	29	37	42	793

* Based on the 781 deaths with sufficient information to code the cause of death. (From ref. 8. with permission.)

Table 47.2. *Comparison of risks of second cancers after all types of childhood cancer from large population-based and treatment-centre based studies*

	Population-based studies								Treatment centre-based studies			
	British registry				Nordic registries				Late effects Study Group			
Type of second cancer	O	E	O/E	95% CI	O	E	O/E	95% CI	O	E	O/E	95% CI
All types	76	13.1	6	(5, 7)	247	69.0	4	(3, 4)	167	11.4	15	(13, 17)
Digestive	9	0.9	10	(5, 20)	20	5.9	3	(2, 5)	12	0.3	38	(20, 67)
Bone	28	0.7	43	(29, 63)	12	1.6	8	(4, 13)	48	0.4	133	(98, 176)
Connective tissue	6	0.4	15	(6, 33)	17	1.2	14	(8, 22)	20	0.4	41	(24, 67)
Breast	3	1.1	3	(0.6, 8)	21	8.7	2	(1.5, 4)	5	0.3	12	(3, 31)
CNS	12	1.7	7	(4, 12)	56	8.4	7	(5, 9)	14	0.9	15	(8, 26)
Thyroid	3	0.2	14	(3, 41)	16	2.2	7	(4, 12)	23	0.4	53	(34, 80)
Leukaemia	6	1.9	3	(1.2, 7)	15	5.3	3	(1.6, 5)	22	1.5	14	(9, 22)

O = Observed; E = Expected; O/E = ratio of observed to expected. (From ref. 6. with permission.)

Key points: second malignancies

■ The commonest primary tumours to develop second malignant neoplasms are lymphomas, soft tissue sarcomas and retinoblastomas

■ Bone cancer is the most commonly occurring second malignant neoplasm

TIME OF ONSET OF SECOND MALIGNANCY

The time at which SMN and leukaemia occur is also of practical importance. Taylor and Potish,[9] reviewing the survival of 341 children treated between 1953 and 1975 and surviving 5 years from diagnosis, noted that the survival of these patients did not parallel that of the general population, even after many years following completion of therapy. Deaths from SMN were occurring as late as 22 years after therapy. Recently, it has been shown that the timing of the occurrence of SMN and secondary leukaemia differs. On average there is a 5-year interval between therapy and the onset of secondary leukaemia, whether the primary tumour is haematological or solid in type (Table 47.3).[10] It should be noted, however, that whereas the maximum incidence of leukaemia occurs at 5 years, this is not the case for solid tumours, whose incidence continues to increase with time.

It is noticeable that after the peak incidence is reached in secondary leukaemia, there is a progressive decrease. This is in contrast with solid tumours, where there is a progressive rise. Van Leeuwen et al.[11] showed that in patients with Hodgkin's disease treated with radiotherapy or chemotherapy, the relative risk of acute leukaemia fell after more than 10 years, whilst the risk of non-Hodgkin lymphoma and lung cancer continually increased (Table 47.4).

TYPE OF SECONDARY MALIGNANCY

The type of SMN varies with the primary tumour. This is probably partly due to an inherent tendency (as yet poorly understood) to develop malignancy. An example is retinoblastoma, which is associated with osteosarcoma, which may arise as an SMN at a site which has not been irradiated. The major determining factor must be the treatment used. For example, radiotherapy in patients with Hodgkin's disease, where the radiotherapy fields have included the thyroid gland or the breast, results in a higher incidence of thyroid or breast cancer.[12] There may be other factors which affect susceptibility. Of particular interest is the fact that when patients have had splenectomy as part of their staging procedure for Hodgkin's disease, there is an increased sus-

ceptibility to breast cancer, for example. In general, radiotherapy is associated with a significant increase in bone tumours, while chemotherapy, and in particular the use of alkylating agents and epipodophyllotoxins such as etoposide and tenoposide, is associated with secondary acute leukaemia. An illustration of the diversity of SMN associated with various primary tumours is given in Table 47.5.[11–20]

CAUSATION

The influence of genetic makeup, type of chemotherapy or extent of radiotherapy in the induction of SMN is complex, and the precise mechanisms at a molecular level are only just beginning to be understood. Nevertheless, enough information is now available to be of value in the clinic, and for those who are involved in the investigation and long-term care of survivors of cancer.

Table 47.3. *Mean time in months and range in a variety of haematological malignancies and solid tumours*

Disease (no. studied)	Mean time (months)	Range (months)
Multiple myeloma (151)	55	15–180
Waldenström's macroglobulinaemia (26)	54	8–168
Hodgkin's disease (457)	76	9–330
Non-Hodgkin's lymphoma (117)	71	7–252
Chronic lymphatic leukaemia (31)	57	24–89
Breast cancer (78)	60	6–312
Ovarian cancer (37)	64	22–372

(From ref. 10. with permission.)

Table 47.4. *Relative risk (observed/expected) numbers of second cancers by interval after start of therapy for Hodgkin's disease*

SMN	Interval (years)	RR (o/e)	95% CI
Leukaemia	<5	32(6/0.19)	11.7–69.5
	5–10	75.5(8/0.11)	32.5–149
	≥10	35.8(2/0.06)	4.3–129
Non-Hodgkin's lymphoma	<5	13.2(2/0.15)	1.6–6.6
	5–10	11.4(1/0.09)	0.29–63.3
	≥10	121(6/0.05)	44.9–266
Lung cancer	<5	1.9(3/1.54)	0.40–5.7
	5–10	6.7(6/0.90)	2.5–14.6
	≥10	11.3 (5/0.44)	3.7–26.3

(From ref. 11. with permission.)

Table 47.5. *Some primary tumours and associated SMNs*

Primary tumour	SMN	Ref.
Hodgkin's disease	Acute leukaemia	[11]
	Non-Hodgkin's lymphoma	[11]
	Breast cancer	[12]
	Lung cancer	[11], [13]
	Thyroid cancer	[14]
Acute lymphoblastic leukaemia	CNS tumours	[15]
	Acute myeloblastic leukaemia	[15], [16]
Wilms' tumour	Acute myeloblastic leukaemia	
	Non-Hodgkin's lymphoma	[17]
	Brain tumours	
	Sarcomas	
	Carcinoma	
Retinoblastoma	Osteosarcoma	
	Soft tissue sarcoma	[18]
	Brain tumour	
	Leukaemia	
	Melanoma	
Ovarian cancer	Leukaemia	[19]
Breast cancer	Leukaemia	[20]

Table 47.6. *Drugs that are carcinogenic in man*

Group I	Diethylstilboestrol
	Melphalan
	Mustine hydrochloride (nitrogen mustard)
Group II	Cyclophosphamide
	Chlorambucil

(Adapted from IARC[21], with permission.)

Key points: timing and type

■ The timing of the occurrence of SMN and leukaemia differs in that whereas the maximum incidence of leukaemia occurs at 5 years, the incidence of solid tumours continues to increase with time

■ The type of SMN varies with the primary tumour which relates mainly to the treatment used

Genetic factors

The role of a genetic abnormality has been investigated in retinoblastoma. This condition is known to be associated with a deletion in band q14 on chromosome 13. The role of this defect was studied in 822 children with retinoblastoma in Britain,[18] who were seen between 1962 and 1977. Three-hundred and eighty-four of these children had the genetic form of the disease. Thirty SMNs were identified, all except four occurring in the genetic disease group. There is a striking difference between the SMN occurring in the genetic and non-genetic types of the disease treated with radiotherapy. Only two tumours were found in 100 children with the non-genetic form treated by

this method. In contrast, 23 of 314 patients with the genetic form of the disease and who received radiotherapy, developed an SMN. This difference is of course due to the fact that in the genetic form of the disease there is already chromosomal damage, and therefore only one further event is needed to produce the damage which will induce a tumour to develop. This inherited genetic damage makes the child more susceptible, for example, to the adverse effects of radiotherapy. The numbers were too small to determine the effect of chemotherapy, which at that time was used infrequently in retinoblastoma.

Chemotherapy

In 1979 the International Agency for Research on Cancer (IARC)[21] published a list of chemical substances including drugs, placed in the order of certainty of their carcinogenic effect in man. An abbreviated list is shown in Table 47.6. Drugs in Group I were those in which there was strong evidence of an association between exposure and cancer. Group II included those which were probably carcinogenic, while Group III contained drugs of undecided/unlikely potential.

This list has now grown considerably, and the order has been rearranged. It would be agreed that Group I should now include the epipodophyllotoxins[22] and anthracyclines (particularly mitoxantrone).[20] Procarbazine should be added, and chlorambucil transferred to Group I.

Much of the evidence for the role of chemotherapy in SMN comes from studies in Hodgkin's disease. This malignancy has had a high response rate and long-term survival for several decades. It has largely been treated in specialist centres where careful data maintenance and follow-up are available. Arsenau et al.[23] were among the first to report an increase in non-lymphomatous tumours. Further reports[24-26] demonstrated that in Hodgkin's disease treated with chemotherapy the commonest SMN was acute myeloblastic leukaemia. Kaldor and colleagues[27] combined the data from 12 population-based cancer registries in Europe and Canada, and six large hospitals in Europe. In a case-controlled study of 163 cases of acute leukaemia following treatment, they were able to show a relative risk of acute leukaemia of 9 (95%

CI 4.1–20), compared to patients treated with radiotherapy alone. Because single-agent therapy is not advocated in Hodgkin's disease, most of the estimates of risk were for drug combinations. For nitrogen mustard and procarbazine, given together for fewer than six cycles, there was a relative risk for SMN of 4.7 (95% CI 2.2–10), whereas with more than six cycles of the same therapy, the relative risk was 14.0 (95% CI 5.1–37), showing a definite relationship between dose and risk. This was also convincingly shown in children in a study by Meadows et al.,[28] who related dose of alkylating agent to risk, as shown in Table 47.7.[28]

From the evidence now available, the most leukaemogenic agents are chlorambucil and melphalan, and least active in the alkylating group of drugs is probably cyclophosphamide. Antimetabolites such as methotrexate or mercaptopurine, and the vinca alkaloids, are relatively safe.

Radiotherapy

From the very earliest reports[1] there appears to have been a relationship between radiotherapy and the occurrence of solid tumours, particularly at the edge of the radiation field. The risks of radiotherapy have been put into perspective by Hawkins and colleagues' study[29] using a population-based National Registry of Childhood Tumours in Britain. They investigated the SMN in a cohort of 13 175 3-year survivors of cancer. Fifty-nine subjects developed bone cancer. When this was analysed, it was found that the majority of these tumours occurred in patients whose primary malignancy had been retinoblastoma, Ewing's sarcoma or other malignant bone tumours. For other primary malignancies the rate was relatively low at 0.9%. This is a reassuring finding for those engaged in long-term follow-up clinics. This study also showed that the relative risk of developing bone cancer was related linearly to the dose of radiotherapy, and they also noted this to be true in the case of alkylating agents.

In an extensive study, Rom et al.[30] analysed several studies of thyroid cancer in irradiated children, resulting from such disparate events as atomic bomb exposure, treatment for tinea capitis, the use of radiotherapy for enlarged tonsils, thymus irradiation, and therapy for cancer. The combined studies involved nearly 120 000 people, of whom 58 000 were exposed to a wide range of doses. A total of three million person-years of follow-up were available for study. Seven hundred thyroid cancers were identified. For childhood exposure, the relationship between thyroid cancer occurrence and dose was linear, with an excess relative risk per Gy of 7.7 (95% CI 2.1–28.7). The risk of developing thyroid cancer remained after 40 years from exposure. It was also found that risk decreased with increasing age from exposure, and there was little risk over the age of 20. Only a small excess was noted in females developing thyroid cancer, and this was attributed to the greater propensity for women to develop

Table 47.7. *Alkylating agent dose (AAD) and risk of leukaemia and non-Hodgkin's lymphoma*

AAD dose	Leukaemia and non-Hodgkin's lymphoma risk
1	0.02
2	0.02
4	0.03
6	0.06
8	1.00
10	1.00

thyroid neoplasms in the general population. They also concluded that the thyroid gland in children had one of the highest risk coefficients of any organ.

In practice, children and adolescents who have had radiotherapy as treatment for Hodgkin's disease should have regular surveillance of the thyroid gland, regular examination of the thyroid for nodularity and thyroid ultrasound to identify active lesions. These procedures will identify carcinoma at a stage where it is operable. The incidence, though small (0.8%) is not negligible, and with early detection this cancer is curable.[31]

Role of gender

The role of gender has been studied recently in relation to the occurrence of SMN in girls and boys after therapy. Although these data will need confirmation, Tarbek et al.[32] in a study of 191 children, noted 15 SMNs in the group, 6–20 years after treatment for Hodgkin's disease. Ten of these tumours occurred in 66 females, but only five occurred among 125 males, giving a risk of 57 times that seen in the general population for females, and only 18 times for males. This was significant at the $p = 0.013$ level. The excess risk in females is now thought probably to be due to a late excess of breast cancer.

Key points: causation

- The causes of SMN and leukaemia are multifactorial and are influenced by the genetic make-up, type of chemotherapy and the extent of radiotherapy

- Currently, the most leukaemogenic agents are chlorambucil and melphalan

- The risk of developing bone or thyroid cancer is related linearly to the dose of radiotherapy

MECHANISMS

The carcinogenic potential of both radiotherapy and chemotherapy has been the subject of intensive study. It has only relatively recently become possible to examine the results, for example, of chemotherapy at the molecular level. Pederssen-Bjergaard et al.[33] reported on chromosomal abnormalities in patients with acute myeloblastic leukaemia occurring as SMN. They found that abnormalities of chromosomes 5 and 7 were the most frequent. Many of these leukaemias developed after a long interval, and some had been preceded by myelodysplastic syndromes so that the relationship was complicated. A much closer association with drug administration was seen in those patients with abnormalities of chromosome 11 — the 11q23 abnormality.[34] It was found that 37 children and adults treated with epipodophyllotoxins had a predominance of monocytic and myelomonocytic leukaemia as SMN, and these showed a high proportion of the 11q23 abnormality. These effects of etoposide and tenoposide have also been demonstrated by Pui.[22] A striking feature was the schedule dependency of SMN production, with weekly or twice-weekly administration of the etoposide or tenoposide being associated with a high degree of risk, while other schedules of administration were safer. These findings are of the utmost value in planning future antileukaemic therapy.

PREVENTION

The increasing knowledge of the intrinsic mechanisms underlying the development of SMN, the role of dosage and schedule, and the sequence of the use of chemotherapy and radiotherapy will do much to reduce the occurrence of SMN in the future. With better understanding, potent drugs will not have to be eliminated from the armamentarium. Identification of particularly harmful drugs such as procarbazine and its replacement has already begun; reduction in the requirement for radiotherapy is now being investigated in childhood tumours. Assessment of the likely propensity of any individual to develop an SMN, the (as yet) ignorance of the role of immunity in their occurrence, and our knowledge of the interplay of the complex factors resulting in SMN, make it vitally important to continue the follow-up of patients, documenting their treatment very carefully and registering all relevant events.

As Aldous Huxley said, 'If hell is paved with good intentions, it is, among other reasons, because of the impossibility of calculating consequences'. We have to make sure we are able to calculate these consequences in the future.

Summary

- Second malignant neoplasms are a consequence of the long-term survival now being seen in children and some adults who have been treated for cancer.

- Radiation usually results in solid tumours within the radiation field, while chemotherapy is commonly associated with leukaemia.

- While a peak incidence of acute leukaemia is reached after about 4–5 years, and then declines, the incidence of solid tumours continues to rise over time.

- The cause is genetic damage induced either by radiotherapy or chemotherapy. The incidence is dose- and schedule-dependent.

- New treatments will have to take into account the possibility of producing late malignancies, and drugs which are heavily implicated, such as procarbazine and the epipodophyllotoxins, will need either to be removed from drug programmes or be given at a greatly reduced dose.

REFERENCES

1. Li F P, Myers M H, Heise H W, Jaffe N. The course of five-year survivors of cancer in childhood. J Pediatr 1978; 93: 185–187

2. Meadows A T, Baum E, Fossati-Bellani F et al. Second malignant neoplasms in children: An update from the Late Effects Study Group. J Clin Oncol 1985; 3: 532–538

3. Hawkins M M, Draper G J, Kingston J E. Incidence of second primary tumours among childhood cancer survivors. Br J Cancer 1987; 56: 339–347

4. Olsen J H, Garwicz S, Hertz H et al. Second malignant neoplasms after cancer in childhood or adolescence. Br Med J 1993; 307: 1030–1036

5. Tucker M A, Meadows A T, Boice J D, Hoover R W, Fraumeni J F. Cancer risk following treatment of childhood cancer. In: Boice J D, Fraumeni J F (eds) Radiation carcinogens: Epidemiology and biological significance. New York: Raven Press, 1984: 211–224

6. Hawkins M M, Stevens M C G. The long-term survivor. Br Med Bull 1996; 52: 900–925

7. Taylor R E. Cancer in children: Radiotherapeutic approaches. Br Med Bull 1996; 52: 875–888

8. Robertson C M, Hawkins M M, Kingston J E. Late deaths and survival after childhood cancer: Implications for cure. Br Med J 1994; 309: 162–166

9. Taylor D D, Potish R A. Late deaths following radiotherapy for pediatric tumours. Am J Clin Oncol 1985; 8: 472–476

10. Rosner F, Grünwald H W. Chemicals and leukaemia. In: Henderson E S, Lister T A (eds) Leukemia (Vth ed). Philadelphia: W B Saunders, 1990: 271–287

11. Van Leeuwen F E, Somers R, Taal B G et al. Increased risk of lung cancer, non-Hodgkin's lymphoma and leukaemia following Hodgkin's disease. J Clin Oncol 1989; 7: 1046–1058

12. Bhatia S, Robison L L, Oberlin O et al. Breast cancer and other second neoplasms after childhood Hodgkin's disease. N Engl J Med 1996; 334: 745–751

13. Coltman C A, Dixon D O. Second malignancies complicating Hodgkin's disease: A South West Oncology Group 10-year follow-up. Cancer Treatment Reports 1982; 66: 1023–1033

14. Bolvin J-F, Hutchison G B, Lyden M et al. Second primary cancers following treatment of Hodgkin's disease. J Nat Cancer Inst 1984; 72: 233–241

15. Neglia J P, Meadows A T, Robison L L et al. Second neoplasms after acute lymphoblastic leukaemia in children. N Engl J Med 1991; 325: 1330–1336

16. Pui C H, Behm F G, Raimondi S C et al. Secondary acute myeloid leukemia in children treated for acute lymphoid leukemia. N Engl J Med 1989; 321: 136–142

17. Breslow N E, Takashima J R, Whitton J A et al. Second malignant neoplasms following treatment for Wilms' tumor: A report from the National Wilms' Tumor Study Group. J Clin Oncol 1995; 13: 1851–1859

18. Draper G J, Sanders B M, Kingston J E. Second primary neoplasms in patients with retinoblastoma. Br J Cancer 1986; 53: 661–676

19. Kaldor J M, Day N E, Petersson F et al. Leukemia following chemotherapy for ovarian cancer. N Engl J Med 1990; 322: 1–6

20. Linassier C, Barin C, Bremond J-L et al. Secondary leukemia in breast cancer patients after exposure to an association of mitoxantrone, fluorouracil and cyclophosphamide and radiotherapy. Proc Am Soc Clin Oncol (abstract 1060) 1996; 15: 360

21. International Agency for Research on Cancer. Evaluation of the carcinogenic risk of chemicals to humans. IARC Monographs (Suppl. 1) Lyon, France: IARC 1979

22. Pui C H, Ribeiro R C, Hancock M L et al. Acute myeloid leukemia in children treated with epipodophyllotoxins for acute lymphoblastic leukemia. N Engl J Med 1991; 325: 1682–1687

23. Arsenau J C, Sponzo R W, Levin D L et al. Non-lymphomatous malignant tumours complicating Hodgkin's disease. N Engl J Med 1972; 287: 1119–1122

24. Glicksman A S, Pajak T F, Gottlieb A et al. Second malignant neoplasms in patients successfully treated for Hodgkin's disease: A Cancer and Leukaemia Group B study. Cancer Treatment Reports 1982; 66: 1035–1044

25. Koletsky A J, Bertino J R, Farber L R et al. Second neoplasms in patients with Hodgkin's disease following combined modality therapy: The Yale experience. J Clin Oncol 1986; 4: 311–317

26. Tucker M A, Coleman C N, Cox R S, Varghese A, Rosenberg S A. Risk of second cancers after treatment for Hodgkin's disease. N Engl J Med 1988; 318: 76–81

27. Kaldor J M, Day N E, Clarke A et al. Leukemia following Hodgkin's disease. N Engl J Med 1990; 311: 7–13

28. Meadows A T, Obringer A C, Marrero O et al. Second malignant neoplasms following childhood Hodgkin's disease: Treatment and splenectomy as risk factors. Med Pediatr Oncol 1989; 17: 477–483

29. Hawkins M M, Kinnear-Wilson M, Burton H S et al. Radiotherapy, alkylating agents and risk of bone cancer after childhood cancer. J Nat Cancer Inst 1996; 88: 270–278

30. Ron E, Lubin J H, Shore R E et al. Thyroid cancer after exposure to external radiation. A pooled analysis of seven studies. Radiat Res 1995; 141: 259–277

31. Constine L S, Donaldson S S, McDougall I R et al. Thyroid dysfunction after radiotherapy in children with Hodgkin's disease. Cancer 1989; 53: 878–883

32. Tarbek N J, Gelber R D, Weinstein H J, Mauch P. Sex differences in risk of second malignant tumours after Hodgkin's disease in childhood. Lancet 1993; 341: 1428–1432

33. Pederssen-Bjergaard J, Philip P, Larsen S O, Jensen G, Byrsting K. Chromosome aberrations and prognostic factors in therapy-related myelodysplasia and acute non-lymphocytic leukemia. Blood 1990; 76: 1083–92

34. Whitlock J A, Greer J P, Lukens J N. Epipodophyllotoxin-related leukemia. Identification of a new subset of secondary leukemia. Cancer 1991; 68: 600–604

Part VII

EFFECTS OF TREATMENT ON NORMAL TISSUE

Chapter 48

Thorax

Herman Libshitz, Revathy Iyer and Evelyne Loyer

INTRODUCTION

Radiotherapy and/or chemotherapy affects all tissues of the thorax. The evidence and the timing of these changes vary, however, from organ to organ. Radiation change is almost always seen in the lungs within weeks of completion of therapy. It is usually far less obvious in bone and takes years to be seen.

The details of the radiotherapy, including the volume and shape of the area treated, dose, time from completion of therapy, possible effects of other treatment including chemotherapy, and the variability of human response are all factors in the appearance of radiotherapy change. The changes secondary to chemotherapy are usually dose related. The radiotherapy changes described are for radiotherapy given with linear accelerators or Co-60 at 180–200 cGy per day with treatment given 5 days a week.

LUNG

Radiologists define radiation pneumonitis as evidence of acute radiotherapy changes in the lungs regardless of the clinical findings. Clinicians require that cough, fever and/or shortness of breath accompany the radiographic changes.[1] It has long been recognized that radiographic changes of radiation pneumonitis are not necessarily accompanied by symptoms.[2]

Radiation pneumonitis is usually evident 6–8 weeks following completion of 3500–4000 cGy. It is generally not apparent below 3000 cGy, variably seen between 3000 and 3500 cGy and almost always evident at doses over 4000 cGy. For each 1000 cGy over 4000 cGy, it presents a week earlier following completion of therapy.

Radiation pneumonitis is most extensive about 3–4 months following completion of radiotherapy. From this point, the changes gradually organize, contract and evolve into radiation fibrosis.

There are no pathognomonic histological findings of radiation pneumonitis.[3] The histological appearance of radiation pneumonitis is that of diffuse alveolar damage.[4] Similarly, the histological appearance of radiation fibrosis is that of organizing diffuse, alveolar disease or end-stage

fibrosis. This lack of histological specificity can result in difficulty in separating radiation effects from toxic effects of chemotherapeutic agents and/or infectious agents.

Key points: radiation pneumonitis

- Radiographic changes of radiation pneumonitis are not necessarily accompanied by symptoms

- Radiation pneumonitis is usually evident 6–8 weeks following completion of 3000–4000 cGY

- Radiation pneumonitis is most extensive about 3–4 months following completion of therapy

- On plain film, the fibrotic changes usually become stable 9–12 months following completion of therapy

Plain film findings

Radiation pneumonitis when extensive has sharp, well-defined areas of consolidation with borders that conform to the radiation portals, not anatomic boundaries.[5–7] Less extensive radiation pneumonitis may present as patchy consolidation in the irradiated fields (Fig. 48.1) or when early or minimal in extent, indistinctness of vessels. Familiarity with standard portals and the availability of prior radiographs facilitates identification of minimal changes. Reports of radiation change outside the radiation field are usually the result of oblique, rotational or misplaced fields.[8] A possible humoral cause is under investigation.[9]

Our experience indicates that radiation fibrosis or evidence of contraction secondary to fibrosis is seen in virtually all patients who received therapeutic doses of radiotherapy. Fibrosis usually presents as strand-like densities with volume loss.

When extensive, there is significant volume loss with bronchiectatic changes within it. While the fibrosis is usually obvious, it can be subtle (Fig. 48.2). The less obvious findings include minimal pleural thickening, slight elevation of one or both hila or the minor fissure, slight medial

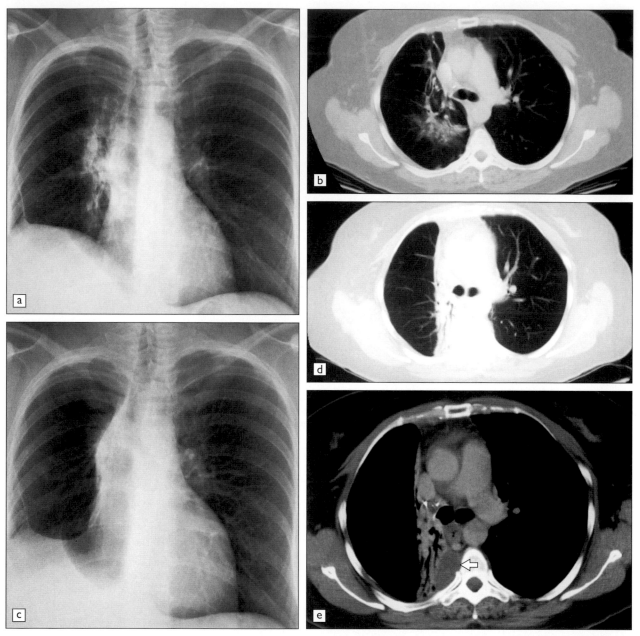

Figure 48.1. *Radiation pneumonitis and fibrosis. (a) Radiation pneumonitis is seen in the right lung 6 weeks following 6000 cGy. A right upper lobectomy had also been performed for bronchogenic carcinoma; (b) CT scan at the same time as (a) showing patchy consolidation in the right lung; (c) radiation fibrosis is present in the right lung 8 months following; (d) CT scan at the same time as (c) showing solid consolidation on lung windows. The sharp margin of the radiation changes is evident; (e) same CT scan as (d) on soft tissue windows showing the bronchiectatic changes to better advantage. A small loculated pleural effusion is present medially (arrow).*

retraction of upper lobe pulmonary vessels, minimal tenting or elevation of a hemidiaphragm, and minor blunting of cardiophrenic angles. The fibrotic changes usually become stable 9–12 months following completion of therapy (Fig. 48.1). Any alteration in stable radiation fibrosis suggests either superinfection or recurrent disease.

The combined effect of radiotherapy and chemotherapy on normal lung is difficult to evaluate. Combined therapy regimens are quite variable and chemotherapy has been given before, during and after radiotherapy. Empiric observation and small animal experimentation[10] has shown that the use of drugs that enhance radiation effect causes greater

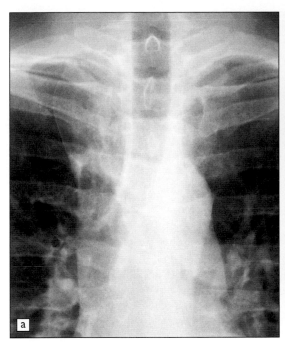
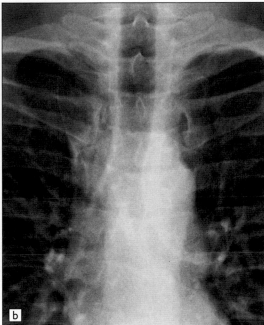

Figure 48.2. *Subtle changes of radiotherapy. (a) Baseline prior to radiotherapy for Hodgkin's disease; (b) 12 months following radiotherapy there is slight retraction of the azygous fissure medially and slight medial contracture of the upper lobe vessels bilaterally as well as minimal elevation of the left hilum.*

radiation damage and a shorter time to the onset of radiation pneumonitis. The radiation-enhancing drugs include:

- Actinomycin D
- Adriamycin
- Bleomycin
- Cyclophosphamide
- Mitomycin C
- Vincristine[10]

Disagreement exists regarding the effect of methotrexate.[10,11]

Bleomycin, busulphan, and methotrexate are recognized to cause pulmonary parenchymal injury independent of associated radiotherapy.[12] Bleomycin is used in the treatment of squamous cell carcinoma, lymphoma and testicular carcinoma. The toxicity is related to accumulation of drug in the lung and is directly related to the cumulative dose administered.[12] The use of concomitant radiation, other chemotherapy or oxygen therapy compounds the pulmonary toxicity. The early changes on chest radiography include a reticulonodular interstitial pattern which is initially seen in the basal segments. Lung injury may be progressive resulting in alveolar damage and eventual pulmonary fibrosis.[13] Gallium-67 is known to accumulate in damaged lung and is helpful in identifying bleomycin toxicity.[14] Busulphan which is used to treat leukaemia may also cause interstitial lung damage resulting in a reticular pattern on conventional radiographs.[13] Methotrexate is also used in the treatment of leukaemia and other malignancies. A hypersensitivity reaction may occur resulting in alveolar infiltrates. Mediastinal adeno-

pathy may also occur. The diffuse alveolar damage may result in fibrosis.[13]

Computed tomography and magnetic resonance imaging findings

Computed tomography (CT), with its greater sensitivity to minimal differences in radiographic density, can identify radiation pneumonitis earlier than conventional radiographs.[15,16] It is also presumed that it can demonstrate radiation pneumonitis at lower radiotherapeutic doses than conventional radiographs. A dose-related effect with greater changes at higher doses has been described with CT.[17]

There have been four patterns of radiation change described at CT:[15]

- Homogeneous consolidation
- Patchy consolidation
- Discrete consolidation
- Solid consolidation

Homogeneous consolidation is thought to be a diffuse, minimal or early radiation pneumonitis that uniformly involves the irradiated lung. The appearance is similar to that of ground-glass consolidation described in thin-section CT with vessels seen through the consolidation that uniformly affects the treated portions of the lungs. It may be seen within 2–3 weeks of completion of therapy. Patchy consolidation (Fig. 48.1) is thought to be the CT analogue of radiation pneumonitis on plain films. The consolidation is contained within the irradiated lung but does not involve the treated area uniformly. Discrete consolidation is defined by the irradiated field with well demarcated borders but does not involve it uniformly (Fig. 48.3). Traction changes may be seen at the boundary of the treated lung. It is felt to represent fibrotic changes in treated lung with areas of relative sparing. It is usually seen in the 3500–4000 cGy range as used in the therapy of Hodgkin's disease rather than in the higher doses used in treating lung cancer. Solid consolidation, which is generally seen at doses of 5000 cGy and higher, more uniformly involves the treated lung causing consolidation and volume loss (Fig. 48.1). Bronchiectatic changes are seen within the area of volume loss in this pattern. It is the CT analogue of a dense radiation fibrosis.

The oedema and inflammatory change of radiation pneumonitis are seen on magnetic resonance imaging (MRI) as increased signal on T2-weighted images and low signal intensity on T1-weighted images.[18] Radiation fibrosis would be expected to demonstrate low signal at both T1- and T2-weighted images. Unfortunately, increased signal on T2-weighted images[19] and contrast enhancement[20] may be seen in irradiated lung at a time when fibrosis would be expected. These observations have made MR evaluation of recurrent disease in irradiated patients problematic.

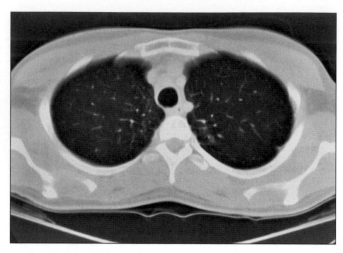

Figure 48.3. *Discrete consolidation is seen in the paramediastinal portions of both lungs 8 years following radiotherapy to the mediastinum for Hodgkin's disease (4000 cGy). The irradiated volume is well-defined with traction changes at the periphery of the field.*

Other imaging findings

Other less common complications include:

- Hyperlucency of an irradiated lung[21]
- Spontaneous pneumothorax[22]
- Pleural effusions secondary to radiotherapy[23]
- Calcification in lymph nodes[24]

Effusions are usually small and more frequently seen with CT (Fig. 48.4). They are indistinguishable from malignant pleural effusions. They usually develop within 6 months of therapy and may resolve spontaneously.[23] Rapid increase or re-accumulation after thoracentesis speaks for a malignant origin. If cytological examination is negative, prolonged follow-up may be necessary.

Calcification may occur in lymph nodes following therapy for lymphoma.[24] This is more frequent in Hodgkin's disease and far more common following radiotherapy than in patients treated only with chemotherapy. The calcification begins about a year after therapy and gradually gets denser over years. Cystic changes that may calcify have been described in the thymus in patients irradiated for Hodgkin's disease (Fig. 48.5).[25] Very rarely, malignant pleural mesotheliomas may develop after radiotherapy.[26]

Evaluation of treated areas

Identification of residual or recurrent malignancy in the thorax may be made more difficult by the superimposition of radiation changes in the areas of concern. In these cases, CT most often provides adequate visualiza-

tion of pulmonary parenchymal masses and/or the mediastinum following radiotherapy. In irradiated lymphoma, a residual mediastinal mass need not represent viable disease and in patients who have been appropriately treated, further therapy is not warranted.[27,28] Enlarging nodes or mass does speak for recurrence. By comparison, a residual mass in bronchogenic carcinoma generally represents residual disease.

Awareness of the timing of radiation change is most helpful in identifying recurrent disease. Routine follow-up studies at 2–3 month intervals following completion of radiotherapy aids in making these observations. Features that should suggest recurrent disease include:

- Alteration in stable contours of radiation fibrosis (Fig. 48.6)
- Failure of contracture of an area of radiation pneumonitis when expected 4 months or more after completion of therapy
- Absence of air-containing ectatic bronchi in an area of solid consolidation at CT, especially if ectatic bronchi were present previously[29]

Infection can usually be distinguished from radiation pneumonitis both by knowledge of the field size and shape, and the date of completion of therapy. However, it is virtually impossible to exclude superimposed infection in an area of radiation pneumonitis with imaging. Further bronchial ectasia or tissue destruction in a treated area suggests superinfection. Recurrent malignancy causing distal pneumonia may be confusing.

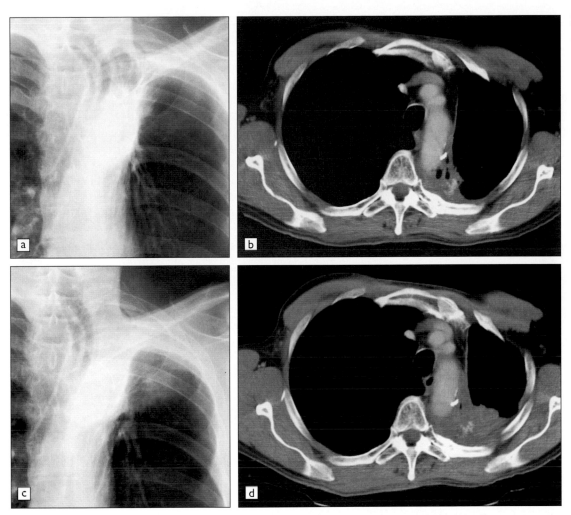

Figure 48.4. *Recurrent lung cancer following radiotherapy. (a) Close-up of left upper chest showing radiation change 9 months following radiotherapy; (b) CT scan at the same time as (a) showing solid consolidation; (c) mass is now seen 3 months following (a) in the left upper chest and the air-containing lung above the aortic knob has been obliterated; (d) CT scan at the same time as (c) showing mass and filling in of bronchiectatic changes.*

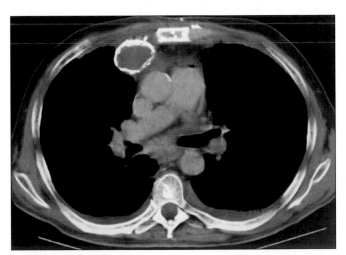

Figure 48.5. *Calcified thymic cyst 30 years following radiation therapy in a patient treated for Hodgkin's disease. The subcarinal adenopathy and small bilateral pleural effusions are related to a current non-small cell lung cancer.*

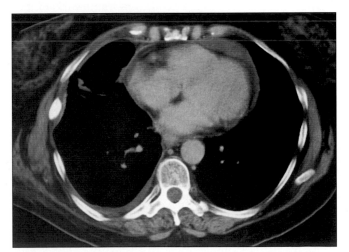

Figure 48.6. *Small right pleural effusion and eccentric small pericardial effusion 8 months following radiotherapy to a non-small cell bronchogenic carcinoma centrally in the right lung.*

HEART

The spectrum of radiation-induced heart disease includes:

- Acute and chronic pericarditis
- Coronary artery disease
- Valvular dysfunction
- Cardiomyopathy
- Conduction abnormalities

The frequency and clinical significance of radiation-induced heart disease, particularly ischaemic disease, are now recognized to be of greater magnitude than had been originally thought.[30,31] Evaluation of myocardial perfusion of asymptomatic long-term survivors, primarily patients treated for Hodgkin's disease, has shown a high incidence of subclinical myocardial lesions.[32]

Pericardial disease

Fajardo et al. have described thickening of the pericardium with fibrosis, fibrin deposition, and protein-rich pericardial effusions. Myocardial fibrosis also occurs but unlike the focal fibrosis seen after infarction, it has a patchy involvement that follows the collagen framework of the myocardium.[33]

The incidence of pericarditis is related to the dose, fraction size, volume irradiated and technique. Below 4000 cGy, the incidence is quite low. At 4000 cGy, it ranges from 2 to 6%[34–37] and has been reported to be as high as 20% at 4500 cGy.[37] Cosset reported an incidence of 4.1% at 3500–3700 cGy, that rose to 10.4% at 4100–4300 cGy.[36] Moderate-sized mediastinal fields have a 1% incidence of pericardial disease that rises to 17% when the fields are larger with treatment of extensive disease.[35] Techniques, previously used, with only anterior fields, gave a 50% greater dose to the pericardium than the dose delivered to the midplane.[38] The dose relationship of coronary artery disease has not yet been demonstrated.[36]

Radiation pericarditis generally presents 6–9 months after therapy and the majority of cases will occur within 12–18 months of therapy, but it may appear many years after radiotherapy. Acute and chronic pericarditis are seen with equal frequency. Both are indistinguishable clinically from other causes of pericarditis.[39]

Symmetrical increase in the size of the cardiac silhouette is the typical appearance of radiation-induced pericardial effusion. Eccentric effusions may occur, presumably because of adhesions in the treated area of the pericardium, that prevent uniform distribution of the fluid (Fig. 48.4).[40] Small pericardial effusions or pericardial thickening are more easily identified with cross-sectional imaging techniques, ultrasound, CT or MR. Far higher incidences of pericardial effusion will be found with these techniques. In a series of breast cancer patients treated with radiotherapy, Ikäheimo found that 33% had pericardial effusions on ultrasound examination.[41]

Evidence of radiation change in the lungs, either pneumonitis or fibrosis depending on the timing following therapy, is almost always present and can raise the possibility of radiation as the cause of cardiac disease. The major differential consideration is malignant pericardial effusion. Nodularity of the pericardium or mediastinal adenopathy may point to this possibility. Cytological evaluation of pericardial fluid is necessary for a definitive diagnosis and is not always positive even in malignant disease. Exclusion of a pericardial effusion as the cause of cardiac enlargement in a patient whose heart has been irradiated raises the question of cardiomyopathy or ischaemic heart disease.

Myocardial disease

The development of cardiomyopathy may also result from the use of chemotherapeutic agents. At a total cumulative dose of 550 mg/m² of doxorubicin, 1–2% of patients have overt congestive heart failure.[42] Non-invasive diagnostic modalities such as echocardiography and radionuclide cine angiogram as well as invasive tests, such as endomyocardial biopsy, aid to assess risk-status of individuals receiving doxorubicin chemotherapy.

Using these techniques, some degree of cardiac injury is demonstrated in more than 50% of asymptomatic patients treated with doxorubicin.[42] While the total dose is the most significant factor contributing to the development of cardiomyopathy, other factors associated with an increased cardiotoxicity are:

- Age
- Pre-existing cardiac disease
- Mediastinal irradiation
- Concomitant administration of cyclophosphamide, actinomycin D and mitomycin C[42]

Stenosis, thrombosis, and aneurysms in vessels such as the aorta, carotid and subclavian arteries have been associated with radiation.[43]

Key points: myocardial disease

■ A high incidence of ischaemic heart disease and impaired myocardial perfusion is induced by radiotherapy, especially in the treatment of Hodgkin's disease

■ Chemotherapy with doxorubicin results in some degree of myocardial disease in 50% of asymptomatic patients

OESOPHAGUS

Radiation-induced injury to the oesophagus may be a limiting factor in therapy of thoracic neoplasms. Doses which result in radiation injury are of the order of 4500 cGy and higher.[44] Chemotherapeutic agents such as Adriamycin exacerbate these effects.

The abnormalities seen on oesophagrams following radiotherapy include:

- Abnormal peristalsis
- Mucosal oedema
- Stricture (Fig. 48.7)
- Ulceration and fistula formation
- Oesophageal dysmotility which is the earliest and most common change

These, generally, occur within 4–12 weeks after completion of therapy. Focal segments with either decreased peristalsis or aperistalsis are seen and correspond to the portals used.[44] A serrated appearance of the oesophageal mucosa is seen when mucosal oedema is present.[45] Marked oesophagitis is usually seen endoscopically.

Cross-sectional imaging may demonstrate thickening of the oesophagus and mucosal enhancement corresponding to the inflammatory changes (Fig. 48.8). The differential diagnosis includes other causes of oesophagitis in the absence of an appropriate history.

Oesophageal strictures corresponding to the portals used are not infrequent and in general develop 4–8 months following therapy.[44] Barium swallow shows narrowing, usually with smoothly tapered margins, although ulceration may also occur. Development of fistulae between the oesophagus and tracheobronchial tree is uncommon and is likely to be related to extrinsic tumour involvement of the oesophageal wall with resultant erosion and fistula formation following therapy.[44] Radiation-induced strictures may be radiographically indistinguishable from those caused by other injury such as ingestion of caustic material or prolonged nasogastric intubation. Oesophageal cancers that respond to radiotherapy also frequently result in stricture formation.

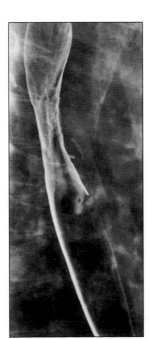

Figure 48.7. *Barium swallow shows slight narrowing of the mid-oesophagus with mucosal irregularity in a patient irradiated 3 months earlier for lung carcinoma. Endoscopy demonstrated oesophagitis.*

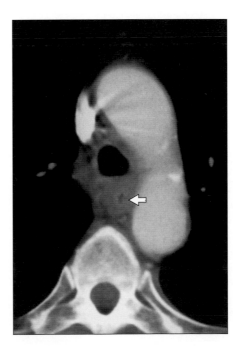

Figure 48.8. *CT scan of the chest demonstrates thickened oesophageal wall and mucosal enhancement (arrow) in a patient who received radiotherapy 4 months earlier for small cell carcinoma of the lung. The patient developed progressive dysphagia and odynophagia.*

A rare but well described complication of therapeutic irradiation is carcinoma of the oesophagus. Squamous cell carcinoma is most common. The mean latency period is 14 years.[46]

Patients with malignancies may also develop infectious oesophagitis as a result of immune compromise due to cytotoxic and/or immunosuppressive drugs or the malignancy itself. The most common pathogen in such patients is Candida albicans, normal flora in the pharynx, that grows in the oesophagus as a result of the altered immunity. Clinical signs include odynophagia and dysphagia. The appearance on double-contrast oesophagrams is usually characteristic.[47] Mucosal plaques are seen which are generally diffuse and in severe cases a shaggy, irregular contour of the oesophagus results. Candida oesophagitis can result in stricture and tracheo-oesophageal fistula formation.[48] Herpes simplex virus also may cause oesophagitis in cancer patients. Discrete superficial ulcers can be seen with oesophagrams.[48]

Key points: oesophageal disease

■ Abnormalities within the oesophagus generally occur within 4–12 weeks after completion of radiotherapy

■ Oesophageal strictures generally develop 4–8 months following radiotherapy and are radiographically indistinguishable from those caused by other injury

■ Carcinoma of the oesophagus is a rare but well-described complication of radiotherapy

■ Immune compromise due to cytotoxic or immuno-suppressive drugs can result in infectious oesophagitis most commonly due to Candida albicans

BONE

A detailed account of changes to the bone marrow following radiotherapy is given in Chapter 49. The radiographic changes in adult bone following radiotherapy follow a temporal pattern. There is a latent period of 12 months or more during which no change is evident.[49] Following this, some degree of demineralization may be seen. With progression, small lytic areas are seen through the cortex with thickening of the remaining trabeculae. This pattern usually develops 2–3 years or more following radiotherapy. These changes can be likened to multiple small foci of aseptic necrosis that are slowly progressive.[50]

Should the radiotherapy changes continue to progress, the lytic areas can reach 1–2 cm in size and may be similar to metastatic disease. It generally takes at least 5 years for the more pronounced changes to occur and in most patients metastatic disease will have developed earlier in the course of disease. The extent of the changes is generally much less with current megavoltage therapy than is seen with orthovoltage irradiation.[49] The presence of similar changes affecting adjacent bones in the irradiated field point to the correct diagnosis.[51] Absence of recurrent mass in the soft tissues with CT or MR speaks against local recurrence or soft tissue sarcoma.

Spontaneous fractures and aseptic necrosis can occur. Radiation-induced fractures may heal quite slowly, taking months to years to heal (Fig. 48.9). Non-union is not uncommon. Abnormal callus formation may be seen. Resorption of fracture fragments may occur. Despite the decreased incidence with current therapy techniques, the changes still occur and long-term survivors from the orthovoltage era remain at risk. Bones subjected to muscular pull or constant weight-bearing tend to fracture more frequently. Radiation-induced fractures may be asymptomatic in non-weight-bearing bones.[52]

Rib fractures are far less common following megavoltage than orthovoltage irradiation[49] and more frequent when higher doses per fraction are used.[53] The current incidence of rib fractures is slightly less than 2%.[54] The fractures may be quite subtle and generally involve the anterior aspects of the ribs included in tangential fields of the chest wall. The abnormal callus at the fractures may simulate a radiation-induced sarcoma. Radiation brachial plexopathy may accentuate demineralization about a treated shoulder joint and may also result in the appearance of a neuropathic-like

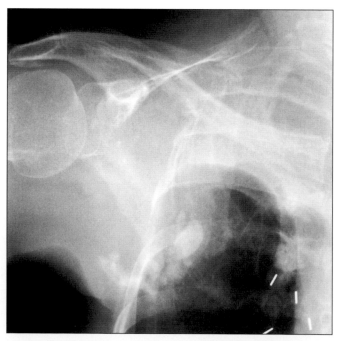

Figure 48.9. *Extensive chest wall changes following postoperative radiation therapy for breast cancer 20 years earlier are present. Multiple rib fractures with resorption, abnormal callus formation and dystrophic calcifications are present. The metallic clips are from coronary artery surgery. Radiation fibrosis is present in the upper right lung.*

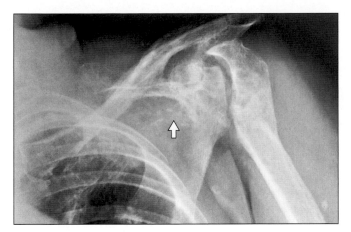

Figure 48.10. *Marked destruction of the left shoulder joint due in part to a radiation-induced brachial plexopathy 16 years following postoperative radiotherapy for breast cancer. Vascular calcification is seen (arrow). Rib and lung changes are also present.*

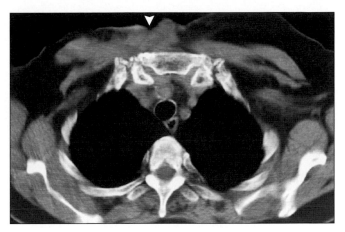

Figure 48.11. *Chest wall ulcer and radiation-induced soft tissue sarcoma. Twenty years earlier, this woman underwent subcutaneous mastectomies and radiotherapy for a right breast cancer. The soft tissue fullness beneath the skin ulcer (arrowhead) proved to be a malignant fibrous histiocytoma rather than inflammation related to the ulcer.*

shoulder joint superimposed on the radiation change (Fig. 48.10). Radiation-induced ulcers of the chest wall may also develop (Fig. 48.11).

Radiation change in the adult spine is not generally obvious on conventional radiographs. However, therapeutic levels of radiotherapy causes conversion of haematopoietic bone marrow to fatty marrow. This is seen at MR as increased signal intensity on T1-weighted images.[55] The transformation begins as early as 2 weeks into a course of radiotherapy at a dose of approximately 1600 cGy.[56]

The effects of therapeutic irradiation on growing bone are far more dramatic than those seen in adult bone because of associated growth impairment (Fig. 48.12). In the spine these changes in progressive order of severity include:

- Growth arrest lines
- End-plate irregularity
- Anterior beaking
- Asymmetry of vertebral development[57]

Significant scoliosis or kyphosis following radiotherapy is rare using modern techniques, but minor scoliotic changes are commonly seen.[58]

Radiation-induced bone tumours

Radiation-induced sarcomas are an infrequent, but well recognized complication of radiotherapy. They are estimated to occur in approximately 0.1% or fewer patients who receive radiotherapy and survive 5 years.[59,60] Radiation-induced sarcomas may occur in either bone or soft tissue. Osteosarcoma is more frequent in bone (Fig. 48.13) and malignant fibrous histiocytoma (Fig. 48.11) more common

in soft tissue.[61-63] Review of Finnish data indicates soft tissue sarcomas are more common than osseous sarcomas.[61]

Radiation-induced sarcomas more commonly occur around the shoulder girdle and pelvis because of the more frequent use of radiotherapy in malignancies in these regions and better survival of patients with those malignancies. A higher incidence in women reflects the malignancies treated more often with radiotherapy.[62]

A long latent period, averaging 10–15 years, is usually present between irradiation and the development of the sarcoma. However, radiation-induced sarcomas have

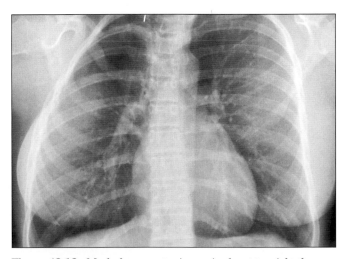

Figure 48.12. *Marked asymmetry is seen in the upper right thorax of a 17-year-old female who received postoperative radiotherapy aged 3 years for a rhabdomyosarcoma. The clavicle spontaneously fractured and resorbed nearly completely several years before.*

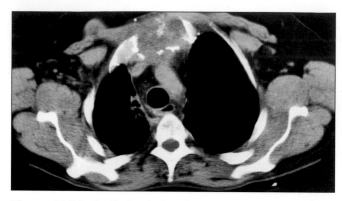

Figure 48.13. *Radiation-induced osteosarcoma of the sternum showing mass and bony destruction. The sarcoma developed 12 years after 3600 cGy mediastinal irradiation for metastases of a testicular seminoma.*

developed as soon as 2–3 years following therapy and as long as 45–55 years after treatment.[61–65]

The appearance of soft tissue sarcomas caused by radiotherapy is not different from the spontaneously developing sarcomas except that evidence of radiotherapy may be seen in adjacent bone or other tissues. They may get quite large if clinically silent.

With conventional radiographs radiation-induced sarcomas, arising in bone, most frequently present as an area of bony destruction.[50] A soft tissue mass may be evident but is better appreciated with CT or MR. Tumour matrix may be seen. An expansile area in a previously irradiated bone is suspect for development of sarcoma. Similarly, an area of lucency that is larger than the background pattern of radiation change is suspect.

At CT, a soft tissue mass and bony destruction are the most common findings.[64] A soft tissue density, rather than

fat, in the marrow cavity of irradiated bones may be the earliest indicator that a sarcoma has developed.

The occasional late metastatic lesion may mimic a radiation-induced sarcoma. Infection that has developed in a treated bone may also mimic radiation-induced sarcoma. Biopsy may be necessary to make the distinction. The absence of a soft tissue mass is helpful in distinguish-ing between extensive benign radiation change and a radiation-induced sarcoma.

Radiation-induced osteochondromas (cartilaginous exostoses) may occur in children until growth stops. The incidence is about 12%.[66] Most are small and asymptomatic. Occasionally, the size and/or location causes symptoms. The appearance is that of the spontaneous osteochondromas and the same concerns apply.

Key points: radiation-induced bone disease

- Bone demineralization results only after 12 months following radiotherapy

- Small lytic areas are seen only 2–3 years following radiotherapy and larger lytic areas 1–2 cm in size occur only after 5 years

- Radiation-induced fractures may take months or years to heal

- Radiation-induced sarcomas occur in about 0.1% of patients who receive radiotherapy

- A latent period of 10–15 years usually exists between radiotherapy and the development of a sarcoma

- Radiation-induced osteochondromas may occur in children until growth stops

Summary

- Radiation pneumonitis is evident 6–8 weeks following completion of radiotherapy and is most extensive 3–4 months after radiotherapy.

- Radiation pulmonary fibrosis usually becomes stable 9–12 months after completion of therapy; any alteration thereafter suggests infection or recurrence.

- Drugs that enhance radiation effect cause greater radiation damage and a shorter time to onset of radiation pneumonitis.

- Bleomycin, busulphan and methotrexate cause pulmonary parenchymal damage independent of radiotherapy.

- Identification of recurrent or residual malignant disease is made difficult by the presence of radiation change, usually requires CT and an awareness of the timing of radiation change and follow-up at 2–3 monthly intervals.

- Radiation-induced heart disease includes pericarditis, coronary artery disease, valvular dysfunction, cardiomyopathy and conduction abnormalities.

- Chemotherapeutic agents, particularly doxorubicin, can result in cardiomyopathy.

- Radiation injury to the oesophagus can result in oedema, dysmotility, stricture, ulceration and fistula formation or carcinoma.

REFERENCES

1. Maasilta P. Radiation-induced lung injury. From the chest physician's point of view. Lung Cancer 1991; 7: 367–384

2. Chu F C H, Phillips R, Nickson J J et al. Pneumonitis following radiation therapy of the breast by tangential technique. Radiology 1955; 64: 642–653

3. Fajardo L F. Respiratory system. In: Pathology of Radiation Injury. New York: Masson Publishing, 1982; 34–46

4. Katzenstein A A, Astin F B. Surgical pathology of non-neoplastic lung disease (2nd ed) Philadelphia: Saunders, 1990; 9–57

5. Libshitz H I, Brosof A B, Southard M E. The radiographic appearance of the chest following extended field radiation therapy for Hodgkin's disease. Cancer 1973; 32: 206–215

6. Libshitz H I, North L B. Lung. In: Libshitz H I (cd) Diagnostic roentgenology of radiotherapy change. Baltimore: Williams & Wilkins, 1979: 33–46

7. Libshitz H I. Radiation changes in the lung. Semin Roentgenol 1993; 28: 303–320

8. Wechsler R J, Ayyangar K, Steiner R M et al. The development of distant pulmonary infiltrates following thoracic irradiation: The role of computed tomography with dosimetric reconstruction in diagnosis. Comput J Imag Graph 1990; 14: 43–51

9. Morgan G W, Briet S N. Radiation and the lung: A re-evaluation of the mechanisms mediating pulmonary injury. Int J Radiat Oncol Biol Phys 1995; 31: 361–368

10. von der Maase H. Experimental drug–radiation interactions in critical normal tissues In: Hill B T, Bellamy S A (eds) Antitumor drug–radiation interactions. (Ch. 11). Boca Raton, FL: CRC Press, Inc., 1990; 191–205

11. Phillips T L. Effects of chemotherapy and irradiation on normal tissues. In: Meyer J L, Vaeth J M (eds) Radiotherapy/chemotherapy interactions in cancer therapy. Front Radiat Ther Oncol. Basel: Karger, 1992; 26: 45–54

12. Cooper J A D, White D A, Matthay R A. Drug-induced pulmonary disease. Part I: Cytotoxic drugs. Am Rev Respir Dis 1986; 133: 321–340

13. Morrison D A, Goldman A L. Radiographic patterns of drug-induced lung disease. Radiology 1979; 131: 299–304

14. Richman S D, Levenson S M, Bunn P A et al. ^{67}Ga accumulation in pulmonary lesions associated with bleomycin toxicity. Cancer 1975; 36: 1966–1972

15. Libshitz H I, Shuman L S. Radiation-induced pulmonary change: CT findings. J Comput Assist Tomogr 1984; 8: 15–19

16. Ikezoe J, Takashima S, Morimoto S et al. CT appearance of acute radiation-induced injury in the lung. Am J Roentgenol 1988; 150: 765–770

17. Mah K, Poon P Y, van Dyk J et al. Assessment of acute radiation-induced pulmonary changes using computed topography. J Comput Assist Tomogr 1986; 10: 736–743

18. Davis S D, Yankelevits D F, Henschke C I. Radiation effects on the lung: Clinical features, pathology and imaging findings. Am J Roentgenol 1992; 159: 1157–1164

19. Glazer H S, Lee J K T, Levitt R G et al. Radiation fibrosis: Differentiation from recurrent tumor by MR imaging. Radiology 1985; 156: 721–726

20. Werthmuller W C, Schiebler M L, Whaley R A et al. Gadolinium-DTPA enhancement of lung radiation fibrosis. J Comput Assist Tomogr 1989; 13: 946–948

21. Wencel M L, Sitrin R G. Unilateral lung hyperlucency after mediastinal irradiation. Am Rev Respir Dis 1988; 137: 955–957

22. Twiford T W, Zornoza J, Libshitz H I. Recurrent spontaneous pneumothorax after radiation therapy to the thorax. Chest 1978; 73: 388–389

23. Bachman A L, Macken K. Pleural effusions following supervoltage radiation for breast carcinoma. Radiology 1959; 72: 699–709

24. Brereton H D, Johnson R E. Calcification in mediastinal lymph nodes after radiation therapy of Hodgkin's Disease. Radiology 1974; 112: 705–707

25. Kim H C, Nosher J, Haas A et al. Cystic degeneration of thymic Hodgkin's disease following radiation therapy. Cancer 1985; 55: 354–356

26. Shannon V R, Nesbitt J C, Libshitz H I. Malignant pleural mesothelioma after radiation therapy for breast cancer. Cancer 1995; 76: 437–441

27. Jochelson M, Mauch P, Balikian J et al. The significance of the residual mediastinal mass in treated Hodgkin's disease. J Clin Oncol 1985; 3: 637–640

28. Radford J A, Cowan R A, Flanagan M et al. The significance of residual mediastinal abnormality on the chest radiograph following treatment for Hodgkin's Disease. J Clin Oncol 1988; 6: 940–946

29. Bourgouin P, Cousineau G, Lemire P et al. Differentiation of radiation-induced fibrosis from recurrent pulmonary neoplasm by CT. J Can Assoc Radiol 1987; 38: 23–26

30. Cosset J M, Henry-Amar M, Meerwaldt J H. Long-term toxicity of early stages of Hodgkin's disease: The EORTC experience. Ann Oncol 1991; 2: 77–82

31. Boivin J, Hutchison G B, Lubin J H et al. Coronary artery disease mortality in patients treated for Hodgkin's Disease. Cancer 1992; 69: 1241–1247

32. Pierga J Y, Maunoury C, Valette H et al. Follow-up thallium-201 scintigraphy after mantle field radiotherapy for Hodgkin's disease. Int J Radiat Oncol Biol Phys 1993; 25: 871–876

33. Fajardo L F, Berthrong M. Radiation injury in surgical pathology. Am J Surg Pathol 1978; 2: 159–199

34. Tarbell N J, Thompson L, Mauch P. Thoracic irradiation in Hodgkin's disease: Disease control and long-term complications. Int J Radiat Oncol Biol Phys 1990; 18: 275–281

35. Cosset J M, Henry-Amar M, Ozanne F et al. Les pericardites radiques: Etudes des cas observes dans une serie de 160 maladies de Hodgkin irradiees en mantelet a l'Institut Gustave-Roussy, de 1976 a 1980. J Eur Radiother 1984; 5: 297–308

36. Cosset J M, Henry-Amar M, Pellae-Cosset B et al. Pericarditis and myocardial infarctions after Hodgkin's disease therapy. Int J Radiat Oncol Biol Phys 1991; 21: 447–449

37. Dana M, Colombel P, Bayle-Weisgerber C et al. Les pericardites apres irradiation du mediastin par grands champs pour la maladie de Hodgkin. J Radiol Electrol 1978; 59: 335–341

38. Kinsella T J, Fraass B A, Glatstein E. Late effects of radiation therapy in the treatment of Hodgkin's disease. Cancer Treat Rep 1982; 66: 991–1001

39. Loyer E M, Delpassand E S. Radiation-induced heart disease: Imaging features. Semin Roentgenol 1993; 28: 321–332

40. Green B, Zornoza J, Ricks J P. Eccentric pericardial effusion after radiation therapy of left breast carcinoma. Am J Roentgenol 1977; 128: 27–30

41. Ikäheimo M J, Niemalä K O, Linnaluoto M M et al. Early cardiac changes related to radiation therapy. Am J Cardiol 1985; 56: 943–946

42. Gerling B, Gottdiener J, Borer J S. Cardiovascular complications of the treatment of Hodgkin's disease. In: Lacher M J, Redman J R (eds) Hodgkin's Disease: The Consequences of Survival. Philadelphia: Lea & Febiger, 1990; 267–295

43. Benson E P. Radiation injury to large arteries: Three further examples with prolonged asymptomatic intervals. Radiology 1973; 106: 195–197

44. Lepke R A, Libshitz H I. Radiation-induced injury of the esophagus. Radiology 1983; 148: 375–378

45. DuBrow R A. Radiation changes in the hollow viscera. Semin Roentgenol 1994; 29: 38–52

46. Ogino T, Kato H, Tsukiyama I et al. Radiation-induced carcinoma of the esophagus. Acta Oncol 1992; 31: 475–479

47. Levine M S, Macones A J, Laufer I. Candida esophagitis: Accuracy of radiographic diagnosis. Radiology 1985; 154: 581–587

48. Yee J, Wall S D. Infectious esophagitis. Radiol Clin North Am 1994; 32: 1135–1145

49. Howland W J, Loeffler R K, Starchman D E et al. Post-irradiation atrophic changes of bone and related complications. Radiology 1975; 117: 677–685

50. Libshitz H I. Radiation changes in the bone. Semin Roentgenol 1994; 29: 15–37

51. de Santos L A, Libshitz H I. Adult bone. In: Libshitz H I (ed) Diagnostic roentgenology of radiotherapy change. Baltimore: Williams and Wilkins, 1979; 137–150

52. Dalinka M K, Neustafler L M. Radiation changes. In: Resnick D, Niwayama G (eds) Diagnosis of bone and joint disorders. Philadelphia: Saunders, 1988; 3024–3056

53. Overgaard M. Spontaneous radiation-induced rib fractures in breast cancer patients treated with post-mastectomy irradiation: A clinical radiobiological analysis of the influence of fraction size and dose–response relationships on late bone damage. Acta Oncol 1988; 27: 117–122

54. Pierce S M, Recht A, Lingos T L et al. Long-term radiation complications following conservative surgery (CS) and radiation therapy (RT) in patients with early stage breast cancer. Int J Radiat Oncol Biol Phys 1992; 23: 915–932

55. Ramsey R G, Zacharias C E. MR imaging of the spine after radiation therapy: easily recognizable effects. Am J Roentgenol 1985; 144: 1131–1135

56. Yankelevitz D F, Henschke C I, Knapp P H et al. Effect of radiation therapy on thoracic and lumbar bone marrow: Evaluation with MR imaging. Am J Roentgenol 1991; 157: 87–92

57. Neuhauser E B D, Wittenborg M H, Berman C Z et al. Irradiation effects of roentgen therapy on the growing spine. Radiology 1952; 59: 637–650

58. Heaston D K, Libshitz H I, Chan R C. Skeletal effects of megavoltage irradiation in survivors of Wilms' tumor. Am J Roentgenol 1979; 133: 389–395

59. Taghian A, de Vathaire F, Terrier P et al. Long-term risk of sarcoma following radiation treatment for breast cancer. Int J Radiat Oncol Biol Phys 1991; 21: 361–367

60. Tountas A S, Fornasier V L, Harwood A R et al. Postirradiation sarcoma of bone: A perspective. Cancer 1979; 43: 182–187

61. Wiklund T A, Blomqvist G P, RŠty J et al. Post-irradiation sarcoma: Analysis of a nationwide cancer registry material. Cancer 1991; 68: 524–531

62. Huvos A G, Woodard H Q, Cahan V G et al. Postradiation osteogenic sarcoma of bone and soft tissues: A clinicopathologic study of 66 patients. Cancer 1985; 55: 1244–1255

63. Laskin W B, Silberman T A, Enzinger F M. Postradiation soft tissue sarcomas: An analysis of 53 cases. Cancer 1988; 62: 2330–2340

64. Lorigan J G, Libshitz H I, Peuchot M. Radiation-induced sarcoma of bone: CT findings in 19 cases. Am J Roentgenol 1989; 153: 791–794

65. Weatherby R P, Dahlin D C, Ivins J C. Postradiation sarcoma of bone: Review of 78 Mayo Clinic cases. Mayo Clin Proc 1981; 56: 294–306

66. Libshitz H I, Cohen M A. Radiation-induced osteochondromas. Radiology 1982; 142: 643–647

Chapter 49

Bone and bone marrow

Lia Moulopoulos

As early as 1926, Ewing[1] reported osseous changes that he believed were related to radiation-induced vascular damage. He introduced the term 'radiation osteitis'[1] to describe these radiation-induced abnormalities. Since that time, many other investigators have described changes related to the effect of radiation on the bones and have introduced many terms, such as osteonecrosis and radionecrosis.

Howland and his colleagues[2] suggested that, since atrophy is the main event that takes place in the radiated bone, the term 'atrophic changes' more accurately defines the expected, uncomplicated postradiation bony changes. All other superimposed conditions, such as fractures, infection, and aseptic necrosis can be considered complications of radiation therapy. The number of complications of radiation therapy that affect the osseous skeleton has been reduced, but not eliminated, since the advent of megavoltage therapy.

PATHOPHYSIOLOGY OF TREATMENT-RELATED OSSEOUS CHANGES

The effect of radiation therapy on the bones has been documented by pathological studies.[3–5] The changes that occur in radiated bones are due to destruction of the cellular bony matrix and the fine vasculature that supplies the bone. Radiation therapy induces an immediate inflammatory reaction in the bone marrow. All cellular elements die early in the postradiation period and, as early as the first week of therapy, the marrow becomes hypocellular with oedema and haemorrhage. Endarteritis occurs later in the postradiation period and is responsible for the late postradiation manifestations observed on radiographic examinations. Destruction of the microvasculature of the bone prevents the migration of haematopoietic elements from contiguous healthy bone marrow. Vascular compromise leads to bone necrosis. Necrotic bone is gradually removed by 'creeping substitution' and new bone is deposited over a period of years.

The development and the severity of postradiation changes of the bones depends on the dose, dose fractionation, field size, and type of radiation treatment. Regeneration of the bone marrow is possible if the microvasculature of the affected bone has not been completely obliterated. Histologically, magnetic resonance (MR) and radionuclide studies[5–11] have not shown recovery of haematopoietic marrow with doses greater than 3000–4000 cGy.

The changes that occur in the *bone marrow* after chemotherapy have been studied on serial bone marrow specimens from patients with acute myelogenous leukemia.[12] Immediately after initiation of chemotherapy, depletion of the cellular elements takes place and the bone marrow becomes oedematous. The vascular sinuses dilate and large, unilocular adipocytes (structured fat) which are produced by multilocular precursor fat cells, appear in the radiated marrow. It is only within these areas of structured fat that foci of regenerating haematopoietic marrow appear after the first week of treatment, suggesting a potential role of structured fat in the proliferation of stem cells.

IMAGING FINDINGS

Postradiation atrophic changes

Local demineralization is the earliest and, most often, the only postradiation change on conventional bone radiographs, together with coarsening of the bony trabecula and thickening of the cortex of the long bones; changes that have been likened to Pagetoid bone.[2] Such changes occur a year after radiation therapy and may become more pronounced with time. Later, both sclerotic and lytic foci representing dead and resorbed bone, respectively, may appear (Fig. 49.1). Postradiation atrophic changes are more obvious on computed tomography (CT) scans because of increased contrast resolution. Occasionally, lytic foci may grow and simulate primary or secondary malignant bone tumours. Appearances that support the diagnosis of postradiation lytic change rather than neoplasm include localization to the radiation portals, absence of an extraosseous mass or periosteal reaction, a sharp transition zone to the uninvolved bone and slow growth of the lesion.[13–15] CT scans should be obtained if review of conventional bone radiographs poses the question of malignancy. If findings are equivocal on CT scans, MR imaging studies may help the detection of extraosseous or bone marrow involvement.

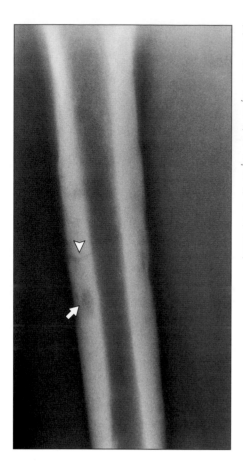

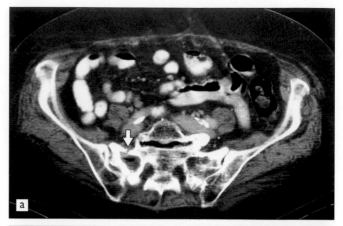

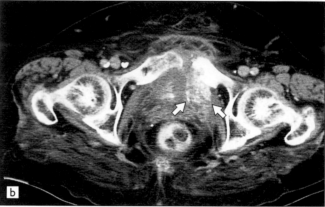

Figure 49.1.
Cortical lucency (arrow) and insufficiency fracture (arrowhead). Anteroposterior tomogram of the femur of a patient with soft tissue sarcoma who received 7000 cGy 5 years ago. (Courtesy of H.I. Libshitz).

Figure 49.2. *Insufficiency fractures of the pelvis. CT scans of the pelvis of a 66-year-old woman who was treated with radiotherapy for vaginal cancer 2 years ago. In (a), the arrow points to a fracture of the right sacral wing. (b) Note healed insufficiency fracture of the left pubic bone and extra-osseous calcifications (arrows).*

Postradiation complications
Fractures

The radiated, atrophic bone is brittle and may fracture, even under physiological stress such as muscular contractions, particularly in weight-bearing bones. The first radiation-induced fracture[16] was described in the femoral neck in 1927. Since the introduction of megavoltage therapy, radiation-induced fractures are seen less often. They are infrequently observed earlier than 2 or 3 years after therapy.[15] They may be discovered incidentally on routine imaging studies or they may present with pain, particularly when weight-bearing bones are involved. Radiation-induced fractures heal more slowly than fractures of healthy bone and formation of abnormal, exuberant callus, non-union of the osseous fragments or bony resorption may occur.

Radiation-induced insufficiency fractures of the pelvis occur earlier than in other parts of the skeleton (Figs 49.2 and 49.3).[15] After treatment with pelvic radiation, the sacrum loses its elasticity and may fracture under the stress of normal activity. A 34% incidence of sacral insufficiency fractures[17] has been reported in patients treated with radiotherapy for cervical cancer. In postmenopausal women, osteoporosis increases the probability of insufficiency fractures of radiated bones. On conventional radiographs,

findings may be absent or very subtle.[18] An H-shaped appearance of increased uptake on radionuclide studies is characteristic of sacral insufficiency fractures which course vertically in the sacral alae.[19,20] The horizontal bar of the 'H' corresponds to a third transverse fracture of the sacrum that need not necessarily be identified on radiographs.

In patients with known malignancies, it may be difficult to differentiate sacral insufficiency fractures, especially unilateral ones, from metastatic disease on conventional radiographs and radionuclide scans alone. Computed tomography or MR imaging can provide a definitive diagnosis in most cases. On T1-weighted MR images of sacral insufficiency fractures,[21] the expected bright signal of radiated marrow is replaced by decreased signal intensity produced by the presence of free water in the oedematous marrow. The water, and consequently the decreased signal, extends well beyond the margins of the fracture (Fig. 49.3). Magnetic resonance imaging studies may demonstrate sacral insufficiency fractures well before any

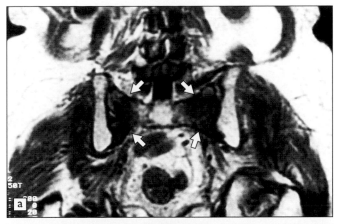

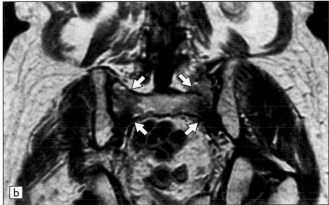

Figure 49.3. *Bilateral insufficiency fractures of the sacrum. T1-weighted (a) and enhanced T1-weighted (b) coronal MR images of the sacrum of a 70-year-old woman who was treated with radiotherapy for cervical cancer 1 year ago. Note oedematous marrow (arrows) with faint enhancement in (b).*

Figure 49.4.
Avascular necrosis of the head of the left femur. T1-weighted (a) and T2-weighted fat-suppressed fast spin-echo (b) coronal MR images of the left proximal femur of a 51-year-old man with a history of lymphoma and radiation treatment to the pelvis, show changes of early avascular necrosis (arrow). Note double line sign in (b).

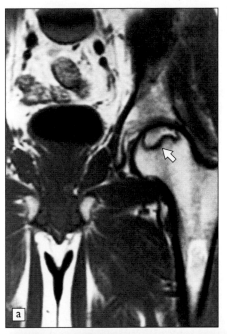

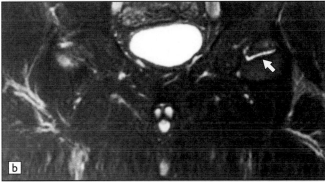

changes appear on CT images because of the higher contrast resolution and capability for multiplanar image acquisition.

Avascular necrosis

Radiation therapy and steroids are known causes of avascular necrosis. Avascular necrosis develops years after radiation treatment and more frequently affects the femoral than the humeral head. Before the introduction of MR imaging, radionuclide examination was the procedure of choice for the diagnosis of avascular necrosis. With this modality, as many as 18% false-negative radionuclide scans have been reported.[22] Radionuclide studies failed to detect 10% of cases of avascular necrosis that had positive MR studies.[23]

The presence of the double-line sign on T2-weighted MR images is characteristic of avascular necrosis (Fig. 49.4) This consists of an outer dark line which is produced by reactive sclerosis at the interface of the lesion with the healthy marrow, and a bright inner line which corresponds to areas of hyperaemia and inflammation at the periphery of the ischaemic marrow.[23] Recognition of the presence of avascular necrosis before the occurrence of a subchondral fracture is important for the success of conservative treatment. Magnetic resonance imaging can detect avascular necrosis within days of the vascular insult. Current research focuses on even earlier recognition of avascular necrosis.[24] With the use of dynamic contrast-enhanced MR images, non-perfused, dead tissue was detected within 3 hours from devascularization in animal models.[24] MR imaging has also been shown to identify those patients at particular risk of developing avascular necrosis when exposed to known predisposing factors. The presence of a sealed-off epiphyseal scar in the femoral head has been associated with an increased risk of avascular necrosis.[25] Magnetic resonance imaging can also reliably assess the extent and the location of the necrotic bone relative to the weight-bearing area, factors that influence the course of avascular necrosis and affect the management of the patient.[26] There is no doubt that MR imaging is the most sensitive and most specific modality for the diagnosis of avascular necrosis.

Key points: fractures and aseptic necrosis

■ Radiation-induced fractures occur earlier in the pelvis than in other parts of the skeleton

■ Sacral insufficiency fractures may be difficult to distinguish from metastases on conventional radiographs and radionuclide scans

■ Magnetic resonance imaging is the most sensitive and most specific technique in the detection of aseptic necrosis

EFFECTS OF RADIATION ON THE GROWING SKELETON

The effect of radiation therapy on the osseous skeleton depends on the type of bone involved, the dosage and, in particular, the patient's age at the time of therapy. The younger the child at the time of radiation therapy, the more pronounced the radiation-induced osseous changes because of the impairment of bone growth. The epiphysis, which is radiosensitive, may show signs of radiation-induced changes with doses as low as 400 cGy. Widening of the epiphyseal plate, and irregularity and sclerosis of the metaphysis are common findings in the growing skeleton exposed to radiation.[15] They may appear quite early after therapy and may resemble the osseous changes observed in rickets. In the diaphyses, changes are minimal and include narrowing of the shaft and some degree of osteoporosis.

Slipped capital femoral epiphysis and, less frequently, slipped capital humeral epiphysis represent a serious complication, occur 1–7 years after treatment and at an earlier age than its idiopathic counterpart.[15,17,27,28] Administration of chemotherapy increases the possibility of epiphyseal slippage. Slipped epiphysis may be accompanied by avascular necrosis of the femoral or humeral head.[29] Because of the late manifestations of postradiation epiphyseal injuries, it is obvious that long-term follow-up is warranted for patients with a history of radiation therapy.

Radiation-induced changes of the growing spine are more pronounced in patients treated before the age of 6 years or at puberty, both being periods of increased skeletal growth.[29] Growth arrest lines, which are dense lines parallel to the vertebral end-plates, are a common manifestation of growth arrest related to prior radiotherapy.

They appear within a year from therapy with doses greater than 1000 cGy and may actually cause a 'bone within bone' appearance. Doses greater than 2000 cGy are associated with more pronounced changes of growth disturbance that become apparent within 5 years of completion of therapy.[30] Such changes include short vertebral bodies, irregularity of the end-plates and, less frequently, contour abnormalities[31] which may resemble changes observed in mucopolysaccharides (Fig. 49.5). Mild scoliosis is a common complication when the spine is included in the radiation field. With the advent of megavoltage therapy, it is unusual for scolioses greater than 5° to occur,[29,30] because of more even distribution of the radiation beam to the vertebrae. Kyphosis may accompany scoliosis but it is extremely rare for it to occur alone.

Osteochondroma is the only benign tumour associated with a history of radiotherapy. While the incidence of spontaneous osteochondromas is less than 1%, the incidence of osteochondromas developing within a previously irradiated field has been reported to be up to 12%.[32] The tumours occur in patients who received radiotherapy during childhood and, histologically, they do not differ from those that occur spontaneously. They appear at an average of 8 years after radiotherapy[32] and should be treated according to the same guidelines as those that occur spontaneously.

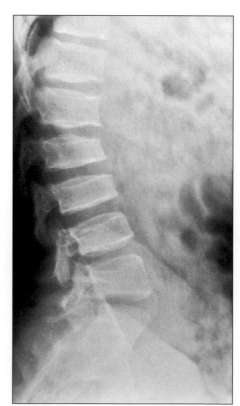

Figure 49.5.
Loss of vertebral body height and irregularities of the vertebral end-plates. Lateral radiograph of the lumbar spine of a 17-year-old boy who received radiation therapy for Wilms' tumour at age 2 years. (Courtesy of H. I. Libshitz)

Key points: effects on the growing skeleton

- In children, epiphyseal changes can occur with doses as low as 400 cGY

- Slipped epiphyses occur 1–7 years after radiation and warrant long-term follow-up

- Spinal changes are more pronounced in patients treated before age 6 or at puberty, both periods of increased skeletal growth

- Osteochondromas occur about 8 years after radiotherapy

RADIATION EFFECT ON THE BONE MARROW

Magnetic resonance imaging has provided a means of recording in vivo the changes that occur in the radiated bone marrow. Immediately after initiation of radiotherapy, the signal intensity of the bone marrow on T1-weighted MR images decreases. This drop in the signal intensity of the marrow reflects an increase in free water that occurs because of oedema and necrosis of the marrow. As early as

2 weeks into therapy, and with doses as low as 800 cGy, the signal intensity of the bone marrow begins to rise as the number of adipocytes within the radiated bone marrow grows (Fig. 49.6).[8,9,33] Conversion of the radiated marrow to fatty marrow is completed before the end of radiotherapy.[34] This 'bright' marrow is due to the short T1 value of adipose tissue and it is sharply delineated from bone marrow outside the radiation portals. Regeneration of the haematopoietic elements of the bone marrow[10] has been reported to occur with doses lower than 3000 cGy, 2–23 years after radiotherapy.[10] With higher doses, however, conversion to fatty marrow appears to be irreversible.[7,9,10] Blomlie et al.[34] reported changes on MR images of non-irradiated bone marrow during radiation therapy. These changes consist of an increase in fatty marrow and, according to the authors' conclusions, they are probably due to an indirect effect of radiation therapy rather than to scattered radiation.

EFFECT OF CHEMOTHERAPY ON MR IMAGES OF THE BONE MARROW

During the first days after the administration of chemotherapy regimens, a drop in the signal intensity of the bone marrow is observed on spinal T1-weighted MR images together with increased brightness on T2-weighted images.

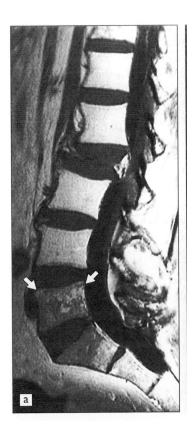
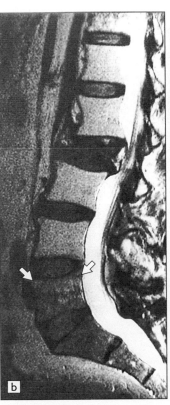
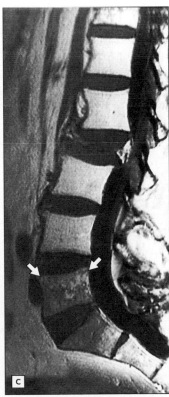

Figure 49.6. *Postradiation changes of the spine. Sagittal T1-weighted (a), T2-weighted (b), and enhanced T1-weighted (c) MR images of the lumbar spine of a 56-year-old man who received radiotherapy for Ewing's tumour at L2. Note bright signal of postradiation change (L4 to lower half of T11) which is sharply delineated from red marrow (arrows) outside the radiation field; there is no perceptible enhancement of the intact red marrow or of the affected, compressed L2 vertebra. On the T2-weighted image the delineation of red and yellow marrow is less obvious; absence of areas of increased signal is in keeping with lack of recurrence or metastases.*

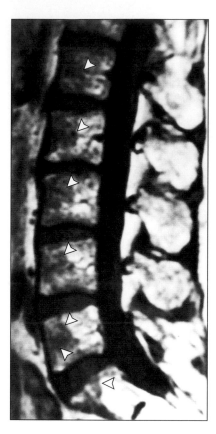

Figure 49.7.
Postchemotherapy changes of the spine. T1-weighted sagittal MR image of the lumbar spine shows islands of regenerating red marrow (arrowheads) in a 50-year-old man who is receiving chemotherapy for melanoma.

factors are administered during chemotherapy. Fletcher et al. reported changes of reconversion in the femoral diaphyses of children receiving haematopoietic growth factors in addition to chemotherapy for musculoskeletal tumours.[35] No such changes were observed in children who did not receive growth factors. Haematopoietic activity induced by growth factors may simulate malignant dissemination to the bone marrow. Awareness of the treatment regimens is necessary for the accurate interpretation of post-therapy MR images.

Magnetic resonance imaging has also been applied to the evaluation of bone marrow after transplantation. Patients who have undergone stem cell transplantation are currently assessed with serial bone marrow biopsies and aspirations. Prospective MR studies are being carried out in an attempt to introduce a potential non-invasive means of following the changes that occur in the marrow of these patients. Stevens and his colleagues[33] reported a characteristic band pattern which was present on T1-weighted images of all but one of 15 patients who received bone marrow transplants. This band pattern consisted of a bright central zone of fatty marrow and a peripheral dark zone of haematopoietic cells. This band-like distribution of red and fatty marrow in the vertebral body may be explained by the pattern of vascular flow into the vertebra, which in turn determines the distribution of the proliferating blood cells.

It becomes obvious from the above that today an MR study is the most accurate imaging modality for the evaluation of large volumes of bone marrow and that this modality provides information complementary to the bone marrow biopsy. Close cooperation of the radiologist and the clinician, and knowledge of the expected changes in the bone marrow under different conditions, is important in order to reach the correct diagnosis.

The changes that occur in the bone marrow immediately after initiation of chemotherapy, reflect the increase in free water in the con-gested bone marrow and vary, depending on the effect of the chemotherapy on the bone marrow. Later, an increase in fatty material is observed on MR images of the bone marrow. When haematopoietic recovery occurs, about 3 to 4 weeks into chemotherapy, the marrow becomes dark again on T1-weighted MR images because of the presence of regenerating red marrow (Fig. 49.7). At this stage, differentiation of regenerating red marrow from malignant infiltration of the marrow may be difficult. Absence of an increase in signal on T2-weighted images and faint or no enhancement on enhanced T1-weighted images favour the presence of red marrow recovery.

Reconversion of fatty to red marrow occurs in the opposite direction to marrow conversion, that is, from the axonal skeleton to the periphery. When there is an increased need for additional haematopoiesis, red marrow will appear in the proximal metaphyses of the femur and humerus. In extreme cases, red marrow may appear at other parts of the peripheral skeleton which are occupied by fatty marrow in healthy adults.

Changes related to increased haematopoiesis on MR images of the bone marrow are accentuated when growth

Key points: bone marrow changes

■ Changes in the bone marrow can be seen on T1-weighted MR images immediately after initiation of radiotherapy due to an increase in free water

■ Within 2 weeks of the start of radiotherapy, fat starts to replace the red marrow; these changes can be irreversible with high doses

■ Chemotherapy results in an increase in water within the bone marrow within days; within a week, there is an increase in fat; about 3–4 weeks later, regenerating marrow appears. All these changes can be monitored on MRI

Summary

■ Radiation therapy results in an immediate inflammatory reaction and hypocellularity in the bone marrow. Endarteritis occurs later and results in bone necrosis.

■ Local demineralization is the earliest, most often the only radiographic change following radiotherapy. Lytic foci may grow and simulate neoplastic lesions.

■ Radiation-induced fractures are seldom seen less than 2–3 years after therapy, are most common in the pelvis and are best detected on MRI.

■ Avascular necrosis occurs years after radiation treatment. It is important to recognize its presence before the development of subchondral fractures.

■ In the growing skeleton subjected to radiotherapy, slipped epiphysis is a serious complication and is made more likely by the addition of chemotherapy.

■ Both radiotherapy and chemotherapy produce serial changes in the bone marrow that can be monitored on MRI.

REFERENCES

1. Ewing J. Radiation osteitis. Acta Radiol 1926; 5: 399–412
2. Howland W J, Loeffler R K, Starchman D E, Johnson R G. Post-irradiation atrophic changes of bone and related complications. Radiology 1975; 117: 677–685
3. Rubin P, Casarett G W. Clinical radiation pathology, vol II. Philadelphia: Saunders, 1968: 557–608
4. Fajardo L F. Locomotive system, in Pathology of Radiation Injury. New York, NY: Masson, 1982; 176–186
5. Knospe W H, Blom J, Crosby W H. Regeneration of locally irradiated bone marrow. I. Dose dependent, long-term changes in the rat, with particular emphasis upon vascular and stromal reaction. Blood 1966; 28: 398–415
6. Sykes M P, Chu F C H, Savel H, Bonadonna G, Mathis H. Long-term effects of therapeutic irradiation upon bone marrow. Cancer 1964; 17: 1144–1148
7. Kauczor H U, Dietl B, Brix G, Jarosch M S, Knopp M V, van Kaick G. Fatty replacement of bone marrow after radiation therapy for Hodgkin disease: Quantification with chemical shift imaging. JMRI 1993; 3: 575–580
8. Remedios P A, Colletti P M, Raval J K. Magnetic resonance imaging of bone after radiation. Mag Reson Imaging 1988; 6: 301–304
9. Yankelevitz D F, Henschke C I, Knapp P H et al. Effect of radiation therapy in thoracic and lumbar marrow: evaluation with MR imaging. Am J Roentgenol 1991; 157: 87–92
10. Casamassima F, Ruggiero C, Caramella D et al. Hematopoietic bone marrow recovery: MRI evaluation, Blood 1989; 73: 1677–1681

11. Sacks E L, Goris M L, Glatstein E, Gilbert E, Kaplan H S. Bone marrow regeneration following large field radiation: Influence of volume, age, dose, and time. Cancer 1978; 42: 1057–1065

12. Islam A, Catovsky D, Galton D. Histological study of bone marrow regeneration following chemotherapy for acute myeloid leukemia and chronic granulocytic leukemia in blast transformation. Br J Hematol 1980; 45: 535–540

13. de Santos L A, Libshitz H I. Adult bone, In: Libshitz H I (ed) Diagnostic radiology of radiotherapy change. Baltimore, MD: Williams and Wilkins, 1979: 137–150

14. Paling M R, Herdt J R. Radiation osteitis: A problem of recognition. Radiology 1980; 137: 339–342

15. Libshitz H I. Radiation changes in bone. Semin Roentgenol 1994; 29: 15–37

16. Baensch W. Knochenschadigung nach Rontgen-bestrahlung. Fortschr Geb Roentgenstr 1927; 36: 1245–1247

17. Abe H, Nakamura M, Takahashi S et al. Radiation-induced insufficiency fractures of the pelvis: Evaluation with ^{99m}Tc-methylenediphosphonate scintigraphy. Am J Roentgenol 1990; 158: 599–602

18. Lundin B, Bjorkholm E, Lundell M, Jacobsson H. Insufficiency fractures of the sacrum after radiotherapy for gynecological malignancy. Acta Oncol 1990; 29: 211–215

19. Ries T. Detection of osteoporotic sacral fractures with radionuclides. Radiology 1983; 146: 783–785

20. Cooper K L, Beabout J W, Swee R G. Insufficiency fractures of the sacrum. Radiology 1985; 156: 15–20

21. Blomlie V, Lien H H, Iversen T, Winderen M, Tvera K. Radiation-induced insufficiency fractures of the sacrum: Evaluation with MR imaging. Radiology 1993; 188: 241–244

22. Bieber E, Hungerford D S, Lennox D W. Factors in diagnosis of avascular necrosis of the femoral head. Adv Orthop Surg 1985; 9: 93–96

23. Mitchell D G, Rao V M, Dalinka M K et al. Femoral head avascular necrosis: Correlation of MR imaging, radiographic staging, radionuclide imaging, and clinical findings. Radiology 1987; 162: 709–715

24. Nadel S N, Debatin J F, Richardson W J et al. Detection of acute avascular necrosis of the femoral head in dogs: Dynamic contrast-enhanced MR imaging vs spin-echo and STIR sequences AJR 1992; 159: 1255–1261

25. Lafforgue P, Dahan E, Chagnaud C et al. Early-stage avascular necrosis of the femoral head: MR imaging for prognosis in 31 cases with at least 2 years of follow-up. Radiology 1993; 187: 199–204

26. Jiang C C, Shih T T F. Epiphyseal scar of the femoral head: Risk factor of osteonecrosis. Radiology 1994; 191: 409–412

27. Dickerman J D, Newberg A H, Moreland M D. Slipped capital femoral epiphysis (SCFE) following pelvic irradiation for rhabdomyosarcoma. Cancer 1979; 44: 480–482

28. Edeiken B S, Libshitz H I, Cohen M A. Slipped proximal humeral epiphysis: A complication of radiotherapy to the shoulder in children. Skeletal Radiol 1982; 9: 123–125

29. Probert J C, Parker B R. The effects of radiation therapy on bone growth. Radiology 1975; 114: 155–162

30. Heaston D K, Libshitz H I, Chan R C. Skeletal effects of megavoltage irradiation in survivors of Wilms' tumor. Am J Roentgenol 1979; 389–395

31. Riseborough E J, Grabias S L, Burton R, Jaffe N. Skeletal alterations following irradiation for Wilms' tumor. J Bone Joint Surg [Am] 1976; 58: 526–536

32. Libshitz H I, Cohen M A. Radiation-induced osteochondromas. Radiology 1982; 142: 643–647

33. Stevens S K, Moore S G, Kaplan I D. Early and late bone-marrow changes after irradiation: MR evaluation. Am J Roentgenol 1990; 154: 745–750

34. Blomlie V, Rofstad E K, Skjonsberg A, Treva K, Lien H H. Female pelvic bone marrow: Serial MR imaging before, during and after radiation therapy. Radiology 1995; 194: 537–543

35. Fletcher B D, Eall J E, Hanna S L. Effect of hemato-poietic growth factors on MR images of the bone marrow in children undergoing chemotherapy. Radiology 1993; 189: 745–751

Chapter 50

Abdomen and pelvis

Richard Johnson, Bernadette Carrington and Paul Hulse

INTRODUCTION

Treatment of abdominopelvic malignancy is usually with surgery, radiotherapy or chemotherapy, either singularly or in combination. This chapter will deal mainly with the effect on normal tissues of radiotherapy in the gastro-intestinal tract, genito-urinary tract and musculoskeletal system. However, pertinent comments will also be made in relation to changes following surgery and chemotherapy.

Radical (curative) radiotherapy is often the treatment of choice for pelvic tumours, particularly cervical, bladder and prostate cancer. Although radical radiotherapy as a single modality treatment is infrequently used for abdominal tumours it may be applied for the treatment of carcinoma of the bile duct and gall bladder, ductal carcinoma of the pancreas and lymphoma. Abdominal lymph nodes may be treated in patients with testicular cancer and in patients with primary pelvic tumours who have metastatic abdominal lymphadenopathy. The solid organs which are injured by abdominal radiotherapy are usually the liver, spleen and pancreas.

RADIATION INJURY

Incidence and susceptibility

Even with modern treatment-planning techniques, a radical course of radiotherapy will result in significant radiation exposure to adjacent normal structures. However, clinically significant pelvic radiation damage occurs in only 5–10% of patients.[1,2] Individual organs demonstrate different sensitivities, with the small bowel being most susceptible and the urinary tract, particularly the ureters, relatively tolerant. Moreover, the onset of clinical symptoms, overall severity and progression of changes vary considerably from patient to patient.

Several constitutional factors affect individual susceptibility to radiation damage:

- Hypertension, atherosclerosis and diabetes mellitus have been implicated, each acting through a mechanism of relative ischaemia[3,4]

- Localized pelvic inflammatory disorders and infection[5,6]
- Adhesions from prior surgery may cause prolonged exposure of immobilized small bowel loops within a treatment field[7]

In addition, certain treatment parameters are known to affect the risk of radiation damage:

- Total radiation dose
- Volume of irradiated tissue
- Size of radiation fractions
- Duration of therapy[8,9]
- Radiation tolerance is reduced by combination treatment with surgery and/or chemotherapy

Biological effects of radiation

The biological effect of ionizing radiation is to damage intracellular DNA, which is rendered incapable of replication, and this results in cell death. Hence, those tissues with a rapid cell turnover, such as the epithelium of the bowel and bladder, manifest radiation injury before cells which divide more slowly, for example vascular endothelium and connective tissue. Early radiation reactions stem from epithelial necrosis, whereas chronic radiation injury results from damage to vascular and stromal cells, and is the dose-limiting factor in radiotherapy.[8] Vessels of all sizes and types are affected. Changes usually affect the entire vessel wall, but always start with endothelial cell damage. Fibrin may occupy the lumen or extend out into the damaged subendothelial layers to produce fibrinoid necrosis. The presence of intraluminal thrombus reduces blood flow, with the thrombus also releasing thromboxane which leads to vascular constriction, further decreasing blood supply to the distal tissues. The vessels may show transmural inflammation, with fibrinoid necrosis and inflammation healing by fibrosis. The vessels may then not be able to withstand normal or increased local blood pressure, with the result of local aneurysm formation and vessel rupture with interstitial haemorrhage.

The vascular damage leads to ischaemia which produces a characteristic tissue fibrosis. This fibrosis is compounded by the direct effect of radiotherapy on the stromal tissues and the healing of interstitial haemorrhages which leads to further ischaemia due to an obliterative vasculopathy, and thereby initiating a vicious cycle. The ischaemia often produces tissue necrosis leading to fistula and abscess formation.[10]

Key points: biological effects of radiation

- ▪ Ionizing radiation damages intracellular DNA

- ▪ Those cells with a rapid turnover show signs of damage in the early phase post-treatment, e.g. epithelial cells

- ▪ Vascular damage occurs later and results in ischaemia which leads to fibrosis

Radiation features: patterns of disease

Clinical radiation reactions are divided into three groups, acute, subacute and chronic, depending on the time interval from start of treatment:

- • Acute reactions occur in the first 3 months
- • Subacute reactions occur from 3 months to 1 year
- • Chronic (late) effects are seen more than 1 year following therapy

However, these definitions are somewhat arbitrary and late presentation may be acute both clinically and pathologically. Patients who have a severe acute radiation reaction are more likely to progress to serious chronic radiation damage. In addition, morbidity and mortality are increased when radiation damage involves multiple organs, as occurs in 15–30% of affected patients.[11]

Although all tissues within a radiation field are susceptible to radiation damage, clinically significant changes are most frequently encountered in the gastro-intestinal and genito-urinary tracts. These post-treatment effects need to be recognized, and if possible a distinction made between treatment effect, other complications which may be superadded (e.g. infection) and residual/recurrent tumour. Accurate localization of the radiation changes is essential in evaluation of these patients.

Symptoms of chronic radiation bowel disease (RBD) occur earlier than the symptoms of radiation urinary tract disease (RUTD). There is little data on the long-term morbidity and survival of patients after surgical treatment of radiation bowel disease, but a major cause of morbidity and mortality in these patients is further radiation disease, most commonly affecting the urinary tract.[3] There is some evidence that patients with RBD have a better prognosis as far as their primary tumour is concerned[12,13] which may balance the increased mortality from radiation-induced disease.

Because of the frequent occurrence of RBD and RUTD in the same patient, we would advocate concurrent assessment of the urinary tract in patients with demonstrable bowel injury.

GASTRO-INTESTINAL SYSTEM

Postsurgical changes

Surgery to the gastro-intestinal tract can alter the appearance and position of the remaining gut, adjacent organs and tissues and result in immediate or delayed postoperative complications.

The radiographic and cross-sectional imaging appearances of postoperative complications are well documented. The complications include:

- • Abdominal wall complications, e.g. haematoma, hernias
- • Postoperative fluid collections, e.g. abscess formation, anastomotic leakages, pancreatitis
- • Bowel obstruction
- • Retained surgical foreign bodies

In oncological radiology practice computed tomography (CT) is commonly used to assess the response to adjuvant treatment, particularly chemotherapy, for gastro-intestinal tract malignancy. In this situation patients will have a baseline scan prior to treatment and then further CT examinations at defined intervals during and after treatment. The radiologist interpreting the images should be aware of modern surgical practice in relation to the malignancy under investigation and the type of operation that an individual patient has had; the latter may need recourse to the operation notes!

An illustrative example of the postoperative appearances which cause most interpretive difficulties in relation to large bowel surgery is described.

After abdominopelvic resection (APR) for rectal or anal carcinoma the bladder, seminal vesicles and to a lesser extent the base of the prostate are retracted into the rectal bed, there being a variable degree and extent of associated fibrosis. The appearances are more complicated if there has been reconstructive surgery of the perineum, for example with a myocutaneous flap.

The seminal vesicles are commonly retracted posteromedially, producing a characteristic appearance. The seminal vesicles are fixed in position due to concurrent fibrosis, the fibrosis being of variable appearance, either amorphous, band-like or as a mass (Fig. 50.1). It may not be possible on

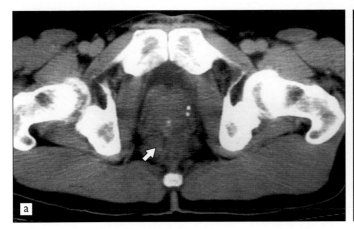

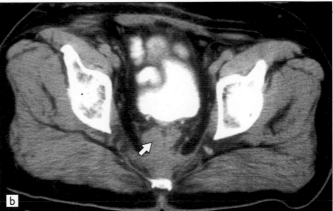

Figure 50.1. *(a) CT scan through the pelvis in a patient who has had a previous abdominopelvic resection (APR). The seminal vesicles have been retracted posteriorly into the rectal bed (right seminal vesicle arrowed). There is little fibrosis present. (b) CT scan through the pelvis in a patient who has had a previous APR and perioperative radiotherapy. The seminal vesicles (right vesicle arrowed) are retracted posteromedially and there is a large presacral soft tissue mass. This mass has been unchanged in appearance over several years. Previous biopsy had not identified tumour and the mass is not invading adjacent structures. These features indicate the mass is due to post-treatment fibrosis.*

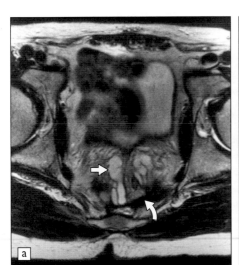

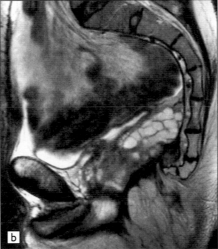

Figure 50.2. *High resolution turbo spin-echo T2-weighted MR images through the pelvis in the transaxial (a) and sagittal (b) planes in a patient who has had a previous APR. The seminal vesicles (right vesicle arrowed) have been retracted posteromedially by a band of fibrous tissue (curved arrow). On the sagittal image the base of the prostate is seen to be displaced posteroinferiorly, with the prostate and seminal vesicles being fixed to the pelvic floor. Note the bladder is also being distorted. These T2-weighted images enable discrimination between anatomical structures, bands of fibrosis and/or soft tissue 'masses'.*

the CT scan to delineate the anatomical structures and identify areas of fibrosis and these interpretive difficulties can often be resolved on magnetic resonance imaging (MRI) (Fig. 50.2). Similar interpretive difficulties occur when patients have undergone a Hartman's procedure (Fig. 50.3).

A major problem is the distinction of fibrosis from recurrent tumour. The important points to consider are:

- The morphology of the lesion
- Evidence of invasion of adjacent structures
- The MRI characteristics of the lesion on different pulse sequences
- The contrast enhancement pattern of the lesion, both on CT and MRI
- Change in the appearance of the lesion over time
- Other evidence of tumour or whether other lesions have appeared, e.g. lymphadenopathy
- The amenability of the lesion to radiologically guided biopsy

Distinction between fibrosis and recurrence may be possible on morphological grounds, especially if there is invasion of local structures. Recurrent tumour and fibrosis can both appear as a mass lesion and CT-guided biopsy is useful to distinguish between the two.

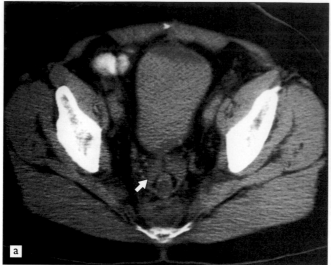

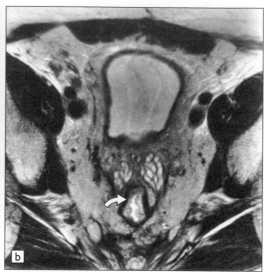

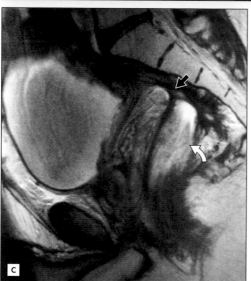

Figure 50.3. *The patient has had a Hartman's procedure, i.e. bowel has been resected and an end-colostomy fashioned. A significant portion of the rectum remains, with the proximal end having been oversewn. On the CT scan (a) the seminal vesicles (right vesicle arrowed) are displaced and distorted and lie in an anterolateral relationship to the residual rectum on MR images (curved arrow [b, c]). Amorphous, abnormal, soft tissue is present in the presacral space. The anatomy is better appreciated on the transaxial high resolution T2-weighted MR image (b). The seminal vesicles are clearly identified and are associated with bands of fibrous tissue. Layers of the rectal wall can be identified and the amorphous soft tissue in the presacral space is of low signal intensity in keeping with fibrosis. The sagittal T2-weighted MR image (c) demonstrates the full length of the remaining rectum and anal canal and the fibrous tissue which is fixing the proximal end to the sacrum (black arrow). The distorted bladder, a seminal vesicle and the prostate gland can be clearly identified.*

Several studies have reported higher specificity for MRI compared with CT in distinguishing between recurrent tumour and surgical fibrosis based on the signal intensity appearances of the lesion on T1- and T2-weighted images. Contrast enhancement patterns can also be confusing, as it is recognized that postoperative changes, including fibrosis, will continue to enhance for several years after treatment.[14] This topic is discussed further on page 989.

Monoclonal antibody labelled isotope scanning and positron emission tomography (PET) with 2-[F-18] fluoro-2-deoxy-D-glucose (18-FDG) may be of value in distinguishing fibrosis from recurrent tumour. Studies using radiolabelled monoclonal antibodies to carcinoembryonic antigen (CEA) or tumour associated glycoprotein have reported a greater sensitivity than CT in the detection of extrahepatic metastases, especially within the

pelvis, both in primary and recurrent tumour. This technique may be of most value in detecting recurrence in patients with raised CEA levels when CT is negative. However, tumour recurrence may be present with a normal CEA level. False-positive localization has been reported in up to 12% of patients and the causes include degenerative joint disease, abdominal aneurysms, postoperative adhesions and local inflammatory changes secondary to surgery or radiotherapy.[15–19]

Positron emission tomography scanning using 18-FDG has been reported to be both sensitive and specific in distinguishing recurrence from fibrous tissue and more accurate than immunoscintigraphy. However, increased uptake of 18-FDG is known to occur and persist after radiotherapy which may limit the use of this technique in patients who have received perioperative radiotherapy.[20–23]

Key points: tumour versus surgical fibrosis

- Distinction between recurrent rectal cancer and postsurgical fibrosis can be made on CT particularly if there is invasion of adjacent structures

- Recurrent tumour and fibrosis can both appear as a mass lesion and CT-guided biopsy may be required

- Magnetic resonance imaging has a higher specificity than CT in distinguishing recurrent tumour from fibrosis, but considerable overlap of signal intensity on T2-weighted images does occur

- Postcontrast enhancement patterns may be confusing

- Monoclonal antibody-labelled isotope scanning and 18-FDG-PET may also be valuable for distinguishing fibrosis from recurrent tumour following surgery

Radiotherapy changes

The liver, spleen and pancreas

Liver

Primary radiotherapy to the whole liver is uncommon, and radiation changes within the liver are usually due to the treatment of adjacent organs or structures. The changes are most commonly seen or investigated by cross-sectional imaging, usually CT.

Acute radiation toxicity occurs if the whole liver is irradiated, there being a reported 10% incidence in patients treated with a dose of 24–29 Gy over $2\frac{1}{2}$ weeks using a moving-strip technique.[24] Patients develop abdominal pain, the liver enlarges and there is ascites; these signs and symptoms develop between 2 and 6 weeks after therapy. Complete recovery may occur or there may be progression with varying degrees of hepatic insufficiency and eventual cirrhosis. The basic pathological process is the occlusion of small veins, which can progress to vessel fibrosis and subsequent tissue fibrosis.

In the acute phase following whole liver irradiation the findings on CT are of an enlarged, hypodense liver. Essentially, the liver is congested due to small hepatic venous occlusions. Following intravenous contrast medium injection, enhancement is heterogeneous and the major hepatic veins and inferior vena cava are seen to be compressed by the congested liver.

If only part of the liver has been irradiated patients are usually asymptomatic. The sequential appearances on CT can be complex. Changes can be observed 1–4 weeks after treatment is completed. The irradiated liver is hypodense with the border of the hypodense area correlating to the radiation field. Contrast enhancement may be normal or the irradiated area may enhance to a greater degree than the normal liver; this exaggerated enhancement is caused either by increased arterial flow secondary to decreased portal perfusion, which in turn is secondary to hepatic vein occlusion, or by delayed clearance of the contrast medium secondary to hepatic vein occlusion.

The chronic changes are of a loss of volume and fibrosis in the irradiated region. The density of this area may vary and can be accentuated if the unirradiated liver is fatty (Fig. 50.4).

The key feature of diagnosis is recognition of the characteristic boundaries corresponding to the radiation field. This boundary can occasionally be simulated by segmental portal and hepatic venous obstruction.

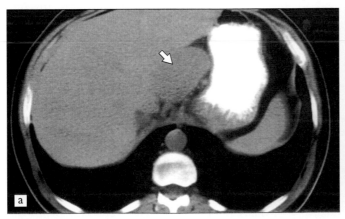
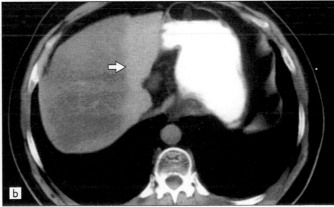

Figure 50.4. *CT scans through the liver in a patient with lymphoma. (a) Demonstrates a large nodal mass in the gastrohepatic ligament (arrowed) which was irradiated. On the post-treatment scan (b), several months following the completion of therapy, the nodal mass has decreased significantly in size. The left lobe of the liver is now smaller than on the pretreatment scan and there is a clear, straight line of demarcation between the irradiated liver and the hypodense unirradiated liver (arrowed). The unirradiated liver now shows evidence of fatty infiltration. The straight line represents the right lateral edge of the treatment field and is the hallmark of previous radiotherapy.*

Postradiation changes in the liver on MRI have been reported.[25] In the acute phase the irradiated liver is of low signal intensity on T1-weighted and high signal intensity on T2-weighted images, reflecting the increased water content due to liver congestion. The late changes of fibrosis are characterized by low signal intensity on both T1- and T2-weighted images. As with CT, knowing that the patient has been previously irradiated, and recognizing the characteristic border configuration are the keys to diagnosis.

Spleen

The spleen may be included in the radiation fields for treatment of lymphoma. Radiotherapy is used to reduce splenic size in patients with hypersplenism and leukaemia. The effects of splenic radiation are usually not clinically significant, although functional hyposplenism has been reported in patients irradiated as part of the treatment of lymphoma, and some patients have developed fulminant pneumococcal sepsis.[26,27]

The spleen is very radiosensitive and a dose of 4–8 Gy will destroy the lymphoid tissue within hours, with phagocytosis occurring rapidly and clearing the dead cells within 24 hours. Regeneration of lymphoid tissue occurs within a week. Higher doses (35–40 Gy over 5–6 weeks) may result in fibrosis and atrophy.

Pancreas

The pathological changes in the irradiated pancreas are similar to those of chronic pancreatitis. The difficulty arises as there are often changes of chronic pancreatitis in patients with carcinoma pancreas and therefore it may not be possible to determine if the changes are disease or treatment-related.

The acinar epithelium is more radiosensitive than the islet cells and necrosis and fibrosis are the features of radiation damage.[28]

Imaging findings are either non-specific or similar to those of chronic pancreatitis.

Stomach, duodenum, small and large bowel

Although the small bowel is more radiosensitive than the large bowel, radiation damage is seen most commonly in the rectum and rectosigmoid region. This is because the rectum and rectosigmoid are fixed in position and are included in whole, or in part in the radiation fields in patients treated for carcinoma of the rectum, cervix, bladder and prostate. The radiation dose to the small bowel is less than to the rectum and rectosigmoid when these cancers are treated. The small bowel is not fixed, unless there are adhesions, and undergoes peristalsis. Additional measures can be undertaken to reduce the dose to small bowel by mobilizing the omentum into the pelvis, or inserting an absorbable synthetic mesh into the pelvis and thereby moving the small bowel out of the radiation field. The ileum is the most frequently damaged portion of the small bowel. Acute bowel reactions are due to epithelial cell damage, with this damage being reversible and with the mucosa becoming histologically normal within a few weeks of completion of therapy.

As indicated, chronic (late) radiation damage is due to the combined effect of radiation on the blood vessels and connective tissue. In the investigation of late radiation bowel disease awareness of the possibility of the diagnosis, and clinical assessment of the patient are of paramount importance. Investigations are directed towards:

- Assessing the general state of the patient
- The accurate localization of the radiation change
- The differentiation between radiation change and recurrent tumour

Localization of radiation changes requires endoscopic examination and/or diagnostic imaging.

Stomach and duodenum

Radiotherapy to retroperitoneal lymphadenopathy and for carcinoma pancreas can produce damage to the stomach and duodenum.

In the stomach two radiological patterns are seen. One is of a fixed narrowing and deformity of the antrum and pylorus which can lead to outlet obstruction and the appearances being similar to primary gastric carcinoma. The second is of ulceration similar to that seen in benign peptic ulcer disease but with the ulcers being resistant to medical treatment.

Changes in the duodenum include ulceration, thickening of the mucosal folds and stricture formation.

Small bowel

The patient previously treated for carcinoma of the cervix with radiotherapy, who presents with an acute distal small bowel obstruction and no clinical evidence of pelvic recurrence, is more likely to have radiation disease than tumour as the cause of her symptoms. If the patient is being treated by a surgeon experienced in these problems then plain abdominal radiographs may be sufficient for management and the decision to perform a laparotomy.

Patients who have chronic symptoms of abdominal pain, diarrhoea, malabsorption or intermittent episodes of subacute obstruction require barium studies — ideally a small bowel enema.[29] Particular attention should be paid to small bowel loops within the pelvis and the terminal ileum. One of the earliest changes of radiation damage is fixity of the loops within the pelvis and this can be overlooked unless they are palpated and compressed whilst being assessed fluoroscopically.

Changes detected on barium studies only occur in small bowel that has been within the radiotherapy field. Several radiological features have been described:[7,30–32]

- Mucosal abnormalities
- Bowel loop fixation, separation, angulation
- Reduction in motility
- Mesenteric fibrosis
- Fistulae

The mucosal folds become thickened and straightened so that the valvulae conniventes become more prominent and mucosal nodular filling defects or 'thumb printing' may be seen and are attributed to oedema. Mucosal ulceration, which may be evident microscopically, is rarely seen radiologically. The bowel loops can become fixed and angulated and separated due to wall thickening (Fig. 50.5). These changes are associated with reduced peristalsis and pooling of barium within the loops. Stenosis is usually a late feature and may be overlooked if the adjacent bowel is not adequately distended. Associated mesenteric fibrosis may cause traction on bowel loops and produce appearances similar to those seen in carcinoid tumours. Fistulae occur and these may require a more tailored examination to assess their extent (see below). No individual feature is specific for radiation damage, and neoplasia, inflammatory bowel disease and infection can all produce these signs. A relevant clinical history and associated changes in the large bowel and/or genito-urinary tract are important pointers to radiation damage.

Changes in the small bowel can be identified on cross-sectional imaging and include altered calibre, variations in wall thickness and diameter of the lumen, abnormal angulations, fistula formation and the presence of ascites (Fig. 50.6).

The large bowel

Following pelvic radiotherapy, damage to the large bowel is essentially confined to the rectum and sigmoid colon. During and immediately after treatment it is usual for patients to have a mild rectal reaction which settles spontaneously. In patients with previous inflammatory bowel disease or diverticular disease an acute exacerbation may occur, as may peritonitis due to an exacerbation of gynaecological inflammatory disease. Bowel perforation is extremely uncommon at this time. After 6 months the main symptoms of radiation damage are rectal bleeding, anal or perineal pain, abdominal pain or symptoms of chronic perforation with abscess formation or fistulae.

Radiological features of large bowel radiation damage include:

- Spasm and strictures
- Mucosal abnormalities
- Bowel fixation
- Widening of presacral space

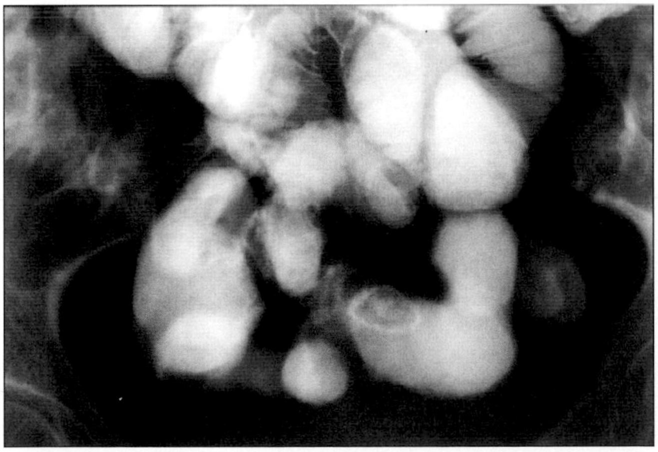

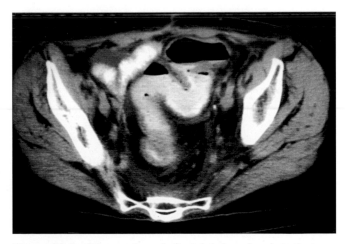

Figure 50.5. *Small bowel enema in a female patient previously treated by radiotherapy for carcinoma of the cervix. The distal ileum is abnormal, with a variation in calibre of the barium filled loops. These also demonstrate abnormal angulation because they are fixed within the pelvis and there is also separation of several of the loops, due to wall thickening and fixation.*

Figure 50.6. *CT scan through the pelvis in a female patient who has had previous radiotherapy. The distal ileal loop in the right iliac fossa is tethered/fixed, which is causing an acute angulation in the loop. The valvulae conniventes are irregularly thickened and there is a small amount of ascites lying anterior to the loop. The sigmoid colon is abnormal, being dilated and has an irregularly thickened wall. In addition, there is soft tissue stranding in the pelvic fat and a presacral soft tissue band. All these findings are due to previous radiotherapy.*

Radiological investigation is usually by double contrast barium enema (DCBE) unless there are fistulae present when the examination will need to be tailored. The DCBE usually underestimates the extent of disease when compared with surgical findings. The earliest sign is spasm but this is a non-specific finding and can be confused with a postradiation stricture. Therefore, the routine use of a smooth muscle relaxant is recommended when assessing these patients.[33] The commonest abnormality is a stricture which is typically smooth and tapered. Strictures usually involve the mid-sigmoid colon or upper rectum and may be multiple or contain more than one area of narrowing (Fig. 50.7). Some of the lesions have a configuration where there is narrowing over a distance of several centimetres but within which there is a much shorter segment of more severe stenosis (Fig. 50.8).[32] These appearances are probably related to a non-uniform radiation dose to the bowel. Short strictures have been described, with an abrupt transition to normal-calibre bowel and these may cause problems in differential diagnosis.

Characteristically the mucosal pattern in the affected segment is effaced, producing a smooth, featureless appearance. Mucosal irregularity can occur (Fig. 50.7b) with either fine surface ulceration, deep focal ulcers or generalized mucosal thickening and irregularity producing a 'cobble stone' pattern. Narrowing may occur without alteration of the mucosal or haustral pattern. Fixity of the large bowel occurs but is more difficult to appreciate than in the small bowel and may only be evident on repeat examination. Extrinsic compression from collections as a result of previous perforation is an uncommon finding. A more common extrinsic change is widening of the presacral space. This is due to traction on the rectum as a result of peri-pararectal fibrosis, but again is a non-specific sign occurring in several conditions including inflammatory bowel disease, neoplasia, abscess formation and obesity.

The appearances on CT of radiation changes in the pelvis are well documented, particularly in relation to the perirectal tissues. Changes can also be recognized in the bowel (Figs 50.6a and 50.9a, b).[34,35] The first evidence of radiotherapy change in the rectum on MR images is an increase in signal intensity of the submucosa and inner (circular) muscle layer on T2-weighted images with the outer muscle layer retaining its normal low signal intensity. With progression of radiation damage the rectal wall becomes thicker (greater than 6 mm in the distended state) and the outer muscle layer demonstrates high signal intensity on T2-weighted images, with consequent loss of differentiation between the different layers of the rectal wall. After intravenous gadolinium-DTPA administration rectal tissue enhances but there is no distinction between the component layers. The perirectal fascia becomes thickened, measuring greater than 3 mm at the S4/5 vertebral level, and the presacral space, which normally has a maximum diameter of less than 1.5 cm at the S4/5 vertebral level, shows increased width. The space may be occupied by fat, with or without areas of fibrosis, or fluid.

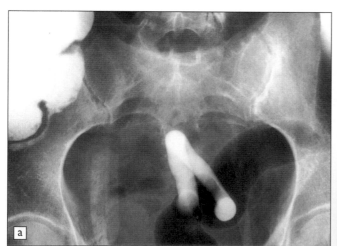

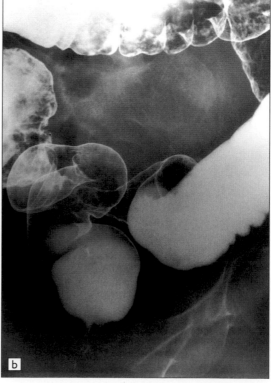

Figure 50.7. *(a) Hypotonic barium enema in a patient treated for carcinoma of the cervix by radiotherapy. There is a long segment, barium filled, radiation stricture of the sigmoid colon. This is of uniform calibre with a tapered transition to normal calibre bowel at either end. The stricture has a smooth featureless inner wall. (b) A patient who has also been treated for carcinoma of the cervix by radiotherapy. The distal sigmoid radiation stricture is shorter and there is mucosal irregularity. The metal clip superimposed on the rectum lies within the vaginal vault.*

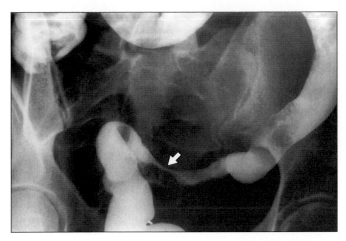

Figure 50.8. *Barium enema demonstrating a variable calibre stricture in the sigmoid colon. Overall there is a long segment stricture, within which there is a short segment, very tight stricture (arrowed). This area of the sigmoid colon received a greater dose than the more proximal sigmoid stricture.*

Fistulae

The ischaemic nature of late radiation bowel disease can lead to necrosis of the bowel wall with fistulation. The common fistula is from the rectum to the vagina, but colovesical, colocolic or colo-enteric fistulae occur. The bowel can communicate with skin, either on the anterior abdominal wall or perineum. Complex fistulae occur with involvement of bowel, bladder and vagina essentially producing an iatrogenic 'cloaca'.

The diagnosis is usually clinical with the patient often requiring an examination under anaesthesia and biopsy to determine if the fistula is due to recurrent tumour or radiation disease alone.

Key points: radiation injury to bowel

- ▪ Acute bowel reaction to radiotherapy is frequently reversible

- ▪ Chronic radiation damage is frequently irreversible

- ▪ Radiological signs include mucosal abnormalities, bowel wall thickening, strictures, intestinal obstruction and fistulae

- ▪ Widening of the presacral space and thickening of the perirectal fascia is seen following pelvic irradiation

- ▪ Barium studies show characteristic features of radiation damage but CT is also valuable for demonstrating changes in the bowel wall, mesentery and perirectal tissues

- ▪ Magnetic resonance imaging may also demonstrate radiation damage to the bowel wall, and adjacent tissues and provides a non-invasive method of investigating fistulae

The radiological demonstration of the fistula/ae requires a tailored examination, with the majority of fistulae being defined by using a catheter and contrast technique (Fig. 50.10).

Magnetic resonance imaging enables fistulae to be defined in a non-invasive manner (Fig. 50.11). Magnetic resonance imaging studies of fistulae have used a variety of pulse sequences, most commonly spin-echo T1- and T2-weighted, fat-suppressed spin-echo T2-weighted and short tau inversion recovery (STIR) sequences. Gadolinium-DTPA

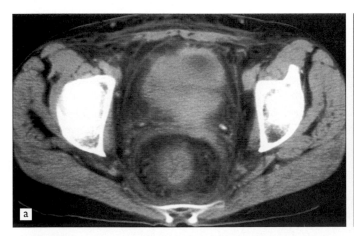

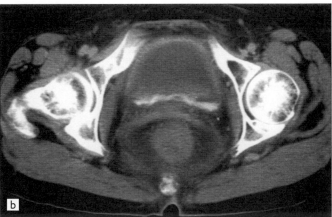

Figure 50.9. *CT scans through the pelvis in a patient who has received pelvic radiotherapy. (a) There is extensive soft tissue stranding in the perirectal space, together with thickening of the perirectal fascia. Oedema is present in the anterior abdominal* wall and there is a general increase in density of the pelvic fat. *(b) At this level of the bladder contrast medium outlines the mucosal thickening, and irregularity on the posterior bladder wall. These are all characteristic effects of radiotherapy.*

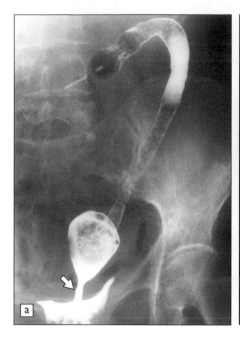
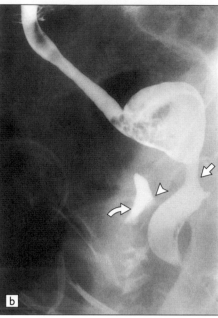

Figure 50.10. *Barium enema. The left hemicolon has been defunctioned and an antegrade barium enema performed via a Foley catheter. The patient has had previous pelvic radiotherapy for carcinoma of the cervix. (a, b) There is a radiation stricture in the rectum (arrow) and a fistula between the rectum and vagina. Contrast is present in the vagina (curved arrow) and a small fistulous tract (arrowhead) can be identified.*

has been used in conventional and dynamic mode and MR fistulography has been undertaken with the installation of saline or contrast medium into the fistulous tract.[36–39]

GENITO-URINARY SYSTEM

Surgery, radiotherapy and chemotherapy may all affect the genito-urinary system, producing transient or permanent effects which may occasionally lead to progressive organ damage. When more than one form of treatment is used, for example surgery and radiotherapy in cervical cancer, morbidity may be further increased.[41]

Treatment changes must be distinguished from residual/recurrent tumour or infection since each has a different clinical management and prognosis. While postsurgical effects are usually readily apparent, radiotherapy change can cause diagnostic difficulty. Chemotherapy may give rise to severe and even life-threatening acute complications or may produce more insidious long-term damage, for example to fertility. Both chemotherapy and radiotherapy are associated with an increased risk of second neoplasms.

Postsurgical changes

The effects of radical surgery and its complications are usually recognizable on cross-sectional imaging. Therefore in the genito-urinary tract, nephro-ureterectomy, cystectomy and urinary diversion are readily identified. However, other procedures may be more confusing, for example bladder augmentation or ureteric re-implantation with a psoas hitch, and auxiliary procedures,

for example omental transposition, can cause diagnostic difficulties. The most commonly encountered postsurgical appearances are discussed below.

Transurethral prostatic resection

In male patients transurethral prostatic resection results in an obvious urine-filled cavity in the position of the prostatic urethra. The bladder base is re-anastomosed to the membranous urethra during radical prostatectomy (Fig. 50.12) and postsurgical strictures occur at this level. After orchidectomy there are easily recognizable changes in the ipsilateral groin but a potential diagnostic problem is a swollen, retracted spermatic cord or thrombosed gonadal vein which may mimic pelvic side wall lymphadenopathy.

Hysterectomy

Most gynaecological procedures are easily discernible. After total hysterectomy and bilateral salpingo-oophorectomy there are characteristic appearances at the vaginal vault and often on the pelvic side walls. The residual vagina is oversewn and this results in a flattened central portion and sutured fornices which are bulbous but symmetrical. During surgery the round ligaments are divided and, in the early postoperative period, small bilateral pelvic side wall 'masses' may be seen continuous with the residual round ligaments. These can occasionally be mistaken for residual tumour masses, especially if they are asymmetrical (Fig. 50.13).[42] The nature of these lesions is unknown; they may possibly represent residual haematomata, but they usually decrease in size or disappear on follow-up imaging.

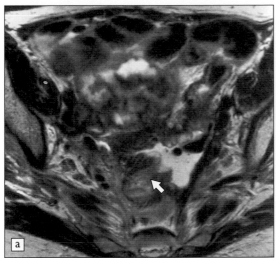

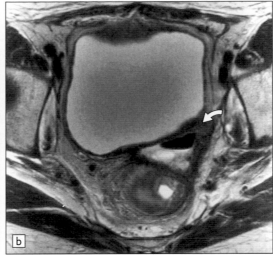

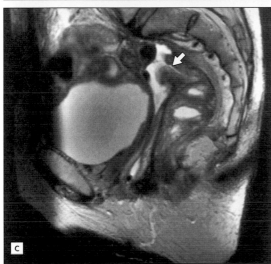

Figure 50.11. *High resolution turbo spin-echo T2-weighted MR images in the axial (a, b) and sagittal (c) planes. The patient has recurrent cervical tumour on the left side of the pelvis involving the bladder (curved arrow) and pelvic side wall. The recurrent tumour is associated with a cavity containing fluid and air and there is a fistulous tract between the rectosigmoid junction through the recurrent tumour to the vault of the vagina. The communication with the large bowel is clearly seen on the transaxial and sagittal images (a, c) (straight arrow). The vagina is clearly defined on the sagittal image, with a small amount of air being present at the introitus.*

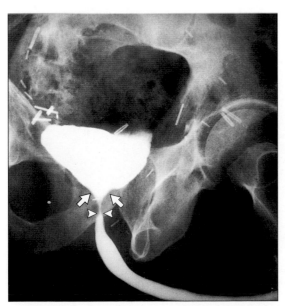

Figure 50.12. *Micturating cystourethrogram in a patient who has undergone a radical prostatectomy. The bladder base (arrows) is low, lying behind the symphysis pubis due to its anastomosis with the membranous urethra. There is mild narrowing at the anastomotic site (arrowheads). Multiple surgical clips are present in the pelvis from the associated lymph node dissection.*

After subtotal hysterectomy the cervix remains in situ and may be mistaken for a tumour mass if there is inadequate clinical information. Similarly, transposed ovaries can cause diagnostic problems. One or both ovaries may be repositioned in the iliac fossae after a modified radical hysterectomy, where their size and attenuation or signal intensity are helpful imaging features (Fig. 50.14).[43,44]

Lymph node dissection

Lymphocoeles are a recognized complication of radical lymph node dissection, particularly when a wholly retroperitoneal surgical approach is used. They are typically unilocular, thin-walled fluid masses and they lie on the pelvic side walls, immediately adjacent to the vessels, especially the external iliac arteries and veins (Fig. 50.15).[45,46]

Pelvic clearance

For unresponsive or recurrent gynaecological malignancies some women undergo pelvic clearance,[47] of which there are three types:

- Anterior pelvic clearance involves removal of the bladder and urethra together with a radical hysterectomy and removal of pelvic ligaments and connective tissue
- Posterior pelvic clearance is when the rectum is removed with the female sex organs
- Total pelvic clearance, or exenteration, occurs when every central pelvic organ is removed together with adjacent supporting and connective tissue

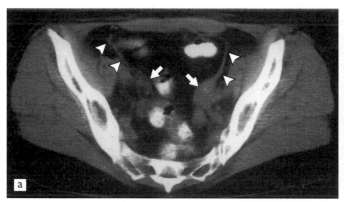
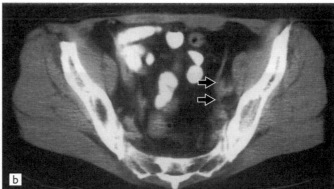

Figure 50.13. *Axial CT scans through the pelvis in the early postoperative period (a) demonstrating bilateral pelvic side wall masses (larrow) continuous with the round ligaments (arrowheads). The left-sided lesion has markedly decreased in size on a follow-up scan 6 months later (black arrows in b) and the right has resolved.*

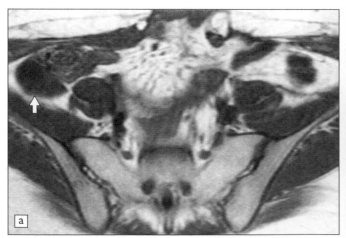
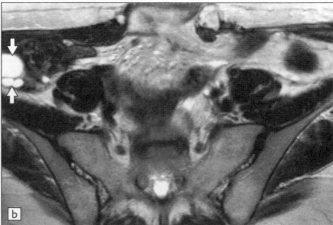

Figure 50.14. *Axial T1-weighted (a) and T2-weighted (b) MR images showing a transposed ovary (arrows) in the right iliac fossa. The ovary is of intermediate to low signal intensity on T1-weighted image and the follicular cysts are of high signal intensity on the T2-weighted image.*

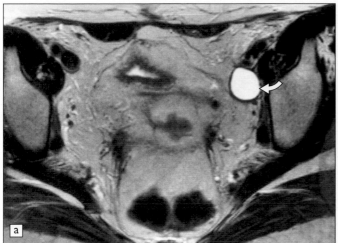

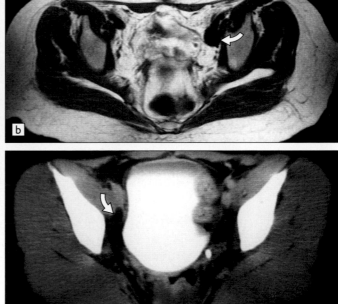

Figure 50.15. *Lymphocoeles on MRI and CT (arrows). Lymphocoeles are of low signal intensity on T1-weighted images (b) and high signal intensity on T2-weighted images (a). On CT they are of uniform low attenuation (c). Most lymphocoeles are unilocular and they are typically located adjacent to the external iliac vessels.*

The effect of massive surgery, often with prior or subsequent radiotherapy, is to cause marked symmetrical fibrosis, particularly in the posterior pelvis, which may be seen on CT but is better evaluated by sagittal MR imaging (Fig. 50.16).

Effects of chemotherapy
Kidneys
Chemotherapy is often nephrotoxic and patients may be investigated after they develop renal failure. Usually ultrasound is performed to exclude any renal obstruction, at which time the kidneys may be enlarged, have increased cortical echogenicity or lack the normal corticomedullary differentiation. Acute drug-induced nephrotoxicity is usually temporary and responds to withdrawal of the responsible drug together with supportive care.

The immunosuppressive effect of cytotoxic drugs may result in renal infection with an increased risk of atypical organisms or fungi, and occasionally thrombocytopenic patients present with haematuria. When there is a large tumour burden, cytotoxic chemotherapy may cause hyperuricaemia which can produce renal failure even when patients have received allopurinol.

Bladder
Haemorrhagic cystitis is a dramatic and sometimes life-threatening complication of cyclophosphamide or ifosfamide treatment. It manifests as a grossly thickened bladder with large intravesical clots and ultrasound is often adequate to confirm the clinical impression (Fig. 50.17).

Fertility
The other principal effect of chemotherapy is on fertility and this depends on the patient's age and the chemotherapeutic agent or regimen used.[48] Children are relatively resistant[48] but in adult females there is age-dependent sensitivity to alkylating agents such as cyclophosphamide.[49] In men, the type of drug and the dose determine the immediate effect on fertility and any potential for long-term recovery.

Radiation therapy change
Kidney
The kidney is radiosensitive and is often the dose-limiting organ during treatment of abdominal malignancies, with the risk of nephrotoxicity increased by prior or concurrent chemotherapy. Radiation-induced nephropathy may appear from months to years after treatment and there is an inverse relationship between the interval and the renal dose.[50] Providing one normally functioning kidney is excluded from the radiation field radiation nephropathy will not develop, but malignant hypertension may occur due to the injured kidney overproducing renin, and in these circumstances, the radiation-damaged kidney may have to be removed. Radiologically, renal compromise results in small, poorly functioning or non-functioning, non-obstructed kidneys.

Ureter
Radiation-induced ureteric injury is uncommon, occurring in less than 5% of those sustaining complications from radiotherapy.[51] It results in stricture formation, or vesico-ureteric

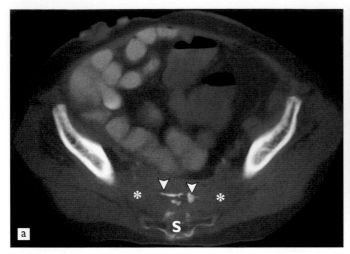

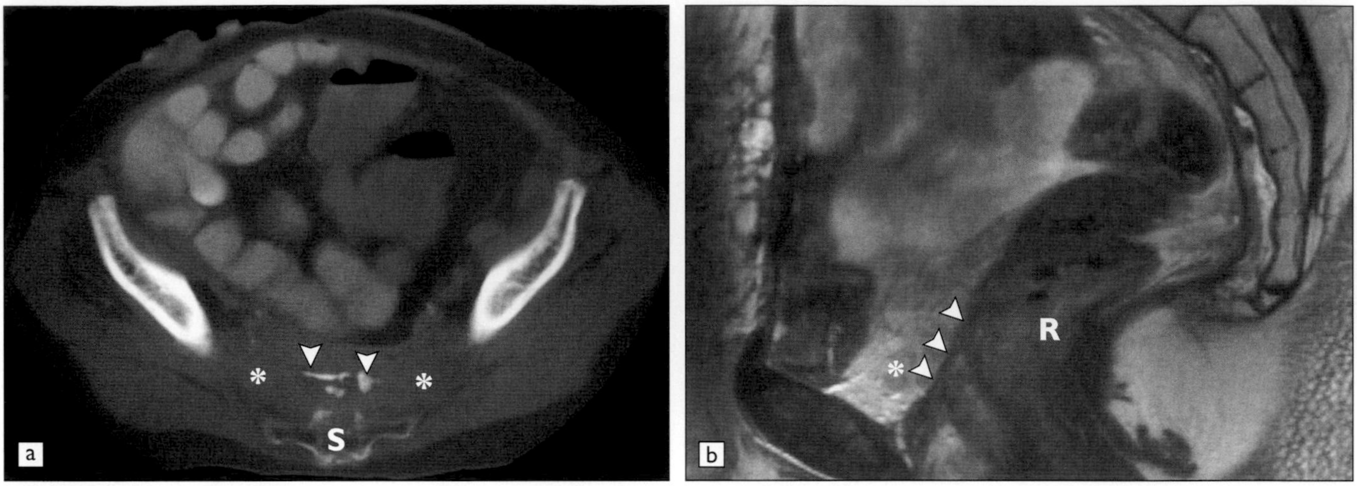

Figure 50.16. *Pelvic clearance: (a) CT scan through the pelvis (on bone settings) demonstrating a symmetrical soft tissue band in the presacral space (asterisks) with associated dystrophic calcification (arrowheads) as a consequence of pelvic surgery and radiotherapy. Note the reduced density of the sacrum (S), a recognized sequel to pelvic radiotherapy; (b)*

sagittal T2-weighted MR image after an anterior pelvic clearance. The anterior pelvis is fat-filled (asterisk) and there is a linear band of fibrous tissue (arrowheads) between the pubic symphysis and the anorectum (R). Postsurgical change is also present in the subcutaneous tissues of the anterior abdominal wall.

reflux secondary to bladder wall fibrosis and vesico-ureteric incompetence. Strictures are more serious since they may cause renal failure but remain clinically silent. They occur most frequently in the distal ureter immediately above the vesico-ureteric junction, extending proximally over a variable length (Fig. 50.18).[32] High strictures have also been demonstrated where the pelvic ureters cross anterior to the iliac vessels.[32] Radiation strictures typically have a smooth

tapering distal margin but the appearances are non-specific and may be seen in patients with tumour recurrence. In some patients strictures are adequately visualized on intravenous urography but in others it may be necessary to perform antegrade pyelography. Isotope renography is valuable since sequential studies will often reveal a deterioration in renal performance before clinical or biochemical abnormalities occur (Fig. 50.18).[52]

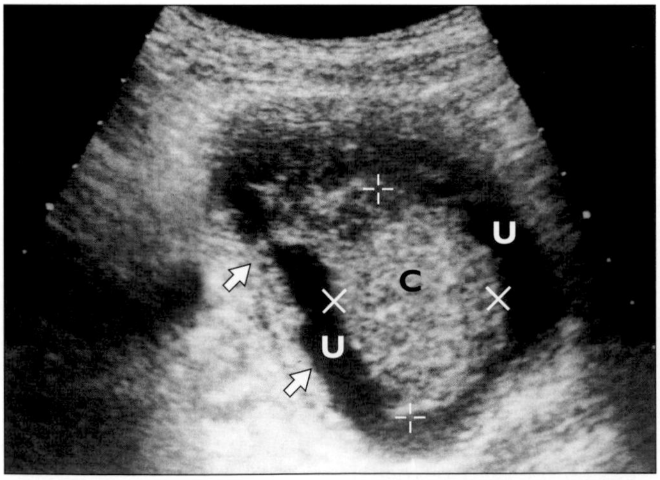

Bladder

The bladder is the most radiation-sensitive organ in the urinary tract[53] and radiation bladder injury may occur in up to 20% of patients, half of whom go on to suffer severe long-term effects.[2] In the acute phase mucosal oedema, haemorrhage and necrosis may produce cystitis and haematuria. With time, fibrosis develops resulting in a small volume non-distensible bladder causing symptoms of frequency and incontinence. Mucosal telangiectasia and ulceration may cause troublesome haematuria.

Ultrasound, CT and MRI may all demonstrate radiation-induced acute mucosal changes and more chronic posterior bladder wall thickening (Fig. 50.19).[34] Adjacent perivesical fibrosis can be identified on CT and MRI. In addition, MRI can identify a spectrum of radiation change corresponding to the severity of clinical symptoms. The earliest abnormality is high signal intensity mucosa on T1- and T2-weighted images probably reflecting haemorrhagic oedema. Initially this may be localized to the posterior wall and trigone[54] but eventually the entire bladder mucosa may become involved. More severe radiation effect causes T2-weighted high signal

Figure 50.17. *Haemorrhagic cystitis. Longitudinal ultrasound examination demonstrating thickened bladder wall (arrows) with a small amount of urine (U) identified in the periphery and a large central hyperechoic clot (C), between the measurement calipers.*

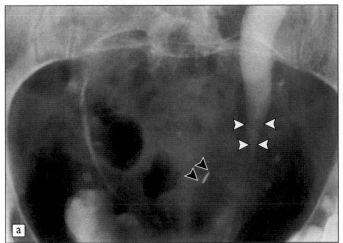

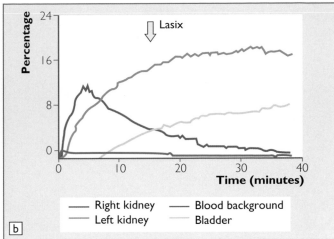

Figure 50.18. *Postradiotherapy ureteric strictures. (a) Fifty-minute film from an intravenous urogram demonstrating a normal right distal ureter and a left hydro-ureter with a smoothly tapering stricture (arrowheads) immediately above the vesico-ureteric junction. Note the marker seed in the cervix* *(black arrowheads); (b) technetium-99m MAG 3 renogram. There is normal uptake and excretion of radionuclide by the right kidney. There is an obstructive curve to the left kidney which does not respond to intravenous Lasix. The patient had developed a radiation stricture of the lower left ureter.*

intensity of the outer bladder wall, increased radial diameter of the wall and poor distensibility. Intravenous gadolinium DTPA may reveal enhancement of the bladder mucosa and patchy or diffuse enhancement of the outer wall, sometimes with variations in signal intensity between different layers of the bladder wall to give a banded or lamellated appearance.[55] With extreme radiation toxicity, fistula formation may occur between the bladder and vagina or bowel and, while the diagnosis is usually clinical, radiographic contrast studies may be required for complex fistulae. Occasionally, cross-sectional imaging reveals hitherto unsuspected fistulae.

Prostate and seminal vesicles

Radiotherapy affects the prostate and seminal vesicles in a similar fashion to any other irradiated organ. In the long term there is increased interstitial fibrosis within normal tissues secondary to an endarteritis obliterans and as a result the prostate atrophies and may develop dystrophic calcification visible on plain films or CT. On MR images the peripheral zone of the gland becomes of a uniformly low signal intensity on T2-weighted images (Fig. 50.20)[54,56], making the diagnosis of recurrent tumour difficult, since most prostate tumours are also low signal intensity on T2-weighted images. The seminal vesicles shrink and develop uniform low signal intensity on T2-weighted sequences[54] (Fig. 50.20). The male urethra is sensitive to radiotherapy especially after prior transurethral resection of the prostate.[57] In severe cases stricture formation occurs, usually in the prostatic or membranous portion of the urethra.

Testis

The adult male testis is an extremely radiosensitive organ and a dose of as little as 0.15 Gy can cause a significant drop in the sperm count[58] and, where possible, the treatment fields are designed to keep testicular doses to an absolute minimum.

Gynaecological organs

In women of child-bearing age, radiotherapy causes uterine atrophy, best appreciated on T2-weighted MR images, where the normal zonal anatomy is lost and the myometrium becomes of uniform low signal intensity often with reduction in width of the endometrium (Fig. 50.21).[59] Rarely, the size of the uterus may be increased when a radiation-induced cervical stenosis causes obstruction with fluid accumulation within the endometrial cavity.[60,61] The vagina also develops low signal intensity of its wall in the chronic phase after radiotherapy, although in the first 3 months after treatment, high signal intensity may be seen within the vaginal submucosa on T2-weighted images and there may be enhancement after gadolinium-DTPA.

After radiation therapy the ovaries shrink, lose their follicular cysts and eventually become fibrotic. The effect of radiation on ovarian function depends on the radiation dose and the age of the patient. Relatively small doses can induce the menopause in middle-aged women, whereas young women require a higher total exposure to induce ovarian failure. Premenarchal girls treated with high doses to the abdomen (in the order of 20 to 30 Gy) will experience premature ovarian failure[62] and the uterus may remain of infantile proportions (Fig. 50.22). In the long term, radiotherapy causes decreased

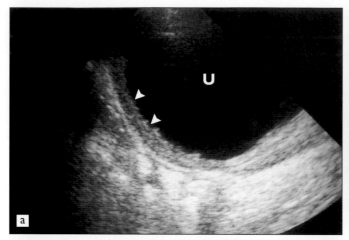

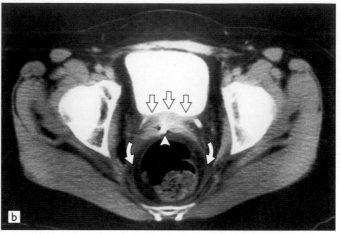

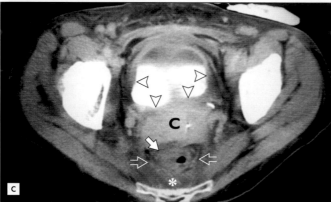

Figure 50.19. *Radiation therapy effect on the bladder. (a) Ultrasound examination demonstrating diffuse mucosal thickening (arrowheads) in the acute phase after radiotherapy treatment on this longitudinal ultrasound scan. Urine (U); (b) contrast-enhanced CT scan demonstrating focal bladder wall thickening in the region of the trigone (straight arrows) in a patient treated for cervical cancer in whom a marker seed is present (arrowhead). Symmetrical thickening of the perirectal fascia is present (curved arrows) and there is stranding within the perivesical fat; (c) contrast-enhanced CT scan demonstrating severe generalized bladder wall thickening (arrowheads) in a patient treated for cervical cancer [a marker seed is present within the cervix (C)]. There is also evidence of generalized radiotherapy change within the pelvis consisting of rectal wall thickening (arrow) and also perirectal thickening (open arrows) with an asymmetrical soft tissue band in a presacral space (asterisk); (d) axial T1-weighted MR image demonstrating high signal intensity bladder mucosa due to haemorrhagic oedema (arrowheads) with a thickened outer bladder wall (arrows) and perivesical stranding anteriorly; (e) large vesicovaginal fistula (arrow) is shown in a patient who has already undergone urinary diversion and colostomy formation.*

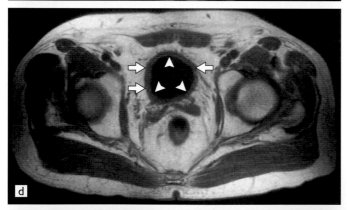

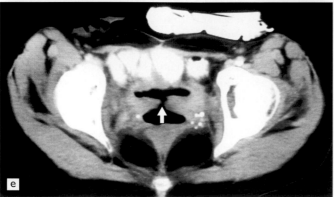

distensibility of the uterus and abdominopelvic connective tissue which probably contributes to the high incidence of miscarriage and premature birth.

RADIATION INJURY VERSUS RESIDUAL/RECURRENT TUMOUR WITHIN THE PELVIS

Clinical assessment of the pelvis may be difficult after surgery or radiotherapy and a major problem in oncological practice is distinguishing residual or recurrent tumour from radiation effect. Computed tomography relies on the presence of a discrete mass, thus more infiltrative tumour recurrences can be indistinguishable from radiation therapy effect (Fig. 50.23). Theoretically, MRI is at an advantage in identifying tumour

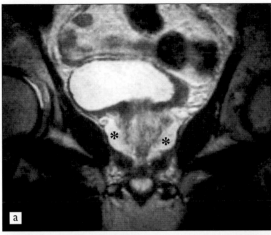

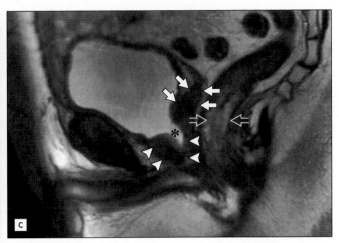

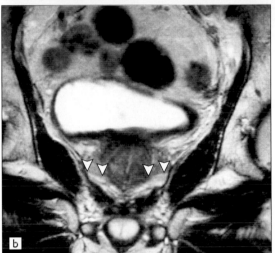

Figure 50.20. *Effects of radiotherapy on the prostate and seminal vesicles. Coronal T2-weighted MR images (a) before treatment and (b) after treatment for a bladder tumour. The normal high signal intensity of the prostate peripheral zone is apparent in (a) (asterisks) but in (b) there is a well demarcated low signal intensity component to the superior aspect of the peripheral zone bilaterally (arrowheads) which corresponds to the inferior margin of the radiotherapy field used to treat the basal bladder lesion; (c) sagittal T2-weighted MR image demonstrating uniform low signal intensity of the prostate (arrowheads) and seminal vesicle (arrows) after radiotherapy for prostate cancer. There is also abnormally thickened high signal intensity mucosa in the lower rectum and anus (open arrows) due to radiotherapy. The patient had undergone a prior transurethral resection of the prostate (TURP) and the urine-filled TURP cavity is seen (asterisk).*

since it offers superior tissue contrast resolution compared with CT or ultrasound. In some instances the signal intensity characteristics of the lesion can be helpful,[55,63,64] for example fibrosis demonstrates low signal intensity on T1- and T2-weighted images and shows little, if any, enhancement after intravenous gadolinium-DTPA. On the other hand, tumour demonstrates intermediate signal intensity on T1-weighted images, high signal intensity on T2-weighted images and enhances after injection of gadolinium DTPA.[64–66] However, there is considerable overlap so that small volumes of tumour may be overlooked within a large area of fibrosis, or desmoplastic tumours (for example breast, carcinoid and rectal tumours) may have similar signal intensity characteristics to fibrosis. In addition, radiation therapy effect, with oedema, inflammation and capillary neovascularity, may have MRI features indistinguishable from tumour.[55] Therefore in some patients it is necessary to adopt a wait-and-see approach, rescanning them at regular intervals to identify disease outside the treatment field or the appearance of a mass lesion. In some cases, percutaneous image-guided biopsy may be valu-

able. Where available, PET and monoclonal antibody imaging may have a role in detecting disease recurrence.[67–69] Recently, quantitative dynamic MRI scanning has shown promise in improving the specificity of contrast-enhanced MRI in distinguishing fibrosis from recurrence in rectal cancer.[70]

ABDOMINOPELVIC MUSCULOSKELETAL SYSTEM

Of the cancer treatment modalities, radiotherapy is principally responsible for treatment-induced injury of the normal musculoskeletal tissues, nerves and blood vessels of the abdomen and pelvis.

Bone

This topic is discussed in detail in Chapter 49 but a few points relevant to the pelvis are made here. After therapeutic radiation there is damage to both the cellular elements of bone marrow and the cortical and trabecular bone. Following pelvic irradiation, changes on MR imaging of the

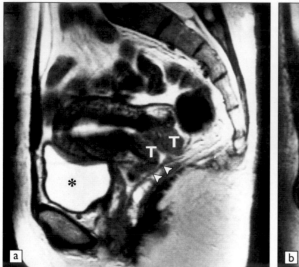
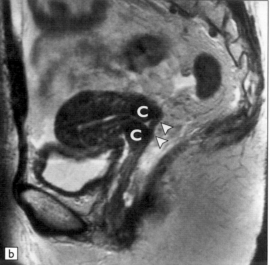

Figure 50.21. *Effects of radiotherapy on the cervix. (a) Sagittal T2-weighted MR image demonstrating a cervical tumour (T) affecting both the anterior and posterior lip. The normal zonal anatomy of the uterus is appreciated and the vaginal wall is of intermediate signal intensity (arrowheads). Urinary bladder (asterisk); (b) 8 months after treatment there has been reconstitution of the low signal intensity cervix (C) but this affects all components of the cervix and in addition there has been a decrease in size of the uterine body which is now of generalized low signal intensity. The endometrial stripe is thinned. The vaginal wall is also of low signal intensity (arrowheads).*

lumbar spine and sacrum may be seen as early as the second week after radiotherapy when STIR images demonstrate an increase in signal intensity of the bone marrow due to oedema and cell necrosis.[71] The boundary of these changes corresponds closely with the radiation field.[72] Progressive ischaemia affects the cortical and trabecular bone, rendering it vulnerable to fracture, infection and impaired healing. The appearances on plain radiographs reflect the initial resorption of dead bone and necrotic tissue followed by the deposition of new bone on unresorbed trabeculae, a process described as creeping substitution.[73] A similar mixed lytic and sclerotic appearance is also seen on CT, but the superior contrast resolution of CT allows more subtle change to be appreciated, particularly in the pelvic bones.

Key points: effects of treatment on the genito-urinary system

- Lymphocoeles are common following radical lymph node dissection and are readily recognized as unilocular thin walled fluid-filled lesions

- Chemotherapy is often nephrotoxic, ultrasound is useful for excluding renal obstruction

- The kidney is radiosensitive and is often the dose-limiting organ during treatment of abdominal malignancy

- The bladder is the most radiation-sensitive organ in the urinary tract, bladder injury occurring in up to 20% of patients following pelvic radiation

- Radiation induces fibrosis of the bladder wall which becomes thickened

- The gynaecological organs, prostate and seminal vesicles show fibrosis and atrophy following radiotherapy

- Radiation fibrosis and tumour may have indistinguishable features on MRI even following contrast enhancement

- Semi-quantitative dynamic contrast-enhanced MRI may improve specificity of MRI in detection of recurrence

- Positron emission tomography and monoclonal antibody imaging may have a role in the distinction of radiation damage and tumour recurrence

As a rule, postradiation atrophy can be differentiated from metastatic disease by noting the absence of abnormality outside the radiation field, the lack of a radiographically recognizable periosteal reaction[74] and the time

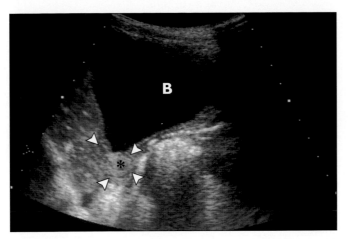

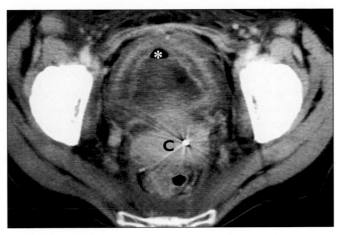

Figure 50.22. *Longitudinal ultrasound scan in a 29-year-old female who had undergone abdominopelvic radiation in childhood for a Wilms' tumour. The uterus (between arrowheads) is of infantile proportions with a cervix (asterisk): body ratio of 1:1. Urinary bladder (B).*

Figure 50.23. *CT scan through the pelvis in a patient presumed to have severe radiation change affecting the bladder, rectum and adjacent pelvic connective tissues. A small locule of air (asterisk) is present within the bladder from a vesico-enteric fistula. However, at surgery there was diffuse malignant infiltration of the pelvic organs. Cervix (C).*

delay before the development of abnormality, as metastases tend to occur earlier in the course of the disease.

Radiotherapy may produce changes in and around joints, for example, the sacro-iliac joints may be wide and irregular following radiotherapy. Plain radiographs show sclerosis of the adjacent joint surfaces, often in a bilateral and symmetrical pattern resembling osteitis codensans illi.[75] Similar sclerotic changes in the pubis resemble osteitis pubis.

Insufficiency fractures of the sacrum, and less commonly the pubis, occur in patients irradiated for gynaecological malignancy in whom postmenopausal osteoporosis, steroid therapy and other metabolic bone diseases may be additional risk factors.[76,77]

Subcapital fractures of the femoral neck previously occurred in approximately 2% of patients receiving pelvic radiation.[78] However, with the abandonment of lateral radiation fields, the change from orthovoltage to supervoltage or megavoltage treatment, and shielding of the femoral neck, these are now seldom seen.

Osteomyelitis is most likely to occur in the pelvis where radiation damage to pelvic bowel loops and surgical intervention increase the risk. The symphysis pubis is most commonly affected and there are usually symmetrical lytic and sclerotic changes in the pubic bones. On CT an associated pelvic abscess is usually seen and a soft tissue mass, fistulae and gas in the symphysis itself are possible additional findings.[79]

Avascular necrosis (AVN) occurs as a complication of chemotherapy,[80] radiotherapy or corticosteroid therapy either alone or in combination. Weight-bearing and trauma are possible additional risk factors accounting for the higher incidence in the femoral than humeral head.[81] Early diagnosis

is critical to allow surgical intervention and modification of therapy. Magnetic resonance imaging is the modality of choice in demonstrating AVN since it is more sensitive than plain radiographs or radio-isotope scans[82,83] and has the ability to identify any associated joint effusion or cartilage abnormality (Fig. 50.24). Initially on T1-weighted images there are diffuse areas of reduced signal intensity in the high signal intensity fatty marrow of the femoral head. Subsequently low signal intensity bands or lines occur within the anterosuperior

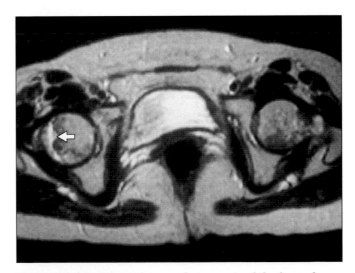

Figure 50.24. *Bilateral avascular necrosis of the femoral head following corticosteroid treatment and chemotherapy for Hodgkin's disease. Note double line sign in right femoral head (arrow) (see text).*

aspect of the femoral head on both T1- and T2-weighted images. On T2-weighted images an additional band of high signal intensity representing the interface between normal and infarcted marrow is seen (double line sign)[82] (Fig. 50.24). Progressive bone necrosis appears of high signal intensity on T2-weighted images and low signal intensity on T1-weighted images and subsequent fibrosis is low signal intensity on both T1- and T2-weighted images. Radiographically the first sign of AVN is a patchy increase in density of the femoral head followed by the development of a subchondral lucency, mirroring the MRI appearances. The joint space is usually preserved but may be reduced if there is eventual collapse and fragmentation of the femoral head.

Skeletal muscle

Injury to skeletal muscle in the radiation field results from vascular damage and may progress for many years following treatment.[84] Muscles undergo necrosis, atrophy and eventual fibrosis. Sigimura et al.[54] noted changes on MR imaging from 3 weeks to longer than 12 months after irradiation for pelvic malignancy. A homogeneous increase in signal intensity on T2-weighted images in a unilateral or bilateral distribution was seen in the pelvic side wall muscles (Fig. 50.25). Chronic atrophic changes are also evident on CT with asymmetry or loss of muscle bulk.

Fat

Irradiated pelvic and mesenteric fat loses its normal homogeneous appearance. On CT there is a diffuse increase in attenuation and on MR imaging a heterogeneous decrease in the normal high signal intensity on T1-weighted images. Fine stranding appears on both CT and T1- and T2-weighted MR images. Following pelvic radiotherapy there may be proliferation of the perirectal fat and thickening of the perirectal fibrous tissue giving a halo[34] or target[85] appearance. Secondary widening of the presacral space may also be observed.

Peripheral nerves

Radiation change to the lumbosacral plexus is uncommon but has been reported in patients with gynaecological cancer who received radiation doses in excess of 70 Gy to the whole pelvis.[84] The imaging features have not been clearly defined.

Blood vessels

Radiation damage to blood vessels occurs predominantly in the intimal layer with changes that are indistinguishable from atherosclerosis.[86] The irradiated artery shows focal or diffuse irregularity, stenosis or occlusion angiographically. Aneurysm formation and rupture may occur. Venous changes are infrequently reported but mesenteric venous occlusion has been noted following pelvic irradiation.[87]

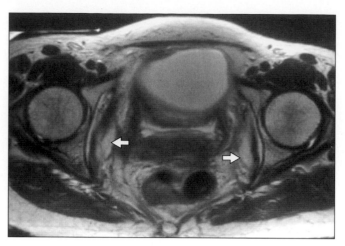

Figure 50.25. *Axial T2-weighted MR image of the pelvis demonstrating bilateral homogeneous increase in signal intensity in the obturator internus muscles (arrows) following pelvic radiotherapy.*

Radiotherapy effects on the growing skeleton

In children skeletal abnormalities result not only from external beam radiation for solid tumours but also from total body irradiation in preparation for bone marrow transplantation.[88] The most striking effect is on growth and may result from damage to nerves, blood vessels, muscles and bones, either alone or in combination.

Changes evident in the pelvis are hypoplasia of the iliac blade and acetabulum, predisposing to hip dislocation. The risk of slipped femoral capital epiphysis is increased and tends to occur at an earlier age than the idiopathic type.[73]

Key points: radiation injury to bone

- Avascular necrosis results from radiotherapy, chemotherapy or corticosteroids used alone or in combination

- Insufficiency fractures of the sacrum occur following RT for gynaecological cancers

- Osteomyelitis is another complication of pelvic irradiation

Radiation-induced interruption of vertebral body growth gives typical radiographic features. The vertebral body height is reduced and there may be anterior beaking resembling the appearance of the mucopolysaccharides. Dense, sometimes multiple growth arrest lines occur parallel to the vertebral end plates and occasionally there is a bone within a bone appearance. The trabecular pattern is coarsened and the end plates irregular.

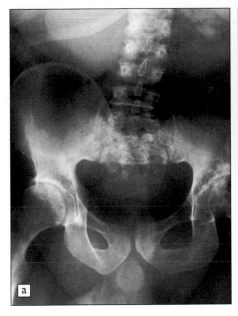
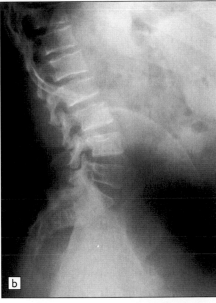

Figure 50.26. *Effects of radiotherapy on the growing skeleton. (a) AP and (b) lateral radiographs of a 26-year-old man, treated with radiotherapy aged 2 years for Wilms' tumour. There is kyphoscoliosis and hypoplasia of the left ribs and left iliac blade. Characteristic vertebral body changes are seen (see text). The sacro-iliac joints are fused. Avascular necrosis of the left femoral head has occurred and there is secondary dysplasia of the acetabulum. Degenerative changes are present in the right hip joint. The left kidney is absent and there is compensatory hypertrophy of the right kidney.*

Asymmetrical vertebral development results in kyphosis and scoliosis particularly when the spine and paravertebral muscles have been unevenly irradiated. The convexity of the scoliosis points away from the irradiated side. Associated rib hypoplasia may also be observed (Fig. 50.26).

SECOND MALIGNANCIES AFTER ABDOMINOPELVIC RADIATION

As more patients become long-term survivors, so the adverse effects of cancer treatment become apparent. Some patients are already genetically predisposed to further malignancy, for example, women who have suffered from ovarian cancer have a higher risk of breast, thyroid, endometrial and lung cancer. Nonetheless, there is also a recognized risk of treatment-induced second malignancies.[89,90] This is highest after treatment for childhood cancer and the overall riskvaries between 2 and 12% in survivors at 20 years.[91] Most tumours are musculoskeletal sarcomas, lymphomas or leukaemia,[92,93] but, in the abdomen, hepatomas may occur in patients who have undergone upper abdominal radiation therapy (Fig. 50.27), and in the pelvis at-risk organs are the bladder and rectum.[94] Therefore, it is necessary to obtain a histological diagnosis of any abnormal mass particularly when there is a long time interval between treatment of the primary lesion and the development of new symptoms.

Radiation-induced sarcomas arise more frequently in soft tissues than in bone[95] usually more than 10 years after radiotherapy, but with a wide time range of 3–55 years.[72] The most common cell types are malignant fibrous histiocytoma and osteosarcoma.[95,96] The cardinal imaging feature is the

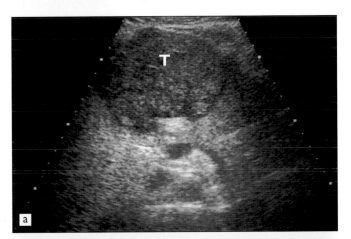
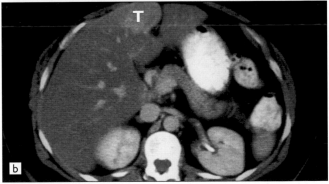

Figure 50.27. *(a) Transverse ultrasound scan and (b) transaxial contrast-enhanced CT scan of the liver in a patient with Hodgkin's disease who received chemotherapy and radiotherapy 10 years previously. There is a large mass (T) within the left lobe of the liver, which is relatively hyperechoic on ultrasound and shows some enhancement on CT within an otherwise fatty liver. Biopsy of this lesion revealed hepatoma.*

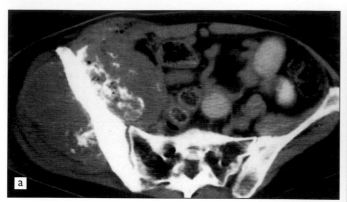

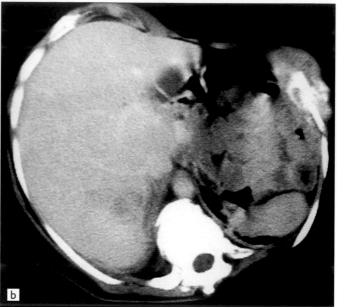

Figure 50.28. *Radiation induced sarcoma. (a) CT scan through the pelvis showing a chondrosarcoma of the right iliac blade following radiotherapy for cervical carcinoma; (b) postcontrast CT scan through the upper abdomen showing an osteosarcoma of the left twelfth rib in an adult irradiated in childhood for Wilms' tumour. (Also note the absent left kidney, vertebral body changes and rib changes).*

presence of a new soft-tissue mass within the radiation field. In bone, focal loss of the expected postradiation high signal intensity fatty marrow on T1-weighted MR images is an early finding. On plain radiographs or CT, a lytic destructive lesion is identified which may extend beyond the area of pre-existing postradiation atrophy (Fig. 50.28).[72] Differentiation from postradiation osteomyelitis can be difficult and require biopsy. The presence of additional lesions outside the radiation field and a short latent period to the development of the lesion are indicative of metastatic disease.

Osteochondroma is the only benign radiation-induced bone neoplasm. It is relatively common occurring in approximately 12% of treated children[97] and is not known to undergo malignant degeneration. The imaging features are indistinguishable from the idiopathic type. This topic is discussed in detail in Chapter 47.

Summary

- Surgery, chemotherapy and radiation all induce changes in normal tissues.

- The biological effect of radiation is to damage intracellular DNA.

- Significant radiation damage occurs in 5–10% of patients and is divided into acute, subacute and chronic reactions.

- Clinically significant damage most frequently occurs in the gastro-intestinal and genito-urinary tracts.

- Radiation damage to the bowel includes mucosal lesions, fixation of bowel loops, motility disturbance, strictures and fistulae.

- Perirectal fascial thickening is associated with increased width of the presacral space due to fat, fibrosis or fluid.

- The bladder is the most radiation-sensitive organ in the urinary tract. Damage is seen in 20% of patients. Oedema, haemorrhage and necrosis lead to fibrosis.

- Distinction of radiation damage from recurrent tumour relies on morphological appearances on CT, ultrasound and MRI. Signal intensity changes on MRI may be helpful but considerable overlap occurs.

- Positron emission tomography and monoclonal antibody imaging may have a role in the detection of recurrent tumour.

- Radiation injury to the musculoskeletal system results in bone marrow atrophy, bone fractures, osteomyelitis, avascular necrosis, muscle atrophy and injury to fat, nerves and blood vessels.

- The development of a second malignancy occurs in 2–12% of survivors following treatment of childhood cancer.

REFERENCES

1. Allen-Mersh T G, Wilson E J, Hope-Stone H F et al. Has the incidence of radiation induced bowel damage following treatment of uterine carcinoma changed in the last 20 years? J R Soc Med 1986; 79: 387–390

2. Schellhammer P F, Jordan G H, El-Mahdi A M. Pelvic complications after interstitial and external beam irradiation of urologic and gynecologic malignancy. World J Surg 1986; 10: 259–268

3. DeCosse J J, Rhodes R S, Wentz W B et al. The natural history and management of radiation-induced injury of the gastrointestinal tract. Ann Surg 1969; 170: 369–384

4. van Nagell R J, Maruyama Y, Parker J C et al. Small bowel injury following radiation therapy for cervical carcinoma. Am J Obstet Gynecol 1974; 118: 163–167

5. Graham J B, Abad R S. Ureteral obstruction due to radiation. Am J Obstet Gynecol 1967; 99: 409–415

6. Stockbrine M F, Hancock J E, Fletcher G H. Complications in 831 patients with squamous cell carcinoma of the intact uterine cervix treated with 3000 rads or more whole pelvis irradiation. Am J Roentgenol 1970; 108: 293–304

7. Mason G R, Dietrich P, Friedland G W et al. The radiological findings in radiation-induced enteritis and colitis. Clin Radiol 1970; 21: 232–247

8. Hellman S. Principles of radiation therapy. In: DeVita V T, Hellman S, Rosenberg S A (eds) Cancer principles and practice of oncology. Philadelphia: Lippincott-Raven, 1989; 247–275

9. Fletcher G H. Parameters involved in radiotherapy complications. In: Libshitz H I (ed.) Diagnostic roentgenology of radiotherapy change. Baltimore: Williams and Wilkins, 1979; 1–2: 85–100, 123–135

10. Haboubi N Y, Hasleton P S. Pathology of radiation injury. In: Schofield P F, Lupton E W (eds) The causation and clinical management of pelvic radiation disease. Berlin, Heidelberg: Springer-Verlag, 1989; 16–35

11. Kimose H H, Fischer L, Spjeldnaes N et al. Late radiation injury of the colon and rectum. Surgical management and outcome. Dis Colon Rectum 1989; 32: 684–689

12. Perez C A, Breaux S, Bebwinek J M et al. Radiation therapy done in the treatment of carcinoma of the uterine cervix. II Analysis of complications. Cancer 1984; 54: 235–246

13. Schofield P F. Treatment of radiation bowel disease. In: Schofield P F, Lupton E W (eds) The causation and clinical management of pelvic radiation disease. Berlin, Heidelberg; Springer-Verlag, 1989; 95–106

14. Mehta S, Johnson R J, Schofield P F. Review staging of colorectal cancer. Clin Radiol 1994; 49: 515–523

15. Buraggi G L, Gasparini M, Seregni E. Immunoscintigraphy of colorectal carcinoma with an anti-CEA monoclonal antibody: A critical review. Int J Radiol App Instrumentation (B) 1991; 18: 45–50

16. Corbisiero R M, Yamauchi D M, Williams L E et al. Comparison of immunoscintigraphy and computerized tomography in identifying colorectal cancer: Individual lesion analysis. Cancer Res 1991; 51: 5704–5711

17. Abdel Nabi H H, Doerr R J. Multicenter clinical trials of monoclonal antibody B72.3-GYK-DTPA ^{111}In (^{111}In-CYT-103; Onco-Scint CR 103) in patients with colorectal carcinoma. Targeted Diagnost Therapy 1992; 6: 73–88

18. Doerr R J, Abdel Nabi H H, Merchant B. Indium 111 ZCE-025 immuno-scintigraphy in occult recurrent colorectal cancer with elevated carcino-embryonic antigen level. Arch Surg 1990; 125: 226–229

19. Abdel Nabi H H, Chan H W, Doerr R J. Indium-labelled anti-colorectal carcinoma monoclonal antibody accumulation in non-tumoured tissue in patients with colorectal carcinoma. J Nucl Med 1990; 31: 1975–1979

20. Lehner B, Schlag P, Strauss L et al. (The value of positron emission tomography in the diagnosis of recurrent rectal cancer.) Die Wertigkeit der Positronen Emissions Tomographie für die Diagnostik des Rektumkarzinom Rezidivs. Zentralblatt für Chirurgie 1990; 115: 813–817

21. Ito K, Kato T, Tadokoro M et al. Recurrent rectal cancer and scar: Differentiation with PET and MR imaging. Radiology 1992; 182: 549–552

22. Schlag P, Lehner B, Strauss L G et al. Scar or recurrent rectal cancer. Positron emission tomography is more helpful for diagnosis than immuno-scintigraphy. Arch Surg 1989; 124: 197–200

23. Engenhart R, Kimmig B N, Strauss L G et al. Therapy monitoring of presacral recurrences after high-dose irradiation: Value of PET, CT, CEA and pain score. Strahlentherapie Onkologie 1992; 168: 203–212

24. Wharton J T, Delclos L, Gallager S et al. Radiation hepatitis induced by abdominal irradiation with the cobalt 60 moving strip technique. Am J Roentgenol 1971; 117: 73–80

25. Unger E C, Lee J K T, Weyman P J. CT and MR imaging of radiation hepatitis. J Comput Assist Tomogr 1987; 11: 264–268

26. Coleman C N, McDougall I R, Dailey M O et al. Functional hyposplenia after splenic irradiation for Hodgkin's disease. Ann Int Med 1982; 96: 44–47

27. Dailey M O, Coleman C N, Fajardo L F. Splenic injury caused by therapeutic irradiation. Am J Surg Pathol 1981; 5: 325–331

28. Friedman N B. Effects of radiation on the gastrointestinal tract, including the salivary glands, the liver, and the pancreas. Arch Pathol 1942; 34: 749–787

29. Nolan D J. Radiological investigation of the small intestine. In: Whitehouse G H, Worthington B (eds) Techniques in diagnostic radiology. Oxford: Blackwell Scientific Publications, 1983: 21–32

30. Rogers L F, Goldstein H M. Roentgen manifestations of radiation injury to the gastrointestinal tract. Gastrointest Radiol 1977; 2: 281–291

31. Mendleson R M, Nolan D J. The radiological features of chronic radiation enteritis. Clin Radiol 1985; 36: 141–148

32. Taylor P M, Johnson R J, Eddleston B E et al. Radiological changes in the gastrointestinal and genitourinary tract following radiotherapy for carcinoma of the cervix. Clin Radiol 1990; 41: 165–169

33. Taylor P M, Johnson R J, Eddleston B. Radiology of radiation injury. In: Schofield P F, Lupton E W (eds) The causation and clinical management of pelvic radiation disease. Springer-Verlag, London, 1989

34. Doubleday L C, Bernardino M E. CT findings in the perirectal area following radiation therapy. J Comput Assist Tomogr 1980; 4: 634–638

35. Ohtomo K, Shuman W P, Griffin B R et al. CT manifestation in the pararectal area following fast neutron radiotherapy. Radiol Medica 1987; 5: 198–201

36. Koelbel G, Schmiedl U, Majer M C et al. Diagnosis of fistulae and sinus tracts in patients with Crohn's disease: Value of MR imaging. Am J Roentgenol 1989; 152: 999–1003

37. Outwater E, Schiebler M L. Pelvic fistulas: Findings on MR images. Am J Roentgenol 1993; 160: 327–330

38. Barker P G, Lunniss P J, Armstrong P et al. Magnetic resonance imaging of fistula-in-ano: Technique, interpretation and accuracy. Clin Radiol 1994; 49: 7–13

39. Spencer J A, Ward J, Beckingham I J et al. Contrast-enhanced MR imaging of perianal fistulas. Am J Roentgenol 1996; 167: 735–741

41. Barter J F, Soong S J, Shingleton H M et al. Complications of combined radical hysterectomy — post-operative radiation therapy in women with early stage cervical cancer. Gynecol Oncol 1989; 32: 292–296

42. Razzaq R, Carrington B M, Hulse P A. CT appearances following surgery for ovarian cancer: Post-operative change or residual disease (Submitted) Radiology Congress, Birmingham 1997

43. Reed D H, Dixon A K, Williams M V. Ovarian conservation at hysterectomy: A potential diagnostic pitfall. Clin Radiol 1989; 40: 274–276

44. Bashist B, Friedman W N, Killackey M A. Surgical transposition of the ovary: Radiological appearance. Radiology 1989; 173: 857–860

45. Ilancheran A, Monaghan J M. Pelvic lymphocyst — A 10-year experience. Gynecol Oncol 29: 333–336

46. van Sonnenberg E, Wittich G R, Casola G et al. Lymphoceles: imaging characteristics and percutaneous management. Radiology 1986; 161: 593–596

47. Lawhead R A, Clark D G C, Smith D H, Pierce V K, Lewis J L. Pelvic exenteration for recurrent on persistent gynecological malignancies: A ten year review of the Memorial Sloan-Kettering cancer experience (1972–1982). Gynecol Oncol 1989; 33: 279–282

48. Sherins R J, Mulvihill J J. Adverse effects of treatment: Gonadal dysfunction. In: DeVita V T, Hellman S, Rosenberg S A (eds) Cancer Principles and Practice of Oncology. Philadelphia: Lippincott-Raven 1989; 591–705

49. Koyama H, Wada T, Nishizaw Y et al. Cyclophosphamide-induced ovarian failure and its therapeutic significance in patients with breast cancer. Cancer 1977; 39: 1403–1409

50. Cassady J R. Clinical radiation nephropathy. Int J Radiation Oncol Biol Phys 1995; 31: 1249–1256

51. Parkin D E. Lower urinary tract complications of the treatment of cervical carcinoma. Obstetric Gynecol Surv 1989; 523–529

52. Johnson R J, Carrington B M. Review: Pelvic radiation disease. Clin Radiol 1992; 45: 4–12

53. Villasanta U. Complications of radiotherapy for carcinoma of the uterine cervix. Am J Obstet Gynecol 1972; 114: 717–726

54. Sugimura K, Carrington B M, Quivey J M et al. Post-radiation changes in the pelvis: Assessment with MR imaging. Radiology 1990; 175: 805–813

55. Hawnaur J M, Johnson R J, Isherwood I et al. Gadolinium-DTPA in magnetic resonance imaging of bladder carcinoma. In: Bydder G, Felix R, Bücheler E et al. (eds) Contrast media in MRI. Medicom Europe, Brinklaan 36, 1404 E W Bussun, The Netherlands, 1990; 357–363

56. Chan T W, Kressel H Y. Prostate and seminal vesicles after irradiation: MR appearance. J Mag Res Imag 1991; 1: 503–511

57. Seymore C H, El-Mahdi A M, Schellhammer P F. The effect of prior transurethral resection of the prostate on post-radiation urethral strictures and bladder neck contractures. Int J Radiat Oncol Biol Phys 1986; 12: 1597–1600

58. Rowley M J, Leach D R, Warner G A et al. Effect of graded doses of ionising irradiation on the human testis. Radiat Res 1974; 59: 665–678

59. Arrivé L, Change Y C F, Hricak H et al. Radiation-induced uterine changes: MR imaging. Radiology 1989; 170: 55–58

60. Scott W W, Rosenshein N B, Siegelman S et al. The obstructed uterus. Radiology 1981; 141: 767–770

61. Grigsby P W, Russell A, Bruner D et al. Late injury of cancer therapy on the female reproductive tract. Int J Radiat Oncol Biol Phys 1995; 31: 1281–1299

62. Wallace W H B, Shalet S M, Crowne E C et al. Ovarian failure following abdominal irradiation in childhood: Natural history and prognosis. Clin Oncol 1989; 1: 75–79

63. Krestin G P, Steinbrich W, Friedmann G. Recurrent rectal cancer: Diagnosis with MR imaging versus CT: Radiology 1988; 168: 307–311

64. Ebner F, Kresel H Y, Mintz M C et al. Tumour recurrence versus fibrosis in the female pelvis: Differentiation with MR imaging at 1.5 T. Radiology 1988; 166: 333–340

65. Hircak H, Swift P S, Campos Z et al. Irradiation of the cervix uteri: Value of unenhanced and contrast-enhanced MR imaging. Radiology 1993; 189: 381–388

66. Weber T M, Sostman H D, Spritzer C E et al. Cervical carcinoma: Determination of recurrent tumor extent versus radiation changes with MR imaging. Radiology 1995; 194: 135–139

67. Cook G J R, Maisey M N. Review — The current status of clinical PET imaging. Clin Radiol 1996; 51: 603–613

68. Wahl R L, Hawkins R A, Larson S M et al. Proceedings of a National Cancer Institute Workshop: PET in oncology — A clinical research agenda. Radiology 1994; 193: 604–606

69. Stomper P C, D'Souza D J, Bakshi S P et al. Detection of pelvic recurrence of colorectal carcinoma: Prospective, blinded comparison of Tc-99m-IMMU-4 monoclonal antibody scanning and CT. Radiology 1995; 197: 688–692

70. Muller-Schimpfle M, Brix G, Layer G et al. Recurrent rectal cancer: Diagnosis with dynamic MR imaging. Radiology 1993; 189: 881

71. Stevens S K, Moore S G, Kaplan I D. Early and late bone marrow changes after irradiation: MR evaluation. Am J Roentgenol 1989; 154: 745–750

72. Remeios P A, Colletti P M, Raval J K et al. Magnetic resonance imaging of bone after radiation. Mag Res Imag 1988; 6: 301–304

73. Libshitz H I. Radiation changes in bone. Semin Roentgenol 1994; 29: 15–37

74. Blumemke D A, Fishman E K, Kuhlman J E et al. Complications of radiation therapy: CT evaluation. Radiographics 1991; 11: 581–600

75. Rubin P, Probhasawat D. Characteristic bone lesions in post irradiated carcinoma of the cervix — metastases versus osteonecrosis. Radiology 1961; 76: 703

76. Rafii M, Fiooznia, Golimbu C et al. Radiation induced fractures of the sacrum: CT diagnosis. J Comput Assist Tomogr 1988; 12: 231–235

77. Blomlie V, Lien H H, Iversen T et al. Radiation induced insufficiency fractures of the sacrum: Evaluation with MR imaging. Radiology 1993; 188: 241–244

78. Bonfiglio M. The pathology of fracture of the femoral neck following irradiation. Am J Roentgenol 1953; 70: 449–459

79. Wignall T A, Carrington B M, Logue J P. Post-radiotherapy osteomyelitis of the symphysis pubis: computed tomographic features. Submitted to Clin Radiol December 1996

80. Harper P G, Trask C, Souhami R L. Avascular necrosis of bone caused by combination chemotherapy without corticosteroids. Br Med J Clin Res Ed 1984; 288: 267–268

81. Mould J J, Adam N M. The problem of avascular necrosis of bone in patients treated for Hodgkin's disease. Clin Radiol 1983; 34(2): 231–236

82. Chan Lam D, Prentice A G, Copplestone J A et al. Avascular necrosis of bone following intensified steroid therapy for acute leukaemia and high grade malignant lymphoma. Br J Haematol 1994; 86: 227–230

83. Gabriel H, Fitzgerald S W, Myers M T et al. MR Imaging of hip disorders. Radiographics 1994; 14: 763–781

84. Gillete E L, Mahler P A, Powers B E et al. Late radiation injury to muscle and peripheral nerves. Int J Radiat Oncol Biol Phys 1995; 5: 1309–1318

85. Frommhold W, Hubener K H. The role of computerised tomography in the aftercare of patients suffering from a carcinomas of the rectum. Comput Tomogr 1981; 5: 161–168

86. Granmayeh M, Libshitz H I. Vascular system. In: Libshitz H I (ed) Diagnostic roentgenology of radiotherapy change. Baltimore: Williams and Wilkins, 1979: 195–201

87. Dencker H, Holmdahl H, Lunderquist A et al. Mesenteric angiography in patients with radiation injury of the bowel after pelvis irradiation. Am J Roentgenol 1972; 114: 476–481

88. Fletcher B D, Crom D B, Krance R A et al. Radiation induced bone abnormalities after bone marrow transplantation for childhood leukaemia. Radiology 1994; 191: 231–235

89. Hutchison G B. Late neoplastic changes following medical irradiation. Cancer 1976; 37: 1102–1107

90. Parker R G. Radiation-induced cancer as a factor in clinical decision making (The 1989 Astro Gold Medal Address). Int J Radiat Oncol Biol Phys 1989; 18: 993–1000

91. Tucker M A, D'Angio G J, Boice J D et al. Bone sarcoma linked to radiotherapy and chemotherapy in children. New Eng J Med 1987; 317: 588–593

92. Messerschmidt G L, Hoover R, Young R C. Gynecologic cancer treatment: Risk factors for therapeutically induced neoplasia. Cancer 1981; 48: 442–450

93. Quilty P M, Kerr G R. Bladder cancer following low or high dose pelvic irradiation. Clin Radiol 1987; 38: 583–585

94. Tucker M A, Fraumeni Jr J F. Treatment-related cancers after gynecologic malignancy. Cancer 1987; 60: 2117–2122

95. Wiklund T A, Blomquist C P, Räty I et al. Post irradiation sarcoma: Analysis of Nationwide Cancer Registry material. Cancer 1991; 68: 524–531

96. Huvos A G, Woodward H Q, Cahan W G et al. Post-irradiation osteogenic sarcoma of bone and soft tissues: A clinicopathological study of 66 patients. Cancer 1985; 55: 1244–1255

97. Libshitz H I, Cohen M A. Radiation induced osteochondromas. Radiology 1982; 142: 643–647

Part VIII

AIDS-RELATED TUMOURS

Chapter 51

Chest

Janet Kuhlman

INTRODUCTION

Worldwide an estimated 10 million people are infected with the human immunodeficiency virus (HIV).[1] As the pandemic continues to spread, no vaccine or cure for acquired immune deficiency syndrome (AIDS) has been developed. Nevertheless, significant strides have been made in the treatment of AIDS-related diseases. Human immunodeficiency virus-infected individuals are living longer, primarily due to prophylactic treatments for opportunistic infections such as pneumocystis pneumonia (PCP).[2,3] New antiretroviral agents may also have slowed the relentless assault of HIV on the body's immune system. Although median survival has improved for HIV-infected patients from the time they reach a CD4 T-cell count of 200 or less, prognosis for these patients once an AIDS-defining illness has occurred remains poor, with median survival of only 17 months.[3,4]

The association between HIV infection and malignancies has been known since the early days of the epidemic.[5] Kaposi's sarcoma (KS) and non-Hodgkin's lymphoma are two AIDS-defining cancers that have a definite increased incidence in HIV-infected individuals. Invasive cervical carcinoma in the HIV-infected woman has recently been added to the list of AIDS-defining neoplasms as well.[5] Other tumours have been reported in association with HIV infection including Hodgkin's lymphoma, testicular cancer, squamous cell cancer of the mouth and anus, lung cancer, and hepatoma, among others, but an increased incidence of these tumours in AIDS has not been demonstrated unequivocally.[6] As HIV-infected patients now survive longer with lower CD4 counts and more severely impaired immune systems, the number of AIDS-related lymphomas is on the rise.[3,7]

NEOPLASMS INVOLVING THE CHEST IN AIDS

Acquired immune deficiency syndrome-defining neoplasms that involve the chest include KS and AIDS-related lymphomas. Other lymphoproliferative disorders such as AIDS-related lymphadenopathy syndromes (ARLS) and lymphocytic interstitial pneumonitis (LIP) are included in this discussion.

Lung cancer and other non-AIDS defining malignancies of the chest are also addressed with respect to their differing manifestations in the HIV-infected individual.

DIAGNOSTIC APPROACH TO PULMONARY/THORACIC NEOPLASMS IN AIDS

Pulmonary disease in AIDS remains extremely common. Radiological diagnosis of thoracic diseases in AIDS is best done as an integrated approach that combines clinical information, radiographic and computed tomography (CT) manifestations with a clear understanding of the natural history of AIDS.[8–13]

Diagnosis of pulmonary disease in AIDS is often challenging. Any number of opportunistic infections or neoplastic processes can present as pulmonary infiltrates, nodules, masses, lymphadenopathy or pleural effusions.[13] Atypical presentations and uncommon features confuse presentations and can delay diagnosis. Multiple pathogens and multifactorial disease often coexist in the lung (i.e. KS with PCP, lymphoma and a bacterial or disseminated fungal infection). Few radiographic features are specific.

Despite these discouraging facts, recognizable patterns of disease are seen in AIDS patients. Combining radiographic and CT pattern recognition with knowledge of the clinical presentation, CD4 count, underlying risk group, sex, race, geographic area, and previous drug treatments narrows the diagnostic possibilities in many cases and expedites management decisions.[9,13,14]

It is perhaps most important to recognize that AIDS encompasses disease states that vary greatly in their degree of immunosuppression, from the asymptomatic HIV-carrier to the end-stage terminal patient with AIDS. The degree of immune suppression often dictates the most likely pulmonary disease or neoplasm present in the patient.

Human immunodeficiency virus causes many defects in the immune system, the most devastating of which is the progressive destruction of CD4 helper T lymphocytes.[15] The CD4 count correlates well with the type of AIDS-related disease that is seen in the chest. Early in the course of HIV disease, when the CD4 count is still normal, virulent pathogens such as *Mycobacterium tuberculosis* and encapsulated pyogenic bacteria successfully infect the lung. At this relatively early stage of AIDS, when immunosuppression is still not severe, KS may also develop.[14] Not until the CD4 count falls below 200–250 cells/mm³ do opportunistic infections like PCP or disseminated fungal infections occur. When severe immunosuppression develops and CD4 counts drop below 50–100 cells/mm³, less virulent pathogens such as cytomegalovirus (CMV) and *Mycobacterium avium* complex (MAC) flourish.[15–17] AIDS-related lymphomas tend to be seen at these later stages of immunosuppression.

When a definitive diagnosis for pulmonary disease is required, diffuse opportunistic lung infections can often be diagnosed with induced sputums or bronchoscopy with bronchoalveolar lavage. More invasive procedures, such as transbronchial and open lung biopsies, are often avoided due to the increased complication rates in AIDS patients.[18] Focal lesions of the lung in the HIV-infected patient, whether due to neoplasm or infection, can be safely diagnosed with transthoracic needle-biopsy aspiration. These techniques have a high diagnostic yield for focal lung lesions in AIDS patients (85%) and carry an acceptable complication rate (28%).[19–21]

Key point

■ The degree of immune suppression in AIDS often dictates the most likely pulmonary disease or neoplasm. While immunosuppression is still not severe, Kaposi's sarcoma may develop, whereas AIDS-related lymphomas tend to develop at later stages of immunosuppression

KAPOSI'S SARCOMA

Kaposi's sarcoma is a vascular neoplasm believed to arise from a mesenchymal cell of origin.[22,23] Its cause is not known,[24] but the histology of KS is characterized by scattered aggregates of spindle cells surrounding slit-like vascular spaces and extravasated red cells. In pulmonary KS, these aggregates proliferate within the interstitium of the lung, demonstrating a predilection for the peribronchial and perivascular lymphatics.[25–27] Several clinical varieties of KS exist:

- The classic form
- The endemic African version
- An acquired form associated with organ transplantation
- The AIDS-related variant

The classic form of the tumour was first described by M. Kaposi, a Hungarian dermatologist, in 1872. He noted most cases to be indolent tumours occurring in older men of Mediterranean or Eastern European heritage or Jewish background.[28,29] Disease was often localized to skin lesions of the lower extremities, but could spread to visceral involvement.[30] A more aggressive, 'endemic' form of the tumour was later recognized in children and young men in central Africa; and an acquired form was found in association with immunosuppression after organ transplantation.[28,30] 'Epidemic' or AIDS-related KS resembles the more deadly form of the tumour and is generally multifocal in its involvement; it affects to various extent:[24]

- The skin
- Mucous membranes
- Lymph nodes
- Gastro-intestinal tract
- Lung
- Visceral organs

In the USA and other industrialized countries, AIDS-related Kaposi sarcoma occurs almost exclusively in HIV-infected homosexual or bisexual men and their sexual partners (~95%). Only an estimated 3–4% of patients with HIV secondary to intravenous drug use or blood transfusion manifest KS and even fewer heterosexual HIV-infected women develop KS.[31–35] Over the last decade, the proportion of AIDS patients presenting with KS has declined from an estimated high of 30–40%[28] of the HIV-infected population to less than 15% of patients.[14,22,35–37] Although the incidence of KS as a presenting diagnosis of AIDS has declined, the prevalence of KS cases continues to increase as the pandemic spreads and AIDS patients live longer with KS from the time of diagnosis.[16,24] Changes in behaviour patterns among homosexual men may explain the decline in the number of new cases of KS;[10,35,37–39] it has long been hypothesized that an environmental or sexually transmitted cofactor is responsible along with HIV for the development of the disease.[14,31,40] In fact, recent discovery of human herpesvirus 8 in all forms of KS, including AIDS and non-AIDS related KS, suggests this may be the causal transmitted agent.[15]

Kaposi's sarcoma however, is still the most common AIDS-related tumour and the most common neoplastic disorder to affect the lung in the patient with AIDS.[26,27,39,41–51] Pulmonary involvement is estimated to occur in anywhere from 3.4 to 40% of patients with KS.[22,26,38–40,52] Pulmonary KS is found to be the cause of lung disease in 8–18% of AIDS patients with lung disorders, and KS is the cause of 10–45% of pleural effusions in AIDS patients.[22] In patients with skin KS and respiratory symptoms, 18–40% are found to have lung KS antemortem while an estimated 38–75% will have evidence of lung KS at autopsy.[22]

When pulmonary KS is present, there is usually widespread multisystem disease with disseminated KS involving the skin, mucous membranes, lymph nodes, visceral organs, bone marrow, and gastro-intestinal tract.[27,40,47–50,53–55] Skin lesions are apparent on physical examination in 95% of AIDS patients with KS.[25,56,57] Exceptions do occur, however, with cases of isolated lung involvement due to KS reported in the literature.[27,40,47,50,52,58] More common, however, is the patient with relatively extensive pulmonary KS, who has limited disease elsewhere, with only a few isolated skin or mucous membrane lesions on physical examination making the diagnosis more difficult to make. An estimated 5–23% of AIDS patients with pulmonary KS do not exhibit skin lesions and patients may have lymph node enlargement from KS without skin involvement.[22]

Definitive diagnosis of pulmonary KS can be problematic.[23] On bronchoscopy, characteristic blue-purple, violaceous, or cherry-red endobronchial papules are seen in only 30–45% of patients with lung KS.[23,31,42,57,59–62] Their absence does not exclude deeper involvement of the lung, since pulmonary KS can be entirely intraparenchymal.[31] More invasive transbronchial biopsies are not commonly performed to confirm suspected KS, however. Unfortunately, transbronchial biopsies are positive in only 10–20% of cases, due to the patchy distribution of the disease.[23,25,31,42–44] Biopsies, even of superficial endobronchial lesions, may prove hazardous with significant bleeding occurring in 30% of attempts.[23,31,40]

Radiological appearances

Fortunately, chest film and CT findings of pulmonary KS often demonstrate a characteristic pattern of involvement that is distinct from opportunistic infections or lymphoma (Figs. 51.1–51.4).[26,38,51] These findings, taken in conjunction with physical examination and evidence of skin or mucous membrane KS, can often substantiate a diagnosis of pulmonary KS without the need for more invasive biopsy procedures.

Kaposi's sarcoma demonstrates a typical bronchovascular distribution of disease on plain films and even more strikingly on CT (Figs. 51.1, 51.2 and 51.4)[26,38,51,63,64] Chest film findings of KS include:

- Reticulonodular infiltrates that are bilateral and more prominent in the perihilar and lower lung zones (Figs. 51.1 and 51.4)
- Thickening of the interstitial markings and septal lines (Fig. 51.5)
- Larger tumoral masses (Fig. 51.3)
- Focal areas of air-space consolidation or collapse as well as rapidly enlarging pleural effusions[23]

The chest film may be normal in 5–20% of patients with pulmonary KS.

Computed tomography findings of pulmonary KS include 'fluffy' or poorly marginated and irregular nodular opacities that are distributed along the bronchovascular bundles (Figs. 51.1, 51.2 and 51.5). Subpleural nodules and

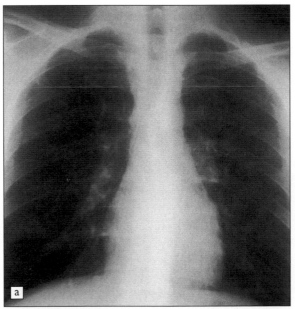
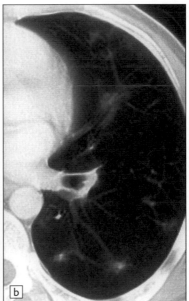
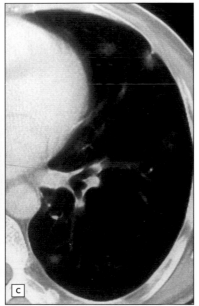

Figure 51.1. *Thirty-two-year-old male homosexual with skin KS and early lung involvement. (a) Chest film shows subtle reticulonodular infiltrates radiating out from both hila, more prominent on the left than the right; (b, c) CT scans show irregular, nodular opacities along the bronchovascular bundles due to pulmonary KS.*

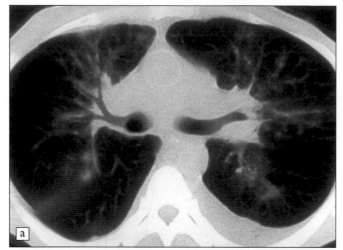

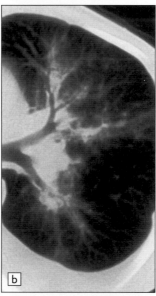

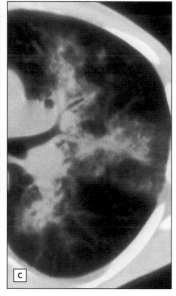

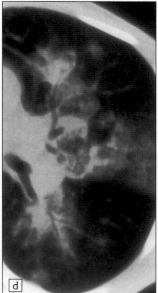

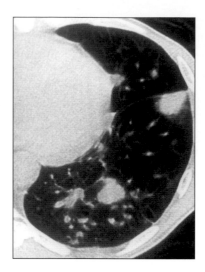

Figure 51.3. *Forty-four-year-old male with AIDS and pulmonary KS. This patient's CT scan demonstrates larger focal masses.*

Figure 51.2. *CT features of pulmonary KS. (a, b) CT shows typical distribution of disease along the bronchovascular interstitium, radiating out from both hila. Note also the bilateral pleural effusions which are quite common in KS. In this patient the disease is more linear and less nodular in appearance; (c, d) more extensive pulmonary KS is present on this CT. The distribution of disease, however, is still strikingly along the bronchovascular bundles. There is also surrounding ground-glass infiltrates due to pulmonary haemorrhage.*

nodular thickening of the interlobular septa are also seen, all due to the tumour's propensity to involve the lymphatics in these locations (Fig. 51.5).[26,38,51,63,65] The pulmonary disease appears to radiate out from the pulmonary hilum and encase the bronchi and vessels[51] (Figs 51.2, 51.5). Parenchymal masses may also be seen, and both nodules and masses may be surrounded by a zone of ground-glass attenuation which is probably due to haemorrhage (Figs 51.2 and 51.3).[65] In one of the larger series of patients with pulmonary KS, reported in the literature, including 53 patients with CT scans, the following findings were made:

- Multiple nodules in 79%
- Larger masses >2 cm in 53%
- A bronchovascular distribution of disease in 66%
- Pleural effusions in 55% (76% bilateral, 24% unilateral)
- Thickening of interlobular septa in 28%[64]

Associated features of thoracic KS include pleural effusions found in 30–67% of patients (Figs 51.2, 51.4 and 51.5).[26,39,51,65] These effusions are frequently bloody on thoracentesis or occasionally chylous due to lymphatic obstruction. The reported frequency of lymph nodes in thoracic KS varies. Lymphadenopathy, in general, is seen in 30–35% of patients with KS.[30,40,65] On chest CT, lymphadenopathy may be identified in the axilla or mediastinum. Mediastinal lymph nodes were observed in 43% of cases in one series, but most nodes in the mediastinum were normal-sized nodes with only 15% of cases demonstrating enlarged mediastinal nodes.[64] In another series, 53% of patients demonstrated axillary lymph nodes; 33% showed mediastinal nodes, 13% hilar nodes, and 6% internal mammary nodes.[51] In general the intrathoracic lymph nodes are not enlarged to the same extent that is seen in cases of lymphoma, mycobacterial or

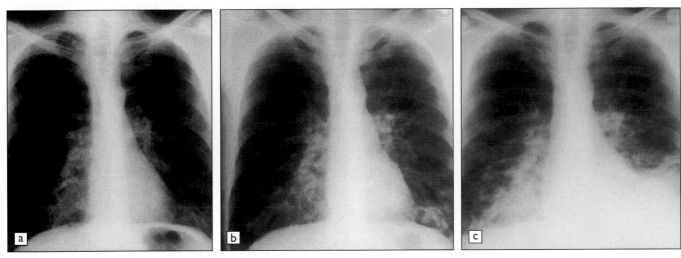

Figure 51.4. *Forty-nine-year-old male with AIDS and progressive shortness of breath over a 6-month period. Chest films in April (a), May (b) and August (c) show the typical pattern of progression of pulmonary KS. Increasing reticulonodular, bibasilar and perihilar disease, more prominent in the lung bases, gradually worsens over the 6-month period. Bilateral pleural effusions appear and increase by August.*

fungal infections in AIDS. Lymphadenopathy due to KS has also been reported to demonstrate enhancement after bolus injection of intravenous contrast that exceeds that of skeletal muscle.[50,66] Other causes of enhancing lymph nodes include Castleman's disease, carcinoid tumour, and angio-immunoblastic lymphadenopathy, but these entities are much less common than KS in AIDS.[66]

Computed tomography scans of the chest may also demonstrate evidence of extrapulmonary disease including: skin and subcutaneous nodules, bone metastases to the ribs, sternum, and thoracic vertebral bodies, and chest wall involvement by larger KS masses. Bone scans may fail to demonstrate osseous lesions due to KS, so radiographs, CT or MRI may be needed to diagnose early bone involvement.[24]

The major differential diagnosis for pulmonary infiltrates in an AIDS patient with KS is opportunistic infection. Differentiating opportunistic infection from KS involving the lung can usually be done by careful examination of the chest radiograph, the CT scan, and correlation with clinical signs and symptoms. In most cases where there is extensive skin KS and typical CT and chest film findings of lung KS, the diagnosis is confirmed with endoscopic visualization of endobronchial lesions and broncho-alveolar lavage (BAL) to exclude superimposed infection.[22] A superimposed infection in patients with pulmonary KS will be present in 17–27% of patients (Fig. 51.5).[22]

Presentation and course of KS in AIDS is highly variable. Patients who develop KS early, at higher CD4 counts, tend to have more indolent disease with slow progression. As the degree of immunosuppression advances, the virulence of KS increases as well, with disease becoming more explosive in some cases.[2]

Patients with pulmonary KS usually present with increasing dyspnoea and/or persistent non-productive cough, that progresses over weeks to months; this is a clinical course more gradual in onset than most cases of opportunistic infection. Recurrent haemoptysis, stridor, or bronchospasm may indicate upper airway or endobronchial disease due to KS.[30] Pleuritic chest pain may indicate pleural or chest wall involvement by KS. Other non-specific symptoms include fever and weight loss which overlap with opportunistic infection.[30,67] Sputum production is not typical of pulmonary KS and is more likely due to opportunistic infection.

Most opportunistic infections in AIDS including PCP, mycobacterial and fungal infections do not demonstrate a striking bronchovascular distribution of disease like KS on plain films or CT. Pleural effusions are rarely seen in PCP infections, but may be seen with mycobacterial or fungal infections, lymphoma, and lung cancer in AIDS patients. Adenopathy is also rare in PCP, unless the infection is disseminated, in which case the lymph nodes show calcification. However, mycobacterial infection, fungal infection, AIDS-related lymphoma, lung cancer, or KS can all cause adenopathy in the chest. Necrotic or low density lymph nodes, demonstrating rim enhancement with intravenous contrast, should suggest infection, particularly tuberculosis (TB), other mycobacterial infection, or fungal infection (Fig. 51.5).

A number of features of KS can also be mimicked by one unusual infection that occurs in AIDS patients: bacillary angiomatosis. Skin nodules, visceral involvement, lytic bone lesions, and hypervascularity with contrast enhancement can be seen in bacillary angiomatosis, a disseminated infection due to Rochalimaea henselae and Rochalimaea quintana,

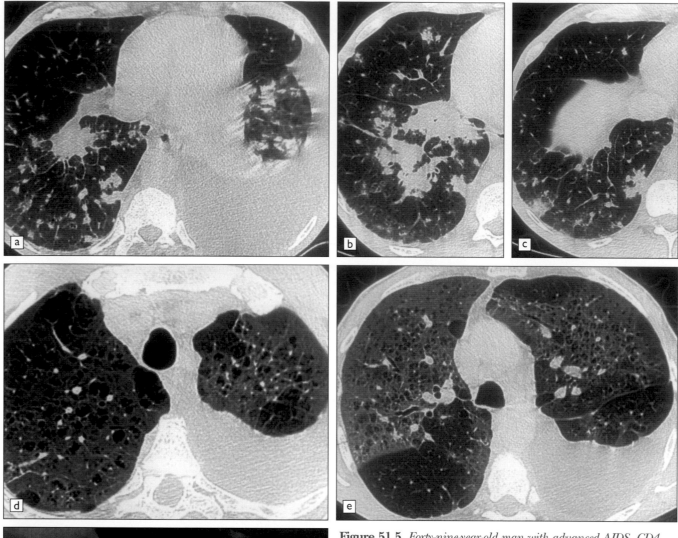

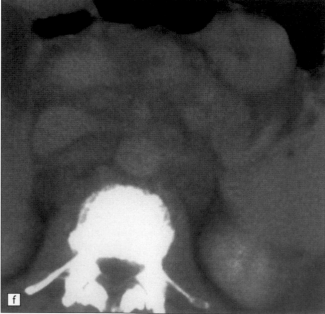

Figure 51.5. *Forty-nine-year-old man with advanced AIDS, CD4 count less than 100, and multifactorial disease due to KS, PCP, and disseminated Mycobacterium avium-intracellulare (MAI). (a–c) CT shows characteristic findings of lung KS with nodular disease encasing the hilum and bronchi, thickening of the interlobular septa, and pleural effusions. On bronchoscopy the patient had bluish-red papules lining the mucosa of the airways compatible with the diagnosis of endobronchial and pulmonary KS; (d, e) upper lung zones show ground glass attenuation bilaterally and cystic changes in the lung parenchyma. These changes are not seen in pulmonary KS, but are typical of PCP in AIDS; (f) CT scan through the upper abdomen revealed retroperitoneal adenopathy. The enlarged lymph nodes are low density on this contrast-enhanced CT scan and proved to be due to disseminated MAI infection. Kaposi's sarcoma does cause adenopathy, but the lymph nodes are not usually of low density after intravenous contrast, and may even demonstrate increased enhancement when compared to muscle. Low density nodes in an AIDS patient should raise the question of mycobacterial infection either due to TB or atypical Mycobacterium, fungal infection, or possibly an AIDS-related lymphoma.*

bacilli in the same family of organisms causing cat-scratch fever.[24,68] Diagnosis of bacillary angiomatosis is made by skin biopsy or positive blood cultures in the presence of bacter-aemia; the infection is effectively treated with antibiotics such as erythromycin or doxycycline.[68]

It is also important to remember that in the more advanced stages of AIDS, multiple diseases coexist simulta-neously in the lung, making it almost impossible to exclude superimposed infection with one or more organisms in addi-tion to involvement of the lung with KS (Fig. 51.5). Thus, bronchoscopy with BAL is often employed in patients with suspected pulmonary KS to exclude other treatable diseases such as superimposed opportunistic infection.

In problem cases, nuclear scintigraphy may provide some additional help. Pulmonary KS is thallium-avid, but does not accumulate gallium tracer. Opportunistic infec-tions in AIDS do not accumulate thallium, but do accumu-late gallium; and lymphoma accumulates both thallium and gallium.[41] Sequential thallium and gallium nuclear scintig-raphy has been used to document the presence of extracu-taneous KS and to non-invasively follow the response of visceral KS to treatment.[41,46]

The role of MRI in the evaluation of patients with KS is limited, but one recent report has stated that pulmonary KS demonstrates enhancement with gadolinium on T1-weighted images, but low signal intensity on the long TE, T2-weighted images.[22,69]

Because the rate of progression of KS and its extent is quite variable, a staging system for KS which incorporates the extent of the tumour, the presence of symptoms, and the CD4 count has been advocated by the AIDS Clinical Trials Group.[70] Prognosis correlates with visceral involve-ment, including the extent of lung disease.[22] The median survival for patients with lung involvement is 6 months.[23]

Patients with longer prognosis are those with tumour limited to the skin, lymph nodes, or minimal oral lesions; a CD4 count greater than 200; no 'B' symptoms or oppor-tunistic infections; and a Karnofsky performance status greater than or equal to 70%.[70]

Treatment of KS is palliative and aimed at slowing the pro-gression of disease.[2,67] Therapy includes local measures and systemic methods.[2] Indications for treatment include: pro-gressive dyspnoea, increasing effusions, impending obstruc-tion of the airway.[23] In the chest, local treatments include pleurodesis of symptomatic pleural effusions and laser or radiotherapy for bleeding or obstructing airway or laryngeal lesions. Systemic methods of treatment include single or multi-agent chemotherapy, whole lung radiation, and alpha-inter-feron.[2] Widespread pulmonary KS has been treated with whole lung radiation therapy or combination chemotherapy. Kaposi's sarcoma is radiosensitive and larger symptomatic masses can be treated with radiation therapy with response rates of 50–80%.[30] Alpha-interferon is often combined with

zidovudine to treat KS early in AIDS because of the suppres-sive effects on both the tumour and viral cofactors. Unfortunately, alpha-interferon works less well as the CD4 count drops below 400 and the response time is relatively slow.[2,22,23,30,67] A number of chemotherapy protocols for treat-ing KS have been used with moderate success in causing tem-porary regression of disease. Unfortunately, relapse always occurs and remissions usually are of short duration.[23] Single agents are employed for early, limited disease and combina-tions of drugs including doxorubicin, vinblastine, vincristine, bleomycin, and etoposide (VP-16) are used for more extensive disease.[30] Because pulmonary KS can cause death due to pro-gressive respiratory failure, it is often treated with combination chemotherapy. Adriamycin, bleomycin, vincristine (ABV) treat-ment in this setting has a reported response rate in the lung of 80%.[30,67,71] New approaches to treatment, including targeting of lesions with liposomal doxorubicin and liposomal daunorubicin, are also being tested.[2,23]

No treatment for KS, however, has been shown to pro-long survival, and all treatments cause myelosuppression increasing the risk of opportunistic infection as a complica-tion.[22,23,30,72] Prophylactic treatment for PCP is mandatory and use of granulocyte-macrophage colony stimulating factor (GM-CSF) with chemotherapy may provide additional haematological support.[17,23] Overall prognosis of patients with pulmonary KS is poor with most patients succumbing to HIV-related infections or progressive respiratory fail-ure.[30,45,73] Serial CT examinations are more accurate than plain films for determining response of the pulmonary KS to treatment on follow-up examinations.

Key points: Kaposi's sarcoma

- AIDS-related KS is of the 'epidemic' variety — the more deadly form of the tumour

- AIDS-related KS occurs almost exclusively in homosexual or bisexual men and their sexual partners

- Skin lesions are present in the majority of AIDS patients with pulmonary KS

- Pulmonary KS can be entirely intraparenchymal, endo-bronchial papules are seen in only 30–45% of patients with lung KS, and transbronchial biopsies are positive in only 10–20% of cases due to the patchy distribution of the disease

- The rate of progression of KS is variable and the prognosis correlates with visceral involvement including the extent of lung disease — if there is lung involvement the median survival is 6 months

AIDS-RELATED LYMPHOMAS

AIDS-related lymphomas are usually seen as a late manifestation of AIDS,[74] often after the CD4 count has fallen below 50–100 cells/mm[3] when the patient is in a state of severe immunosuppression.[16] An estimated 2–5% of AIDS patients are affected by an AIDS-related lymphoma, and the incidence of these tumours is increasing.[40,74–80] As prophylactic and supportive therapies for AIDS patients have prolonged survival, the number of patients developing AIDS-related lymphomas is expected to continue to increase.[2,16,74] AIDS-related lymphomas are mostly non-Hodgkin's B cell lymphomas — poorly differentiated large or anaplastic lymphomas, Burkitt's lymphoma, and immunoblastic sarcomas.[74] The cause of AIDS-related lymphomas is not known, but various cofactors including viral agents have been implicated as possible stimulants of B-cell overproliferation.[77,81]

Acquired immune deficiency syndrome-related lymphomas are aggressive, rapidly growing tumours that present with widespread visceral involvement including extranodal sites (85%) such as bone marrow, bowel, liver/ spleen, kidneys, central nervous system, and skin.[28,76,77,82,83] The reported incidence of thoracic lymphoma in AIDS ranges from 6 to 40%.[81] The lung parenchyma is involved in approximately 10% of patients.[28] Lymphoma is the initial AIDS-defining illness in almost 80% of cases.[83] Characteristics of AIDS-related lymphomas include high-grade, late-stage lymphoma at presentation and severe B symptoms.[74,81]

Thoracic manifestations of AIDS-related lymphomas are varied[28] and differ from the typical findings of lymphoma in the general population. Only 22–25% will demonstrate hilar or mediastinal lymph node involvement, the more typical findings of lymphoma in the general population (Fig. 51.6).[28,40,81] AIDS-related lymphomas also present in atypical patterns with chest wall masses, lytic bone lesions, pulmonary nodules and masses with or without lymphadenopathy (Fig. 51.7).[11,28] Pleural effusions are more common in AIDS-related lymphomas occurring in 30–50% of patients.[81] Lung involvement may take the form of nodules, masses, reticulonodular infiltrates or airspace consolidation.[81] Pulmonary nodules or masses are more common in AIDS-related lymphomas occurring in 10–30% of cases at the time of presentation (Fig. 51.7).[40,81] Lung nodules from lymphoma may be small or large, but they rarely cavitate so enabling differentiation from nodules due to infections; additionally they are usually more well marginated compared to the nodules in KS.[81] Lung masses due to lymphoma may also demonstrate very aggressive growth patterns.[28,81]

Staging of AIDS-related lymphomas includes CT examinations of the head, chest, abdomen, and pelvis. Gallium scanning may also be used. Initial staging also involves bone marrow aspiration and lumbar puncture for cytology.[77]

The prognosis for AIDS-related lymphomas is poor, although some (33–60%) will temporarily respond to chemotherapy.[77] Relapse rates are high and remission usually short-lived with median survival of 5–7 months.[40,77,81] Combination chemotherapy with cyclophosphamide, doxorubicin, vincristine and prednisone (CHOP) is often used in conjunction with GM-CSF in an attempt to lessen myelosuppression while treating the lymphoma.[2]

Whether AIDS patients also have an increased risk for Hodgkin's lymphoma remains uncertain.[74] Some reports have shown an increased incidence in homosexual HIV-infected males, but overall incidence of Hodgkin's disease in AIDS has not been documented.[19] Hodgkin's disease in the setting of HIV infection, however, is atypical in its manifestations; patients present with tumours at more advanced stages of disease and with more aggressive histologies, usually of mixed cellularity types, and they present with more extranodal disease; additionally their Hodgkin's disease responds less well to treatment. Prognosis is significantly

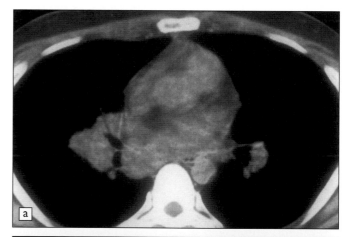

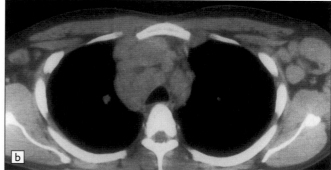

Figure 51.6. *Thirty-five-year-old man with AIDS-related lymphoma. (a, b) Bulky adenopathy is present in both axilla, the right hilum, and the mediastinum including the internal mammary nodes, the anterior mediastinum, the right paratracheal zone, and the subcarinal area. Only 25% of AIDS-related lymphomas will demonstrate this pattern of nodal disease in the chest.*

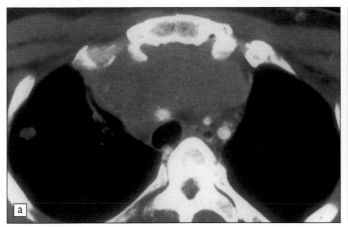

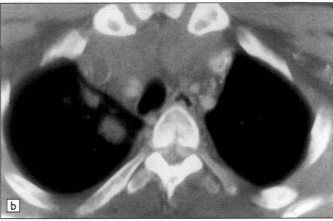

Figure 51.7. *Forty-five-year-old man whose AIDS-defining illness was this aggressive, non-Hodgkin's lymphoma. (a, b) CT scans show a large infiltrative tumour in the anterior mediastinum encasing the vessels and obliterating the fat planes. Note also the multiple right pulmonary nodules found at presentation. Lymphoma in the general population rarely presents with pulmonary nodules, rather pulmonary spread is usually a late manifestation after treatment failure and recurrence. Not so in the AIDS patient who may present with pulmonary disease due to an AIDS-related lymphoma.*

poorer in the HIV-infected patient with Hodgkin's disease than in the general population.[77,81]

Rare primary pulmonary T-cell lymphomas have been reported in HIV-infected patients. These tumours present as slow growing pulmonary masses.[84]

Key points: AIDS-related lymphoma (ARL)

■ ARL is usually seen when the patient is in a severe state of immunosuppression

■ ARLs are most commonly non-Hodgkin's B cell lymphomas, poorly differentiated, Burkitt's or immunoblastic

■ ARL presents with atypical patterns with chest wall masses, lytic bone lesions, pulmonary nodules and masses. Only 22–25% have mediastinal or hilar lymph node involvement

■ The prognosis for ARL is poor, relapse rates are high, remission short-lived and the median survival is 5–7 months

AIDS-related lymphadenopathy syndromes

Other HIV-associated lymphoproliferative disorders include AIDS-related adenopathy. Lymphadenopathy is a common finding in patients with AIDS and may be due to a variety of causes including:

- Infection (secondary to tuberculosis, *Mycobacterium avium* complex, fungal infections, disseminated PCP)
- AIDS-related lymphomas
- The lymphadenopathic form of KS[85]
- Benign lymphoid hyperplasia[86]

Adenopathy due to lymphoid hyperplasia that occurs in the HIV-infected patients without an AIDS-defining illness is part of the AIDS-related complex (ARC) and the persistent generalized lymphadenopathy syndrome (PGL). Persistent generalized lymphadenopathy syndrome is lymphadenopathy present at two or more extra-inguinal, non-contiguous sites that persists for more than 3 months. No other AIDS-defining illnesses, infection, or drug reaction may be present to fit the criteria.[16]

These patients frequently demonstrate moderately enlarged lymph nodes on chest CT scans in the axilla, the supraclavicular region, and the cervical neck region.

Extensive mediastinal adenopathy is not usually a manifestation of lymphoid hyperplasia or the PGL syndrome. When extensive mediastinal adenopathy is detected on CT or plain films the differential diagnosis should include opportunistic infection particularly due to mycobacterial or fungal pathogens, an AIDS-related lymphoma, or rarely the lymphadenopathic form of KS.[11,85–88] Persistent generalized lymphadenopathy syndrome indicates chronic overstimulation of B-cell production and a proportion of these patients will go on to develop an AIDS-related B lymphoma.[74]

Other features of mediastinal and hilar nodes may be helpful in narrowing the differential diagnosis. For example, enlarged lymph nodes due to mycobacterial infection, particularly tuberculosis, often demonstrate necrotic low-density centres and rim enhancement. Such features, however, may also be seen in disseminated fungal infections and lymphoma (Fig. 51.5).[87,88] Lymph nodes involved with KS may show enhancement greater than surrounding muscle or soft tissues when intravenous contrast is administered. Disseminated Pneumocystis infection can cause large bulky mediastinal and hilar lymph nodes that demonstrate significant dystrophic calcification on CT.[89,90]

LYMPHOID INTERSTITIAL PNEUMONITIS

Lymphoid interstitial pneumonitis (LIP) is characterized pathologically by infiltration of the lung interstitium by lymphocytes and plasma cells.[40,91] This is an AIDS-defining pulmonary illness when it occurs in children and adolescents less than 13 years of age (Fig. 51.8). It has also been reported in adult patients with AIDS, primarily in blacks and Haitians.[40,91] On chest radiographs, LIP presents as bilateral reticular or reticulonodular pulmonary infiltrates (Fig. 51.8). Hilar and mediastinal lymphadenopathy may also be seen.[92] Lymphoid interstitial pneumonitis must be distinguished from PCP in the infant with AIDS. Pneumocystis pneumonia usually occurs within the first year of life, between the ages of 3 and 6 months. Lymphoid interstitial pneumonitis, on the other hand, is more likely to occur in

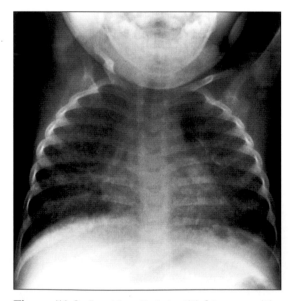

Figure 51.8. *Lymphocytic interstitial pneumonitis (LIP) in a child less than 13 years of age is an AIDS defining illness. Chest film in this 1-year-old girl with AIDS shows typical LIP reticulonodular infiltrates bilaterally. (Reprinted with permission from Kuhlman J E. Pneumocystic infections: The radiologist's perspective, Radiology 1996; 198:623–635.)*

the HIV-positive infant who is older than 1 year of age.[93,94] A closely related disorder is pulmonary lymphoid hyperplasia (PLH) which is in the spectrum of polyclonal B-cell lymphoproliferative disorders (PBLD) seen in HIV-infected children. In cases of PLH, hyperplastic lymphoid follicles proliferate around distal small airways. PLH may be seen with LIP. Epstein–Barr virus has been implicated as the infectious cofactor in both PLH and LIP.[16]

LUNG CANCER IN AIDS

Whether other malignancies such as lung cancer have an increased incidence in AIDS is uncertain.[4,5,95] A few small series of young male patients with AIDS and lung cancer have appeared in the literature, but an increased risk factor for developing lung cancer due to HIV has not yet been documented. Most, if not all patients with lung cancer and AIDS, are long-term smokers (90%) and male (97%) (Figs 51.9 and 51.10).[5,8,96–101] The degree of immunosuppression and the CD4 count do not correlate well with the presence of lung cancer in HIV-infected patients, so if there is an increased association of lung cancer in AIDS it may be due to a direct oncogenic effect of HIV rather than through immunosuppression.[5,102] Lung cancer appears to occur at an earlier age in HIV-infected patients, and present at more advanced stages of disease.[5,8,98–101,103] The most common histology is adenocarcinoma (Fig. 51.9).[4,5,95] Prognosis is very poor with less than 1 year survival after diagnosis.[5,98–101,104–109]

Radiographic manifestations of bronchogenic carcinoma in 30 HIV-infected patients were recently reviewed by Fishman et al.[98] Findings included a peripheral mass (60%) versus a central hilar or mediastinal mass (37%). One patient presented with a pleural mass. Peripheral tumours had a predilection for the upper lobes. Lymphadenopathy was identified in 63%, and pleural effusions in 33%. Peripheral tumours in three patients were mistaken for or hidden by inflammatory disease, so delaying diagnosis.[98] Distribution of cell types was as follows: adenocarcinoma (43%), squamous cell (30%), adenosquamous (7%), small cell (7%), large cell (7%), mixed small and large cell (3%), poorly differentiated non-small cell (3%).[98] Only 20% of tumours were Stage-I at presentation, while 20% were Stage-III and 53% were Stage-IV tumours.[98] Similar findings have been noted in other series, including cases in which pleural disease and effusions were the predominant presenting manifestations of lung cancer (Fig. 51.10).[5,99]

Because delays in diagnosis of lung cancer have occurred when focal lung lesions are assumed to be due to infection in an AIDS patient, any focal lesion which fails to respond to antibiotic treatment should be further evaluated.[101] Peripheral focal lung lesions are amenable to percutaneous transthoracic biopsy which has a high diagnostic yield of 85% for focal lung lesions.[110] Complication rate in this setting is acceptable and not higher than in non-HIV infected patients.[110]

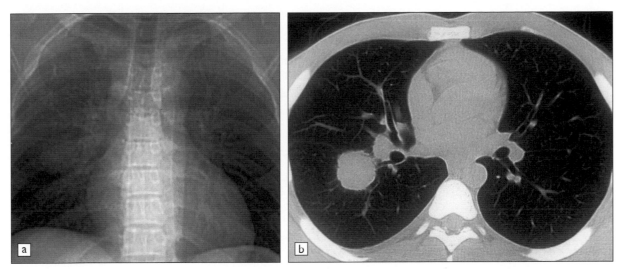

Figure 51.9. *Twenty-seven-year-old HIV-infected man who smokes. (a, b) A 3 cm mass is present in the perihilar region of the superior segment of the right lower lobe. Bronchoscopic biopsy revealed adenocarcinoma of the lung. It is not known whether there is an increased incidence of lung cancer in HIV-infected patients. What is known is that lung cancer occurs at an earlier age, is more aggressive, presents at a more advanced stage, and has a poorer prognosis in the HIV-infected patients. The most common cell type is adenocarcinoma.*

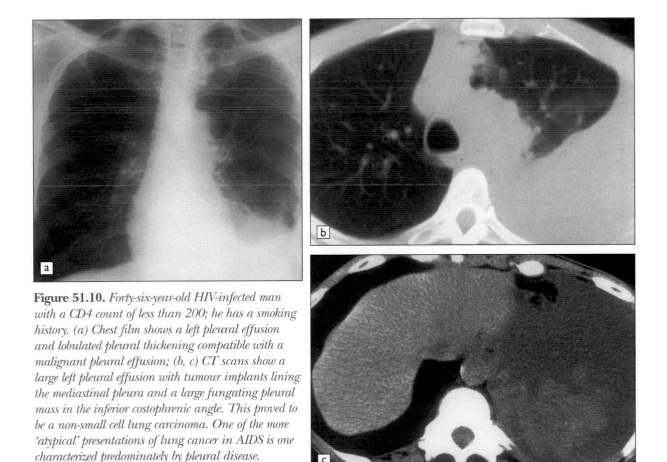

Figure 51.10. *Forty-six-year-old HIV-infected man with a CD4 count of less than 200; he has a smoking history. (a) Chest film shows a left pleural effusion and lobulated pleural thickening compatible with a malignant pleural effusion; (b, c) CT scans show a large left pleural effusion with tumour implants lining the mediastinal pleura and a large fungating pleural mass in the inferior costophrenic angle. This proved to be a non-small cell lung carcinoma. One of the more 'atypical' presentations of lung cancer in AIDS is one characterized predominately by pleural disease.*

Summary

- The degree of immune suppression often dictates the most likely pulmonary neoplasm or disease.

- Kaposi's sarcoma can develop when immunosuppression is still not severe.

- Kaposi's sarcoma is the most common neoplastic disorder to affect the lung in the patient with AIDS, and when present is usually part of a widespread multisystem system.

- The major differential diagnosis for pulmonary infiltrates in an AIDS patient with KS is opportunistic infection — sputum production is not typical of pulmonary KS and is more likely due to opportunistic infection.

- In the more advanced stages of AIDS, multiple diseases coexist simultaneously in the lung, making it almost impossible to exclude superimposed infection with one or more organisms in addition to involvement of the lung with KS.

- ARL is usually a late manifestation of AIDS, often after CD4 counts have fallen below 50–100 cells/mm^3.

- Thoracic manifestations of ARL differ from the typical findings of lymphoma in the general population.

- Causes of lymphadenopathy in AIDS include ARL, KS, lymphoid hyperplasia and opportunistic infection.

- Lymphoid interstitial pneumonitis is an AIDS-defining pulmonary illness where it occurs in children and adolescents of less than 13 years of age.

REFERENCES

1. Mann J M, Welles S L. Global aspects of the HIV epidemic. In: de Vita V T, Hellman S, Rosenberg S A (eds) AIDS: Etiology, diagnosis, treatment and prevention. Philadephia: Lippincott, 1988: 89–98

2. Conant M A. Management of human immunodeficiency virus-associated malignancies. Recent Results in Cancer Res 1995; 139: 423–432

3. Osmond D, Charlebois E, Lang W, Shiboski S, Moss A. Changes in AIDS survival time in two San Francisco cohorts of homosexual men, 1983 to 1993. JAMA 1994; 271: 1083–1087

4. Mitchell D M, Miller R F. New developments in the pulmonary diseases affecting HIV infected individuals. Thorax 1995; 50: 294–302

5. White C S, Haramati L B, Elder K H, Karp J, Belani C P. Carcinoma of the lung in HIV-positive patients: Findings on chest radiographs and CT scans. Am J Roentgenol 1995; 164: 593–597

6. Safui B, Diaz B, Schwartz J. Malignant neoplasms associated with human immunodeficiency virus infection. Cancer J Clin 1992; 42: 74–95

7. Munoz A, Schrager L K, Bacellar H et al. Trends in the incidence of outcomes defining acquired immuno-deficiency syndrome (AIDS) in the multicenter AIDS cohort study: 1985–1991. Am J Epidemiol 1993; 137: 423–438

8. Padhani A R, Kuhlman J E. Pulmonary manifestations of AIDS. Appl Radiol 1993; 22: 13–19

9. Kuhlman J E. Invited commentary. CT pattern recognition in AIDS. Radiographics 1993; 13: 785–786

10. Naidich, D P. Pulmonary manifestations of HIV infection. In Greene R (ed) Syllabus: A categorical course in diagnostic chest radiology. Oak Brook, Illinois: Radiologic Society of North America, Inc, 1992: 135–155

11. Kuhlman J E. CT evaluation of the chest in AIDS. In Thrall J H, Decker B C (eds) Current Practice of Radiology. Mosby-Year Book Inc, 1993: 9–18

12. Gradon J D, Timpone J G, Schnittman S M. Emergence of unusual opportunistic pathogens in AIDS: A review. Clin Infect Dis 1992; 15: 134–157

13. Sider L, Gabriel H, Curry D R et al. Pattern recognition of the pulmonary manifestations of AIDS on CT Scans. Radiographics 1993; 13: 771–784

14. Katz M J, Hessol N A, Buchbinder S P, Hirozawa A, O'Malley P, Holmberg S D. Temporal trends of opportunistic infections and malignancies in homosexual men with AIDS. J Infect Dis 1994; 170: 198–202

15. Weiss R A. Human herpesvirus 8 in lymphoma and Kaposi's sarcoma: Now the virus can be propagated. Nature Med 1996; 2: 277–278

16. Nash G, Said J W, Nash S V, DeGirolami U. Short course: The pathology of AIDS. Mod Pathol 1995; 8: 199–217

17. Wang C Y E, Schroeter A L, Su W P D. Acquired immunodeficiency syndrome-related Kaposi's sarcoma. Mayo Clin Proc 1995; 70: 869–879

18. Trachiotis G D, Hafner G H, Hix W R, Aaron B L. Role of open lung biopsy in diagnosing pulmonary complications of AIDS. Ann Thorac Surg 1992; 54: 898–902

19. Hessol N A, Katz M H, Liu J Y et al. Increased incidence of Hodgkin disease in homosexual men with HIV infection. Ann Int Med 1992; 117: 309–311

20. Gruden J F, Klein J S, Webb W R. Percutaneous transthoracic needle biopsy in AIDS: Analysis in 32 patients. Radiology 1993; 189: 567–571

21. Scott W W Jr, Kuhlman J E. Focal pulmonary lesions in patients with AIDS: Percutaneous transthoracic needle biopsy. Radiology 1991; 180: 419–421

22. Cadranel J, Mayaud C. Intrathoracic Kaposi's sarcoma in patients with AIDS. Thorax 1995; 50: 407–414

23. Denton A S, Miller R F, Spittle M F. Management of pulmonary Kaposi's sarcoma: New perspectives. Br J Hosp Med 1995; 53: 344–350

24. Steinbach L S, Tehranzadeh J, Fleckenstein J L, Vanarthros W J, Pais M J. Human immunodeficiency virus infection: Musculoskeletal manifestations. Radiology 1993; 186: 833–838

25. White D A, Zaman M K. Pulmonary disease. Medical management of AIDS patients. Med Clin North Am 1992; 76: 19–44

26. Davis S D, Henschke C I, Chamides B K et al. Intra-thoracic Kaposi sarcoma in AIDS patients: Radiographic– pathologic correlation. Radiology 1987; 163: 495–500

27. Sivit C J, Schwartz A M, Rockoff S D. Kaposi's sarcoma of the lung in AIDS: radiologic–pathologic analysis. Am J Roentgenol 1987; 148: 25–28

28. Goodman P C. Pulmonary manifestations of AIDS. Curr Probl Diagn Radiol 1988; 17: 81–89

29. Albini A, Mitchell C D, Thompson E W et al. Invasive activity and chemotactic response to growth factors by Kaposi's sarcoma cells. J Cell Biochem 1988; 36: 369–376

30. Cooley T P. Kaposi's sarcoma. In: Libman H, Witzburg R A (eds) HIV Infection: A Clinical Manual (2nd ed) Boston: Little, Brown & Co, 1993: 354–367

31. Mitchell D M, Miller R F. Recent developments in the management of the pulmonary complications of HIV disease. Thorax 1992; 47: 381–390

32. Ognibene F P, Steis R G, Macher A M et al. Kaposi's sarcoma causing pulmonary infiltrates and respiratory failure in the acquired immunodeficiency syndrome. Ann Intern Med 1985; 102: 471–475

33. Zibrak J D, Silvestri R C, Costello P et al. Bronchoscopic and radiologic features of Kaposi's sarcoma involving the respiratory system. Chest 1986; 90: 476–479

34. Wahman A, Melnick S L, Rhame F S, Potter J D. The epidemiology of classic, African, and immunosuppressed Kaposi's sarcoma. Epidemiol Rev 1991; 13: 178–199

35. Beral V, Peterman T A, Berkelman R L, Jaffe H W, Kaposi's sarcoma among patients with AIDS: A sexually transmitted infection? Lancet 1990; 335: 123–128

36. Friedman-Kien A E, Saltzman B R. Clinical manifestations of classical, endemic African and endemic AIDS-associated Kaposi sarcoma. J Am Acad Dermatol 1990; 22: 1237–1250

37. Montaner J S G, Le T, Hogg R et al. The changing spectrum of AIDS index disease in Canada. AIDS 1994; 8: 693–696

38. Naidich D P, McGuinness G. Pulmonary manifestations of AIDS: CT and radiographic correlations. Radiol Clin North Am 1991; 29: 999–1017

39. Naidich D P, Garay S M, Leitman B A et al. Radiographic manifestations of pulmonary disease in acquired immunodeficiency syndrome (AIDS). Semin Radiol 1987; 22: 14–30

40. Heitzman E R. Pulmonary neoplastic and lymphoproliferative disease in AIDS: A review. Radiology 1990; 177: 347–351

41. Lee V W, Fuller J D, O'Brien M J et al. Pulmonary Kaposi sarcoma in patients with AIDS: Scintigraphic diagnosis with sequential thallium and gallium scanning. Radiology 1991; 180: 409–412

42. Hanson P J V, Hancourt-Webster J N, Grazzard B G et al. Fibroscopic bronchoscopy in the diagnosis of pulmonary Kaposi's sarcoma. Thorax 1987; 42: 269–271

43. Lau K Y, Rubin A, Littner M et al. Kaposi's sarcoma of the tracheobronchial tree: Clinical bronchoscopic and pathologic features. Chest 1986; 89: 158–159

44. Pitchenick A E, Fischl M A, Saldoma M. Kaposi's sarcoma of the tracheobronchial tree: Clinical bronchoscopic and pathologic features. Chest 1985; 87: 122–124

45. Gill P J, Akil B, Colletti P et al. Pulmonary Kaposi's sarcoma: Clinical findings and resulting therapy. Am J Med 1989; 87: 57–61

46. Lee V W, Rosen M P, Baum A et al. AIDS-related Kaposi sarcoma: Findings on thallium-201 scintigraphy. Am J Radiol 1988; 151: 1233–1235

47. Garay S M, Belenko M, Fazzini E et al. Pulmonary manifestations of Kaposi's sarcoma. Chest 1987; 91: 39–43

48. Antman K, Nadler L, Mark E J et al. Primary Kaposi's sarcoma of the lung in an immunocompetent 32-year-old heterosexual white man. Cancer 1987; 54: 1696–1698

49. Kornfeld H, Axelrod J L. Pulmonary presentation of Kaposi's sarcoma in a homosexual patient. Ann Rev Respir Dis 1983; 127: 248–249

50. Herts B R, Megibow A J, Birnbaum B A et al. High-attenuation lymphadenopathy in AIDS patients: Significance of findings at CT. Radiology 1992; 185: 777–781

51. Wolff S D, Kuhlman J E, Fishman E K. Thoracic Kaposi sarcoma in AIDS: CT findings. J Comput Assist Tomogr 1993; 17: 60–62

52. Caray S, Belenko M, Fazzini E, Schinella R. Pulmonary manifestations of Kaposi's sarcoma. Chest 1987; 91: 39–43

53. Medur G U, Stover D E, Lee M et al. Pulmonary Kaposi's sarcoma in the acquired immune deficiency syndrome. Am J Med 1986; 81: 11–81

54. Zibrak J D, Silvestri R C, Costello P et al. Bronchoscopic and radiologic features of Kaposi's sarcoma involving the respiratory system. Chest 1986; 90: 476

55. White D A, Stover D E. Pulmonary effects of AIDS. Clin Chest Med 1988; 9: 363–535

56. Franquet T, Gimenez A, Caceres J, Sabate J M, Nadal C. Imaging of pulmonary–cutaneous disorders: Matching the radiologic and dermatologic findings. Radiographics 1996; 16: 855–869

57. Longo D L. Kaposi's sarcoma and other neoplasms. Ann Intern Med 1984; 100: 92–106

58. Nash G, Fligiel S. Kaposi's sarcoma presenting as pulmonary disease in the acquired immunodeficiency syndrome. Diagnosis by lung biopsy. Hum Pathol 1984; 15: 999

59. Meduri G U, Stover D E, Lee M et al. Pulmonary Kaposi's sarcoma in the acquired immune deficiency syndrome. Am J Med 1986; 81: 11–18

60. Pitchenik A F, Fischl M A, Saldana M J. Kaposi's sarcoma of the tracheobronchial tree: Clinical, bronchoscopic and pathologic features. Chest 1985; 87: 122–124

61. Hanson P J V, Hancourt-Webster J N, Grazzard B G, Collins J V. Fibroscopic bronchoscopy in the diagnosis of pulmonary Kaposi's sarcoma. Thorax 1987; 42: 269–271

62. Lau K Y, Rubin A, Littner M, Krauthammer M. Kaposi's sarcoma of the tracheobronchial tree: Clinical, bronchoscopic and pathologic features. Chest 1986; 89: 158–159

63. Naidich D P, Tarras M, Garay S M et al. Kaposi's sarcoma: CT–radiographic correlation. Chest 1989; 96: 723–728

64. Khalil A M, Carette M F, Cadranel J L, Mayaud C M, Bigot J M. Intrathoracic Kaposi's sarcoma: CT findings. Chest 1995; 108: 1622–1626

65. Hartman T E, Primack S L, Muller N L, Staples C A. Diagnosis of thoracic complications in AIDS: Accuracy of CT. AJR 1994; 162: 547–553

66. Herts B R, Megibow A J, Birnbaum B A, Kanzer G K, Noz M E. High-attenuation lymphadenopathy in AIDS patients: Significance of findings at CT. Radiology 1992; 185: 777–781

67. Wagner R P, Farber H W. Pulmonary manifestations. In: Libman H, Witzburg R A (eds) HIV Infection: A Clinical Manual (2nd ed). Boston: Little, Brown & Co, 1993: 124–145

68. Tappero J W, Koehler J E, Berger T G et al. Bacillary angiomatosis and bacillary splenitis in immunocompetent adults. Ann Int Med 1993; 118: 363–365

69. Khalil A M, Carette M F, Cadranel J L et al. Magnetic resonance imaging (MRI) findings in pulmonary Kaposi's sarcoma: A series of 10 cases. Eur Respir J 1994; 7: 1285–1289

70. Krown S E, Metroka C, Werntz J C. AIDS Clinical Trials Group Oncology Committee. Kaposi's sarcoma in the acquired immune deficiency syndrome: A proposal for uniform evaluation, response and staging criteria. J Clin Oncol 1989; 7: 1201–1207

71. Gill P S, Alcil B, Colletti P et al. Pulmonary Kaposi's sarcoma: Clinical findings and results of therapy. Am J Med 1989; 87: 57–61

72. Krigel R L, Friedman-Kien A E. Kaposi's sarcoma. In: de Vita V T, Hellman S, Rosenberg S A (eds) AIDS: Etiology, diagnosis, treatment and prevention. Philadelphia: Lippincott, 1988: 245–261

73. White D A, Matthay R A. Noninfectious pulmonary complications of infection with the human immuno-deficiency virus. Am Rev Resp Dis 1989; 140: 1763–1787

74. Gaidano G, Dalla-Favera R. Molecular pathogenesis of AIDS-related lymphomas. Adv Cancer Res 1995; 67: 113–120

75. Hessol N A, Katz M H, Liu J Y et al. Increased incidence of Hodgkin disease in homosexual men with HIV infection. Ann Intern Med 1992; 117: 309–311

76. Nyberg D A, Jeffrey R B Jr, Federle M P et al. AIDS-related lymphomas: Evaluation by abdominal CT. Radiology 1986; 159: 59–63

77. Cooley T P. Aids-related lymphoma. In: Libman H, Witzburg R A (eds) HIV Infection: A Clinical Manual (2nd ed) Boston: Little, Brown & Co, 1993; 368–375

78. Kaplan L D, Abrams D I, Feigal E et al. AIDS associated non-Hodgkin's lymphoma in San Francisco. JAMA 1989; 261: 719–724

79. Pluda J M et al. Development of non-Hodgkin's lymphoma in a cohort of patients with severe human immunodeficiency (HIV) infection on long-term anti-retroviral therapy. Ann Intern Med 1990; 113: 276–282

80. Moore R D, Kessler H, Richman D D et al. Non-Hodgkin's lymphoma in patients with advanced HIV infection treated with zidovudine (Abstract). 7th International Conference on AIDS, Florence, June 1991.

81. Dodd G D, Greenler D P, Confer S R. Thoracic and abdominal manifestations of lymphoma occurring in the immunocompromised patient. Radiol Clin N Am 1992; 30: 597–610

82. Meduri G U, Stein D S. Pulmonary manifestations of acquired immunodeficiency syndrome. Clin Infect Dis 1992; 14: 98–113

83. Radin D R, Esplin J A, Levine A M, Ralls P W. AIDS-related non-Hodgkin's lymphoma: Abdominal CT findings in 112 patients. AJR 1993; 160: 1133–1139

84. Kohler C A, Gonzales-Ayala E, Rowley P, Malamud F, Verghese A. Primary pulmonary T-cell lymphoma associated with AIDS: The syndrome of the indolent pulmonary mass lesion. Am J Med 1995; 99: 324–326

85. Kuhlman J E, Fishman E K, Knowles M G et al. Disease of the chest in AIDS: CT diagnosis. Radiographics 1989; 9: 827–857

86. Bottles K, McPhaul L W, Volberding P. Fine-needle aspiration biopsy of patients with the acquired immunodeficiency syndrome (AIDS): Experience in an outpatient clinic. Ann Int Med 1988; 108: 42–45

87. Radin D R. Intraabdominal Mycobacterium tuber-culosis vs Mycobacterium avium-intracellulare infections in patients with AIDS: distinction based on CT findings. Am J Roentgenol 1991; 156: 487–491

88. Radin D R. Disseminated histoplasmosis: Abdominal CT findings in 16 patients. Am J Roentgenol 1991; 157: 955–958

89. Groskin S A, Massi A F, Randall P A. Calcified hilar and mediastinal lymph nodes in an AIDS patient with Pneumocystis carinii infection. Radiology 1990; 175: 345–346

90. Radin D R, Baker E L, Klatt E C et al. Visceral and nodal calcification in patients with AIDS-related Pneumocystis carinii infection. Am J Roentgenol 1990; 154: 27–31

91. Travis W D, Fox C H, Devaney et al. Lymphoid pneumonitis in 50 adult patients infected with the human immodeficiency virus: Lymphocytic interstitial pneumonitis versus nonspecific interstitial pneumonitis. Hum Pathol 1992; 23: 529–541

92. Rubinstein A. Pediatric AIDS. Curr Probl Pediatr 1986; 16: 364

93. Marquis J R, Bardeguez A D. Imaging of HIV infection in the prenatal and postnatal period. Clin Perinatal 1994; 21: 125–147

94. Simonds R J, Lindegren M L, Thomas P et al. Pro-phylaxis against Pneumocystis carinii pneumonia among children with perinatally acquired human immunodeficiency virus infection in the United States. N Engl J Med 1995; 332: 786–790

95. Fraire A E, Awe R J. Lung cancer in association with human immunodeficiency virus infection. Cancer 1992; 70: 432–436

96. Braun M A, Killam D A, Remick S C et al. Lung cancer in patients seropositive for human immunodeficiency virus. Radiology 1990; 175: 341–343

97. Moser R J III, Tenholder M F, Redennour R. Oat-cell carcinoma in transfusion-associated immunodeficiency syndrome. Ann Intern Med 1985; 103: 478

98. Fishman J E, Schwartz D S, Sais G J, Flores M R, Sridhar K S. Bronchogenic carcinoma in HIV-positive patients: Findings on chest radiographs and CT scans. Am J Roentgenol 1995; 164: 57–61

99. Braun M A, Killam D A, Remick S C, Ruckdeschel J C. Lung cancer in patients seropositive for human immunodeficiency virus. Radiology 1990; 175: 341–343

100. Sridhar K S, Flores M R, Raub W A Jr, Saldana M. Lung cancer in patients with human immunodeficiency virus infection compared with historic control subjects. Chest 1992; 102: 1704–1708

101. Tenholder M F, Jackson H D. Bronchogenic carcinoma in patients seropositive for human immunodeficiency virus. Chest 1993; 104: 1049–1053

102. Shiramizu B, Hendier B G, McGrath M S. Identification of a common clonal human immunodeficiency virus integration site in human immunodeficiency virusassociated lymphomas. Cancer Res 1994; 34: 2069–2072

103. Unusual malignant tumours in 49 patients with HIV infection. AIDS 1989; 3: 449–452

104. Chan T K, Aranda C P, Rom W N. Bronchogenic carcinoma in young patients at risk for acquired immunodeficiency syndrome. Chest 1993; 103: 862–864

105. Nguyen V Q, Ossorio M A, Roy T M. Bronchogenic carcinoma and the acquired immunodeficiency syndrome. J Ky Med Assoc 1991; 89: 322–324

106. Karp J, Profeta G, Marantz P R, Karpel J P. Lung cancer in patients with immunodeficiency syndrome. Chest 1993; 103: 410–413

107. Fraire A E, Awe R J. Lung cancer in association with human immunodeficiency virus infection. Cancer 1992; 70: 432–436

108. Vaccher E, Tirelli U, Spina M et al. Lung cancer in 19 patients with HIV infection (letter). Ann Oncol 1993; 4: 85–86

109. Biggar R J, Burnett W, Miki J, Nasca P. Cancer among New York men at risk of the acquired immunodeficiency syndrome. Int J Cancer 1989; 43: 979–985

110. Scott W W, Kuhlman J E. Focal pulmonary lesions in patients with AIDS: Percutaneous transthoracic needle biopsy. Radiology 1991; 180: 419–421

Chapter 52

Abdomen and pelvis

Alec Megibow

INTRODUCTION

Acquired immune deficiency syndrome (AIDS) occurs in every part of the world and the epidemic has spared no socio-economic segment of the population. As the disease entity was recognized 'early' in the USA, a large volume of case experience has accrued. Imaging has maintained a peripheral, but important role in the evaluation of these patients. Because of the overlap of radiological findings in neoplastic and non-neoplastic diseases encountered in the patient with AIDS, the major role of imaging has been first to localize sites of disease and second to attempt to guide therapy to the site of disease which is most treatable and has the most significant morbidity.[1] In these patients, neoplastic diseases are not the source of immediate life-threatening clinical situations. Nevertheless, their distribution and appearance must be appreciated so that other foci of diseases are recognizable and treatment therefore expedited.

There are two neoplasms which account for virtually all of the neoplasms in AIDS patients: Kaposi's sarcoma (KS) and non-Hodgkin's lymphoma. The association between AIDS and other cancers is mostly speculative because surveillance biases tend to favour detecting associations that may be spurious. The overall risk of other cancers appears, however, to be only twofold that in the general population, with associations being most convincing for anal (but not cervical) cancer, leiomyosarcoma and possibly also for Hodgkin's disease and testicular cancer.[2] Kaposi's sarcoma preferentially affects homosexual men and risk varies by geographic area, suggesting that there is an environ-mental cofactor for KS in addition to human immunodeficiency virus (HIV). Despite intensive investigation, the responsible cofactor has not been identified conclusively. Human immune deficiency virus-associated non-Hodgkin's lymphoma affects all HIV transmission groups, and non-Hodgkin's lymphoma risk increases with duration of HIV infection and age.[3] The radiological features of each will be described for the abdomen. Differential diagnostic consideration will be catalogued at the end of the chapter.

PATHOLOGY AND CLINICAL BACKGROUND

The unusual appearance of KS in a young homosexual male was the first reported case which led to the recognition of the AIDS epidemic. One of the earliest radiological series was derived from this clinical material.[4]

Ninety-five percent of patients with KS will have cutaneous lesions.[5] After the skin, the organs most frequently involved by KS are lymph nodes and the gastro-intestinal (GI) tract.[6] Extracutaneous spread is common, involving most frequently the oral cavity, GI tract, lungs, and lymph nodes.[7] The tumour is derived from lymphatic endothelia and is associated with luminal lesions in at least 40% of patients. Its presence generally does not alter overall survival in AIDS.[8] A high frequency of GI involvement by KS has been shown, with the most frequently involved site being the small intestine, followed by the stomach and colon. Early stages of KS in the GI tract are not as easily recognized as they are in the skin or lymph nodes.[6]

The incidence of non-Hodgkin's lymphoma continues to increase in the UK and in the USA (see Chapter 28). Improvements in diagnostic techniques, changes in disease classifications, and the increase in AIDS-related lymphomas (ARL) account for only a small percentage of the increase.[9] The incidence of non-Hodgkin's lymphoma is greatly increased in HIV-infected individuals, the vast majority being clinically aggressive B-cell derived neoplasms (similar to Burkitt's lymphoma). Approximately 80% arise systemically (nodal and/or extranodal), and the remaining 20% arise as primary central nervous system (CNS) lymphomas. Extranodal sites of involvement include:[10]

- Gastro-intestinal tract (54%)
- Liver (29%)
- Kidney (11%)
- Adrenal gland (11%)
- Lower genito-urinary tract (11%)
- Spleen (7%)
- Peritoneum and omentum (7%)
- Pancreas (5%)

- Epidural space (4%)
- Bone (3%)
- Muscle (10%)

The GI tract is a common site of involvement in ARL. The most common presentations of GI non-Hodgkin's lymphoma are:

- Abdominal pain (77%)
- Abdominal tenderness (77%)
- Weight loss (77%)
- Gastro-intestinal bleeding (38%)

The most common sites of GI involvement are[11]:

- The large bowel (46%)
- Ileum (39%)
- Stomach (23%)

Gastro-intestinal lymphomas are usually symptomatic and almost always require treatment. Clinical symptoms include change in bowel habits, rectal bleeding, involuntary weight loss, abdominal pain, abdominal tenderness, peripheral lymphadenopathy, cachexia, and hepatosplenomegaly. Obstruction, perforation and bleeding may occur in patients with luminal involvement, whereas hepatic or biliary disease may lead to jaundice. There is a strong correlation with the presence of significant symptomatology and the presence of definable lesions in patients with gastro-intestinal ARL.[8,12]

RADIOLOGICAL IMAGING OF THE ABDOMEN: AN OVERVIEW

The AIDS patient is most frequently referred for imaging to evaluate an acute change in symptomatology. Because the definition of AIDS is partially dependent on the clinical diseases afflicting the patient, the underlying disease(s) will be known at the time of imaging.[13] Computed tomography (CT) has become the most widely used imaging technique for a global overview of the entire abdomen, facilitating the recognition of the distribution and patterns and separating the multiple diseases often present in these individuals.[14,15] Radin[16] evaluated a consecutive series of HIV-positive patients undergoing abdominal CT. Computed tomography scans with abnormal findings in 259 patients with HIV infection were analysed. Diagnoses were mycobacterial infection (n=87), lymphoproliferative disease (n=63), KS (n=17), fungal infection (n=17), hepatocellular disease (n=13), Pneumocystis carinii infection (n=8), other disorders (n=39), or unknown (n=30). Abnormal findings included lymph node enlargement (n=159), hepatomegaly (n=100), splenomegaly (n=62), GI mass or wall thickening (n=61), and low attenuation lesions in the liver (n=50) or spleen (n=55). Diagnoses thought to account for CT findings were made in 247 (95%) of the 259 patients.

Other modalities are reserved for clinically directed studies. *Ultrasound* may be useful in the evaluation of hepatobiliary disease. In a large series (414 patients under-going 684 ultrasound studies) evaluating the use of ultrasound, abnormalities were detected in 264 of the 399 studies available for review. These include splenomegaly (n=124), lymphadenopathy >3 cm (n=83), gallbladder/bile duct abnormalities (n=80), hepatomegaly (n=77), and ascites (n=54). Clinical indications with the highest frequency of abnormal findings included hepatosplenomegaly (n=337) and abnormal liver function tests (n=270).[17] Barium radiography may be used in patients with symptoms directly related to the GI tract and oesophagus.[18] No data is available to assess the role of *magnetic resonance imaging* (MRI) in the evaluation of abdominal disease in AIDS patients.

Radiological technique is critical to successful detection and characterization of abdominal AIDS pathology. All CT scans should be performed with sufficient oral contrast to outline the entire bowel. Intravenous contrast administered with a power injector is critical for the detection of solid organ pathology and characterization of lymph nodes. Barium studies will be requested for the evaluation of intestinal mucosa. In this regard, double-contrast techniques are mandatory. While there may be some increase in the detection of small bowel pathology with enteroclysis techniques, these patients are generally too debilitated to justify nasoduodenal intubation.

KAPOSI'S SARCOMA

Alimentary tract

In AIDS patients, Kaposi's sarcoma (EKS) rarely presents in the GI tract without cutaneous manifestations. Kaposi's sarcoma is associated with luminal lesions in at least 40% of patients. Gastro-intestinal EKS is usually asymptomatic but may rarely bleed, obstruct or become the lead point of an intussusception.[8]

Kaposi's sarcoma is recognized by the presence of nodules of varying size. Careful fluoroscopic evaluation will show these lesions to arise within the submucosa of the alimentary canal. As opposed to classic KS, few of the nodules display the so-called 'bull's eye' appearance. In advanced disease, the nodules coalesce and present as infiltrating lesions which can cause contour abnormalities simulating varices. The lesions are best visualized with double-contrast radiography.

Differential diagnosis is generally not problematic. Multiple submucosal lesions may be seen in a variety of metastatic tumours to the gut wall, but these are not likely in the AIDS patient. Infiltration commonly occurs in the stomach and the appearance can simulate advanced gastric lymphoma. The endoscopic appearance is so characteristic that this problem is rarely encountered clinically.

Liver and spleen

Kaposi's sarcoma affects the liver in approximately one-third of patients with cutaneous disease.[5] The lesions are rarely visualized at CT. Sporadic reports have appeared characterizing the lesions as low attenuation masses against a background of enhanced hepatic parenchyma. They have been reported to present in close association with portal vein branches. Imaging rarely demonstrates EKS in the spleen. Because of the relatively minor importance of EKS splenic involvement, establishing its presence is rarely pursued.

Several types of lesions can produce small lucencies within the liver in the AIDS patient. Most common differential considerations include micro-abscesses,[19] mycobacterial disease[20] and bacillary angiomatosis.[21]

Lymph nodes

Lymphadenopathy is the most frequent abnormality encountered in AIDS imaging. Differential diagnosis of the cause of adenopathy is critical because it may be caused by treatable disease. Kaposi's sarcoma has a distinctive appearance on CT scans on which the lymph nodes show bright enhancement after intravenous contrast medium (Fig. 52.1). This can be ascribed to hypervascular hyperplasia of lymph nodes containing interweaving fascicles of spindle cells, extravasated red blood cells, vascular slits, and deposition of haemosiderin.[6] The positive predictive value of hyperattenuating adenopathy for EKS was shown recently to be 79%; findings statistically significant at the 95% confidence interval.[22]

The distribution of adenopathy is not characteristic. Most cases we have seen involve retroperitoneal and pelvic lymph nodes. There is a high frequency of inguinal and femoral node involvement, relating to lymphatic drainage from the lower extremities. In many patients, CT will show characteristic 'streaky' soft tissue attenuation and infiltration in the inguinal fat. This results in obscuration of the borders of the femoral vessels and nodes (Fig. 52.2).

Key points: Kaposi's sarcoma (KS)

- Gastro-intestinal KS is seldom present without skin KS
- Kaposi's sarcoma of the GI tract usually manifests as nodules
- Liver and spleen involvement is rarely demonstrated on imaging
- Lymph nodes infiltrated with KS typically show intense enhancement following intravenous contrast medium injection

AIDS-RELATED LYMPHOMA

Alimentary tract

There is a wide spectrum of radiological abnormalities seen in the GI tract in patients with ARL. In a large review of CT findings in patients with ARL, the GI tract was shown to be the most common site of the disease.[10] Of interest is the almost mirror-like sites of involvement compared to non-AIDS GI lymphoma (see Chapter 28). In ARL, distal involvement is common with the stomach being least frequently affected.

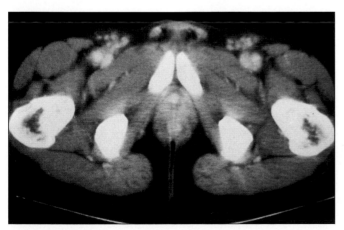

Figure 52.1. *KS: enhanced lymphadenopathy. Brightly enhanced inguinal adenopathy, isodense with pelvic vessels.*

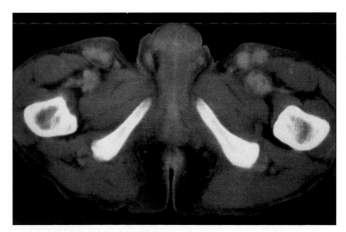

Figure 52.2. *KS: infiltrative changes in inguinal fat. Inguinal and femoral adenopathy, isodense with pelvic vessels. Note the streaky increased density in the inguinal fat. This finding is typical of KS and may persist in the absence of adenopathy.*

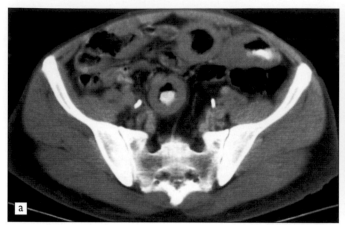
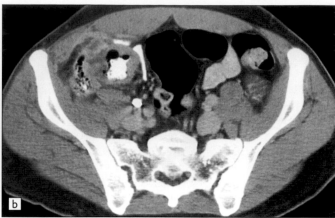

Figure 52.3. *ARL: small bowel. (a, b) Images from CT studies in two different patients reveal focal, variable, segmental, soft tissue attenuating wall thickening indicative of enteric ARL.*

No barium correlation is necessary to establish the aetiology. Note the lack of peritumoral adenopathy frequently accompanying similar lesions in non-ARL cases.

There is no unique pattern of radiological change. One will usually see an obvious thickening of the wall of the affected segment of bowel (Fig. 52.3). Ulceration may occur. Correlation with barium radiological patterns suggests that mural infiltration and irregular fold thickening are the most common manifestations. However, ARL rarely results in mucosal infiltration (as seen in 'Mediterranean lymphomas'), the endo-exoenteric forms, nor in so-called aneurysmal dilatation typically seen in non-AIDS patients.[23] Finally, as opposed to non-AIDS GI lymphomas, the presence of local adenopathy is unusual.

Even though there are no 'typical' appearances to GI lymphomas, the lesions are often large or extensive at presentation. Computed tomography alone can detect the disease and it is rarely necessary to use barium radiography or endoscopy (Fig. 52.4). Barium is used to validate equivocal findings. We find this method to be more cost-effective than endoscopy because when present the disease is usually obvious and subtle, equivocal abnormalities are usually due to misinterpreted, unfilled or undistended loops.

Bulky perirectal lymphomas are virtually unique in ARL. Huge central pelvic masses massively thicken the rectal wall, displacing the lower pelvic viscera (Fig. 52.5). Endoscopic evaluation is limited because the mucosa is not affected. In our experience, patients are often seen by their physician complaining of tenesmus or other related symptomatology suggesting a perianal or perirectal abscess. An apparent fluctuant mass may be palpated. When aspiration fails to reveal pus, the patient is referred for imaging localization and the entire extent of the lesion becomes immediately apparent.

AIDS-related lymphoma may present within the peritoneal cavity (Fig. 52.6). The features are identical to any metastatic lesion within the peritoneal cavity including omental caking.[24] Peritoneal lymphomatosis may be seen in non-AIDS lymphomas as well.

Liver and spleen

The liver is the second most frequent abdominal site of radiologically detectable ARL. Focal splenic and hepatic involvement is more common in both AIDS-related Hodgkin's disease (10%) and non-Hodgkin's lymphomas (26%) than reported in the non-AIDS population.[25] Moderate or marked hepatomegaly (cephalocaudal span >20 cm) and splenomegaly (cephalocaudal span >15 cm) is unusual without demonstrable focal masses.[10] Most hepatic disease is seen in the context of multicentric, extranodal disseminated disease. However, primary hepatic lymphoma has been reported.[26]

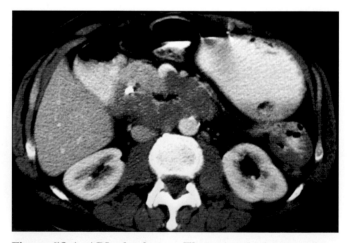

Figure 52.4. *ARL: duodenum. The patient had presented with obstructive jaundice. On the contrast-enhanced CT scan a bulky low attenuation mass surrounds the irregular, ulcerated duodenal lumen. The mass invades the superior mesenteric vein. Notice the discretely defined borders of the enhanced pancreatic parenchyma.*

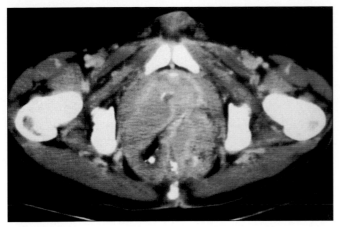

Figure 52.5. *ARL: rectum. This is a typical appearance of ARL involving rectum on CT with lateral spread throughout the pelvis.*

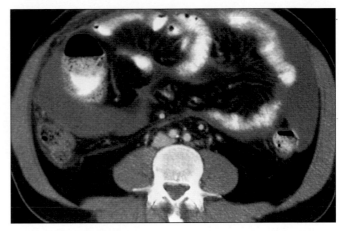

Figure 52.6. *ARL: peritoneal cavity. CT scan showing changes typical of peritoneal carcinomatosis with loculated ascites and omental caking are seen. Bowel appears normal. There is no adenopathy.*

Focal liver lesions in ARL present as well-defined round masses which in our experience range from 1–3 cm in size. We have not seen conglomerate solitary masses. The periphery of the lesion is not sharply circumscribed as in 'typical' metastatic disease. The lesions almost always have a uniform attenuation value slightly less than that of enhanced hepatic parenchyma. Their detection requires contrast-enhanced CT performed during peak hepatic enhancement (Fig. 52.7). In approximately 10% of cases, the lesions will have varying amounts of central low attenuation, presumably necrosis. The presence of this feature does not correlate with the size of the lesions. On sonography, the masses are deceptively hypoechoic (typical of lymphomatous lesions elsewhere), but display poor through-transmission.

Splenic lesions are large (>1.5 cm) masses with a homogeneous attenuation similar to the liver lesions. This is the only radiologically detectable form of the disease. Unlike non-AIDS lymphoma, splenic infiltration and enlargement is uncommon. Diffuse enlargement probably reflects haematopoietic or reticulo-endothelial hyperplastic states as opposed to neoplastic infiltration.

Genito-urinary (GU) disease

Renal lymphoma is usually a manifestation of disseminated disease and is often asymptomatic. Occasionally, the kidney(s) may be the major or only demonstrable site of disease, which may then present with a variety of urological symptoms. The imaging studies should be tailored according to the presenting symptoms and prior history. Currently, CT with intravenous contrast material enhancement is the study of choice for both the evaluation of renal involvement as well as staging of the disease. When necessary, CT or sonography may be used to guide percutaneous needle biopsy of suspicious masses.[27] Most renal disease is

seen in the context of multicentric non-nodal involvement. However, primary renal lymphoma has been reported.[28] Multiple bilateral homogeneously attenuating soft tissue masses, similar to lymphomatous renal involvement seen in non-AIDS related lymphomas, are visualized (Fig. 52.8). We have not seen renal ARL present as diffuse nephromegaly, a well-documented manifestation in non-AIDS related lymphoma (see Chapter 28).

Adrenal enlargement may signal lymphomatous involvement of these structures. The patients do not have clinical or chemical evidence of adrenal malfunction. Function is not compromised during or following systemic treatment.

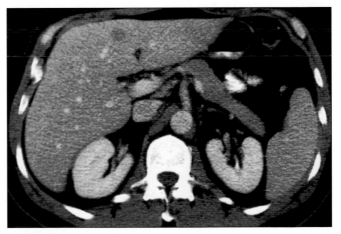

Figure 52.7. *ARL: liver. The lesion seen in the medial segment of the left lobe is typical of hepatic ARL on CT. Note the lack of a discrete border and the minimal contrast against enhanced hepatic parenchyma. Meticulous scanning technique in terms of hepatic enhancement is necessary to detect these findings.*

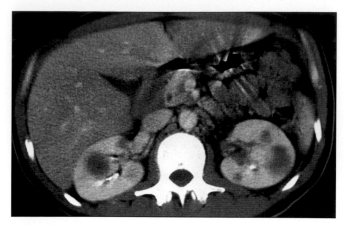

Figure 52.8. *ARL: kidneys. There are bilateral homogeneous soft tissue masses in the kidneys. This is virtually pathognomonic of lymphoma. The appearances of ARL are identical to non-ARL.*

Although lymphomas may affect any portion of the GU tract, focal masses along transitional epithelium are rare. Lower GU involvement, when seen, manifests as sheet-like infiltration of the lower pelvic viscera. The fat planes between the bladder, seminal vesicles and prostate are blurred by the dense soft tissue sheets of infiltrating neoplasm. As the disease is treated, follow-up imaging will show the normal visceral contours emerging from the pelvic infiltration.

Lymph nodes

Although extranodal involvement is the hallmark of ARL, nodal disease does occur. Radin et al. found lymphadenopathy in 41 of 72 patients with ARL and with focal abdominal abnormalities on CT scanning.[10] However, these authors did not establish that the adenopathy was due to lymphoma. In our experience, one must be wary of assuming that adenopathy in patients with extranodal abdominal ARL is due to lymphoma. When confronted with this finding, we recommend biopsy of an accessible node to confirm that the patient is not harbouring a second disease (most frequently mycobacterial). Gallium scanning is also useful in identifying the nodes as lymphomatous. Conversely, if clinical symptomatology and laboratory data do not support infection, one could treat the lymphoma and monitor nodal response. A more complete discussion of lymphadenopathy is presented in the previous section on KS.

Key points: AIDS-related lymphoma (ARL)

- The gastro-intestinal tract is the most common site of involvement

- The appearances are non-specific; distal GI tract involvement is common and the disease is usually bulky

- Bulky perirectal lymphoma is almost unique to AIDS

- Focal liver and spleen abnormalities are common in ARL and usually range in size from 1–3 cm

- Renal ARL is most commonly manifest as multiple masses

- Even in visceral involvement by ARL, lymphadenopathy may be due to other causes

Summary and differential diagnosis

The major differential diagnosis confronting the clinician caring for the patient with AIDS is between infectious or neoplastic disease. Based on imaging findings alone, differentiation is frequently impossible, and often imaging serves as a guide for needle aspirations or tissue biopsies. There are several 'rules' which may direct the investigation:

■ Most visceral masses greater than 1 cm are due to ARL. Liver lesions such as tuberculosis, micro-abscesses, bacillary angiomatosis, etc. produce lesions in the 0.3–10 mm range. Involvement of solid organs with these entities will produce a myriad of lesions, whereas lymphomas produce only few.

■ Organ enlargement is not typical of ARL.

■ Lymphadenopathy is rare in ARL in marked contra-distinction to non-ARL. Lymphadenopathy is common in mycobacterial diseases and in KS. In the latter entity, one may see high attenuation in the nodes in approximately 80% of cases.

■ Kaposi's sarcoma rarely produces significant masses in the GI tract.

■ Liver and spleen involvement are well established at autopsy, but rarely produce disease recognizable by current imaging methods.

■ Virtually all patients suspected of KS lesions by imaging will have cutaneous manifestations of the disease.

■ Although the hallmark of GI pathology on CT scanning is mural thickening, non-neoplastic disease can be separated from neoplastic abnormalities by visualization of oedema in the bowel wall; its visibility is enhanced by intravenous contrast administration.

■ The radiologist must be aware that, more often than not, multiple diseases will be present in the same individual.

REFERENCES

1. Wyatt S H, Fishman E K. The acute abdomen in individuals with AIDS. Radiol Clin North Am 1994; 32: 1023–1043

2. Bigger R J, Rabkin C S. The epidemiology of AIDS-related neoplasms. Hematol Oncol Clin North Am 1996; 10: 997–1010

3. Rabkin C S. Epidemiology of AIDS-related malignancies. Curr Opin Oncol 1994; 6: 492–496

4. Rose H S, Megibow A J, Horowitz L, Laubenstein L. Alimentary tract involvement in Kaposi sarcoma: radiographic and endoscopic findings in 25 homosexual men. Am J Roentgenol 1982; 139: 661–666

5. Federle M P, Nyberg D A, Hulnick D H, Jeffrey R Jr. Malignant neoplasms: Kaposi's sarcoma, lymphoma, and other diseases with similar radiographic features. In: Federle M P, Megibow A J, Naidich D P (eds) Radiology of AIDS. New York: Raven, 1988: 77–105

6. Amazon K, Rywlin A M. Systemic manifestations of Kaposi's sarcoma. In: Gottlieb G, Ackerman A (eds) Kaposi's sarcoma: A text and atlas. Philadelphia: Lea & Febiger, 1988: 113–127

7. Dezube B J. Clinical presentation and natural history of AIDS-related Kaposi's sarcoma. Hematol Oncol Clin North Am 1996; 10: 1023–1029

8. Friedman S L. Kaposi's sarcoma and lymphoma of the gut in AIDS. Baillière's Clin Gastroenterol 1990; 4: 455–475

9. Palackdharry C S. The epidemiology of non-Hodgkin's lymphoma: Why the increased risk? Oncology 1994; 8: 67–73

10. Radin D R, Esplin J A, Levine A M, Ralls P W. AIDS-related non-Hodgkin's lymphoma: Abdominal CT findings in 112 patients. Am J Roentgenol 1993; 160: 1133–1139

11. Knowles D M. Etiology and pathogenesis of AIDS-related non-Hodgkin's lymphoma. Hematol Oncol Clin North Am 1996; 10: 1081–1091

12. Cappell M S, Botros N. Predominantly gastrointestinal symptoms and signs in 11 consecutive AIDS patients with gastrointestinal lymphoma: A multicenter, multiyear study including 763 HIV-seropositive patients. Am J Gastroenterol 1994; 89: 545–549

13. Pantongrag-Brown L, Nelson A M, Brown A E, Buetow P C, Buck J L. Gastrointestinal manifestations of acquired immunodeficiency syndrome: Radiologic pathologic correlation. Radiographics 1995; 15: 1155–1178

14. Jeffrey R Jr. Abdominal imaging in the immuno-compromised patient. Radiol Clin North Am 1992; 30: 579–596

15. Megibow A J, Wall S D, Balthazar E J, Rybak B J. Gastrointestinal radiology in AIDS patients. In: Federle M P, Megibow A J, Naidich D P (eds) Radiology of AIDS. New York: Raven, 1988: 77–105

16. Radin R. HIV infection: Analysis in 259 consecutive patients with abnormal abdominal CT findings. Radiology 1995; 197: 712–722

17. Smith F J, Mathieson J R, Cooperberg P L. Abdominal abnormalities in AIDS: detection at US in a large population. Radiology 1994; 192: 691–695

18. Wall S D. Gastrointestinal imaging in AIDS-luminal gastrointestinal tract. Gastroenterol Clin North Am 1988; 17: 523–533

19. Murray J G, Patel M D, Lee S, Sandhu J S, Feldstein V A. Microabscesses of the liver and spleen in AIDS: Detection with 5 MHz sonography. Radiology 1995; 197: 723–727

20. Schneiderman D J. Hepatobiliary abnormalities of AIDS. Gastroenterol Clin North Am 1988; 17: 615–630

21. Mohle-Boetani J C, Koehler J E, Berger T G et al. Bacillary angiomatosis and bacillary peliosis in patients infected with human immunodeficiency virus: Clinical characteristics in a case-control study. Clin Infect Dis 1996; 22: 794–800

22. Herts B B, Megibow A J, Birnbaum B A, Kanzer G K, Noz M E. High-attenuation lymphadenopathy in AIDS patients: significance of findings at CT. Radiology 1992; 185: 777–781

23. Levine M S, Rubesin S E, Pantongrag-Brown L, Buck J L, Herlinger H. Non-Hodgkin's lymphoma of the gastro-intestinal tract: Radiographic findings. Am J Roentgenol 1997; 168: 165–172

24. Maya M M, Fried K, Gendal E S. AIDS-related lymphoma: An unusual case of omental caking [letter]. Am J Roentgenol 1993; 160: 661

25. Nyberg D A, Jeffrey R Jr, Federle M P, Bottles K, Abrams D I. AIDS-related lymphomas: Evaluation by abdominal CT. Radiology 1986; 159: 59–63

26. Scerpella E G, Villareal A A, Casanova P F, Moreno J N. Primary lymphoma of the liver in AIDS. Report of one new case and review of the literature. J Clin Gastroenterol 1996; 22: 51–53

27. Eisenberg P J, Papanicolaou N, Lee M J, Yoder I C. Diagnostic imaging in the evaluation of renal lymphoma. Leuk Lymphoma 1994; 16: 37–50

28. Tsang K, Kneafsey P, Gill M J. Primary lymphoma of the kidney in the acquired immunodeficiency syndrome. Arch Pathol Lab Med 1993; 117: 541–543

Index

A

abdominal abscess drainage 869
abdominal complications of treatment 936-9
abdominal treatment effects 975-97
    radiation injury 975-6
    second malignancies 995-6
acoustic schwannoma (neuroma) 558-9
ACTH production
    mediastinal carcinoid tumours 72
    pituitary micro-adenomas 563, 564
actinomycin D 957
acute radiation reactions 37, 976
    liver irradiation 979
adamantinoma 354
adenocarcinoma of unknown origin 854-5
    radiological investigations 855-6
adrenal adenoma 832, 835
adrenal cortical carcinoma 329-30
    adrenal mass differential diagnosis 832,
        833, 835
    clinical features 329-30
    computed tomography (CT) 331, 332
    hormone overproduction 329
    incidence 329
    magnetic resonance imaging (MRI) 333
    pathology 329
    prognosis 330
    radionuclide imaging 334
    staging 335-6
    staging system 331
    treatment 330
    ultrasound 334
adrenal gland
    diffuse enlargement 838
    leukaemic infiltration 648
    primary malignant tumours 329-36
    radiological appearances 831
adrenal lymphoma 610
adrenal metastases 831-8
    breast cancer 408
    computed tomography (CT) 831-2, 835
    differential diagnosis 832, 833, 835
    fluorine-18 fluorodeoxyglucose positron
        emission tomography (FDG PET)
        837
    incidence 831
    influence on staging 834-5
    lung cancer 58
    magnetic resonance imaging (MRI) 832,
        833, 835
        chemical-shift imaging 836-7
        gadolinium-enhancement 836
    oesophageal cancer 95
    percutaneous biopsy 837
    radionuclide imaging 837
    renal cell carcinoma 196, 201-2
    sites of origin 831
adrenal myelolipoma 832
adriamycin 116, 937, 957, 1009
adult T-cell leukaemia/lymphoma 635
    HTLV-1 in aetiology 636
    mediastinal lymphadenopathy 645
aerodigestive tract anatomy 430

aerodigestive tract tumours 429-54
    imaging methods 432
    lymph node involvement 431
        staging 447-50
        surgical management 431-2
    prognosis 430-2
    recurrence 452-3
    treatment 430-2
    see also nasopharyngeal cancer
AIDS-related lymphadenopathy syndromes
    1011-12
AIDS-related lymphoma 584, 602, 1003, 1004
    abdominopelvic sites 1019-20
    adrenal 1023-4
    brain involvement 818
    central nervous system 544, 545
    chest 1010-11
    clinical features 1020
    gastro-intestinal tract 1021-2
    genito-urinary tract 1023, 1024
    liver 1022-3
    lymphadenopathy 1024
    prognosis 1010
    spleen 1023
    staging 1010
AIDS-related tumours
    abdominopelvic region 1019-24
    chest 1003-11
        diagnostic approach 1003-4
    computed tomography (CT) 1020
    ultrasound 1020
alcohol intake 20, 482
alkylating agents 38, 39
alpha-1-antitrypsin deficiency 707
α-foetoprotein (AFP) 28, 29
    endodermal sinus tumours 719
    germ cell tumours 283, 340, 549
        mediastinal 73
        testicular 260
    hepatoblastoma 707
    hepatocellular carcinoma 169
alpha-interferon 1009
anaplastic astrocytoma 520
anaplastic thyroid carcinoma 486
    clinical presentation 486
    pathology 486
    prognosis 484, 486
    treatment 508
anaplastic Wilms' tumour 683
androblastoma *see* Sertoli-Leydig cell
    neoplasms
androgen-secreting adrenal cortical
    carcinoma 329
aneurysmal bone cyst 361, 373
angiography
    meningiomas 558
    pancreatic cancer staging 164
    paragangliomas 562
    skull base chordomas 570
    Wilms' tumour 677-8
angiosarcoma
    bone 354
    computed tomography (CT) 341
    mediastinum 75

retroperitoneum 338
aniline dyes 215
anthracyclines 38
antibody therapy 38
APUDoma
    carcinoid tumours 72
    localization with venous sampling 884-5
aromatic amine carcinogens 215
arytenoid cartilages 460
asbestos exposure 79
ascites 841
    image-guided drainage procedures 869
    ovarian cancer 293, 294
        cytology 288
    pancreatic cancer 160
Askin tumours 353
aspergillosis 935, 939, 940
astrocytoma 518-23
    anaplastic 520
        prognosis 525
    fibrillary 518-19
        brain stem 537
        hypothalamic/optic chiasma 536-7
        prognosis 519, 525
    pilocytic 535-6
        brain stem 537
        cerebellar 535
        hypothalamic/optic chiasma 536-7
    spinal cord 572
    treatment 525-6
        postsurgical change evaluation 526-30
atypical mycobacterial infection 934
automatic image analysis 252
avascular necrosis 652, 653, 962, 969-70, 993
azacitidine 937
azathioprine 932, 937

B

bacilliary angiomatosis 1007, 1009
bacterial pneumonia 934
barium studies
    ovarian cancer 302
    peritoneal metastases 841, 844, 847, 849
Barrett's oesophagus 112
basal cell naevus 377
basisphenoid bone tumour, primary 571, 572
Beckwith-Wiedemann syndrome 671, 672,
    707
Bence-Jones proteins 28, 625, 626
benign prostatic hypertrophy 239
β human chorionic gonadotrophin (HCG)
    28, 29
    embryonal carcinoma 719
    germ cell tumours 283, 340, 549
        mediastinal 73
        testicular 260
    gestational trophoblastic tumours 325
β₂ microglobulin 632
bile duct cancers *see* cholangiocarcinoma
biliary atresia 707
biliary cystadenocarcinoma 183, 185
biopsy 35

adrenal metastases 837
bone tumours 371-2, 882-3
breast cancer 883-4
image-guidance
  gastro-intestinal 866-9
  thoracic 861-2
intra-operative ultrasound 885
Kaposi's sarcoma endobronchial lesions 1005
liver 867
lung metastases 755
lymph node 744, 745, 867
lymphoma 618
paediatric oncology 663
pleural effusion 758
soft tissue sarcomas 378
transcaval 869
Wilms' tumour 679
bischloroethyl nitrosourea (BCNU; carmustine) 668, 931, 932
bladder
  biopsy 218
  post-chemotherapy changes 987
  post-irradiation changes 988-9, 990
bladder cancer 215-36
  aetiology 215
  clinical features 217
  grade of malignancy 216
  imaging rationale 215
  incidence 215
  Jewett-Strong-Marshall classification 218
  lumbosacral plexus pathology 827
  lymph node involvement 216, 217, 220, 235
  metastatic disease 216, 217
  pathology 215-16
  patterns of spread 216
  pelvic CT examination technique 220-1
  predisposing factors 215
  prognosis 217
  radiotherapy 35
    treatment planning 890
  reconstructive surgery 35
  recurrence 216
  relapse 235
  restaging 235
  staging
    accuracy of imaging techniques 230, 233-5
    computed tomography (CT) 221-4, 230, 233-5
    cystoscopic evaluation with biopsy 218
    lymph nodes 220
    magnetic resonance imaging (MRI) 224-30, 233-5
    pelvic organ invasion 222, 223, 224, 230, 231, 232, 235
    perivesical spread 222, 228, 229-30
    primary tumour 219
    ultrasound 218-20, 230
  staging classification 218
  treatment 217
bladder lymphoma 608, 609
bladder rhabdomyosarcoma 712, 713, 714
bleomycin 668, 931, 932, 933, 957, 1009
bone lesion biopsy 882-3
bone leukaemic infiltration 649-52
bone lymphoma 614, 615, 616
bone marrow 765-6
  adult pattern of distribution 766

chemotherapy effects 967, 971-2
  examination for staging 27
  magnetic resonance imaging (MRI) 765, 774, 775, 776, 777, 971-2
    metastatic involvement 779, 780
    normal features 778, 779
    technique 778
  radiation effects 971
bone marrow lymphoma 614, 615, 616
bone marrow metastases 779, 780
  neuroblastoma 697, 698-700
bone metastases 765-83
  bladder cancer 216
  breast cancer 406-7, 771
    radionuclide imaging 405-6, 407
  cholangiocarcinoma 185
  clinical features 766-7
  computed tomography (CT) 773
    comparative aspects 781
    lytic lesions 773
    sclerotic lesions 773
  distribution 767
  endometrial carcinoma 320
  evaluation flow diagram 768
  fractures 772
  imaging modalities 765
  imaging rationale 783
  incidence 767
  lung cancer 59
  magnetic resonance imaging (MRI) 773-4, 775, 776, 777, 779
    comparative aspects 781
    technique 778
  neuroblastoma 697, 698-700, 771
  oesophageal cancer 95
  ovarian cancer 284
  pathological features 767-8
  plain radiography 770-2, 773, 781
    osteoblastic lesions 771, 772
    osteolytic lesions 771, 772
  prostate cancer 242, 252, 771
  radionuclide imaging 765, 768-9, 770
  renal cancer 196, 771
  rhabdomyosarcoma 714
  small cell lung cancer 61
  spinal cord compression 820
  thyroid cancer 771
  tumour response assessment 783, 905
  vascular embolization 883
  vertebral collapse 773, 774, 781-3
bone, radiation effects 962-4, 967-73, 991-4
  atrophic changes 967, 968, 992
  avascular necrosis 969-70, 993
  bone tumours 963-4
  fractures 968-9, 993
  growing skeleton 963, 970, 971, 994
  pathophysiology 967, 991-2
bone scintigraphy
  bone metastases 252, 698, 699, 765, 768-9, 770
  breast cancer metastatic disease 405, 407
  chondrosarcomas 364
  leukaemic bone lesions 650
  lung cancer metastases 59
  primary bone tumours 363-5
  small cell lung cancer staging 61
bone tumours, primary 351-74
  age associations 357
  chondroid origin 353
  classification 351-2

clinical features 352-4
colour Doppler ultrasound 366-7
computed tomography (CT) 365, 369
epidemiology 32
fibrous origin 353
imaging procedures 356
location in bone 357
location in skeleton 357
magnetic resonance imaging (MRI) 365-7, 368-70
malignant round cell tumours 353-4
notochordal origin 354
osteosarcomas 352-3
pattern of osseous destruction 357-9
  geographic lesions (grade I) 357-8
  moth-eaten (grade II) 358
  permeative (grade III) 358-9
percutaneous biopsy 371-2
periosteal response 359-61
plain radiography 351, 356, 359
radiological diagnosis 354-67
  principles 356
  rate of growth 356-7
radionuclide scintigraphy 363-5
recurrence detection 373-4
soft tissue extension 362-3
specific diagnostic features 357
staging 368-71
synovial origin 354
therapeutic response monitoring 372-3, 905
tumour matrix 361-2
vascular origin 354
brachial plexus pathology 410-12, 827-8
brachytherapy 37-8
brain abscess 643
brain lymphoma 610-11, 818
brain metastases 811-18
  bladder cancer 216
  breast cancer 408, 812, 816-17
  clinical presentation 811-12
  colorectal cancer 818
  computed tomography (CT) 812-13, 814
  differential diagnosis 814-15
  distribution within brain 812
  endometrial carcinoma 320
  lung cancer 58-9, 813, 816
  magnetic resonance imaging (MRI) 813, 814
  malignant melanoma 812, 817
  oesophageal cancer 95
  pathophysiology 812
  primary sites 811
  renal cell carcinoma 196
  screening for asymptomatic tumours 813
  small cell lung cancer 61
  testicular germ cell tumours 270
  trophoblastic teratomas 263, 264
brain, post-treatment changes
  chemotherapy 530, 532, 939
  paediatric patients 667
  postsurgical change evaluation 526-30
    contrast-enhanced computed tomography 526
    contrast-enhanced magnetic resonance imaging 526
    dural enhancement 527, 528-30
    parenchymal enhancement 526, 527
  radiotherapy late effects 530-4, 644
    focal radiation necrosis 532, 815

major vessel occlusion 532
mineralizing micro-angiopathy 531-2
necrotizing leukoencephalopathy 531, 644
pituitary gland 533
second malignancy 533-4
telangiectasia 533
white matter changes 530-1, 644
brain stem gliomas 537-9
diffuse 537-8
focal 538-9
brain tumours, primary 515-71
cerebropontine angle tumours 559, 560
factors assisting diagnosis 515-16
germ cell tumours 548-52
glial-cell 517-42
haemangioblastomas 552-3
histological classification 516
imaging techniques 515, 516-17
incidence 518
interventional radiology 886
jugular foramen masses 562
lymphoma 544-5
meningeal metastases 825-6
meningiomas 554-8
nerve tumours 558-60
non-glial 542-71
paragangliomas 562
pineal region 548-52
radiotherapy treatment planning 890, 891, 896
sella region 562-9
skull base 569-70
WHO grading system 543
branchial cysts 443
BRCA1 277, 395, 408
breast cancer 5, 395-412
aetiology 395
arm swelling/neurological symptoms 410
baseline chest X-ray 405
biopsy techniques 883-4
brachial plexus pathology 410-12, 827
carcinoma classification 396
chemo-endocrine neo-adjuvant therapy
response assessment 402-4
coexistent ovarian cancer 408
ductal carcinoma 396
epidemiology 395
genetic factors 395
histopathology 396
incidence/mortality trends 13, 15, 395
inflammatory carcinoma 396
interventional radiology 883-4
intraductal component (EIC) detection
401, 402
lobular carcinoma 396
lymph node involvement 404-5, 406, 407
metastatic disease 405-9
abdomen 408
adenocarcinoma of unknown origin
855
adrenal 831
bone 405-6, 407, 767, 771
brain 408, 816-17
computed tomography (CT) 406, 407, 408
diagnosis at follow-up 406
intracranial meningeal disease 818
intrathoracic 406, 407
liver 406, 408

meninges/spinal cord 408, 825
peritoneal 849
positron emission tomography (PET)
409
pleural effusions 757
pTN classification 399
radiological diagnosis 396-7
radiotherapy 35
treatment planning 891, 896
recurrent locoregional disease 409-12
imaging methods 409, 410
screening 13
second malignancies 947
spinal cord compression 820
staging 28
lymph nodes 399
magnetic resonance imaging (MRI)
401, 402
metastatic disease 405-9
primary tumour 398, 400-2
prognostic relevance 25
stage grouping 399, 400
surgical 27
staging classification 397, 399
surgical treatment 34
survival trends 18
synchronous carcinoma in second breast
405
treatment 24, 399-400
tumour response assessment 905, 906
ultrasound 397
X-ray mammography 397
breast lymphoma 601
breast-ovarian familial cancer syndrome 277
Brenner tumour 278, 280, 281
imaging 290
bronchial arteriography and embolization
866, 867
bronchoscopic tracheobronchial stenting
864-5
Budd-Chiari syndrome
drug-induced 937
renal cell carcinoma venous invasion 202, 203
Burkitt's lymphoma 584, 616, 635
stomach 604
testis 608
busulphan 668, 931, 932, 957

C

CA 19.9 28
CA-125 28
ovarian cancer 277, 283
with breast cancer 408
residual disease assessment 303, 304
screening 289
calcitonin 28, 29
medullary thyroid carcinoma 487
immunohistochemical staining 502
cancer pathogenesis 3-5
Candida infection 935, 937, 962
carboplatin 40, 288
carcinoembryonic antigen (CEA) 28
immunoscintigraphy
colorectal cancer 140
lymph node evaluation 743
postsurgical abdominopelvic fibrosis
978

medullary thyroid carcinoma 487
immunohistochemical staining 502
ovarian cancer 283
carcinogenesis 3
bladder cancer 215
gastric cancer 111
carcinoid syndrome 72
carcinoid tumour
mediastinum 72
ovarian germ cell tumours 282
thymus 71, 72
tumour markers 28
carcinomatous meningitis 27
cardiotoxic chemotherapy 668, 936
cardiovascular function, post-cancer
treatment 668, 936
carmustine (bischloroethyl nitrosourea;
BCNU) 668, 931, 932
catecholamine tumour markers 28
neuroblastoma 691
catheter device complications 925
embolic catheter fragments 925
fibrin sheaths 928
investigation 863
algorithm 864
local trauma during insertion 925
malposition 925, 926, 927
catheter tip 928
mural thrombus 928-31
occlusion 927
paediatric patients 664
sepsis 931
superior vena cava erosion 925
cauda equina compression see spinal cord
compression
cell cycle regulation 3
central nervous system complications 939-40
drug toxicity 939
infections 939-40
central nervous system primary tumours
515-75
diagnostic imaging 515
central neurocytoma 543-4
central venous catheter insertion 862-3, 865
thoracic interventional radiology 862-3
central venous obstruction 863-4
cerebellar medulloblastomas 545, 546-8
pre-operative staging 547-8
prognosis 548
cerebellar mutism 547-8
cerebellar pilocytic astrocytoma 535
cerebral haemorrhage 815
cerebral radiation necrosis 815
cerebropontine angle tumours 559, 560
cervical cancer 20, 309-19
aetiology 309
baseline chest X-ray 324
clinical features 309-10
FIGO classification 310
incidence 13, 15, 309
intravenous urography 324
local recurrence 311
lumbosacral plexus pathology 827
pathology 309
patterns of spread 310
prognosis 311
radiotherapy 35
recurrence detection 318-19
screening 13
staging 310-11

computed tomography (CT) 314-15
Doppler ultrasound 314
lymph nodes 310
magnetic resonance imaging (MRI) 315-18
metastatic disease 312, 313
primary tumour 311, 312, 313
transvaginal/transrectal ultrasound 311, 314, 315
treatment 311
cervical intra-epithelial neoplasia 309, 310
cervical lymphoma 609
chemodectoma, mediastinal 75, 76
chemotherapy 38-41
acute lymphoblastic leukaemia (ALL) 639
acute myeloid leukaemia (AML) 639
bladder cancer 217
bladder changes 987
breast cancer 399
cervical cancer 311
chronic leukaemias 639
combination 39
complications
bone marrow toxicity 39-40
cardiotoxicity 668
central nervous system 939
in children 668
gastrointestinal system 937
liver 937
nephrotoxicity 668, 703
pancreas 937
pulmonary toxicity 668, 931-3, 934
urinary tract 937
dose intensity 39
dose response 39
drug resistance 38
fertility following 987
gastric cancer 116
germ cell tumours 288
high-dose 40
Hodgkin's disease 589
intracranial post-treatment changes 530-2
Kaposi's sarcoma 1009
locoregional 885-6
multiple myeloma 625
nasopharyngeal cancer 430
neuroblastoma 694
new drug trials 40-1
Non-Hodgkin's lymphoma 589
oesophageal cancer 95, 96
ovarian cancer 277, 288
paranasal sinus neoplasms 419
renal changes 987
second malignancies 947, 948-9
small cell lung cancer 60
staging 24
testicular germ cell tumours 264
therapeutic response assessment for clinical trials 904-5
chest wall ulcers, radiation-induced 963
chest X-ray
breast cancer metastatic disease 405
cervical cancer 324
endometrial cancer 324
Kaposi's sarcoma 1005
lung cancer staging 50-1
lung metastases 750, 752
malignant pleural mesothelioma 80-2
diagnosis 80-1
staging 81-2

ovarian cancer 289, 302
pleural effusion 757, 758
pulmonary drug reactions 931
pulmonary infection 933-4
radiation pneumonitis 955-6
soft tissue sarcomas 390
testicular germ cell tumours 259, 268, 271
tumour response assessment 905
tumour volume 906
Wilms' tumour 678, 679
chlorambucil 932, 948, 949
chloroma see granulocytic sarcoma
cholangiocarcinoma 169, 178-85
extrahepatic 180, 181
intrahepatic 179, 181
imaging appearances 179-80
metastatic disease 183, 185
pathology 181
predisposing conditions 178-9
staging 181-5
lymph node involvement 185
primary tumour 184
vascular involvement 183
choledochal cyst 178
chondroblastoma 361
chondroma
larynx 461
tumour matrix 361
chondromyxoid fibroma 358
chondrosarcoma 353, 365, 369
extraskeletal 380
larynx 462
paranasal sinuses 422, 423
periosteal response 360
radionuclide scintigraphy 364
skull base 571, 572
tumour matrix 361
chordoma 354
imaging 570
skull base 570
surgical removal 570-1
choriocarcinoma 260, 282, 283, 325, 716
mediastinal 73
primary extragonadal 340
tumour markers 283
choroid plexus tumour 542
chromium exposure, occupational 415
chromosomal abnormalities
leukaemia 636
Wilms' tumour 671
cirrhosis 789, 876
hepatocellular carcinoma 165, 169, 170-1
cisplatin 116, 264, 266, 288, 668, 937
clear cell ovarian tumour 278, 280, 281
imaging 290
clear cell sarcoma 387
kidney 682
clinical staging 26-7
clinical trials 8
drug trials 40-1
therapeutic response assessment imaging strategy 902-5
objective response definitions 903-4
Clonorchis sinensis 178
Codman's triangle 360, 362
coeliac plexus percutaneous neurolysis 878
colonic lymphoma 604
colorectal cancer 129-45
Dukes' classification 129
follow-up goals 131, 132

hepatic metastases detection 142-5
image-guided biopsy 867
immunoscintigraphy 140-1, 142
incidence/mortality trends 13, 15, 129
local extension 133, 134
metastatic disease
brain metastases 818
intraperitoneal seeding 846
liver metastases preoperative assessment 803-5
peritoneal invasion 843
positron emission tomography (PET) 141-2
postsurgical appearances 976-8
radio-immuno-guided surgery (RIGS) 141
recurrence detection 132, 918, 919
computed tomography (CT) 135-6, 137
endoscopic ultrasound 140
magnetic resonance imaging (MRI) 135, 137-8
screening 13
staging 28, 129-30
computed tomography (CT) 132-5, 137
endoscopic ultrasound 139-40, 142
goals 129
imaging rationale 129
lymph node involvement 131, 133, 135, 137, 139
magnetic resonance imaging (MRI) 136-7, 138
primary tumour 131, 132-3, 136-7, 139
surgical treatment 34, 129
survival trends 17
therapeutic response assessment 900, 901
colour Doppler ultrasound
bone tumours 366-7
cervical cancer staging 314
colorectal cancer
liver metastases detection 145
local recurrence detection 140
endometrial carcinoma staging 321
liver metastases 796, 798
Doppler perfusion index 801
ovarian mass characterization 292
paediatric hepatic neoplasms 708
prostate cancer staging 245
echo-enhancing agents 252
neovascularity 250
renal cell carcinoma venous invasion 207
tumour response assessment 906
tumour composition 911
complications of treatment 925-41
abdomen 936-9
central nervous system 939-40
pelvis 936-9
thorax 925-36
computed tomography arterial portography (CTAP) 876, 877
cholangiocarcinoma 182
hepatocellular carcinoma 173, 176
liver metastases 143, 792, 803
paediatric hepatic neoplasms 710
computed tomography arteriography (CTA)
hepatocellular carcinoma 173, 176
liver metastases 792
computed tomography (CT)
adrenal cortical carcinoma 331, 332
adrenal gland appearances 831

adrenal imaging technique 331
adrenal metastases 831-2, 835
aerodigestive tract tumours 432
AIDS-related abdominopelvic tumours 1020
angiosarcoma 341
ascites detection 841
astrocytoma
    anaplastic 520
    cerebellar 535
    fibrillary 519
    hypothalamic/optic chiasma 536
    pilocytic 535
biliary cystadenocarcinoma 183, 185
bladder cancer staging 218, 221-4
    accuracy 230, 233-5
    lymph node involvement 235
bone metastases 773
    comparative aspects 781
    lytic lesions 773
    sclerotic lesions 773
bone tumours, primary 365
    staging 369
brain neoplasms 515, 516, 517
    metastases 812-13, 814
breast cancer
    abdominal metastases 408
    liver metastases 122
    locally recurrent disease detection 410
    lymph node involvement 405, 406, 407
cerebellar medulloblastomas 546
cervical cancer
    recurrence detection 318
    staging 314-15
cholangiocarcinoma
    extrahepatic 180
    intrahepatic 179-80
    staging 181, 182
colorectal cancer
    liver metastases detection 142-3
    local recurrence detection 135-6, 137
    peritoneal invasion 844
    staging 132-5, 137
craniopharyngiomas 568
dysgerminoma of ovary 290, 291
endometrial carcinoma staging 321-2
epithelioid haemangioendothelioma 187
fibrolamellar hepatocellular carcinoma 178
fibrosarcoma 341
gastric cancer
    direct invasion 843, 844
    staging 117-22, 125
germ cell tumours
    mediastinal 74
    primary extragonadal 341-2
glioblastoma multiforme 521, 522
gliomatosis cerebri 524-5
granulocytic sarcoma 640, 641
    bone 650
haemangioblastoma 552
haemangioma 802
haemangiopericytoma 341
hepatic angiosarcoma 186
hepatoblastoma staging 708-10
hepatocellular carcinoma
    appearances 169, 170, 176
    paediatric neoplasms 708-10
    staging 171, 173-4
hypopharyngeal cancer staging 443-4

Kaposi's sarcoma 1005-6
Krukenburg tumours 847
laryngeal cancer 474-5
    post-treatment evaluation 476
leiomyosarcoma 340
leukaemia
    intracranial abscess 643
    intracranial haemorrhage 643
    meningeal/dural disease 640
    paranasal sinus infections 643, 644
liposarcoma 340, 382
liver cysts 802
liver focal fatty change 803
liver metastases 122, 408, 698, 714, 789, 791-4, 803
    appearances 793-4
    delayed images 791
    dual-phase 791
    hypervascular 794
    intravascular contrast enhancement 789-90
    single-phase volumetric 791
    small lesions 801-2
liver post-irradiation changes 979
lung cancer metastases
    adrenal glands 58
    brain 58-9
    liver 58
lung cancer staging 49, 50, 51-3, 61
    regional lymph node involvement 55, 56
lung metastases
    accuracy 752-4
    indications 755
    paediatric testicular cancer 718
    rhabdomyosarcoma 714
    soft tissue sarcomas 391, 392
    solitary nodule assessment 754
    technique 755
lymph node evaluation 406, 407, 731
    accuracy 742
lymphoma
    adrenal glands 610
    bladder 608, 609
    brain 544, 610
    kidney 607, 608
    liver 602
    lung 599
    neck 592
    nodal disease 589, 590-1
    pancreas 605
    pericardial effusions 600
    pleural effusions 600
    residual mass assessment 617
    small bowel 603-4
    stomach 603
    therapeutic response monitoring 617
    thorax 593-5, 596
    thymus 600
malignant fibrous histiocytoma 340-1
malignant mesenchymoma 341
malignant peripheral nerve-sheath tumour 341
malignant pleural mesothelioma 82-5
    diagnosis 82-4
    staging 84-5
mediastinal lymphadenopathy 714
meningeal metastases, intracranial 819
multiple myeloma 627, 628
    therapeutic response monitoring 630

nasopharyngeal cancer staging 435-6, 437
neck imaging after treatment 452
neuroblastoma 695
    liver metastases 698
    staging 697
oesophageal cancer 96
    recurrence following surgery 104, 105
    staging 97-9, 103-4
oligodendroglioma/oligo-astrocytoma 523
optic gliomas 536
oral cavity/oropharyngeal carcinoma staging 438, 439, 442
ovarian cancer
    intraperitoneal seeding 847
    residual disease assessment 303-4
    staging 289, 293-8, 299, 301, 304
ovarian mass characterization 290, 292-3, 304
paediatric imaging 662, 663
paediatric ovarian germ cell tumours 719-20, 721
pancreatic cancer
    direct invasion 843, 844
    staging 154-60, 162, 163, 165
paragangliomas 562
paranasal sinus neoplasms
    post-treatment recurrence 425
    staging 419, 420, 424
    technique 420-2
pelvic assessment, post radiotherapy 990-1
pelvic examination technique 220-1
peritoneal metastases 841
    accuracy 850
    direct invasion 843-4
    embolic metastases 849
    intraperitoneal seeding 847
phaeochromocytoma 332
pineal germinoma 550
pineal parenchymal tumours (pineoblastoma/pineocytoma) 552
pleomorphic xantho-astrocytoma 539
pleural effusion, malignant 759, 760
post-surgical abdominopelvic fibrosis 978
posterior fossa ependymoma 540
prostate cancer staging 246
    fine-needle aspiration cytology 252
    pelvic lymph node involvement 251
pseudomyxoma periotnei 847
radiation pneumonitis 957-8
radiotherapy treatment planning 36, 893-4
    image fusion 895, 896
    image handling 895
renal cell carcinoma staging 196-202
    accuracy 196
    lung metastases 202
renal transitional cell carcinoma staging 209-10
    accuracy 210
retroperitoneal sarcomas 340-1
rhabdomyosarcoma staging 714
sacrococcygeal teratoma staging 721, 724
skull base chordomas 570
small cell lung cancer staging 61
soft tissue sarcomas 379, 380
    local recurrence detection 389
spinal cord compression 821
supratentorial ependymoma 541
testicular cancer metastatic disease 717

testicular germ cell tumours 259, 268-70
  stage I tumour surveillance 271-2
  therapeutic response monitoring 272, 273
thymic lymphoma/leukaemia 71
thymoma staging 69-70
thyroid cancer 506, 507
trigeminal neuromas 560
tumour response assessment 899, 905
  for clinical trials 904, 905
  tumour composition 911-12
  tumour volume 907-9
vertebral collapse 773, 781
Wilms' tumour 675-6
  chest imaging 678
computed tomography myelography (CT myelography), spinal cord compression 821
conformal therapy 891-2, 893
congenital mesoblastic nephroma 684-5
Conn's syndrome 330
  tumour localization with venous sampling 885
constrictive pericarditis, radiotherapy-induced 668
convexity meningiomas 554
core biopsy 35
Cotswold classification 587
Cowden's syndrome 485
craniopharyngiomas 562-3, 567-9, 570
  differential diagnosis 569
  imaging 568-9
  prognosis 569
  sites 567
  treatment 569
cricoid cartilage 457
Cryptococcus infection 935, 939, 940
cryptorchidism 259
Cushing's syndrome 72, 329, 330
cyclophosphamide 931, 932, 936, 937, 957, 987
cyclophosphenol 668
cyclosporin 644, 931, 933, 937, 939
cystectomy 217
cystic hygroma 443
cystinosis 707
cystitis 215, 216
cystoscopy 218
cytomegalovirus 936, 937
  encephalitis 940
cytosine arabinoside 644, 931, 932, 937, 939
cytotoxic drugs 38
  classification 38, 39

D

dacarbazine 937
'dancing eyes' syndrome (myoclonic encephalopathy of infancy) 704
Denys-Drash syndrome 671
dermatofibrosarcoma protuberans 378
desmoid tumour
  mediastinum 74
  oral cavity/oropharynx 443
desmoplastic infantile ganglioglioma 543
diagnosis 8
diagnostic impact 6-7
diagnostic performance 6
  statistical analysis 7-8

diaziquone 937
diffuse lung disease
  drug reactions 932
  infections 935-6
digital rectal examination, prostate cancer staging 242, 244
Doppler perfusion index (DPI) 801
  liver metastases detection 145
Down's syndrome 636
doxorubicin 1009
drug trials 40-1
Dukes' classification 129
duodenal post-irradiation changes 980
Durie and Salmon classification 626, 628
dysembryoplastic neuro-epithelial tumour 544
dysgerminoma, ovarian 282, 719
  imaging 290, 291

E

embryonal brain tumour 545-6
embryonal carcinoma 5, 260, 283, 716
  mediastinal 73
  paediatric ovarian tumours 719
  primary extragonadal 340
  tumour markers 283, 719
embryonal sarcoma 707
  paediatric hepatic tumours 712
  paratesticular 259
endodermal sinus tumour 282, 716
  mediastinal 73
  paediatric ovarian tumours 719
  tumour markers 283, 719
endometrial carcinoma 319-24
  baseline chest X-ray 324
  clinical features 319
  epidemiology 319
  FIGO classification 320
  imaging accuracy 323-4
  intravenous urography 324
  lymph node involvement 320
  metastatic disease 320
  pathology 319-20
  patterns of spread 320
  prognosis 319
  staging 320-1
    computed tomography (CT) 321-2
    magnetic resonance imaging (MRI) 322-3, 324
    primary tumour 321-4
    transvaginal ultrasound 321, 322
  treatment 320
endometrioid cancers 279, 280, 281
  imaging 290
  prognosis 285
endorectal coil MRI, prostate cancer staging 246, 247, 248
endoscopic retrograde cholangiopancreato-graphy (ERCP) 872-3
endoscopic ultrasound
  colorectal cancer
    local recurrence detection 140
    staging 139-40, 142
  gastric cancer staging 122-4, 125
    lymph node involvement 124
  image-guided gastro-intestinal biopsy 867
  oesophageal cancer
    lymph node involvement 102

metastatic disease 102
  recurrence following surgery 104, 105
  staging 100-4
pancreatic cancer staging 162-3, 165
ependymoma 517, 540-1
  posterior fossa 540-1
  spinal cord 572-3
  supratentorial 541
epidemiology 11-21
  adrenal cortical carcinoma 329
  bladder cancer 215
  bone tumours, primary 32
  brain tumours, primary 518
  breast cancer 395
  cervical cancer 309
  colorectal cancer 129
  endometrial carcinoma 319
  gastric cancer 111
  hepatoblastoma 707
  hypopharyngeal tumours 430
  incidence rates 6
  laryngeal cancer 457
  leukaemia 636
  lung cancer 45-6
  lymphoma 583
  malignant pleural mesothelioma 79, 81
  multiple myeloma 625
  nasopharyngeal cancer 429
  neuroblastoma 691
  oesophageal cancer 93
  oral cavity/oropharyngeal tumours 430
  ovarian cancer 277, 278
  pancreatic cancer 151
  paranasal sinus neoplasms 415
  phaeochromocytoma 330
  prostate cancer 239-40
  renal cell carcinoma 191
  soft tissue sarcomas 377
  testicular germ cell tumours 259
  thyroid cancer 481
  Wilms' tumour 671
epidermoid, cerebropontine angle 560
epidural space metastases, prostate cancer 242
epiglottic tumours 447, 469
epiglottis 460
epiphyseal slippage 970, 994
epipodophyllotoxins 38
epirubicin 116, 876
epithelioid cell sarcoma 387
epithelioid haemangioendothelioma 187
Epstein-Barr virus 583-4
esthesioneuroblastoma (olfactory neuroblastoma) 419, 422
ethmoid tumours 416
  staging 416, 417
etoposide 40, 947, 1009
EUROCARE 12, 13, 17, 18, 19
evaluation of imaging 6-7
  diagnostic impact 6-7
  diagnostic performance 6
  impact on health 7
  statistical analysis 7-8
  technical performance 6
  therapeutic impact 7
Evans classification 692, 693
Ewing's sarcoma 5, 353-4
  atypical 353
  Codman's triangle 360, 362
  extraskeletal 378

periosteal response 360-1
radiological diagnosis 379, 380
staging 27
treatment 353-4
tumour matrix 362
external beam radiotherapy 37

F

familial medullary thyroid carcinoma 486
fat, post-irradiation changes 994
feminization 330
ferritin serum level 691
fertility
following chemotherapy 987
following radiotherapy 989-90
fibrillary astrocytoma 518-19
brain stem 537
hypothalamic/optic chiasma 536-7
prognosis 519, 525
fibrolamellar hepatocellular carcinoma 177-8
computed tomography (CT) 178
paediatric neoplasms 707
staging 178
fibroma
imaging 291
ovarian 281, 288
fibrosarcoma 353
bone 360
computed tomography (CT) 341
paratesticular paediatric neoplasms 718
retroperitoneal sarcomas 337, 338
soft tissue 378
thyroid 487
fibrosing mediastinitis 74
FIGO classification
cervical cancer 310
endometrial carcinoma 320
ovarian cancer 285, 286
paediatric ovarian germ cell tumours 719
financial aspects 6
fine-needle aspiration cytology 35
bone tumours, primary 372
breast cysts 883
lung cancer regional lymph node
involvement 56
prostate cancer pelvic lymph node
involvement 252
soft tissue sarcomas 378-9
solitary thyroid nodule 505, 506, 509
staging 27
thoracic 861
thyroid nodules 481
fistulae, post-irradiation bowel damage 983-4,
985
fluorine-18 fluorodeoxyglucose positron
emission tomography (FDG PET)
adrenal metastases 837
brain neoplasms 515
breast cancer metastatic disease 409
colorectal cancer 142
gliomas (glial-cell tumours) 523
laryngeal cancer post-treatment
evaluation 476
lung cancer regional lymph node
involvement 56, 57
lymphoma
nodal disease 590
residual mass assessment 618

multiple myeloma 627
neuroblastoma 704-5
oesophageal cancer 104
paranasal sinus neoplasms staging 424
pilocytic astrocytoma 535
pituitary micro-adenomas 564
postsurgical abdominopelvic fibrosis 978
small cell lung cancer staging 61
thyroid cancer 72, 499
tumour response assessment 906
for clinical trials 904
tumour composition 916-17
fluoroscopy
laryngeal cancer 474
tracheobronchial stenting 864-5
5-fluorouracil 116, 876, 937, 939
focal radiation necrosis 532, 815
foetal alcohol syndrome 707
follicular thyroid carcinoma 485, 486
clinical presentation 485
pathology 485
prognosis 484, 485
treatment 508
radio-iodine ablation 494
fractures 993
irradiated bone 962, 968-9
free fluid cytology 27
fungal infection
AIDS opportunistic infection 1007
lung infections 935

G

gallium nitrate 937
gallium-67 citrate imaging
bleomycin pulmonary toxicity 957
lymph node evaluation 742-3
thyroid cancer 498-9
ganglioglioma 543
ganglioneuroblastoma
mediastinum 75, 76
myoclonic encephalopathy association
704
ganglioneuroma
mediastinum 75, 76
myoclonic encephalopathy association
704
gastric cancer 111-25
advanced disease 112
in Barrett's oesophagus 112
chemotherapy 116
early disease 112
surgical resection 115
image-guided biopsy 867
imaging rationale 117
incidence/mortality trends 13, 111
intra-operative ultrasound 124
Lauren classification 111, 112
magnetic resonance imaging (MRI) 125
metastatic disease
intraperitoneal seeding 846
peritoneal invasion 843
pathology 111-12
predisposing factors 111
stage grouping 115
staging 112-15
computed tomography (CT) 117-22,
124, 125
endoscopic ultrasound 122-4, 125

lymph node involvement 113, 114,
121-2, 124
metastatic disease 113, 122
primary tumour 113, 114, 118, 119,
122-3
recommendations 125
surgery 115-16
survival 18, 115
gastric lymphoma 603
gastric outlet obstruction 870, 871, 872
post-irradiation damage 980
gastric polyps 111
gastric ulceration, post-irradiation damage
980
gastro-enterostomy feeding tube insertion
871-2, 874
gastro-intestinal interventional radiology
866-79
biopsy techniques 866-9
gastro-intestinal strictures 869-71
gastrostomy/gastro-enterostomy feeding
tube insertion 871-2, 874
inferior vena caval stent/filters insertion
878
obstructive jaundice management 872-5
percutaneous drainage procedures 869
percutaneous neurolysis 878
tumour ablation techniques 879
visceral arteriography 875-8
gastro-intestinal leukaemic infiltration 647
gastro-intestinal lymphoma 603-5
gastro-intestinal strictures
lower gastro-intestinal tract 871, 873
upper gastro-intestinal tract 869-71
gastro-intestinal tract
drug-related complications 937
post-irradiation changes 980-4
fistulae 983-4, 985
post-surgical changes 976-8, 979
gastrostomy feeding tube insertion 871-2
gender differences
second malignancies 949
survival trends 17, 18
genito-urinary paediatric tumours 712-15
genito-urinary system treatment changes
984-90
postsurgical changes 984-7
genito-urinary tract lymphoma 605
germ cell tumours
brain 548-52
meningeal metastases 825
pineal region 550-1
high-dose chemotherapy 40
mediastinal 67, 73-4
clinical features 73
imaging 74
pathology 73
pattern of spread 73
treatment 73, 74
ovarian 279, 282-3, 718-21
follow-up evaluation 721
imaging 290, 719-20
lymph node involvement 720
metastatic disease 720
peritoneal implants 720
prognosis 286
staging 719
treatment 288
primary extragonadal 336, 340
computed tomography (CT) 341-2

magnetic resonance imaging (MRI) 344
 staging 344, 346
 testicular *see* testicular germ cell tumours
 therapeutic response assessment 272, 273, 718, 721, 901-2, 903
  tumour composition 912
 tumour markers 283, 340, 549, 719
 see also sacrococcygeal teratoma
germinoma, intracranial/pineal region 549
 treatment 551
gestational trophoblastic tumours 325
giant cell hepatitis 707
giant cell tumour, bone 354, 359
 vascular embolization 883
Gleason grade 240, 250
glioblastoma multiforme 520-3
glioma (glial-cell tumour) 517-18, 814
 astrocytoma 518-20
 glioblastoma multiforme 520-3
 gliomatosis cerebri 524-5
 malignant grades differentiation 523
 oligo-astrocytoma 523-4
 oligodendroglioma 523-4
 WHO grading system 518
gliomatosis cerebri 524-5
 prognosis 525
glomus jugulari tumour 562
glycogen storage disease type I 707
gonadal dysfunction, treatment-related 668, 686
graft versus host disease 665-6
 abdominopelvic disease 938
 leukaemia 647, 648
 pulmonary disease 936
granulocytic sarcoma (chloroma) 638
 bone 650
 intracranial 640, 641
 orbit 645
 spinal 642
granulosa-theca cell tumour 279, 281, 282
 imaging 291
 paediatric tumours 719
 prognosis 286
gynandroblastoma 279, 281

H

haemangioblastoma, brain 552-3
haemangio-endothelioma
 bone 354
 paediatric hepatic tumours 712
 thyroid 487
haemangioma
 bone 366, 367
 liver 802
 mediastinum 75
 oral cavity/oropharynx 443
 supraglottic 461
 testicular paediatric neoplasms 718
haemangiopericytoma
 bone 354
 computed tomography (CT) 341
 mediastinum 75
 paranasal sinuses 422
 retroperitoneal sarcomas 338
haemango-epithelioma, mediastinum 75
haemoptysis management 865-6
haemorrhagic complications

leukaemia 643, 646, 648
 paediatric patients 666
Hashimoto's thyroiditis 487
Hayes classification 692, 693
head and neck tumours 429
 aerodigestive tract 429-54
  imaging methods 432
  lymph node involvement 431, 432
  lymph node staging 447-50
  surgical management 431-2
 clinical assessment 26
 imaging neck after treatment 451-3, 476
 lymphoma 611, 613
 metastases of unknown primary site 854
 radiotherapy 35, 36
 see also laryngeal cancer; paranasal sinus neoplasms
heart disease
 cardiotoxic chemotherapy-induced 668, 936
 radiation-induced 960-1
Helicobacter pylori 111
hemihyperplasia 671, 672, 679, 707
hemorrhagic cystitis 987, 988
hepatic adenoma 712
hepatic angiosarcoma 186
hepatic venous sampling 884
hepatitis B 20
hepatoblastoma 707-12
 diagnosis 708
 epidemiology 707
 imaging 708
 metastatic disease 710
 pathology 707
 staging 708-10
  clinical grouping 708, 709
 treatment 708
 treatment follow-up 710-11
 tumour markers 707
hepatocellular carcinoma 169-78
 α-foetoprotein (AFP) levels 169
 fibrolamellar tumours 177-8
 imaging appearances 169-71, 176
 lymph node involvement 177
 metastatic disease 177
 mortality 169
 paediatric neoplasms 707-12
  clinical grouping 708, 709
  diagnosis 708
  imaging 708
  incidence 707
  pathology 707
  staging 708-10
  treatment 708
  treatment follow-up 710-11
 pathology 169
 staging 170-7
  computed tomography (CT) 171, 173-4
  magnetic resonance imaging (MRI) 174-5
  primary tumour 171-6
  ultrasound 175-6
 treatment 171
 vascular invasion 176
 visceral arteriography with chemo-embolization 876-7
hepatotoxic drugs 937
herpes simplex virus
 encephalitis 815, 940
 oesophagitis 962

hilar lymphadenopathy, leukaemia 645
Hodgkin's disease 583
 AIDS patients 1010-11
 clinical features 587, 590
 Cotswold classification 587
 Epstein-Barr virus association 583-4
 extranodal disease 597-616
  chest wall 600
  gastro-intestinal tract 603
  liver 602
  lung 598-600
  musculoskeletal system 613
  pericardial effusions 600
  spinal leptomeningeal involvement 611
  spleen 601-2
  thymus 600
 high-dose chemotherapy 40
 incidence/mortality trends 16, 17, 583
 intraperitoneal dissemination 849
 nodal disease 589-97
  abdomen 595-7
  imaging techniques 589-91
  neck 592
  pelvis 595-7
  thorax 592-5, 596
 pathology 584
 prognosis 588
 radiotherapy 35
 residual mass assessment 617-18
 Rye classification 584
 second malignancies 947, 948, 949
 staging 30
  surgical 35
 staging system 585, 587
 therapeutic response assessment 617, 902, 909
 treatment 588-9
 tumour markers 28
hormonal therapy 38
 breast cancer 399
 early prostate cancer 250
Horner's syndrome 433
HTLV-1 584, 636
human papilloma virus (HPV) 20, 309, 314
hydatidiform mole, complete 325
hydatidiform mole, partial 325
5-hydroxyindoleacetic acid (5 HIAA) 28
hypopharyngeal cancer 443-7
 anatomical aspects 443
 clinical features 443
 incidence 430
 pathology 430
 pyriform fossa tumours 443, 444, 446
 staging 443-7
  computed tomography (CT) 443-4
  magnetic resonance imaging (MRI) 443-4, 446-7
  primary tumour 445
 treatment 470
hysterectomy 288, 320
 post-surgical changes 984, 986

I

ifosfamide 668, 685, 686, 703, 937
imaging strategies 8-9
immunoglobulin tumour markers 28
immunoscintigraphy
 colorectal cancer 140-1, 142

liver metastases 800
lymph node involvement evaluation 743
ovarian cancer 301-2
postsurgical abdominopelvic fibrosis 978
small cell lung cancer staging 61
impact on health 7
In-111 pentetreotide (octreotide) 699, 700
incidence of cancer 6, 11
   data 11-12
      analytical approach 12
   trends 13-16
indirect portography 876
inferior vena cava filters insertion 878, 879
inferior vena cava obstruction 338, 864
inferior vena cava stent insertion 878
inferior vena cava thrombus
   magnetic resonance imaging (MRI) 204,
      205, 206
   renal cell carcinoma 196, 197-200, 204-6,
      207
   ultrasound 204, 205, 207
   Wilms' tumour 674, 678
inferior vena cava transcaval biopsy 869
interferon alpha (INF-a) 639
interleukin-2 (IL-2) 931, 932, 937
interstitial (Leydig cell) tumours 259, 716
interventional radiology 861-86
   breast cancer 883-4
   gastro-intestinal 866-79
   locoregional chemotherapy 885-6
   musculoskeletal 882-3
   neurological tumour imaging 886
   parathyroid tumour ablation 885
   percutaneous retrieval techniques 885
   thoracic 861-6
   tumour localization with venous sampling
      884-5
   urinary tract 879-82
intra-operative ultrasound 885
   biopsy 885
   gastric cancer 124
   liver metastases 144, 145, 799-800, 803,
      885
intravenous urography
   cervical/endometrial cancer 324
   ovarian cancer 302
      staging 289
   Wilms' tumour 673, 674
intravesical ultrasound, bladder cancer 230
   staging 219
inverted papilloma, paranasal sinuses 422,
   423

J

jugular foramen masses 562
juvenile angiofibroma 433, 436

K

Kaposi's sarcoma 1003, 1004-9
   clinical variants 1004
   gastrointestinal involvement 1019, 1020-1
   liver involvement 1021
   lymph node involvement 1021
   prognosis 1009
   pulmonary involvement 1005
      bacilliary angiomatosis differentiation

      1007, 1009
   biopsy 1005
   lymphadenopathy 1006-7, 1012
   opportunistic infection differentiation
      1007, 1009
   pleural effusions 1006
   radiological appearances 1005-9
   spleen involvement 1021
   staging system 1009
   treatment 1009
kappa statistics 7, 8
Klatskin tumour 180, 181
Krukenberg tumour 113, 283, 291
   computed tomography (CT) 847
kyphosis 963, 970, 995

L

lactic dehydrogenase 28
   neuroblastoma 691
   testicular germ cell tumours 260
laparoscopy, ovarian cancer residual disease
      assessment 302
laparotomy
   ovarian cancer residual disease
      assessment 302-3
   staging 27, 28
large bowel post-irradiation changes 981-2
laryngeal anatomy 457-61
   cartilage 457, 460
   glottic region 461
   ligaments 460
   magnetic resonance imaging (MRI) 458,
      459
   mucosa 460
   muscles 460
   spaces 460
   subglottic region 461
   supraglottic region 461
laryngeal benign neoplasms 461
laryngeal cancer 457-77
   cartilage invasion 472, 473
   clinical blind spots imaging 472
   computed tomography (CT) 474-5
   fluoroscopy 474
   imaging rationale 472-4
   incidence/mortality trends 17, 457
   magnetic resonance imaging (MRI) 475
   pathology 462, 463
   positron emission tomography (PET) 475
   post-treatment neck imaging 476
   prognosis 463
   staging
      glottic tumours 465
      subglottic tumours 466
      supraglottic tumours 464
   staging classification 463
   treatment 463, 467-71
      glottic tumours 469-70
      hypopharyngeal tumours 470
      subglottic tumours 470, 471
      supraglottic tumours 468-9
   ultrasound 475
   vascular invasion 474
   vocal cord paralysis 476-7
laryngeal cysts 461
laryngeal papillomatosis 461
laryngectomy
   supraglottic (voice-sparing partial) 467,

      468, 476
   total 467, 470, 476
laryngocoele 461, 462
leiomyoma of larynx 461
leiomyosarcoma 325
   computed tomography (CT) 340
   magnetic resonance imaging (MRI) 343,
      344
   paratesticular paediatric neoplasms 718
   retroperitoneal sarcomas 337, 338
   soft tissue 378
leptomeningeal leukaemia 640
leukaemia 635-54
   abdominal involvement 647-8
   aetiology 636
   central nervous system involvement 640-2
      meningeal/dural disease 640
      parameningeal disease 640, 641
   cerebral infarction 643
   chromosomal abnormalities 636
   classification 635
   clinical features 636-8, 639
   graft versus host disease 647, 648
   granulocytic sarcoma (chloroma) 638
      bone 650
      intracranial 640, 641
      orbit 645
      spinal 642
   head and neck involvement 645
   imaging 640
   incidence/mortality trends 13, 636
   intra-abdominal haemorrhage 648
   intra-abdominal infection 649
   intracranial haemorrhage 637, 638, 643
   intracranial infection 643
   intrathoracic disease 645-6
   lymphadenopathy 637, 638
   mediastinal widening 646
   meningeal infiltration 825
   paranasal sinus infections 643, 644
   pelvic involvement 647-8
   post-treatment bone changes 652-3
   pulmonary infection 646
   pulmonary infiltration/oedema 646-7
   second malignancies 947, 948
   sinovenous thrombosis 643
   skeletal involvement 649-52
   staging, prognostic relevance 25
   thymic involvement 71
   treatment 639
   treatment-related complications 643-5
leukaemia, acute lymphoblastic (ALL) 635
   central nervous system involvement 640
   clinical features 637
   incidence 636
   lytic bone lesions 650, 651, 652
   mediastinal lymphadenopathy 645, 646
   treatment 639
   treatment-related complications 644
leukaemia, acute myeloid (AML) 635
   clinical features 637
   incidence 636
   lytic bone lesions 650
   secondary following cancer therapy 636
   survival trends 17
   treatment 639
leukaemia, chronic lymphocytic (CLL) 635
   clinical features 637
   incidence 636
   lymphadenopathy 637, 638, 645

leukaemia, chronic myelocytic (CML) 635
  acute blastic transformation 639
  clinical features 637
  lytic bone lesions 650
Leydig cell tumours 259, 716
Li-Fraumeni syndrome 377, 395
lifetime risk 13
lipiodol-CT 173-4
lipoma
  mediastinum 74, 75
  oral cavity/oropharynx 443
  testicular paediatric neoplasms 718
liposarcoma
  bone 354
  computed tomography (CT) 340, 382
  magnetic resonance imaging (MRI)
        342-3, 382, 383
  mediastinum 74
  oral cavity/oropharynx 443
  pathology 337
  soft tissue 377, 378
        radiological diagnosis 380
        radiological features 380, 382, 383
Listeria meningitis 940
liver cancer 20, 169, 188
  epithelioid haemangioendothelioma 187
  image-guided biopsy 867
  lymphoma 187, 602, 603
  paediatric neoplasms 707-12
        differential diagnosis 712
  tumour markers 28
  see also hepatocellular carcinoma
liver cysts 802
liver focal fatty change 803
liver, leukaemic infiltration 647
liver lymphoma 187, 602, 603
liver metastases 787-806
  benign focal lesions differentiation 802-3
  bladder cancer 216
  breast cancer 406
  cholangiocarcinoma 185
  colorectal cancer 142-5
        preoperative assessment 803-5
  computed tomography arterial
        portography (CTAP) 143, 792, 803
  computed tomography arteriography
        (CTA) 792
  computed tomography (CT) 142-3, 698,
        789, 791-4, 803
        appearances 793-4
        delayed images 791
        dual-phase 791
        single-phase volumetric 791
        small lesions 801-2
  Doppler perfusion index 801
  early detection 802
  endometrial carcinoma 320
  follow-up evaluation 806
  gastric cancer 113, 122
  hypervascular 794
  imaging objectives 790
  imaging strategy 803-6
  immunoscintigraphy 800
  incidence 787
  intra-operative ultrasound 885
  intravascular contrast enhancement
        789-90
  lung cancer 58
  magnetic resonance imaging (MRI) 143,
        144, 698, 789, 794-6, 797, 798, 803

dynamic gadolinium-enhanced
      imaging 796
liver-specific contrast media 796
opposed-phase imaging 796
small lesions 801-2
superparamagnetic iron oxide (SPIO)
      contrast enhancement 795, 796,
      803
technique 795, 796
transient hepatic attenuation defects
      796, 798
malignant pleural mesothelioma 80
mechanisms of development 787-9
      blood supply 789
      growth rates 788-9
      route of spread 788
neuroblastoma 697, 698
occult metastases detection 800-1
oesophageal cancer 95
ovarian cancer 284
paediatric ovarian germ cell tumours 720
pancreatic cancer 152, 160
percutaneous ablation techniques 879
physical limitations of imaging 801-2
positron emission tomography (PET) 800
preoperative assessment 803-4
primary tumour sites 787, 788
prostate cancer 242
radionuclide imaging 800
      scintigraphic hepatic perfusion index
      801
renal cell carcinoma 202
rhabdomyosarcoma 714
sacrococcygeal teratoma 723
somatostatin receptor imaging 800
testicular germ cell tumours 271
tumour response assessment 912, 913
ultrasound 144, 145, 271, 789, 796,
      798-800, 803
      colour-flow Doppler 796, 798
      power Doppler 799
      small lesions 802
      vascular contrast agents 799
visceral arteriography with
      chemo-embolization 876, 877
liver, radiotherapy changes 979-80
liver veno-occlusive disease, drug-induced
      937
locoregional chemotherapy 885-6
lumbosacral plexus pathology 827, 828, 994
lumpectomy 402
lung cancer 45-61
  AIDS patients 1012, 1013
  clinical features 46
  imaging rationale 45, 57
  incidence/mortality 13, 14, 45
  lifetime risk 13
  metastatic disease 57-60
        adrenal glands 58, 831
        bone 59
        brain 58-9, 816, 818
        brain screening 813
        frequency 57-8
        intracranial meningeal disease 818
        liver 58
        lung 60
        meningeal 818, 825
        peritoneal 849
        preoperative screening policy 60
  pathology 45-6

pleural effusions 757
radiotherapy 35
      treatment planning 896
regional lymph nodes
      classification 54
      involvement detection 55, 56
      mediastinal biopsy 56-7
      prognostic significance of involvement
      54-5
spinal cord compression 820, 824
staging 46-7
      chest wall invasion 50-3, 54
      extrathoracic disease 57-60
      lymph nodes 53, 54-7
      mediastinal invasion 49, 50, 51
      primary tumour 47-9
surgical treatment 34, 45
survival trends 17, 18
tracheobronchial stenting 864-5
tumour response assessment 905
see also small cell lung cancer
lung metastases 749-56
  biopsy 755
  bladder cancer 216
  breast cancer 406, 751, 752
  bronchogenic carcinoma 60
  chest X-ray 750, 752
  cholangiocarcinoma 185
  chondrosarcoma 751
  clinical features 750
  colorectal cancer 751, 752
  computed tomography (CT)
        accuracy 752-4
        indications 755
        solitary nodule assessment 754
        technique 755
  endometrial carcinoma 320
  incidence 749
  lymphangitis carcinomatosis 752, 756
  malignant pleural mesothelioma 80
  metastatic pathways 749-50
  oesophageal cancer 95, 99, 100
  osteosarcoma 751
  ovarian cancer 284, 751
  paediatric ovarian germ cell tumours 720
  paediatric testicular cancer 718
  pathology 750
  prostate cancer 242
  radiological appearances 750-2
  renal cell carcinoma 196, 202, 752
  retroperitoneal germ cell tumours 340
  rhabdomyosarcoma 714
  sacrococcygeal teratoma 723
  soft tissue sarcomas 390, 391
  surgical resection 756
  synovial sarcomas 751
  testicular germ cell tumours 263
        chest X-ray 271
        computed tomography (CT) 270, 272
  thyroid cancer 751, 752
  tumour response assessment 905
  Wilms' tumour 678, 679
luteinizing hormone-releasing hormone
      (LHRH) agonists 38
lymph node biopsy 744, 745, 867
lymph node involvement 5, 729-45
  accuracy of imaging 742
  aerodigestive tract tumours 431, 447-50
        surgical management 431-2
  bladder cancer 216, 217, 220, 235

breast cancer 399, 404-5, 406, 407
cervical cancer 310
cholangiocarcinoma 185
colorectal cancer 131, 135, 137, 139
computed tomography (CT) 268, 406, 407, 731
endometrial carcinoma 320
gastric cancer 113, 114, 121-2, 124
hepatocellular carcinoma 177
identification of disease sites 732, 733
immunoscintigraphy 743
intravenous contrast medium in assessment 741-2
Kaposi's sarcoma 1021
leukaemic abdominal infiltration 647
lung cancer staging 53, 54-7
lymphangiography 744
magnetic resonance imaging (MRI) 731-2
malignant pleural mesothelioma 80
mechanisms of spread 729-30
misdiagnosis 732, 734, 735
neuroblastoma 697
oesophageal cancer 94, 98, 100, 102
ovarian cancer 284, 285, 288
paediatric ovarian germ cell tumours 720
pancreatic cancer 152, 153, 158-9
paranasal sinus neoplasms 416, 420, 422, 424
positron emission tomography (PET) 743
prostate cancer 242, 244, 251-2
radiological criteria of abnormality 736-41
    extracapsular tumour spread 741
    nodal number 738
    size of nodes 736
    tissue characteristics 738-40
    tumour drainage site 737
radionuclide imaging 742-3
renal cell carcinoma 192, 195, 196, 200-1, 206
rhabdomyosarcoma 387, 713
sentinel node imaging 744
soft tissue sarcomas 387
synovial sarcomas 387
testicular germ cell tumours 260, 261, 262-3, 267, 268, 717
thyroid cancer 490
    papillary thyroid carcinoma 483
lymph node sampling 27, 28
lymph nodes
    anatomy 729, 730
    factors influencing size 736
lymphangiography
    lymph node evaluation 744
    lymphoma 590-1
    testicular germ cell tumours 271
lymphangioma
    mediastinum 74
    oral cavity/oropharynx 443
lymphangitis carcinomatosis 752, 756
lymphatic system 729
lymphocoele 986, 987
lymphoid interstitial pneumonitis 1012
lymphoma 583-618, 635
    adrenal glands 610
    aetiology 583-4
    bladder 608
    bone 353, 354
    bone marrow 614, 615, 616
    breast 601
    central nervous system 610-11

brain 544-5
    secondary cerebral involvement 610-11
    spinal leptomeningeal involvement 611
chest wall 600
classification 584
clinical assessment 26
clinical features 587–588
extranodal disease 597-616
female genitalia 609
gastro-intestinal tract 603-5, 606
genito-urinary tract 605-9
head and neck 611, 613
high-dose chemotherapy 40
imaging rationale 583
incidence 583
kidney 607-8
larynx 462
liver 187, 602, 603
lung 598-600
musculoskeletal system 613-16
mycosis fungoides 601
nodal disease 589-97
    abdomen 595-7, 598
    imaging techniques 589-91
    neck 592
    pelvis 595-7, 598
    thorax 592-5, 596
orbit 612-13
pancreas 605, 607
paranasal sinuses 421
pathology 584-5
percutaneous biopsy 618
pericardium/heart 600
pleural disease 600
prostate 608
radiotherapy 35, 36
residual mass assessment 617-18
salivary glands 613
soft tissues 616
spinal cord compression 824-5
spleen 601-2
staging 27
staging classification 585, 587
testis 259, 608-9
therapeutic response monitoring 617
thymus 71, 600
thyroid 487, 613, 614
see also Hodgkin's disease; Non-Hodgkin's lymphoma
Lynch-II syndrome (multiple site cancer family syndrome) 277

M

magnetic resonance angiography, Wilms' tumour 678
magnetic resonance imaging (MRI)
    acoustic schwannomas (neuromas) 559
    adrenal cortical carcinoma 333
    adrenal gland appearances 831
    adrenal imaging technique 332-3
    adrenal metastases 832, 833, 835
        chemical-shift imaging 836-7
        gadolinium-enhanced imaging 836
    aerodigestive tract tumours 432
    astrocytoma
        anaplastic 520
        cerebellar 535-6

fibrillary 519
hypothalamic/optic chiasma 536
pilocytic 535
spinal cord 572
bladder cancer staging 218, 227-30
    accuracy 230, 233-5
    intraveous contrast medium 226, 234
    lymph node involvement 235
bladder imaging 227
bone marrow 765, 774, 775, 776, 777
    chemotherapy effects 971-2
    metastatic involvement 779, 780
    normal features 778, 779
    technique 778
bone metastases 773-4, 775, 776, 777, 779
    breast cancer 406-7
    comparative aspects 781
    neuroblastoma 699, 700
    technique 778
    therapeutic response monitoring 783
bone tumours, primary 365-7, 368
    contrast enhancement 366
    examination technique 36
    sequences 369-70
    staging 368-70
    therapeutic response monitoring 372
brain neoplasms 515, 516-17
    haemangioblastoma 552-3
    metastases 408, 813, 814
breast cancer
    brachial plexus investigation 410-12
    chemo-endocrine neo-adjuvant therapy response assessment 404
    locally recurrent disease detection 409, 410, 411
    metastatic disease 405, 408
    staging 401, 402
    tumour size assessment 401
cerebellar meduloblastomas 546-7
cervical cancer
    recurrence detection 318-19
    staging 317-18
chemical shift imaging (CSI) 226
cholangiocarcinoma
    intrahepatic 180
    staging 181, 182
colorectal cancer
    liver metastases detection 143, 144
    local recurrence detection 135, 137-8
    staging 136-7, 138
craniopharyngiomas 568-9
endometrial carcinoma staging 322-3, 324
ependymomas, spinal cord 572-3
epithelioid haemangioendothelioma 187
examination technique 380
fistulae, post-irradiation bowel damage 983-4, 985
gastric cancer 125
germ cell tumours
    paediatric ovarian 719-20, 721
    primary extragonadal 344
    testicular 259, 268, 271, 717
glioblastoma multiforme 521, 522-3
gliomatosis cerebri 524-5
hepatic angiosarcoma 186
hepatic haemangioma 802
hepatoblastoma staging 708-10
hepatocellular carcinoma
    appearances 169, 170, 176
    paediatric neoplasms 708-10, 711

staging 174-5
hypopharyngeal cancer staging 443-4, 446-7
imaging coils 225
Kaposi's sarcoma 1009
laryngeal anatomy 458, 459
laryngeal cancer 475
    cartilage invasion 472, 473
leiomyosarcoma 343, 344
leukaemia
    bone lesions 650
    bone marrow evaluation 652
    granulocytic sarcoma 640, 642
    intracranial abscess 643
    intracranial haemorrhage 643
    meningeal/dural disease 640
    post-treatment bone changes 652-3
liposarcoma 382, 383
liver cysts 802
liver focal fatty change 803
liver metastases 58, 143, 144, 698, 789, 794-6, 797, 798, 803
    dynamic gadolinium-enhanced imaging 796
    intravascular contrast enhancement 789-90
    opposed-phase imaging 796
    small lesions 801-2
    superparamagnetic iron oxide (SPIO) contrast enhancement 795, 796, 803
    technique 795, 796
    transient hepatic attenuation defects 796, 798
liver post-irradiation changes 980
lung cancer metastases
    adrenal glands 58
    bone 59
    brain 58-9
    liver 58
lung cancer staging 49, 50, 51-3, 61
    regional lymph node involvement 55, 56
lymph node evaluation 731-2
    accuracy 742
    contrast-enhanced imaging 742
lymphoma
    bone marrow 614, 615
    brain 544, 610
    chest wall 600
    head and neck 613
    liver 602
    nodal disease 590, 594, 597
    pancreas 605, 607
    residual mass assessment 618
    soft tissues 616
    thymus 600
malignant fibrous histiocytoma 343-4
malignant peripheral nerve-sheath tumour 345, 385
malignant pleural mesothelioma 85
meningeal metastases
    intracranial 819
    spine 408, 825, 826
meningioma 573, 574
multiple myeloma 628-9, 630
    prognostic value 631-2
    therapeutic response monitoring 630-1
nasopharyngeal cancer staging 435-6, 437

neck imaging after treatment 452
neuroblastoma 696
    liver metastases 698
    staging 697
oesophageal cancer 96
    staging 99-100
oligodendroglioma/oligo-astrocytoma 524
optic gliomas 536
oral cavity/oropharyngeal carcinoma staging 439-40, 442
osteosarcoma 362, 363
ovarian cancer 298-9, 304
    residual disease assessment 304
    staging 289
ovarian mass characterization 290, 300-1
paediatric imaging 662, 663
pancreatic cancer staging 160-2, 163, 165
    accuracy 162
paragangliomas 562
paranasal sinus neoplasms
    post-treatment recurrence 425-6
    staging 423-4
pelvic assessment, post radiotherapy 990-1
pelvic examination technique 225, 226, 299-300, 315
pelvic imaging coils 315-16
pelvic imaging planes 226-7
pelvic imaging sequences 225-6
peritoneal metastases 841
phaeochromocytoma 76, 334
pineal germinoma 550
pineal parenchymal tumours (pineoblastoma/pineocytoma) 552
pituitary macro-adenomas 565-6
pituitary micro-adenomas 563-4
pleomorphic xantho-astrocytoma 539
pleural effusion, malignant 760
posterior fossa ependymoma 540-1
postsurgical abdominopelvic fibrosis 978
prostate cancer staging 246-8, 251, 252, 253
    dynamic gadolinium-DTPA imaging 248, 249
    endorectal coils (ERC MRI) 246, 247, 248
    pelvic lymph node involvement 251
radiation pneumonitis 957-8
radiotherapy treatment planning 897
    image fusion 895
renal cell carcinoma staging 202-6
retroperitoneal examination 342
retroperitoneal sarcomas 342-4
rhabdomyosarcoma 345
    staging 714
sacrococcygeal teratoma staging 721, 723
schwannomas
    lower cranial nerve 561, 562
    spinal cord 574
skull base chordomas 570
small cell lung cancer staging 61
soft tissue sarcomas 379, 380, 381
    local recurrence detection 389
spinal cord compression 821
spinal intramedullary deposits 827
STIR technique 226
supratentorial ependymoma 541
synovial sarcoma 384
thymic lymphoma 71, 72
thymoma staging 70

thyroid cancer 507, 508
transitional cell carcinoma 211
trigeminal neuromas 560
tumour response assessment 899, 905
    for clinical trials 904, 905
    tumour composition 913-15
    tumour volume 909-11
uterine anatomy 316-17
uterine/cervical examination 316
vertebral collapse 774, 781, 782, 783
Wilms' tumour 676-7
magnetic resonance spectroscopy
    cerebellar medulloblastomas 548
    tumour response assessment 906
    tumour composition 917
malignant fibrous histiocytoma
    bone 353, 362, 363
    computed tomography (CT) 340-1
    larynx 462
    magnetic resonance imaging (MRI) 343-4
    radiation-induced 963, 995
    retroperitoneal sarcomas 337, 338
    soft tissue 377, 378, 380, 381, 382
malignant melanoma
    brain metastases 817
    Clark level staging 30
    incidence/mortality trends 13
    intracranial meningeal disease 818
    paranasal sinuses 423
    peritoneal metastases 849
malignant mesenchymoma
    computed tomography (CT) 341
    retroperitoneal sarcomas 337, 338
malignant peripheral nerve-sheath tumour
    computed tomography (CT) 341
    magnetic resonance imaging (MRI) 345, 385
    retroperitoneal sarcomas 337, 338
    soft tissue 378, 380, 385
malignant pleural mesothelioma 79-88
    chest X-ray 80-2
        diagnosis 80-1
        staging 81-2
    computed tomography (CT) 82-5
        diagnosis 82-4
        staging 84-5
    epidemiology 79, 81
    historical aspects 79
    lymph node involvement 80
    magnetic resonance imaging (MRI) 85
    pathology 79-80, 81
    patterns of spread 80
    staging classifications 85-8
        primary tumour 88
    thoracoscopic appearances, prognostic significance 86, 87
    TNM descriptors of extent 85, 86
MALT lymphomas, lung 600
mammography
    chemo-endocrine neo-adjuvant therapy response assessment 403-4
    locally recurrent disease detection 409
    synchronous carcinoma in second breast 405
    tumour diagnosis 397
    tumour response assessment 905
    tumour size assessment 401, 402
mastectomy 35, 400
maxillary antral tumour staging 416, 417
    primary tumour 418

mediastinal biopsy 56-7
mediastinal invasion, oesophageal cancer 97,
    99
mediastinal lymph nodes 67
    Kaposi's sarcoma involvement 1006
    lung cancer involvement 54, 55
    lymphoma involvement 593, 600
    malignant pleural mesothelioma
        involvement 80
    oesophageal cancer involvement 98
    renal cell carcinoma involvement 200
    rhabdomyosarcoma involvement 714
mediastinal lymphadenopathy
    AIDS-related 1011
    leukaemia 645
mediastinal lymphoma 905
mediastinal mass 900-1, 902
mediastinal sarcoma 74, 75
mediastinal tumours 67-76
    germ cell tumours 73-4
    mesenchymal 74-5
    neurogenic 75-6
    primary 67
    secondary 67
    thymic tumours 67-72
    thyroid carcinoma 72, 73
medullary thyroid carcinoma 486-7
    clinical presentation 487
    familial form 486
    imaging agents 500-2
    immunohistochemical staining 502
    pathology 487
    prognosis 484
    treatment 508
    tumour markers 487
medulloblastoma 825
Meigs' syndrome 281
melphalan 625, 932, 949
meningeal leukaemia 640, 825
meningeal lymphoma 825, 826
meningeal metastases
    breast cancer 408
    intracranial 818-19
    spinal meningeal disease 825-6
meningioma 554-8
    angiography and embolization 558
    computed tomography (CT) 555, 556,
        557
    convexity 554
    magnetic resonance imaging (MRI) 556,
        557-8
    olfactory groove 554
    parasagittal 554
    parasellar 555
    posterior fossa 555
    prognosis 558
    sphenoid ridge 554
    spinal cord 573, 574
    treatment 558
    WHO classification 554
6-mercaptopurine 932
mesenchymal hamartoma 712
mesenchymal mediastinal tumours 74-5
mesothelioma see malignant pleural
        mesothelioma
meta-iodobenzylguanidine (MIBG)
    bone metastases imaging 699, 700
    medullary thyroid carcinoma imaging 500
    neuroblastoma treatment 694
    phaeochromocytoma 76, 334-5

metastases of unknown primary site 853-7
    adenocarcinoma 854-5
    definition 853
    histology 853-4
    radiological strategy 855-6
    sites of presentation 853
    squamous carcinoma 854
    treatment potential 855
metastasis 4, 5
metastatic disease
    bladder cancer 216, 217
    breast cancer 405-9
    cholangiocarcinoma 183, 185
    endometrial carcinoma 320
    gastric cancer 113
    hepatoblastoma 710
    hepatocellular carcinoma 177
    lung cancer 57-60
    neuroblastoma 697-8
    oesophageal cancer 95, 98-9, 102
    ovarian cancer 284, 302
    paediatric ovarian tumours 720
    prostate cancer 242, 252
    renal cell carcinoma 196, 201-2, 206
    rhabdomyosarcoma 714
    sacrococcygeal teratoma 723
    small cell lung cancer 61
    soft tissue sarcomas 390-2
    surgical treatment 35
    testicular germ cell tumours 263, 264
    testicular paediatric tumours 717-18
    therapeutic response monitoring 25
    Wilms' tumour 678, 679
methotrexate 116, 668, 931, 932, 937, 939,
        957
    intrathecal 639, 644
mineralizing micro-angiopathy 531-2
minor salivary gland tumours 415, 422, 423
    larynx 462
    oral cavity/oropharynx 441
mitomycin 931, 932, 937, 957
mitoxantrone 948
mixed epithelial ovarian tumour 279, 280
mixed germ cell tumour 260
    mediastinal 73
mixed Müllerian sarcoma 324-5
mortality 11
    data 11-12
        analytical approach 12
        trends 13-16
mucinous ovarian tumour 278, 279, 280, 281
    prognosis 285
mucocoele, paranasal sinuses 422
mucosal cyst, larynx 461
multinodular goitre 509
multiple endocrine neoplasia (MEN)
        syndromes 482
multiple endocrine neoplasia type I (MENI),
        mediastinal carcinoid tumours 72
multiple endocrine neoplasia type IIa
        (MENIIa) 330
    medullary thyroid carcinoma 486, 500,
        501
    phaeochromocytoma 501
multiple endocrine neoplasia type IIb
        (MENIIb) 330
    medullary thyroid carcinoma 486
multiple field biopsies 27-8
multiple myeloma 625-33
    bone metastases differentiation 627, 628

clinical features 625
complications 632
computed tomography (CT) 627, 628
Durie and Salmon staging system 626,
    628
epidemiology 625
extra-osseous variant 632-3
laboratory tests 632
magnetic resonance imaging (MRI)
    628-9, 630
plain film radiography 626
prognostic value of radiographic findings
    631-2
radionuclide imaging 626-7
sclerotic variant 633
spinal cord compression 820
staging 27, 626
    prognostic relevance 25
therapeutic response monitoring 630-1
treatment 625
tumour markers 28
multiple site cancer family syndrome
        (Lynch-II syndrome) 277
muscle metastases 828
muscle, post-irradiation changes 994
musculoskeletal interventional radiology
        882-3
    percutaneous skeletal biopsy 882-3
    percutaneous vertebroplasty 883
    vascular embolization 883, 884
myasthenia gravis 68
mycobacterial infection, AIDS opportunistic
        infection 1007, 1011-12
mycosis fungoides 601
myelodysplasia 636
myocardial disease, radiation-induced 960-1
myoclonic encephalopathy of infancy
        ('dancing eyes' syndrome) 704
myocutaneous flaps 35
myxoid liposarcoma 378, 389

N

N-myc 691
N-nitroso compounds 111
nasopharyngeal cancer 432-7
    anatomical aspects 432, 433
    clinical assessment 26-7
    clinical features 432-3
    incidence 429
    pathology 429
    staging 433-7
        angiography 436-7
        computed tomography (CT) 435-6,
            437
        magnetic resonance imaging (MRI)
            435-6, 437
        primary tumour 433, 434
    survival trends 17
    treatment 430-1
neck tumours see head and neck tumours
necrotizing leukoencephalopathy 531, 644
negative predictive value 7
neovascularization 3, 5
    liver metastases 789
nephrectomy 196
nephroblastoma, cystic partially
        differentiated 683
nephroblastomatosis 680, 681

nephrostomy, percutaneous 879-80
nerve plexus pathology 827-8
neurilemmoma *see* schwannoma
neuroblastoma 691-705
 antenatal 704
 clinical features 693
 complications 703
 diagnosis 691, 693, 694-5
 extra-abdominal tumours 701-2, 703
  cerebral 702
  cervical 702
  pelvic 701
  thoracic 701-2
 genetic aspects 691
 imaging
  computed tomography (CT) 695, 697
  magnetic resonance imaging (MRI)
   696, 697
  plain radiograph 696
  ultrasound 694-5, 696
 incidence 691
 intraspinal extension 697
 local disease 697
 lymph node involvement 697
 mediastinum 75, 76
 metastatic disease 697-8
  bone 697, 698-700, 771
  bone marrow 697, 698-700
  liver 697, 698
 myoclonic encephalopathy association
   704
 oral cavity/oropharynx 443
 paratesticular 718
 pathology 691
 presacral 724
 prognosis 691, 694
 recurrent disease 703
 soft tissue 378
 spinal cord compression 824
 staging 27, 693-4, 696
 staging systems 692, 693
  Evans 692, 693
  Hayes 692, 693
  INSS 693
  TNM 692, 693
 treatment 694
  late effects 703
  response 702-3
 tumour markers 28, 691
 tumour response assessment 909
neurofibroma
 mediastinum 75, 76
 spinal cord 574
 spinal cord compression 823, 824
 testicular paediatric neoplasms 718
neurofibromatosis 330, 377, 573
neurogenic tumours, mediastinal 67, 75-6
neurological complications 811-29
 classification 812
 intracranial meningeal disease 818-19
 major nerve plexuses 827-8
 peripheral nerves 828
 spinal cord compression 820-5, 826
 spinal intramedullary deposits 826-7
 spinal meningeal disease 825-6
 see also brain metastases
neurolysis, percutaneous 878
neuroma *see* schwannoma
neuronal-glial tumours 542-4
neurone specific enolase (NSE) 28

neuroblastoma 691
neurotoxic drugs 939
neutropenic colitis 664-5
nickel exposure, occupational 415
Nocardia lung infection 935
Non-Hodgkin's lymphoma 6, 583
 bone 353, 354, 614, 615, 616
 bone marrow 614, 615
 chest wall 600
 classification 584, 585
 clinical features 587–588, 590
 extranodal disease 597-616
 female genitalia 609
 gastro-intestinal tract 603-5
 head and neck 613
 high-dose chemotherapy 40
 incidence 583
 intracranial meningeal disease 818
 intraperitoneal dissemination 849
 liver 602
 lung 598-600
 musculoskeletal system 613
 nasopharyngeal tumours 436
 nodal disease 586, 589-97
  abdomen 595-7, 598
  imaging techniques 589-91
  neck 592
  pelvis 595-7, 598
  thorax 592-5, 596
 oral cavity/oropharyngeal carcinoma 438,
   441
 orbit 612-13
 pathology 585
 prognosis 589
 REAL classification 587
 residual mass assessment 617-18
 spinal cord compression 824-5
 spinal leptomeningeal involvement 611
 spleen 601
 staging system 587
  Murphy's system 588
 testis 608, 609
 thyroid 613, 614
 treatment 589
 tumour response assessment 617-18
  tumour composition 913, 914
non-specific interstitial pneumonitis 936

O

objective response criteria 903-4
obstructive jaundice 872-5, 876
 endoscopic retrograde
   cholangiopancreatography (ERCP)
   872-3
 percutaneous transhepatic
   cholangiography (PTC) 873, 874
 stent insertion 873, 874, 875, 876
oesophageal cancer 5, 93-106
 image-guided biopsy 867
 imaging rationale 96
 imaging techniques 96
 incidence 93
 lymph node involvement 94, 98, 100, 102
  prognosis 95
 mediastinal invasion 67, 97, 99
 metastatic disease 95, 98-9, 100, 102
 pathology 93
 positron emission tomography (PET) 104

recurrence detection 104-5, 106
 restaging 104-5
 staging 93-5
  algorithm 103
  computed tomography (CT) 97-9,
   103-4
  endoscopic ultrasound 100-4
  lymph nodes 94
  magnetic resonance imaging (MRI)
   99-100
  primary tumour 94
  surgical 99, 102
 survival 17, 95
 therapeutic irradiation association 962
 treatment 95-6
oesophageal injury, radiation-induced 961-2
oesophageal lymphoma 605
oesophageal strictures 869-71, 961
 dilation 869
 stenting 869, 870, 871
oesophagitis, infectious 962
olfactory groove meningioma 554
olfactory neuroblastoma
   (esthesioneuroblastoma) 419, 422
oligo-astrocytoma 523-4
oligodendroglioma 517, 523-4
 postsurgical change evaluation 526-30
 prognosis 525
 treatment 525-6
oncocytoma 191
oncogenes 3
operability 24
operative risk 33
opportunistic infection 933-6, 937, 962
 AIDS patients 1003, 1004, 1007
 central nervous system 939-40
optic glioma 536-7
 computed tomography (CT) 536
 magnetic resonance imaging (MRI) 536
 prognosis 537
 treatment 537
oral cavity/oropharyngeal cancer 437-43
 anatomical aspects 437-8
 benign neoplasms 443
 clinical features 438
 incidence/mortality trends 13, 430
 minor salivary glands 441
 pathology 429
 soft palate 438, 441
 staging 438-43
  computed tomography (CT) 438, 439,
   442
  magnetic resonance imaging (MRI)
   439-40, 442
  primary tumour 439
 tongue 438, 439
 tonsillar fossa 438, 441
oral contraceptive pill 316, 317
orbital granulocytic sarcoma 645
orbital lymphoma 612-13
oropharyngeal tumours *see* oral
   cavity/oropharyngeal tumours
osteoblastoma 362
osteochondroma
 radiation-induced 964, 970, 996
 Wilms' tumour treatment association 685
osteogenic sarcoma 379, 380
osteoid osteoma 366
osteoma 362
osteomyelitis 359, 360, 361, 993

osteoporosis, leukaemic 649
osteosarcoma 352
  conventional intramedullary 352
  high grade surface variant 353
  low grade central variant 353
  magnetic resonance imaging (MRI) 362, 363, 370
  Paget's sarcoma 352
  paranasal sinuses 422
  parosteal 352, 363, 371
  periosteal 352, 368
  prognostic features 362
  radiation-induced 963, 995
  radionuclide scintigraphy 364
  recurrence detection 373
  small cell 353
  soft tissue extension 362
  surgical treatment 34
  telangiectatic 352
  therapeutic response monitoring 372
  treatment strategy 24
  tumour matrix 362
ovarian cancer 277-305
  characterization of masses 290-3
    computed tomography (CT) 290, 292-3, 304
    magnetic resonance imaging (MRI) 300-1, 304
    plain abdominal radiograph 302
    ultrasound 290, 291-2, 304
  chemotherapy 277
  chest X-ray 289, 302
  clinical features 277-8
  coexistent breast cancer 408
  common epithelial tumours 278, 279, 280, 281
  epidemiology 277, 278
  FIGO classification 285, 286
  germ cell tumours see germ cell tumours
  hereditary forms 277, 278
  histological classification 278, 279
  imaging rationale 304
  immunoscintigraphy 301-2
  intravenous urography 302
  lymph node involvement 284, 285, 292, 297
  metastatic disease 284, 294-6, 298
    adenocarcinoma of unknown origin 855
    barium studies 302
  metastatic tumours 283
  paediatric tumours 718-21
  pathology 278, 279, 280
  patterns of spread 283-4, 285
    transcoelomic 283
  peritoneal metastases 283, 292, 296, 297
    intraperitoneal seeding 846, 847
    peritoneal invasion 843
  residual disease assessment 302-4
    restaging accuracy 304
  screening 289
  sex cord stromal tumours 279, 281
  site-specific 277
  sites of origin 278, 279
  staging 28
    accuracy 301
    computed tomography (CT) 293-8, 299, 301, 304
    imaging 289-90
    lymph nodes 288
    metastases 287
    primary tumour 287
    prognostic significance 285-6
    surgical 288, 301
    ultrasound 289
  staging classifications 285, 286
  survival 277
  TNM classification 285, 286
  treatment 286-9
    chemotherapy 288
    radiotherapy 288
    surgery 286, 288
  tumour markers 28, 283, 304
ovarian lymphoma 609
ovarian metastases 283
  gastric cancer 113
  imaging 291
ovaries, radiotherapy damage 989-90

P

P53 tumour suppressor gene mutations 395
paediatric oncology 661-8
  abdominal malignancies 707-25
  acute complications 664-6
    chest infection 666
    graft versus host disease 665-6
    haemorrhage 666
    neutropenic colitis 664-5
    pseudomembranous colitis 665
  diagnostic imaging 662
  equipment 661-2
  genito-urinary tumours 712-15
  heat loss management 661
  information for children 661
  information for parents 663
  injections management 661
  intravenous long line access 661
    complications 664
  liver tumours 707, 712
  long-term treatment effects 666-8, 685-6
    cardiopulmonary function 668, 685
    central nervous system 667
    gonadal dysfunction 668, 686
    musculoskeletal disease 667-8, 685
    nephrotoxicity 668, 685
    thyroid dysfunction 668
  radiographers 662
  research aspects 663
  staging 662-3
  tissue diagnosis 663
Paget's sarcoma 352
palliative radiotherapy 38
palliative surgery 34-5
pancreas, radiotherapy changes 980
pancreatic cancer 151-65
  epidemiology 151
  image-guided biopsy 867
  imaging rationale 152, 154, 165
  imaging techniques 154
  liver metastases 152
  local invasion 158
  pathology 151-2
  peritoneal metastases 160
    intraperitoneal seeding 152, 846
    peritoneal invasion 843
  prognosis 152, 154, 165
  staging
    arteriography 164
    computed tomography (CT) 154-60, 162, 163, 165
    endoscopic ultrasound 162-3, 165
    extrapancreatic spread 155-8
    lymph node involvement 152, 153, 158-9
    magnetic resonance imaging (MRI) 160-2, 163, 165
    metastatic disease 160
    primary tumour 153, 154-5
    transabdominal ultrasound 163-4
  staging classification 152
  surgical treatment 152, 154, 165
  vascular involvement 155-8, 164
pancreatic drug complications 937
pancreatic lymphoma 605
pancreaticoduodenectomy 154
papillary thyroid carcinoma 483-5
  aetiology 483
  clinical presentation 485
  lymph node involvement 483
  microcarcinomas 484
  pathology 483
  prognosis 484-5
  treatment 508
    radio-iodine ablation 494
  variants 483-4
paraganglioma 562
  larynx 461
  mediastinum 76
paranasal sinus metastases 421
paranasal sinus neoplasms 415-26
  imaging rationale 419-20
  incidence 415
  intracranial spread 423, 424
  pathology 415-16
  perineural extension 423, 424
  post-treatment assessment 425-6
  prognosis 416
  staging 416, 419
    computed tomography (CT) 419, 420-2, 424
    lymph nodes 416, 420, 422, 424
    magnetic resonance imaging (MRI) 419, 420, 421, 423-4
    plain radiography 419
    positron emission tomography (PET) 421, 424
    primary tumour 418, 421-2, 423
  treatment 419
parasagittal meningioma 554
parasellar meningioma 555
paratesticular lymphoma 718
paratesticular paediatric neoplasms 718
parathyroid adenoma 885
parathyroid tumours
  ablation 885
  mediastinal mass 67
pelvic abscess drainage 869
pelvic clearance 986-7
pelvic embolization 881-2
pelvic treatment complications 936-9
  radiation injury 975-6
pelvis, post-radiotherapy assessment 990-1
pentavalent technetium dimercaptosuccinic acid (Tc(V)DMSA) 500
pentostatin 937
percutaneous nephrostomy 879-80
percutaneous neurolysis 878
percutaneous retrieval techniques 885

percutaneous skeletal biopsy 882-3
percutaneous transhepatic cholangiography
  (PTC) 873, 874
percutaneous tumour ablation 880
percutaneous vertebroplasty 883
pericardial disease, radiation-induced 960
pericardial effusions
  Hodgkin's disease 600
  image-guided drainage procedures 862,
    863
  sclerotherapy 862
periosteal response 359-61
peripheral blood examination 28-9
peripheral neuropathy 828
peritoneal anatomy 841, 842, 843
peritoneal metastases 841-50
  barium studies 841, 844, 847, 849
  breast cancer 849
  cholangiocarcinoma 185
  colorectal cancer 843, 844, 846
  computed tomography (CT) 841, 843-4,
    849
    accuracy 850
  direct invasion 843-4, 845, 846
  embolic metastases 849
  gastric cancer 113, 122, 124, 843, 844, 846
  intraperitoneal seeding 846-9
  lung cancer 849
  lymphatic metastases 849
  magnetic resonance imaging (MRI) 841
  malignant melanoma 849
  ovarian cancer 283, 296, 297, 843, 844,
    846, 847
    paediatric ovarian germ cell tumours
      720
  pancreatic cancer 152, 160, 843, 844, 846
  radionuclide imaging 841
  ultrasound 841
peritoneal washings 288
Perlman syndrome 671, 672
phaeochromocytoma 330-1, 832
  clinical features 330-1
  computed tomography (CT) 332
  hormone production 330
  incidence 330
  intravenous contrast medium use 332
  magnetic resonance imaging (MRI) 334
  mediastinum 75, 76
  MIBG imaging 501
  pathology 330
  prognosis 331
  radionuclide imaging 334-5
  staging 335-6
  treatment 331
  tumour localization with venous sampling
    885
  tumour markers 28
  ultrasound 334
pharyngeal cancer 429-54
  incidence/mortality trends 14
  lymph nodes 448
Philadelphia chromosome 636
pilocytic astrocytoma 535-6
  brain stem 537
  cerebellar 535
  hypothalamic/optic chiasma 536-7
  postsurgical imaging 536
  prognosis 536
pineal germinoma 549-50
  imaging 550

treatment 551
pineal parenchymal tumours 552
pineal teratoma 550
  treatment 551
pineal tumours 548-52
pineoblastoma 548, 549, 552
  meningeal metastases 825
pineocytoma 548, 552
pituitary adenomas 562, 563-7
  hormone secretion 563
  macro-adenomas 563
    follow-up 566-7
    imaging 565-6
  micro-adenomas 563, 568
    follow-up 565
    imaging 563-4
  tumour localization with venous sampling
    885
placental alkaline phosphatase (PLAP) 28
plain radiography
  bone metastases 698, 770-2, 773, 781
    osteoblastic lesions 771, 772
    osteolytic lesions 771, 772
  breast cancer metastatic disease 405
  multiple myeloma 626
  neuroblastoma 696, 698
  ovarian cancer 302
  thyroid cancer 502
  Wilms' tumour 673, 674
plasmacytoma
  larynx 462
  paranasal sinuses 422, 423
pleomorphic adenoma, larynx 461
pleomorphic xantho-astrocytoma 539
pleural effusion, malignant 27, 756-60
  biopsy 758
  breast cancer 406
  computed tomography (CT) 759, 760
  exudates/transudates 757, 760
  image-guided drainage procedures 862,
    863
  Kaposi's sarcoma 1006
  lymphocytic 757
  lymphoma 600
  magnetic resonance imaging (MRI) 760,
    761
  mechanism 757
  pathology 757
  pleural cytology 758
  prognosis 757
  radiography 757, 758
  sclerotherapy 862
  thoracoscopy 758
  ultrasound 759
pleural mesothelioma see malignant pleural
    mesothelioma
pleural metastases 284
pleural tumours 79
  see also malignant pleural mesothelioma
plicamycin 937
Plummer-Vinson syndrome 443
pneumatosis intestinalis 937, 938
Pneumocystis carinii pneumonia 935
  AIDS opportunistic infection 1007, 1012
polyposis coli 35, 707
positive predictive value 7
positron emission tomography (PET)
  aerodigestive tract tumours relapse 453
  bone metastases 699, 700
  brain neoplasms 515

metastases 813
  breast cancer metastatic disease 409
  colorectal cancer 141-2
  gliomas (glial-cell tumours) 523
  laryngeal cancer 475
    post-treatment evaluation 476
  liver metastases 800
  lymph node evaluation 56, 743
  lymphoma, residual mass assessment 618
  neuroblastoma 704
  oesophageal cancer 96, 104
    recurrence following surgery 104, 105,
      106
  paranasal sinus neoplasms
    post-treatment recurrence 426
    staging 421, 424
  therapeutic response assessment for
    clinical trials 904
  thyroid cancer 72, 499
  see also fluorine-18 fluorodeoxyglucose
    positron emission tomography
    (FDG PET)
posterior fossa ependymoma 540-1
  prognosis 541
  treatment 541
posterior fossa meningioma 555
postsurgical abdominopelvic fibrosis 976-8
prednisolone 625
presacral lymphoma 724
primary sclerosing cholangitis 178, 179
  imaging 181-2
primitive neuro-ectodermal tumours
    (PNET), intracranial 545, 546, 549
  meningeal metastases 825
  supratentorial 548
procarbazine 931, 932, 948, 949
programmed cell death (apoptosis) 3
progressive multifocal leucoencephalopathy
    815, 940
prostate cancer 239-53
  anatomical zones of prostate 240, 241
  clinical features 240
  diagnostic techniques 19
  epidemiology 239-40
  Gleason grade 240, 250
  histopathology 240
  incidence/mortality trends 13, 18-19
  localized tumour treatment 250
    imaging strategies 250-1
  lumbosacral plexus pathology 827
  lymph node involvement 242, 244, 251-2
  metastatic disease 242, 767
    adenocarcinoma of unknown origin
      855
    bone metastases 771
  microscopic tumours 239
  neovascularity 250
  patterns of spread 242
  predisposing factors 239
  prostate specific antigen (PSA) 239, 244,
    251
  radiotherapy 35
    treatment planning 890
  relapse detection 917
  spinal cord compression 820
  staging 242-50
    computed tomography (CT) 246, 251
    digital rectal examination 242, 244
    limitations 248, 250, 251
    lymph nodes 244, 251-2

magnetic resonance imaging (MRI) 246-8, 249, 251, 252, 253
  metastatic disease 252
  pathological 248
  primary tumour 243
  prognostic variables 248, 250
  prostate specific antigen (PSA) 244, 251
  seminal vesicle involvement 245, 246, 247
  transrectal ultrasound 244-5, 246, 251, 252, 253
  staging classifications 242
  tumour markers 28, 29
  tumour volume 250
prostate leukaemic infiltration 648
prostate lymphoma 608
prostate, radiotherapy changes 989
prostate rhabdomyosarcoma 712, 713, 714, 715, 716
prostate specific antigen (PSA) 28, 29
  prostate cancer 239
    staging 244, 251
prostatectomy 250, 984, 985
prostatitis 239
pseudomembranous colitis 665, 937
pseudomyxoma peritonei 294
  computed tomography (CT) 847
pulmonary drug toxicity 931-3, 934, 957
  diffuse air-space shadowing 932
  diffuse interstitial opacities 932
  pulmonary nodules 933
  radiation pneumonitis exacerbation 956-7
pulmonary function, cancer treatment effects 668, 685
pulmonary haemorrhage 936
pulmonary infection 933-6
  chest X-ray 933-4
  leukaemia 646
  lobar/segmental consolidation 934-5
  paediatric patients 666
  pulmonary nodules 935
pulmonary lymphoma 598-600
pulmonary nodules
  bacterial infections 935
  drug reactions 933
  fungal infections 935
pulmonary treatment effects 955-60
  pulmonary drug toxicity 957
  radiation pneumonitis 955-6
    cytotoxic drug interactions 956-7
pyriform fossa tumours 443, 444, 446

Q

quadrantectomy 400

R

radiation bowel disease 976
radiation hepatitis 685
radiation necrosis of brain 532, 815
radiation pneumonitis 955
  computed tomography (CT) 957-8
  evaluation of treated areas 958, 959
  magnetic resonance imaging (MRI) 957-8
  plain film findings 955-6
radiation-induced heart disease 960-1

radiation-induced leukaemia 636
radiation-induced oesophageal injury 961-2
radiation-induced sarcoma 963-4, 995
radiation-induced urinary tract damage 976
radio-immuno-guided surgery (RIGS) 141
radio-iodine ablation therapy, thyroid cancer 494-6, 508
radio-iodine imaging, thyroid cancer 491
radionuclide imaging
  adrenal cortical carcinoma 334
  adrenal metastases 837
  bone metastases 252, 765, 768-9, 770
    neuroblastoma 698, 699
  bone tumours, primary 363-5
  breast cancer metastatic disease 405, 407
  chondrosarcomas 364
  leukaemic bone lesions 650
  liver metastases 58, 800
    scintigraphic hepatic perfusion index 801
  lung cancer metastases 58, 59
  lymph node evaluation 742-3
    lung cancer 55, 56
  lymphoma 590
    residual mass assessment 618
  multiple myeloma 626-7
  paediatric imaging 662
  peritoneal metastases 841
  phaeochromocytoma 334-5
  small cell lung cancer staging 61
  thyroid cancer 72, 487-8
    diagnostic applications 491-4
    follow-up imaging 496
    gallium-67 citrate 498-9
    medullary thyroid carcinoma 500-2
    post-thyroidectomy ablation therapy 494-6
    radio-iodine 491
    technetium-99m methoxyisobutylisonitrile (Tc-99m MIBI) 496, 497
    technetium-99m pertechnate 488, 490
    technetium-99m tetrofosmin 497
    thallium-201 (Tl-201) 498
  thyroid nodules 481
  tumour response assessment 905
    tumour composition 916-17
  Wilms' tumour 678
radiosensitivity 36
radiotherapy 35-8
  abdominopelvic radiation injury 975-6
  accelerated schedules 36
  acute radiation reactions 37, 976, 979
  biological effects 36, 975-6
    bone tissue 967, 991
  bladder cancer 217, 235
  bladder changes 988-9, 990
  brachytherapy 37-8
  breast cancer 400
  cervical cancer 311
  complications in children 667-8
  conformal therapy 889
  early prostate cancer 250
  endometrial carcinoma 320
  external beam 37
  fractional schedules 37
  Hodgkin's disease 587–588-9
  imaging 36
  intracranial with intrathecal methotrexate 644

intracranial, late effects see brain, post-treatment changes
Kaposi's sarcoma 1009
laryngeal cancer 467, 468, 470
  post-treatment late changes 476
late side-effects 37, 476
leukaemia 639, 644
liver changes 979-80
multiple myeloma 625
nasopharyngeal cancer 430
nephrotoxicity 668
neuroblastoma 694
neurotoxic side-effects 644
Non-Hodgkin's lymphoma 589
oesophageal cancer 95, 96
ovarian cancer 288
ovarian damage 989-90
palliative 38
pancreatic changes 980
paranasal sinus neoplasms 419
pineal germ cell tumours 551
prostate changes 989
radiation pneumonitis see radiation pneumonitis
radiosensitivity 36
renal changes 987
second malignancies 947, 949
seminal vesicle changes 989
seminoma 266
skeletal tissue effects 967-73, 991-5
small cell lung cancer 60
soft tissue sarcomas 387, 388
spleen changes 980
staging 24
testicular damage 989
thymoma 68
thyroid cancer 508
tissue damage 37
ureteric injury 987-8
uterine atrophy 989
radiotherapy treatment planning 889-97
  computed tomography (CT) techniques 893-4
    image fusion 895, 896
    image handling 895
  conformal therapy 891-2, 893
    multileaf collimator 892
    tumour sites 895
  gross tumour volume definition 890
  immobilization devices 891, 892
  magnetic resonance imaging (MRI) 897
  organ movement effects 890-1
  patient alignment 892, 893
  planning steps 889
  target volumes 889-91
    sources of error 891
  tumour classification 890
REAL classification 587
receiver-operator characteristics (ROC) 7-8
reconstructive surgery 35
rectal cancer
  lumbosacral plexus pathology 827
  radiotherapy 35
  see also colorectal cancer
rectal lymphoma 604, 606
relapse detection 917-18
  baseline staging 25
renal artery embolization 881, 882
renal cell carcinoma 191, 212
  clinical features 191-2

epidemiology 191
metastatic disease 196, 201-2, 206
   bone 771
paediatric tumours 683
renal artery embolization 881, 882
Robson's classification 192, 194
staging
   computed tomography (CT) 196-202
   lymph node involvement 192, 195,
     196, 200-1, 206
   magnetic resonance imaging (MRI)
     202-6
   metastatic disease 201-2, 206
   perinephric spread 192, 196-7, 198,
     203-4
   primary tumour 193
   prognosis 192, 195-6
   for surgery 196
   ultrasound 206-7
   venous invasion 192, 196, 197-200,
     204-6, 207
staging classifications 192
survival 192, 195
synchronous tumour in second kidney
   202, 206
renal clear cell sarcoma 682
renal irradiation changes 987
renal leukaemic infiltration 647
renal lymphoma 605, 607-8
paediatric tumours 683
renal metastases 284
renal post-chemotherapy changes 987
renal rhabdoid tumour 682
renal tumours 191-212
collecting system neoplasms 207-11
pathology 191
surgical treatment 34
survival trends 17
renal vein thrombus 196, 197-200, 204-6, 207
Ret oncogene activation 483
retinoblastoma 947, 948
retroperitoneal lymph node involvement
diagnostic problems 269-70
testicular germ cell tumours 260, 261,
   262-3
   computed tomography (CT) 268-9
retroperitoneal lymphadenectomy 266
retroperitoneal primary tumours 336-47
retroperitoneal sarcoma 336-7
clinical features 339
computed tomography (CT) 340-1
magnetic resonance imaging (MRI) 342-4
pathology 336-8
prognosis 339
staging 344, 346
staging system 339
treatment 339
retroperitoneal tumours 329-47
staging 344, 348
rhabdoid tumour of kidney 682
rhabdomyoma, larynx 461
rhabdomyosarcoma 378, 712, 713
clinical features 713
diagnostic imaging 713
follow-up evaluation 714
heart 75
lymph node involvement 387, 713, 714
magnetic resonance imaging (MRI) 345
metastatic disease 714
nasopharyngeal tumours 433

oral cavity/oropharynx 443
paranasal sinuses 421
paratesticular 718
patterns of spread 713
staging 713
   imaging findings 714
treatment 713
rib fracture, radiation-induced 962
Robson classification 192, 194
Rye classification 584

S

sacrococcygeal teratoma 721-4
classification 721, 722
diagnostic imaging 721, 723
differential diagnosis 724
follow-up evaluation 723
metastatic disease 723
staging 721
salivary gland lymphoma 613
salpingo-oophorectomy 288
sarcoma
radiation-induced 963-4, 995
radiotherapy 35
tumour grade 378
schistosomiasis 215
schwannoma
acoustic 558-9
intracranial 558
larynx 461
lower cranial nerves 560-2
mediastinum 75, 76
paranasal sinuses 422, 423
spinal cord 574
trigeminal 560
scintigraphic hepatic perfusion index 801
scoliosis 685, 703, 963, 970, 995
screening
breast carcinoma 13
colorectal cancer 13
ovarian cancer 289
uterine cervix cancer 13
second malignancies 945-51
abdominopelvic irradiation 995-6
acute myeloid leukaemia (AML) 636
associated primary tumours 948
brain 533-4
causation 947-9
chemotherapy associations 947, 948-9
gender associations 949
genetic factors 948
incidence 945, 946
mechanisms 950
neuroblastoma treatment 703
prevention 950
radiotherapy associations 947, 949
time of onset 947, 948
types 947, 948
Wilms' tumour treatment 686
seminal vesicle radiotherapy changes 989
seminoma 259, 716
mediastinal 73, 74
primary extragonadal 340
radiotherapy 35, 36, 266
recurrence 265
tumour markers 260
tumour response assessment 907, 908
sensitivity 7

sentinel node imaging 744
serous ovarian tumour 278, 280, 281
Sertoli cell tumour 259, 716
Sertoli-Leydig cell neoplasm
     (androblastoma) 281, 282
imaging 291
paediatric ovarian tumours 719
prognosis 286
treatment 288
serum tumour markers 28
sex cord stromal tumours 279, 281, 282
prognosis 286
treatment 288
silent interval 5-6
single photon emission computed
     tomography (SPECT)
brain neoplasms 515
   metastases 813
colorectal cancer 140
lung cancer regional lymph node
   involvement 56
ovarian cancer 301
paranasal sinus neoplasms staging 424
small cell lung cancer staging 61
thyroid cancer imaging 490
skin metastases 697
skin tumours
radiotherapy 35
surgical treatment 34
skull base tumours 569-70
imaging 570
slipped capital femoral epiphysis 970, 994
slipped capital humeral epiphysis 970
small bowel lymphoma 603-4, 606
small bowel post-irradiation changes 980-1
small cell lung cancer 45
bone metastases 59
brain metastases 816
high-dose chemotherapy 40
pathology 45
staging 60-1
therapeutic strategies 60
tumour markers 28
small cell osteosarcoma 353
soft palate tumours 438, 441
soft tissue lymphoma 616
soft tissue sarcoma 377-92
biological behaviour 378
biopsy 378
clinical diagnosis 378-9
computed tomography (CT) 379, 380
epidemiology 377
local recurrence
   detection 389
   management 390
lymph node involvement 387
magnetic resonance imaging (MRI) 379,
   380, 381
metastatic disease 390-2
pathology 377-8
plain radiography 379
radiation-induced 963, 964, 995
radiological diagnosis 379-80
radiological features 380-4
retroperitoneal 336, 388-9
staging 386-7
treatment 387-9
tumour grade 378
tumour response assessment 910
soft tissue tumour vascular embolization 883,

884
solitary bone cyst 357, 367
solitary plasmacytoma 28
solitary thyroid nodule
  fine-needle aspiration cytology 505
  preoperative imaging 509
  radionuclide imaging 491
  ultrasound 502-5
somatostatin receptor imaging
  liver metastases 800
  medullary thyroid carcinoma imaging 500
sonoelastic imaging 252
sonohystrography 321
specificity 7
sphenoid ridge meningioma 554
spinal cord compression 820-5, 826
  clinical presentation 820
  computed tomography (CT)/CT
    myelography 821
  differential diagnosis 823-5
  imaging 821, 823
  magnetic resonance imaging (MRI) 821,
    823
  pathophysiology 821, 822
spinal cord metastases 408
spinal intramedullary deposits 826-7
spinal meningeal disease 825-6
spinal tumours 571-5
  extradural 571, 572
  intradural 572
    extramedullary 573-4
  intramedullary 572
  mediastinal mass 67
spleen, leukaemic infiltration 647
spleen, radiotherapy changes 980
splenic lymphoma 601-2
squamous carcinoma of unknown origin 854
stage migration 9, 26
staging 8-9, 23-31
  for chemotherapy 24
  clinical assessment 26-7
  medical imaging 29
  methods 25-31
  peripheral blood examination 28-9
  prognostic relevance 25
  purposes 23
  for radiotherapy 24
  for surgery 23-4
  surgical 27-8, 35
  therapeutic response standardization 24-5
  TNM nomenclature 29-31
  tumour marker assays 28-9
statistical analysis 7-8
stent insertion
  gastric outlet obstruction 870, 871, 872
  inferior vena cava 878
  lower gastro-intestinal tract strictures 871,
    873
  obstructive jaundice 873, 874, 875, 876
  oesophageal strictures 869, 870, 871
  tracheobronchial stenting 864-5
  ureteric stenting 879-80, 881
stomach, post-irradiation changes 980
Stouffer's syndrome 192
streptozocin 937
struma ovarii 282
subependymal giant cell astrocytoma 539-40
subependymoma 541-2
superior vena cava obstruction 863-4, 928
  stent insertion 863, 865

superparamagnetic iron oxide (SPIO)
  contrast enhancement 795, 796,
    803
supraglottic laryngectomy (voice-sparing
  partial) 467, 468
supratentorial ependymoma 541
supratentorial primitive neuro-ectodermal
  tumours 548
surgical staging 27-8, 35
  oesophageal cancer 99, 102
  ovarian cancer 301
surgical treatment 33-5
  breast cancer 399, 400
  cervical cancer 311
  diagnosis/staging 35
  early prostate cancer 250
  endometrial carcinoma 320
  gastric cancer 115-16
  historical developments 34
  laryngeal cancer 467-8, 469, 470
  lung metastases 756
  metastatic disease 35
  neuroblastoma 694
  oesophageal cancer 95, 96
  operative risk 33
  ovarian cancer 286, 288
  palliative 34-5
  pancreatic cancer 152, 154
  paranasal sinus neoplasms 419
  primary curative 34
  reconstructive 35
  renal cell carcinoma 196
  soft tissue sarcomas 387-9
    local recurrence 390
  thymoma 68
surveillance 9
  colorectal cancer follow-up goals 131, 132
  testicular germ cell tumours 271-2
survival 8, 9, 11, 19, 20
  data 12-13
  international differences 17-18
synovial sarcoma 354, 378
  lymph node involvement 387
  magnetic resonance imaging (MRI) 384
  radiological diagnosis 379, 380
  soft tissue 380, 382

T

TAG-72 immunoscintigraphy 140
tamoxifen 38
technetium-99m radionuclide imaging
  bone metastases 769, 770
    neuroblastoma 698, 699
  multiple myeloma 626
  thyroid cancer 488, 490, 496, 497
    diagnostic applications 491-4
technical performance 6
tenoposide 947
teratocarcinoma 716
teratoma 260
  immature 282
  intracranial/pineal region 550, 551
  mature 282
  monodermal 282
  ovarian 282, 290, 718, 719
  paediatric tumours 718, 719, 721
  primary extragonadal 340
  see also sacrococcygeal teratoma

testicular benign lesions 718
testicular cancer
  clinical assessment 26
  incidence/mortality trends 13, 16
  lymphoma 259, 605, 608-9, 716
  paediatric tumours 716-18
    diagnostic imaging 717
    differential diagnosis 718
    follow-up evaluation 718
    lymph node involvement 717
    metastatic disease 717-18
    staging 716, 717
    treatment 716
  pathology 259-60
  surgical staging 27
  survival trends 17, 18
  tumour markers 28
  see also testicular germ cell tumours
testicular carcinoma in situ 259
testicular germ cell tumours 259-74, 716
  aetiology 259
  brain metastases screening 813
  chest X-ray 268, 271
  classification 259-60
  clinical features 264
  computed tomography (CT) 268-70
    stage I tumour surveillance 271-2
    therapeutic response monitoring 272,
      273
  imaging rationale 259
  imaging techniques 268
  incidence 259
  lymph node involvement 260, 261, 262-3,
    268-9
    diagnostic problems 269-70
    staging 267
  lymphangiography 271
  magnetic resonance imaging (MRI) 268,
    271
  metachronous tumour in second testis
    259
  metastatic disease 263, 264, 270, 271
  micrometastases 272
  pathology 259-60
  patterns of spread 260-3, 264
  prognostic features 264
  recurrence 265, 266
  relapse detection 918, 920
  retroperitoneal metastases 340
  Royal Marsden Hospital classification 266,
    267
  serum markers 260
  staging classifications 263, 265
  TNM classification 265
  treatment options 264, 266
  tumour response assessment 907, 908
  ultrasound 271
testicular leukaemic infiltration 716
testicular lymphoma 259, 605, 608-9, 716
testicular radiotherapy damage 989
thallium-201 (Tl-201) imaging 498
thecoma 281, 288, 291
therapeutic response assessment 8, 899-905
  baseline examinations 24-5, 899
  computed tomography (CT) 899
  germ cell tumours 272, 273, 718, 721,
    901-2, 903
  Hodgkin's disease 902
  imaging strategies 900-5
    clinical research support 902-5

curable disease assessment 901
   individual patient management 900-1
magnetic resonance imaging (MRI) 899
metastatic disease 25, 783, 806
neuroblastoma 702-3
oesophageal cancer 104-5
rhabdomyosarcoma 714
sacrococcygeal teratoma 723
staging for standardization 24-5
WHO criteria 24
thioguanine 937
thoracic interventional radiology 861-6
   biopsy techniques 861-2
   central venous obstruction 863-4
   drainage procedures 862
   haemoptysis management 865-6
   tracheobronchial stenting 864-5
   venous access 862-3
thoracic tissue treatment effects 955-64
   bone 962-4
   heart 960-1
   lung 955-60
   oesophagus 961-2
thoracic treatment complications 925-36
   catheter device complications 925-31
   drug reactions 931-3
   graft versus host disease 936
   non-specific interstitial pneumonitis 936
   opportunistic lung infections 933-6
   pulmonary haemorrhage 936
thoracic venous anatomy 926
thorotrast 178, 186
thymic carcinoid tumours 71
thymic carcinoma 71
thymic lymphoma 71, 600
thymic tumours 67-72
thymoma 67-70
   epidemiology 68
   pathology 68
   patterns of spread 68
   staging 69
      imaging 69-70
   treatment options 68
thyroglobulin 28
thyroglossal cyst 443, 461
thyroid cancer 72, 73, 481-510
   aetiology 481-2
   anaplastic (undifferentiated) carcinoma
      484, 486
   bone metastases 771
   computed tomography (CT) 506, 507
   epidemiology 481
   follicular carcinoma 484, 485, 486
   follow-up 509-10
   histological classification 483
   lymph node ultrasound 505
   lymphoma 487
   magnetic resonance imaging (MRI) 507,
      508
   medullary carcinoma 484, 486-7
      imaging agents 500-2
   occult 505
   papillary carcinoma 483-5
   plain radiography 502
   positron emission tomography (PET) 499
   preoperative imaging 509
   radiation exposure association 481, 482,
      483, 506
   radio-iodine ablation therapy 508
   radionuclide imaging 487-8

follow-up imaging 496
gallium-67 citrate 498-9
post-thyroidectomy ablation therapy
   494-6
radio-iodine 491
technetium-99m
   methoxyisobutylisonitrile (Tc-99m
   MIBI) 496, 497
technetium-99m pertechnate 488, 490
technetium-99m tetrofosmin 497
thallium-201 (Tl-201) 498
second malignancies 947
staging
   lymph nodes 490
   primary tumour 489
staging classification 487, 488
treatment 508
tumour markers 28
ultrasound 502-6
thyroid cartilage 457
thyroid dysfunction, treatment-related 668
thyroid gland anatomy 482
thyroid gland lymphatic drainage 482
thyroid lymphoma 613, 614
thyroid mass 67
thyroidectomy 494, 508
   follow-up 509-10
TNM classification 29-31
   adrenal cortical carcinoma 331
   bladder cancer 218
   breast cancer 397
   cholangiocarcinoma 181, 182, 183
   colorectal cancer 129-30
   fibrolamellar hepatocellular carcinoma
      178
   gastric cancer 112-15
   hepatocellular carcinoma 170, 171
   lung cancer 46, 47
   malignant pleural mesothelioma 85, 86
   neuroblastoma 692
   oesophageal cancer 93
   ovarian cancer 285, 286
   pancreatic cancer 152
   paranasal sinus neoplasms 416, 417
   prostate cancer 242
   renal cell carcinoma 192
   renal transitional cell carcinoma 208
   retroperitoneal sarcomas 339
   rhabdomyosarcoma 713
   soft tissue sarcomas 339, 386
   testicular germ cell tumours 265
   thyroid cancer 487, 488
tobacco use 20, 215, 216, 239
tongue tumours 438, 439
tonsillar fossa tumours 438, 441
toxoplasmosis 544, 545
tracheobronchial invasion 97
tracheobronchial stenting 864-5
transabdominal ultrasound
   bladder cancer staging 218
   endometrial carcinoma 320
   ovarian cancer screening 289
   ovarian mass characterization 290, 291-2
transhepatic portal venous sampling 884
transitional cell carcinoma 191, 207-11, 212,
   215, 216
   clinical features 208
   imaging techniques 208
   intravenous urography 208-9
   magnetic resonance imaging (MRI) 211

multiplicity 207
pathology 207
percutaneous tumour ablation 880
staging
   computed tomography (CT) 209-10
   primary tumour 209
   prognosis 208
   treatment 208
transoesophageal ultrasound 56
transrectal ultrasound
   bladder cancer staging 218, 219
   cervical cancer staging 311, 314, 315
   image-guided gastro-intestinal biopsy 867
   ovarian cancer residual disease
      assessment 303
   prostate cancer staging 244-5, 246, 252,
      253
      automatic image analysis 22
      sonoelastic imaging 252
transurethral prostatic resection, postsurgical
   changes 984
transurethral ultrasound 218
transvaginal ultrasound
   bladder cancer staging 218
   cervical cancer staging 311, 315
   endometrial carcinoma staging 320, 321,
      322
   image-guided gastro-intestinal biopsy 867
   ovarian cancer screening 289
   ovarian mass characterization 290, 291-2
treatment modalities 33-41
trephine biopsy 372
trigeminal neuroma 560
tuberculosis 934, 940
tumour growth imaging 5-6
tumour growth rates 5-6
tumour invasion 5
tumour markers 28
   germ cell tumours 260, 283, 340, 549, 719
   hepatoblastoma 707
   medullary thyroid carcinoma 487
   neuroblastoma 691
   ovarian cancer 283
   serum 28
   staging 28-9
   urine 28
tumour response assessment 905-17
   tumour composition 905, 911-17
      computed tomography (CT) 911-12
      magnetic resonance imaging (MRI)
        913-15
      magnetic resonance spectroscopy 917
      radionuclide imaging 916-17
      ultrasound 911
   tumour volume 905, 906-11
      chest X-ray 906
      computed tomography (CT) 907-9
      magnetic resonance imaging (MRI)
        909-11
      ultrasound 906-7
tumour suppressor gene mutations 3, 395
typhlitis 938
tyrosinaemia 707

U

ultrasound
   adrenal gland appearances 831
   adrenal tumours 334

aerodigestive tract tumours 432
AIDS-related tumours 1020
bladder cancer staging 218-20
breast cancer
    chemo-endocrine neo-adjuvant
        therapy response assessment 404
    diagnosis 397
    metastatic disease 405, 408
    staging 401, 402
    tumour size assessment 401
cholangiocarcinoma
    intrahepatic 180
    staging 181, 182
haemangioma 802
hepatocellular carcinoma
    appearances 169, 176
    staging 175-6
laryngeal cancer 475
leukaemic abdominal infiltration 647
liver cysts 802
liver focal fatty change 803
liver metastases 58, 144, 145, 789, 796,
        798-800
    intraoperative 799-800
    small lesions 802
    vascular contrast agents 799
lung cancer 58
    chest wall invasion 52
lymphoma
    liver 602
    nodal disease 589-90
    testis 609
neuroblastoma 695
    staging 696
ovarian cancer
    residual disease assessment 303
    staging 289-90
ovarian mass characterization 290, 291-2,
        304
paediatric hepatic neoplasms 711
paediatric imaging 662
paediatric ovarian germ cell tumours 719
pancreatic cancer staging 163-4
    accuracy 164
pericardial effusions guided drainage
        procedures 862
peritoneal metastases 841
pleural effusions 759
    guided drainage procedures 862
renal cell carcinoma staging 206-7

testicular germ cell tumours 259, 271
    paediatric tumours 717, 718
thyroid cancer 502-6
thyroid nodules 481
tumour response assessment 906
    tumour composition 911
    tumour volume 906-7
    Wilms' tumour 674-5
ureteric radiation injury 987-8
ureteric stent insertion 879-80, 881
ureteroscopic tumour ablation 880
urinary tract drug complications 937
urinary tract infection 215, 216
urinary tract interventional radiology 879-82
    percutaneous nephrostomy 879-80, 881
    percutaneous tumour ablation 880
    renal artery embolization 881, 882
    therapeutic pelvic embolization 881-2
    ureteric stent insertion 879-80, 881
    ureteroscopic tumour ablation 880
urine tumour markers 28, 691
uterine anatomy 316-17
uterine atrophy, post-irradiation 989
uterine leukaemic infiltration 648
uterine lymphoma 609

V

vaginal rhabdomyosarcoma 712, 713, 714
vascular contrast agents 799
vascular mediastinal tumours 74, 75
vascular sarcoma 337
vertebral collapse 773, 774, 781-3
    computed tomography (CT) 773, 781
    magnetic resonance imaging (MRI) 774,
        781, 782, 783
vertebroplasty, percutaneous 883
vertical hemilaryngectomy 468, 470, 476
vinblastine 931, 1009
vincristine 931, 937, 957, 1009
vinyl chloride 186
virilisation 329, 330
visceral arteriography 875-8
vocal cord paralysis 476-7
vocal cords 460, 461
voice-sparing partial laryngectomy 467, 468
von Hippel-Lindau syndrome
    phaeochromocytoma 330
    renal cell carcinoma 191, 202

W

WAGR syndrome 671
Wilms' tumour 671-80
    anaplastic 683
    associated syndromes 671-2
    bilateral 681
    chest computed tomography (CT) 678,
        679
    chest X-ray 678, 679
    chromosomal abnormalities 671
    clinical features 672
    diagnostic imaging 673-8
        angiography 677-8
        computed tomography (CT) 675-6
        intravenous urography 673, 674
        magnetic resonance imaging (MRI)
            676-7
        plain abdominal radiograph 673, 674
        radionuclide imaging 678
        ultrasound 674-5
    epidemiology 671
    follow-up radiology 679
    hereditary form 671
    intrapelvic 683
    metastatic disease 678, 679
    percutaneous biopsy 679
    predisposing factors 671
    staging 672, 673
    treatment complications 685-6
    ultrasonic monitoring of at risk child 679
    with unfavourable histology 682
    variants 683
Wilson's disease 707
wood workers 415

Y

yolk sac tumour 260, 282, 716
    primary extragonadal 340

Z

zidovudine 1009